Biochemistry
of
Steroids
and Other
Isopentenoids

Biochemistry
of
Steroids
and Other
Isopentenoids

by

William R. Nes, Ph.D.
W. L. Obold Professor of Biological Sciences
Drexel University

and

Margaret Lee McKean, Ph.D.
Postdoctoral Fellow
Department of Biological Sciences
Drexel University

University Park Press
Baltimore · London · Tokyo

UNIVERSITY PARK PRESS
International Publishers in Science and Medicine
Chamber of Commerce Building
Baltimore, Maryland 21202

Copyright © 1977 by University Park Press

Typeset by Action Comp Co., Inc., and Alpha Graphics, Inc.
Manufactured in the United States of America by Universal Lithographers, Inc.,
and The Optic Bindery Incorporated

Library of Congress Cataloging in Publication Data

Nes, William R.
  Biochemistry of steroids and other isopentenoids.
  Includes indexes.
  1. Steroids. 2. Steroid metabolism.
I. McKean, Margaret Lee, joint author. II. Title.
III. Title: Isopentenoids.
QP752.S7N47   574.1'9243   77-7186
ISBN O-8391-1127-4

Contents

Preface.. vii

Chapter 1 **Historical Introduction** 1

Chapter 2 **Structure and Nomenclature**............................... 37

Chapter 3 **Analytical Procedures** 85

Chapter 4 **The Formation of the Isopentenoid Unit** 147

Chapter 5 **Polymerization of the C_5 Unit**............................... 171

Chapter 6 **Head-to-Head Coupling of Isopentenoid Polymers** 205

Chapter 7 **The Cyclization of Squalene** 229

Chapter 8 **Cyclization of Other Isopentenoids** 271

Chapter 9 **Metabolism of Lanosterol and Cycloartenol to Δ^5-Sterols**......... 325

Chapter 10 **Occurrence, Physiology, and Ecology of Sterols**................ 411

Chapter 11 **The Function of Steroids**.................................... 535

Author Index 631
Subject Index 663

Preface

The development of our knowledge of steroids and biosynthetically related molecules known collectively as isopentenoids has clustered into three major periods. The first, which lasted a bit more than a century after the discovery of cholesterol in 1815, was characterized by the isolation and purification of a variety of isopentenoids, the recognition that they are widely distributed in nature, and elucidation of the structures of the simpler representatives. In addition, a basis for later structural and biochemical examination was formulated in the "isoprene rule." The more complex structures existing in the steroids and higher terpenoids, together with stereochemical phenomena, were then resolved in the second period, which ensued during the next thirty-five years or so, culminating in the total synthesis of cholesterol in the 1950s. The writings of Louis and Mary Fieser, especially in their book *Steroids*, have elegantly covered these early phases, and the conciseness with which they summarized the depth and breadth of the subject greatly facilitated movement into the third period, biosynthesis. Since the structural period also coincided with the development of a biological concept centered on enzymology, as well as with the evolution of tracer methodology, elucidation of the main aspects of biosynthesis and metabolism was able to follow very rapidly. It is this fascinating period of biochemical activity, currently ending, that is the main subject of our book. The fourth period, already strongly overlapping with the third, will undoubtedly be concerned with the physiology of the compounds and can be expected to lead to a sophisticated understanding of their significance in ecology, phylogeny, and evolution. We have included the principal aspects of these subjects to the extent that they are presently investigated and have also brought up to date the structural story in a way that will allow the nonchemist to appreciate its meaning, such as by including rules for stereochemical and other designations and a discussion of the fundamentals of three-dimensional phenomena in polycyclic and acyclic systems, both of which apply to, and unfortunately complicate, an understanding of the subject. Although our emphasis is on steroids, the reader will find that the more important elements of the structure, biosynthesis, and function of other compounds, such as the terpenes, have also been reviewed.

One of us (W.R.N) has had the pleasure of working in the field since the time, more than a quarter of a century ago, when the second and third periods were interfaced. It has been a most exciting adventure to have lived through this entire historical phase. This book, which summarizes an intellectual quest to understand the subject as a whole, has its origins in the opportunity and stimulation provided to W.R.N. by the late Dr. Edward C. Kendall, with whom he worked on the partial synthesis of cortisone at the Mayo Clinic in 1950–1951. Succeeding nurture was given by the late Dr. Erich Mosettig at the National Institutes of Health and by Dr. Ralph I. Dorfman at the Worcester Foundation for Experimental Biology. Without them and without inquisitive and productive students over the years, and the continuing financial support of NIH research grants, the assimilation and collation of the material presented here would never have been possible. All are most gratefully thanked, as is Mrs. Velma Moultrie for her untiring and meticulous efforts in typing the manuscript and making the drawings. It was our hope, which time did not allow to materialize, to have each chapter reviewed by at least one person active in the field. Several people did, however, carefully examine various parts of the manuscript, and we are especially pleased to acknowledge the efforts of Dr. Konrad Bloch and Dr. John H. Adler.

To
Estelle

Biochemistry
of
Steroids
and Other
Isopentenoids

Chapter 1

Historical Introduction

A. Orienting Survey 2
B. Early Observations 3
    1. *Biological Experimentation* 3
    2. *Biochemical Experimentation* 4
C. Isoprene Rule 7
    1. *C_5 Concept* 7
    2. *Wallach's Proposal* 8
    3. *Problem of Regularity* 9
    4. *Ruzicka's Extension* 12
D. Structural Period 13
    1. *Introduction* 13
    2. *Wagner-Meerwein Rearrangements* 13
    3. *Monoterpene Structure* 14
    4. *Sesquiterpene Structure* 16
    5. *Diterpenes* 17
    6. *Triterpenes and Steroids* 18
E. Nobel Prizes 19
    1. *In 1910 to Otto Wallach (1847–1931) of Germany "for his Innovative Work in the Field of Alicyclic Substances"* 20
    2. *In 1927 to Heinrich Wieland (1877–1957) of Germany "for his Research on Bile Acids and Analogous Substances"* 20
    3. *In 1928 to Adolf Windaus (1876–1959) of Germany "for his Studies on the Constitution of the Sterols and Their Connection with the Vitamins"* 21
    4. *In 1937 to Paul Karrer (1889–1971) of Switzerland "for his Investigations on Carotenoids, Flavins and Vitamins A and B_2," and Walter N. Haworth (1883–1950) of England "for his Investigations on Carbohydrates and Vitamin C".* . . 22
    5. *In 1938 to Richard Kuhn (1900–1967) of Austria and Germany "for his Work on Carotenoids and Vitamins"* 22
    6. *In 1939 to Adolf Butenandt (1903–   ) of Germany "for his Work on Sex Hormones" and to Leopold Ruzicka (1887–   ) of Yugoslavia and Switzerland "for his Work on Polymethylenes and Higher Terpenes"* 23
    7. *In 1943 to Henrik Dam (1895–1976) of Denmark "for his Discovery of Vitamin K" and to Edward A. Doisy (1893–   ) of the United States "for his Discovery of the Chemical Nature of Vitamin K".* 25

8. *In 1947 to Sir Robert Robinson (1886-   ) of England "for his Investigations on Plant Products of Biological Importance"* 26
9. *In 1950 to Edward Calvin Kendall (1886-1972) of the United States, Philip Showalter Hench (1896-1965) of the United States, and Tadeus Reichstein (1897-   ) of Poland, Russia, and Switzerland "for their discoveries Concerning the Suprarenal Cortex Hormones, Their Structure and Biological Effects"*. 27
10. *In 1950 to Otto Paul Hermann Diels (1876-1954) of Germany and Kurt Alder (1902-1958) of Germany "for the Development of the Diene Synthesis"* .. 30
11. *In 1964 to Konrad Bloch (1912-   ) of Germany and the United States and to Feodor Lynen (1911-   ) of Germany "for their Discoveries Concerning the Mechanism and Regulation of Cholesterol and Fatty Acid Metabolism"*. 30
12. *In 1965 to Robert Burns Woodward (1917-   ) of the United States "for his Outstanding Achievements in the Art of Organic Synthesis"* 32
13. *In 1969 to Derek H. R. Barton (1918-   ) of England and to Odd Hassel (1897-   ) of Norway "for their Contributions to the Development of the Concept of Conformation and Its Application in Chemistry"* 32
14. *In 1975 to John W. Cornforth (1917-   ) of England "for his Researches on the Stereochemistry of Enzyme-Catalyzed Reactions" and to Vladimir Prelog (1906-   ) of Switzerland "for his Researches on the Stereochemistry of Organic Molecules and Reactions"*. 33
    Literature Cited 34

A. ORIENTING SURVEY

This book is concerned with the nature, origin, and function of steroids and other compounds which are derived biologically from an isopentenoid unit. All organisms, ranging from various bacteria to man, which have been carefully examined, biosynthesize, or require these substances. They are formed by the polymerization of an appropriately functionalized C_5

$$C$$
$$|$$
$$C—C—C—C$$

Carbon Skeleton of Isopentenoid Unit

unit. However, they differ from other biological polymers in several important ways: 1) The union between the units is a C—C bond, and the isopentenoids are not readily depolymerized by hydrolysis. In fact, there are no known examples of biological depolymerization of isopentenoids comparable to the conversion of proteins to amino acids or of polysaccharides to monomeric carbohydrates. 2) A major characteristic of isopentenoid metabolism once polymerization has occurred is the further formation of C—C bonds. These new bonds are frequently formed intramolecularly with concomitant carbon rearrangements. 3) Superimposed upon this is a set of oxidative processes that remove carbon atoms in many instances. Consequently, 4) the final result often is a molecule that bears little or no resemblance either to a linear polymer or to the other isopentenoids.

Thus it is that the history of isopentenoids has a number of different lines. Over many years there developed a "feeling" that these lines converged at some point, but it was not until the mid-1950s and entirely through an accident that the point of convergence was reached. The solution to the problem lay in the discovery of mevalonic acid, which proved to be the ubiquitous precursor of the C_5 unit. Through incubations of radioactively labeled mevalonic acid, it has been possible to prove in the last 15 years or so that the diverse groupings of isopentenoid compounds are indeed members of a single biosynthetic family. In what follows we trace the development of the field, ending with a summary of the lives and work of 19 Nobel Laureates whose efforts epitomize the dramatic and complicated history of this subject.

B. EARLY OBSERVATIONS

1. Biological Experimentation

Among the biological properties of the isopentenoids, there are some that are especially evident and attracted early attention. One of these has to do with sexual characteristics and behavior, in particular, the so-called "secondary sex characteristics," e.g., growth of the penis, development of pubic hair, and certain aspects of sexual desire. Since the male gonads of man and many animals are externally located, they were easily accessible for experimentation. As early as 1400 B.C. it was recommended in the Ayur-Veda of India that testis tissue be used as a treatment for impotence. Still more importantly, Aristotle (384–322 B.C.) in Book 9 of Volume 4 of the *Historia Animalium* carefully described the effect of castration in the bird and made a number of observations in man. Aristotle's work probably represents the first serious study that could be assumed to have anything to do with isopentenoids, but, as was true for early science in general, experimentation proceeded at an agonizingly slow pace. Finally, the collapse of the Greco-Roman world ended significant work until the rise of modern science. Then in 1849 an entirely different observation was made. Addison discovered 11 cases in which diseased human adrenal glands were linked to a clinical condition comprising pigmentation, marked weakness, anorexia, nausea, vomiting, anemia, and emaciation. Subsequent work demonstrated that human beings cannot live more than six or seven days after complete failure or surgical removal of the adrenals, and comparable findings have been documented with experimental animals. We now know that the life-maintaining properties of the adrenal glands and the control of "secondary sex characteristics" by the gonads, both result from secretion of the isopentenoidal steroids. The foundation for this knowledge was being laid at about the same time by the rise of chemical investigations and their association with biological phenomena.

2. Biochemical Experimentation

a. Transition in the Eighteenth Century In the eighteenth century an association of biological phenomena with chemical substances developed through the efforts of such men as Lavoisier (who in the 1770s showed that animals convert carbon compounds to CO_2 with consumption of oxygen), Priestley (who, after discovering oxygen in 1774, demonstrated the assimilation of CO_2 and production of oxygen by plants), and Ingenhonsz and Engelman (who showed that chlorophyll and light were in some way controlling the things that Priestley had observed). With this conceptual basis, the succeeding generations began to look in earnest for chemicals in living systems and to concern themselves with problems of purity and of chemical structure and properties. Although it was not until the present century that the early biological observations were associated with a defined chemical entity, isopentenoids began to be isolated in pure form shortly after 1800.

b. Discovery of Steroids In 1815 Chevreul (*1*) concerned himself with some crystals that Vallisnieri, nearly a century before, and, after him, Poulletier de la Salle had obtained from an alcoholic solution of gallstones. By demonstrating that saponification failed to alter the crystals, Chevreul was able to show that the gallstone substance was quite different from other biological materials, notably waxes, which also were alcohol- but not water-soluble. He named the substance "cholesterine," from the Greek "chole" for bile and "stereos" for solid. After the passage of another generation, Berthelot in 1859 (*2*) showed that "cholesterine" was itself chemically an alcohol by the preparation of esters. From this derives our present English name, cholesterol, and this compound has the distinction of being the first pure isopentenoid to have been isolated from nature. From it the generic term "steroids" is derived (see Chapter 2).

Since cholesterol, unlike ethanol, is a solid, Berthelot's proof of its alcoholic nature aroused a great deal of attention, and the full elucidation of it structure, achieved in the 1930s and confirmed by synthesis in the 1950s, has played a large role over the years in the whole development of chemistry. The progress made both with its structure as well as with those of many other isopentenoids has been a measure of and integrally associated with progress in understanding generally how atoms can be joined together in such large numbers. In 1888 Reinitzer (*3*) arrived at the correct empirical formula for cholesterol, $C_{27}H_{46}O$, after an approximation had been established by Berthelot. Even this feat was monumental, for there were no easy methods for obtaining formula numbers at the level of accuracy needed. It was not until many years later that Pregl (Nobel Laureate, 1923) developed the modern technique of combustion microanalysis, and he proudly discussed in his Nobel Address (*4*) how good his method was by virtue of the results obtained by Windaus on cholesterol derivatives. He also took pains "to mention that one of the first results was the discovery that the yellow coloring matter in corpora lutea of cattle ovaries was by micro-analytical carbon hydrogen determination found to be carotin." "Carotin" is an older name for the isopentenoidal carotene.

c. Discovery of Bile Acids   Following earlier observations of Liebig, Berzelius, and others, Strecker in 1848 (5) obtained an acid (cholic acid) from ox bile (Greek, chole) hydrolyzates. It proved to have the formula $C_{24}H_{40}O_5$. Thirty-seven years later, Mylius (6) obtained another acid (desoxycholic acid) containing one less oxygen atom, and subsequently still others were isolated. These large-molecular-weight acids occurring in the gastrointestinal tract are called "bile acids." The similarities of their origin and empirical formulas with those of cholesterol suggested that they were steroids, and Wieland and Windaus and others working in the first quarter of the present century succeeded in establishing that such a relationship does in fact exist.

d. Discovery of Terpenes   Parallel with the studies of animal constituents, other workers were investigating plants. They were motivated by various unusual odors and useful medicinal and physical properties that had slowly become apparent over the long course of history. Several groups of plant materials are of special significance to us. They are the distillable exudate of conifers (turpentine), the residue (rosin or colophony), and the expressable or steam-volatile oils (essential or ethereal oils), usually of angiosperms. As early as 1592 the *Dispensatorium Valeri* listed no less than 60 kinds of essential oil, and the use of conifer exudates for caulking boats and weatherproofing ropes is an age-old process (from which the term "naval stores" for the whole exudate is derived). The water-insolubility and volatility of both turpentine and the essential oils suggested a structural relationship between the two. The German word for turpentine is "terpentine" and, although turpentine and the essential oils are mixtures, by the mid to late nineteenth century the word "terpene" was already being applied to the few defined components separated from either source. The validity for the assumption of common structural features became apparent in the 1880s, when heating or acid treatment of turpentine or certain ethereal oils or of various substances isolated from them yielded the same compound, dipentene. In some cases the dipentene was an artifact, yet the fact that constituents of both classes of oil yielded it proved the presence of similar materials. Still more important, at about the same time true constituents of both classes were shown to be identical.

To Wallach goes the honor of having first carefully purified terpene hydrocarbons. In three classic papers (7-9) he showed that of the many supposed compounds which had been "isolated," most were still mixtures. He concluded (9) that there were really only eight components (pinene, camphene, limonene, dipentene, terpinolene, sylvestrene, terpinene, and phellandrene) that were sufficiently pure to allow analysis. He began then a remarkably fruitful investigation of their structures that laid the basis for all later isopentenoid considerations. By 1887 he was able to suggest structures that were fundamentally right, if not correct in every detail. How he was able to achieve this is so important to the basic biochemistry of isopentenoids that it is amplified in Section C. Twenty-three years later, with equally brilliant work intervening, he was awarded the Nobel Prize (Section E). With Wallach, isopentenoids entered the modern era, but, when Wallach undertook his work, a relationship of terpenes to steroids was still far from imagined.

While Wallach's work on the terpene hydrocarbons holds special significance, other investigations of the period were also important. As early as 1853, a terpene was isolated that proved to be an alcohol (linalool) (*10*). In 1871 Palmarosa oil (Turkish geranium oil) yielded another one (geraniol) (*11*). Then in 1877 Tilden introduced the use of nitrosylchloride as a means of obtaining solid derivatives (*12*), and henceforth the isolation, purification, and analysis of alcholic terpenes moved at a rapid pace.

   e. Discovery of Carotenoids   Because the world is filled with color, men began to investigate natural pigments as soon as it became evident that living systems are chemical systems. In 1831 the orange coloring matter (carotene) of carrot roots was isolated by Wackenroder (*13*), and 16 years later Zeise (1847) (*14*) approximated its empirical formula as $(C_5H_8)_n$; however, it was not until 1907 that Willstätter and Mieg established the fully correct formula as $C_{40}H_{56}$ (*15*). Similarly, Willstätter and Escher (1910) (*16*) showed that the red coloring matter of tomatoes (lycopene) has the same empirical formula, $C_{40}H_{56}$, but again it was in the earlier work of Hartsen (1873) (*17*) and Millardet (1875) (*18*) that the substance was first obtained. The name carotenoids is applied to this class of pigment in deference to carotene, which was the first one isolated.

   f. Discovery of Rubber   The diverse threads of history and chance that have affected the field of isopentenoids are perhaps no more clearly illustrated than by man's discovery of rubber and by its introduction to the European mind. Rubber, like "naval stores," is an exudate of plants. It has been found in many species, belonging notably to the families Euphorbiaceae, Moraceae, Apocynaceae, Compositae, and Asclepiadaceae. These include trees, shrubs, vines, and smaller plants. But it was the South and Central American Indian who first widely collected it and perceived a useful and interesting property, namely, its elasticity. They took advantage of this property in making figures and playing games. The Mayans, for instance, developed a major sport in which a rubber ball was bounced around from the shoulders or thighs of players until it went through a stone loop high on a wall. The game was accompanied by betting of the spectators, and the playing fields in Mexico remain visible today as a result of archeological excavations. A modern version known as "hulama" is still played near the village of Mazatlan.

   This remarkable material is an isopentenoid, and studies of its structure and origin have had a major bearing on the development of the field, as is discussed in Section C. The history of its introduction to Europe, where scientific examination could proceed, begins with Columbus, who, during his second voyage in 1493–1496, saw the natives of Haiti playing the same sort of game the Mayans played. Nearly three hundred years later, Charles de la Condamine was sent to South America by the Paris Academy of Science to measure a meridian of the equator. This took him eight years (1736–1744), and during his stay he discovered the Indians' source of rubber. It was a tree they called "heve," and our botanical name *Hevea* is derived from it. The Mayan Indian word for rubber was "caoutchouc," meaning "to flow or weep," and variations of this word, which was introduced into European languages, still exist, e.g., Kautschuk, a German word for rubber. In 1762 Fresneau pursued the source of rubber in greater detail and described and named the Brazilian rubber tree, *Hevea guianensis*. An Amazon relative, *Hevea brasiliensis*, growing about 60 feet tall, now is the principal (97%) commercial source of natural rubber. Both trees belong to the family *Euphorbiaceae*. Ten million acres of *Hevea brasiliensis* were under cultivation in 1957, mainly in Malaya, Indonesia, Ceylon, and the southeast Asian peninsula. The tree was introduced to Asia from Brazil, but Roxburgh noted in 1801 in his *Flora Indica* that natives of eastern Asia also obtained rubber from an indigenous tree, *Ficus elastica*, and used it for weatherproofing and making torches.

C. ISOPRENE RULE

1. C₅ Concept

As has been described in Section B, serious discovery of isopentenoids only began in the nineteenth century, and it was not until the twentieth century approached that adequate means for determining the atomic content of molecules were available. It is particularly remarkable, therefore, that as early as 1826 Faraday (*19*) arrived at the correct empirical formula for the macromolecule rubber. He showed it to be $(C_5H_8)_n$, which led to the recognition that it was a polyunsaturated polymer of a pentadiene. By the time Wallach began his investigations in the early 1880s, it had also been established that carotene was a $(C_5)_n$ compound and that the terpene hydrocarbons had formulas represented by $C_{10}H_{16}$. Furthermore, plants were beginning to yield compounds bearing 15 carbon atoms, the so-called sesquiterpenes. Thus, in 1840 Souberain and Capitaine (*20*) isolated a hydrocarbon from *Piper cubeba* that Wallach (*21*) later called cadinene ($C_{15}H_{24}$). In 1888 Bruhl (*22*) had sufficient physical data on it to conclude it must contain two double bonds and be bicyclic. In 1885 Vesterberg (*23*) isolated pure dextropimaric acid from rosin. This substance proved to have 20 carbon atoms. Thus, there seemed to be a series of naturally occurring compounds having two, three, four, and by virtue of rubber (with a molecular weight in the thousands) many more C_5 units linked together.

During the same period, Bouchardat (24), Williams (25), Tilden (26), and others actively pursued the chemical nature of rubber. Of tremendous importance was their finding that rubber, on pyrolysis at 300–350°, gives isoprene and dipentene. From the work of Gladziatsky (1887) (27) and others, it became known that isoprene has the structure shown in Scheme 1.1. It was also known at that time that isoprene could be polymerized to give dipentene and trimers as well as higher polymers with rubber-like properties. From this the correct structure of rubber was deduced (Scheme 1.2).

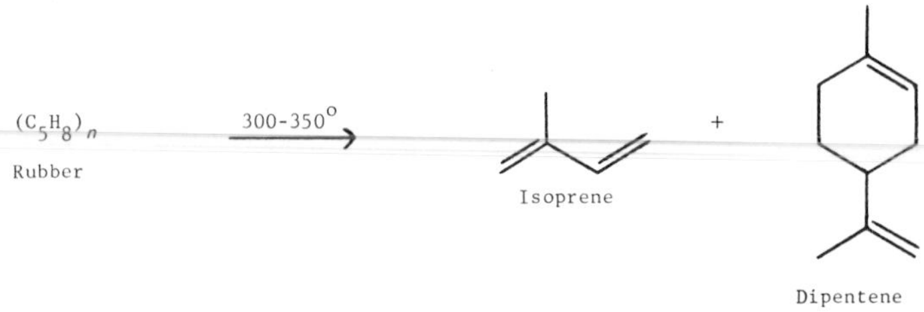

Scheme 1.1. Pyrolysis of rubber.

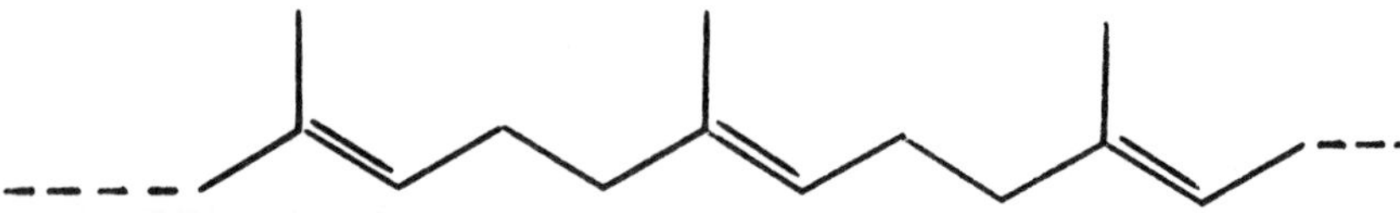

Scheme 1.2. Segment of *trans*-rubber.

In 1884, with these facts and ideas just breaking forth, Tilden (28) made the remarkable suggestion that a natural terpene (terpilene) probably was constructed of two symmetrical C_5 halves.

2. Wallach's Proposal

As seen from the previous section, the idea that there is something fundamental in nature about a C_5 unit did not develop in a single stroke. Nevertheless, it is because of one man, Wallach, that it reached its first general significance. Considering the facts outlined in Section B, Wallach (29) wrote in 1887, "Such a structure for isoprene...allows a polymerization to terpenes, sesquiterpenes, etc., to appear reasonable, as a look at the following shows in which the C-atoms arising from the different isoprene molecules are apparent by the numbering." While his structures (Scheme 1.3) were not exactly right, they did reflect clearly the basis of his proposal.

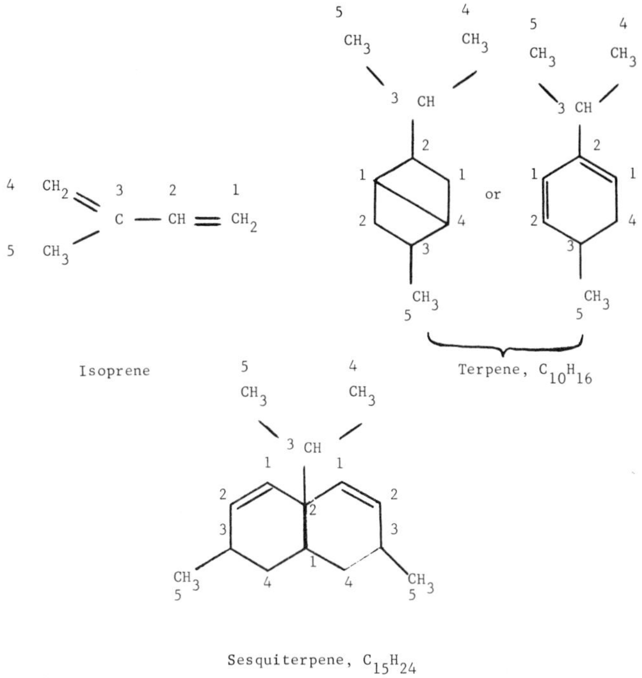

Scheme 1.3. Wallach's proposal (1887).

This has come to be known as *the isoprene rule,* which states in its simplest form that certain substances are constructed of isoprene skeletons and therefore probably arise by the natural polymerization of isoprene. Compounds following the isoprene rule were then called isoprenoid.

3. Problem of Regularity

As time moved on, the isolation and elucidation of more than just a few structures made it evident that there were several different ways in which a compound could follow the isoprene rule. They are:

1. By head-to-tail (or *regular*) union
2. By some other (or *irregular*) way

Farnesol is an example of a compound following the isoprene rule in a regular way. It is composed of three C_5 units (shown by dashed lines) with each unit joined to another so that the isopropyl ends of all the C_5 units are directed toward the same side of the chain (Scheme 1.4). This arrangement is also seen in the structures of the cyclic compounds, dipentene and cadinene, in which a single, regular chain of C_5 units is present despite cyclization. The linear "backbone" of this series of C_5 units is numbered 1–8 in the former case and 1–12 in the latter (Scheme 1.5).

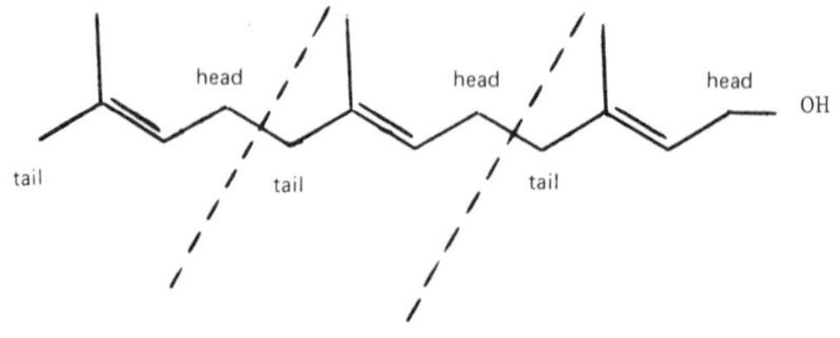

Farnesol

Scheme 1.4. Farnesol.

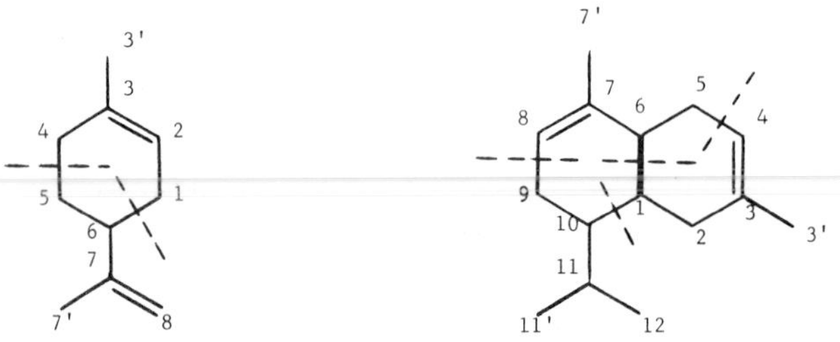

Dipentene

Cadinene

Scheme 1.5.

An example of a compound that fails to follow the regular arrange-ment is abietic acid. In dipentene, cadinene, and rimuene it will be seen that it is possible to have a series of consecutively numbered C atoms such that every other odd-numbered carbon atom bears a protruding C atom (a characteristic of regular arrangement). With abietic acid it is not possible to achieve this. Although this is a tricyclic substance, reference to the regular arrangement in rimuene, which is also tricyclic, will show that the tricyclic character has nothing intrinsic to do with irregularity (Scheme 1.6).

Another problem that arose after more and more structures became known is that, despite a close relationship to obvious isopentenoids, some compounds failed to have formulas with an even multiple of five carbon atoms. An example is santene (C_9H_{14}), the structure of which was eluci-dated by Semmler and Bartelt in 1907–1908 (30-33). It is tantalizingly similar to camphene (Scheme 1.7) ($C_{10}H_{16}$), which is isomeric with α-pinene (Berthelot, 1858) and strictly isopentenoid, following the isoprene rule in a regular manner; however, santene lacks a carbon atom. For a thorough discussion of these and related terpenes, see de Mayo (34). Much more serious was the steroid structure. Cholesterol has 27 carbon atoms, estrone has 18, etc. (Scheme 1.8). Nevertheless, it soon became apparent that cholesterol contained at least some isopentenoid character. In 1872 Loebisch

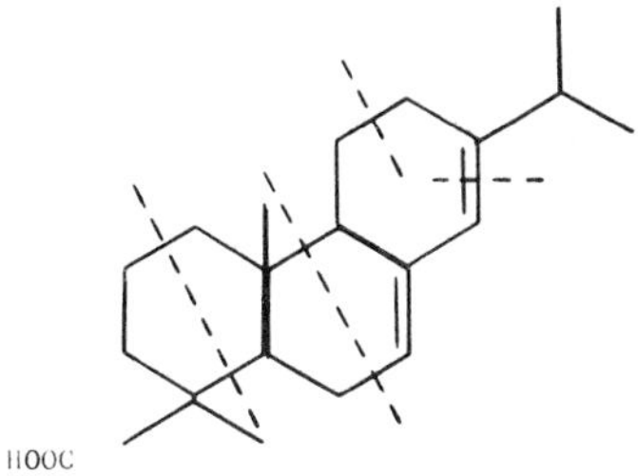

Abietic acid 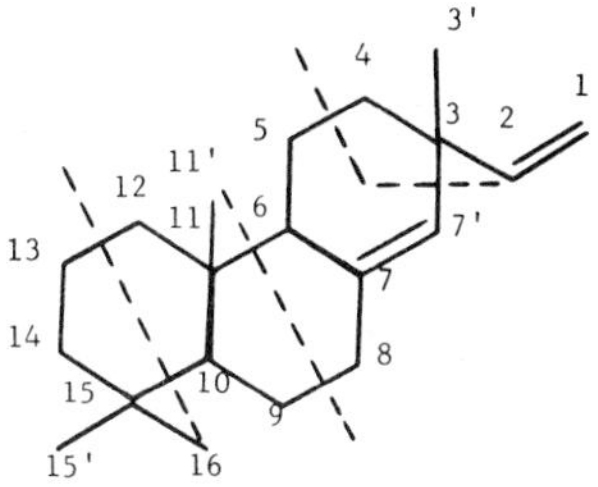   Rimuene

Scheme 1.6.

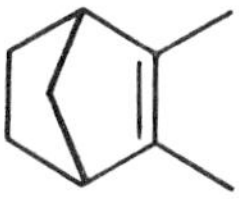

Santene 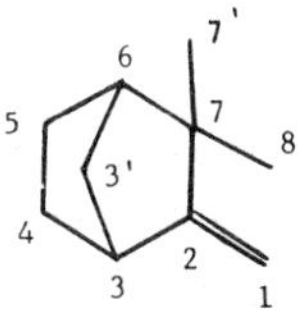   Camphene

Scheme 1.7.

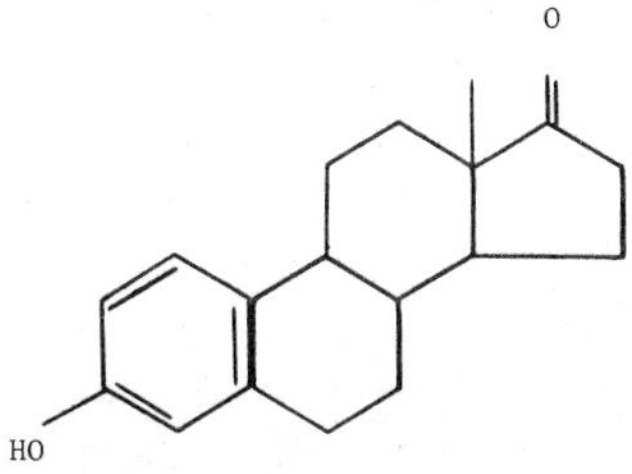

Estrone 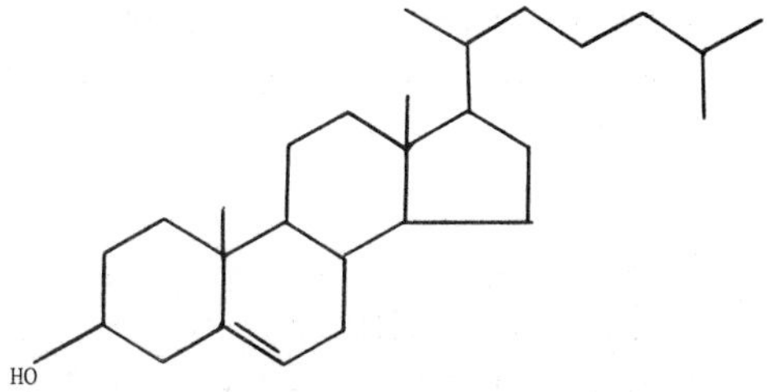   Cholesterol

Scheme 1.8.

(35) obtained a volatile and pleasant-smelling substance from oxidation of cholesterol. This fragment was identified by Windaus and Resau (1913) (36) as methyl isohexyl ketone (Scheme 1.9). It represents the side chain of cholesterol and clearly has an isopentenoid terminus. Then, after the structure of cholesterol was established in the 1930s, other isopentenoid parts of the molecule were evident. However, the structure failed both to have an even multiple of C_5 units and to follow the isoprene rule in what C atoms there were. Thus, it and its apparent relatives, such as estrone, were placed in a more or less separate category illustrated by the name steroid.

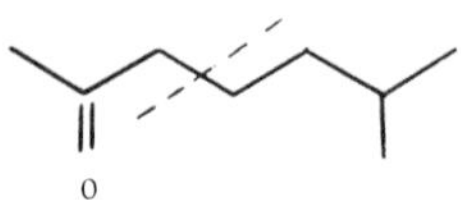

Scheme 1.9 Methyl isohexyl ketone.

4. Ruzicka's Extension

Despite the excessive simplicity of the isoprene rule, it was used in a remarkably fruitful way by Leopold Ruzicka, who deduced the structure of many an isopentenoid with its help, suggested on its basis that previously proposed structures for others were wrong, and then went on to prove his thoughts experimentally. Facing what finally became a bewildering array of substances, he attempted to extend the original idea of "isopentenoid" character so that it would accommodate all the known compounds. This was a formidable undertaking. How can steroids, terpenes, rubber, carotenoids, etc., all be brought together under one roof? As a group they have formulas that only approximate $(C_5)_n$. They contain every kind of functionality. Some are cyclic. Some are acyclic. Some are small and some are large. And neither Ruzicka nor anyone else could find isoprene in nature! The solution to the problem was to consider reaction mechanisms, more or less to ignore the precise character of the biological precursor, and only to assume it to have an "isopentenoid" structure during reaction. He further assumed that biosyntheses involve electrophilic attack, e.g., of a proton, on a double bond. The electrophilic species produced by the initial attack then proceeds by various further condensations and, in many cases, rearrangements to a final charged species. The latter, by elimination of a proton or addition of a nucleophile, e.g., OH⁻ from water, yields the observed products. This proposal is contained particularly in two papers (*37, 38a*), and can be summarized in the following way, which Ruzicka calls the *biogenetic isoprene rule:* a compound is "isoprenoid" if it is derived biologically with or without rearrangements from an "isoprenoid" precursor. This differs from Wallach's proposal in its emphasis on biosynthesis instead of on structural characteristics, and it therefore encompasses compounds regardless of whether or not they follow Wallach's isoprene rule. The more profound contribution that Ruzicka and his colleagues made, though, was to show in considerable detail how one could actually arrive at the known structures of a large number of compounds using the mechanistic considerations discussed above. Coupled to the *de novo* origin of the compounds is now the obvious fact that many other kinds of metabolism can be superimposed on the biosynthetic pattern. The latter explains why many of the compounds lack carbon atoms.

Ruzicka, of course, was not entirely alone in arriving at these ideas. It is of particular importance to mention Robinson (Nobel Laureate, 1947), who many years earlier had dramatically shown how tropinone could arise in nature by known chemical processes. In so doing he really set the stage for the more sophisticated mechanistic extrapolations. Robinson's summary of his more recent ideas in 1955 (*386*) must be considered a classic in science. Similarly, simultaneous with Ruzicka's mechanistic proposals were those of Woodward (Nobel Laureate, 1965), whose insights explained, among other things, the cyclization leading to steroids (*39*). Still other investigators were using such ideas significantly, but with less success. Nevertheless, to Ruzicka belongs the credit for having concentrated his efforts on the isopentenoids and for having systematized a large share of the field using the powerful combination of structure and mechanism.

D. STRUCTURAL PERIOD

1. Introduction

With the turn of the twentieth century, the isopentenoid field entered the great period of structure determination. The challenges that were met spawned the equally important endeavor of searching widely for new substances to investigate. It also ushered in our modern methods of separation and identification. While the 1880s could only muster perhaps two dozen reasonably pure compounds, mostly with unknown structures, the present decade witnesses many hundreds of isopentenoids with constitutions understood in great detail. This is a remarkable achievement in 90 years. Its history is completely entwined in the concomitant development of organic and of physical organic chemistry, and it would be impossible to follow it all through here. More detailed accounts are available, especially those of Rodd (*40*), and Fieser and Fieser (*41, 42*). There are, however, some major aspects that deserve mention.

2. Wagner-Meerwein Rearrangements

As early as 1802, Kindt (*43*) had found that anhydrous hydrogen chloride furnished a crystalline material from turpentine. It was known as "artificial camphor" or later as "pinene hydrochloride," because it was also obtained in a similar manner from the more defined terpene, pinene. Berthelot (1859,1862) (*44, 45*) showed that, on treatment with bases, "pinene hydrochloride" yielded camphene, which itself was isolable from nature. Furthermore, Riban (1875) (*46*) showed that hydrogen chloride converted camphene to isobornyl chloride. C,H analyses demonstrated that all of these compounds had the same empirical formula except for the addition or elimination of HCl. Thus isomerism was being introduced during the various reactions. This and a number of other similar observations were finally explained by the work of Wagner (1899) (*47*) and Meerwein (1910, 1914, 1918) (*48-50*) and subsequent workers. The process has therefore come to be known as a Wagner-Meerwein rearrangement. It has found fundamental significance throughout organic chemistry and for our purposes, still more importantly, it forms much of the basis of Ruzicka's mechanistic "biogenetic isoprene rule" (Section C.4). In principle, what is involved is the formation of a positively charged species, which, by transfer of a pair of electrons (together with its accompanying carbon or hydrogen atom) to the charged site, results in a rearrangement of the structure. The incoming atom, as we know, approaches generally from the side opposite to the leaving atom, which produced the charge. When a proton attacks α-pinene (Scheme 1.10), it does so on the nucleophilic π-electrons of the

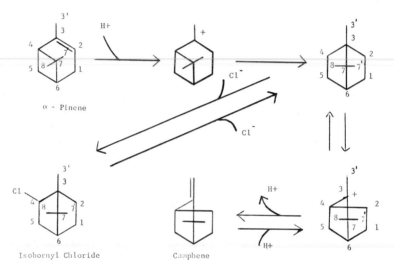

Scheme 1.10. Wagner-Meerwein rearrangement of α-pinene.

double bond creating a stabilized tertiary carbonium ion with the charge on C-3. The electrons of C-7 then feed into this charged center, breaking the C-4,7 bond and producing a charge on C-4. The C-2 electrons then do the same thing, yielding, after elimination of a proton, the rearranged and isomeric compound, camphene. Alternatively, the species with a charge on C-4 can add a chloride ion, yielding isobornyl chloride, which by treatment with base loses first a chloride ion, giving back the C-4 charged species, which proceeds then to camphene by further rearrangement and proton loss. In the presence of HCl the product is the hydrochloride, while in base it is the hydrocarbon purely from equilibrium conditions imposed by the reagent.

3. Monoterpene Structure

Geraniol, the simplest of the monoterpenes (C_{10}), was recognized by Semmler (51) in 1890 to be a primary alcohol. Five years later the structure of its aldehyde (the naturally occurring citral-a) and hence of itself was deduced by Tiemann and Semmler (1895) (52) from oxidations; shortly afterward it was confirmed by ozonolysis and synthesis. The structures of various other acyclic monoterpenes soon followed, e.g., of the isomeric linalool, which was synthesized by Ruzicka and Fornasir in 1919 (53) (Scheme 1.11).

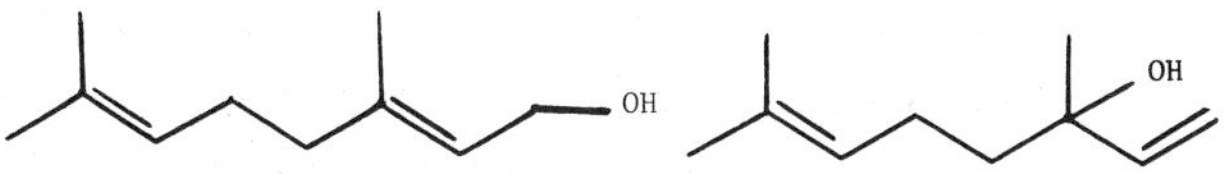

Geraniol   Linalool

Scheme 1.11.

α-Pinene, dipentene, and the latter's optical isomers, (+)- and (−)-limonene, have played an unusually large role in the elucidation of cyclic terpene structures, because of their ready availability in both turpentines and essential oils. From brominations, oxidations, and many other reactions and interconversions carried out by Wallach, Tilden, von Baeyer, Tiemann, Semmler, and others just before the turn of the century, a multitude of products were obtained. Their interrelationships were interpreted in the 1890s to mean that they must have the structures shown in the accompanying formulas (Scheme 1.12), and subsequent work has fully verified them. As early as 1904, limonene was obtained by synthesis (54).

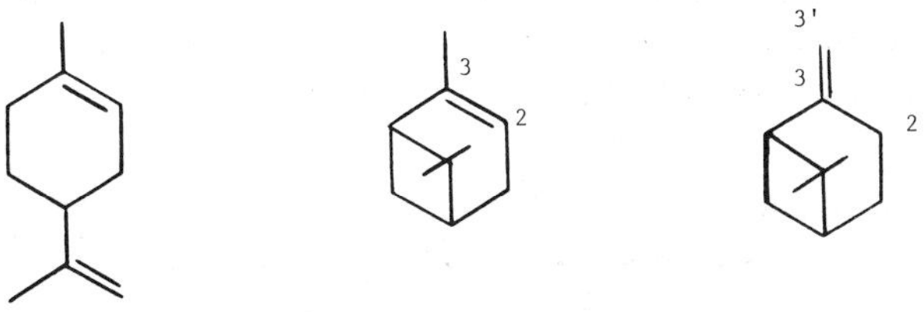

Dipentene α - Pinene β - Pinene
   or
Limonene

Scheme 1.12.

The elucidation of these structures was a major accomplishment, for the intellectual trial and error and the accumulation of facts and compounds produced in their investigation opened the door to structural definition of other compounds. A simple example is α-pinene's frequently co-occurring isomer (Scheme 1.12), β-pinene. β-Pinene, which has the double bond at C-3,3′ (instead of C-2,3), came to be understood during the next decade or so when it was shown, among other things, that both α- and β-pinene furnish the same hydrocarbon on hydrogenation (55, 56), that β-pinene can be isomerized to α-pinene by hydrogen-saturated platinum black (*57*), and that β-pinene on oxidation yields a monocarboxylic monohydroxy acid in which the rings are still intact (*58*). This information proved that the isomers had the same carbon skeleton and that the double bond of α-pinene must be at the carbon atom protruding from the six-membered ring.

The introduction of noble-metal catalysis after about 1900 had a tremendous effect on structural elucidation, because fundamental carbon skeletons became available for comparisons through hydrogenation. Similarly, an increasing catalog of carboxylic acids derived from terpene oxidations and unequivocal proof of their structures by synthesis allowed these reference materials also to enter the field. With such methods, together with a growing understanding of mechanism, the next 50 years saw all of nature's principal monoterpenes brought to structural definition.

4. Sesquiterpene Structure

Because the ability to understand structure was itself developing parallel with and in part because of research on terpenes, the chronological history of structural elucidation of these compounds follows roughly the size and complexity of the molecule. The C_{10} compounds came first. These were then followed by the C_{15} compounds (sesquiterpenes). The sesquiterpenoid cadinene and perhaps a few others were known early, but it was not until the 1920s that their chemistry was placed on a satisfactory basis. Before this, only one such terpene, farnesol, had yielded its structure (Scheme 1.13). This important feat (Kerschbaum, 1913) (*59*) was made unequivocal by the ozonolysis work of Harries and Haarmann (1913) (*60*).

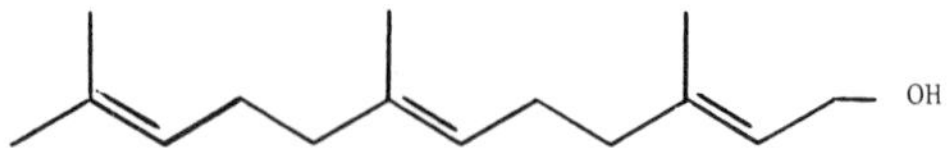

Scheme 1.13. Farnesol.

At this point Ruzicka entered the scene and masterfully began to solve the problem. One of his first contributions (Ruzicka and Meyer, 1921) (*61*) was a dehydrogenation with sulfur that converted cadinene to a naphthalenic hydrocarbon, cadalene (Scheme 1.14.). He then proved the structure of cadalene by synthesis (Ruzicka and Seidel, 1922) (*62*). This proved that Wallach's suggestion of 1887 (*21*) that sesquiterpenes such as cadinene have a naphthalenic skeleton (see Section C.2) was essentially correct. However, it was not until 1948 that Campbell and Soffer (*63*) arrived at the completely correct structure. Nevertheless, during this and subsequent periods, Ruzicka, Semmler, and more recently many others arrived at the structures of a large number of sesquiterpenes.

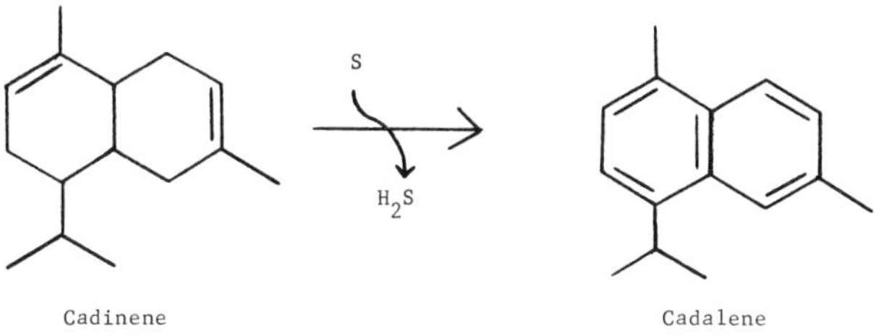

Cadinene   Cadalene

Scheme 1.14. Dehydrogenation of cadinene to a naphthalenic hydrocarbon.

5. Diterpenes

Probably the earliest diterpene (C_{20}) to be investigated seriously was phytol. It was isolated by Willstätter (Nobel Laureate, 1915) in the period 1907–1909 by cleavage from the chlorophyll molecule (*64–66*). He also carried out some important degradations of phytol (*67, 68*) (Scheme 1.15), which ultimately led in 1928 to a final solution of its structure through the synthetic work of F. G. Fischer (*69*).

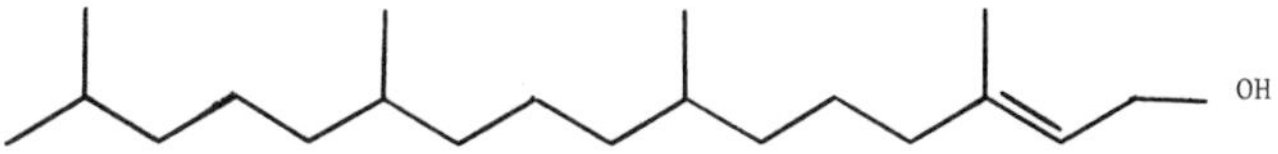

Scheme 1.15. Phytol.

Shortly thereafter, representatives of the cyclic diterpenes yielded their structures. The first clue came from Vesterberg (*70*), who converted abietic acid to retene by dehydrogenation with sulfur in 1903 (Scheme 1.16). In

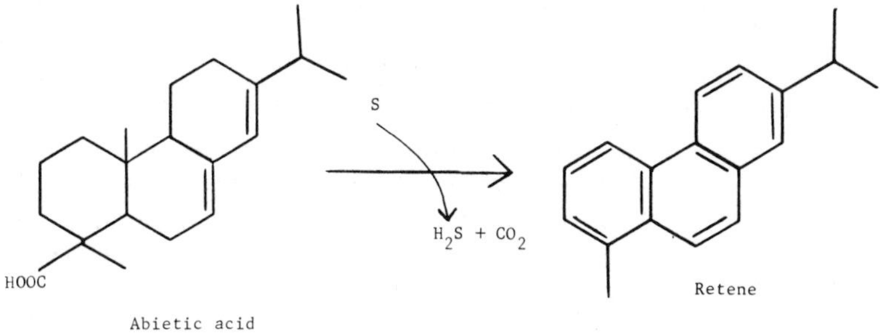

Scheme 1.16. Dehydrogenation of abietic acid to a hydrocarbon with a phenanthrene skeleton.

so doing he introduced this important kind of experiment to the isopentenoid field. As mentioned in the preceding section, Ruzicka made good use of it later for sesquiterpenes, as did Diels for steroids (Section D.6).

In the early 1930s the structures of retene and some related phenanthrenes were rigidly established by synthesis, and this and other extensive work occurring at the same time led to the correct formulation of not only abietic acid but several other diterpenes. In the following two decades, many more became known.

6. Triterpenes and Steroids

Because no C_{25} compounds had been discovered up to the time of the great flurry of activity in the terpene field taking place during the second quarter of the present century, no name has ever been given to these compounds as a class. However, the next larger molecules, the C_{30} compounds or triterpenes, were known. Of immense importance was the discovery of squalene (Scheme 1.17) in the liver of sharks, as early as 1916, by Chapman (1917)

Scheme 1.17. Squalene.

(71) and Tsujimoto (1916) (72). Being acyclic and symmetrically composed of two farnesyl residues linked head-to-head, this molecule was amenable to relatively easy structural elucidation principally through degradation at the double bonds carried out by Heilbron (73-75) in the late 1920s, and a few years later squalene yielded to synthesis from farnesol, a feat achieved by Karrer and Helfenstein (76). The all *trans*-character of the double bonds was demonstrated some years later through x-ray crystallography (77). The cyclic triterpenes and their relatives, the steroids, proved to be much more formidable structures to attack. Indeed, Wieland's steroidal structure, which formed a basis for his Nobel Prize in 1927, was wrong, illustrating the great complexity of the molecule. Later, in the 1950s, steroids were made industrially by total synthesis. This was the most complicated synthesis ever attempted on a commercial basis; in fact, it was so complicated that it was soon abandoned in favor of steroids that are preformed by plants and are only chemically modified. In the case of 11-oxygenated steroids of the corticoid type, which are so important to clinical medicine, even the industrial modification involves a step left to microbial metabolism.

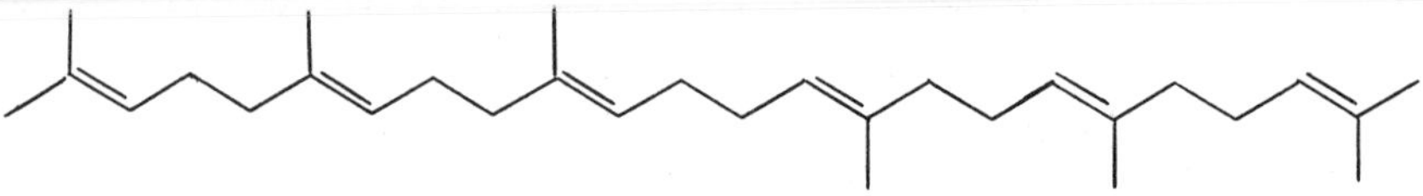

Much of the complication lies in the stereochemistry of these substances. Naturally occurring steroids can have as many as 11 asymmetric centers with 2^{11} or 2,048 stereoisomers. While this number is extreme, one of the most common steroids, sitosterol, still has nine asymmetric centers with 512 isomers, and cholesterol and cortisol have only one and two asymmetric centers less, respectively. Only two isomers of sitosterol exist and only one of cholesterol. Much of the earliest work in the 1920s and 1930s was therefore done on the stereochemically simpler steroids that bear double bonds in rings A and B that not only had fewer asymmetric centers but also had precise points (π-electron) that could be chemically attacked or formed. The estrogens, especially the naphthalenic equilenins isolated from horse urine, and vitamin D played a large role. The efforts of Bachmann (78, 79) and of Robinson (80–82) in the former case and those of a variety of workers in the latter were especially successful (for a thorough discussion, see Ref. 42). This, together with Diels' studies of the dehydrogenation of steroids to polycyclic aromatic hydrocarbons (83, 84), laid the basis for our understanding of the steroidal tetracyclic nucleus. A detailed account, especially of the stereochemical aspects, is beyond the scope of this discussion, but it is described in depth by Fieser and Fieser (42). Some appreciation of the events can be had from perusal of the biographies of the Nobel Laureates that follow in the next section. For a key to the literature on the structural elucidation of the triterpenoids, the books by de Mayo (85) and Ourisson et al. (86) should be consulted. The work of Ruzicka, Barton, Spring, and Jones was especially important.

The structures of most of the steroids and triterpenoids were determined in the quarter century between 1925 and 1950. In the next 25 years, just preceding the present writing, the major aspects of biosynthesis and distribution were worked out. It is this that is the subject of the remainder of this book, and in subsequent chapters the important steroid and triterpenoid structures are found at appropriate places, together with reference to their discovery. As we shall see, an intimate knowledge of the structures, especially of the simple ones described in this chapter, is crucial to an understanding of the biosynthesis, and Wallach's isoprene rule, Ruzicka's attention to electrophilic attacks on and reactions of double bonds, and the rearrangements of Wagner and Meerwein set the stage for the analysis of how nature makes these remarkable molecules. Since we now begin to perceive the purpose of their biosynthesis, which is discussed in the last chapter, the next 25 years should witness the elucidation of function in as great detail as the preceding two quarter centuries have seen structure and biosynthesis elucidated. Chapter 2 describes these fundamental structures, their classifications, and convention of nomenclature. Chapter 3 presents analytical methods used currently in research, and our biosynthetic story begins with Chapter 4.

E. NOBEL PRIZES

In one way or another work on the isopentenoids has been intermingled throughout the history of science with great discoveries and achievements. This is beautifully illustrated by the Nobel Prizes. Few other fields have had as many awards made. The Nobel prize has been given to no less than

19 scientists for work specifically with isopentenoids or for work utilizing these compounds at some stage. A brief biographical description of the Nobel Laureates and a summary of their achievements are discussed in this section.

1. In 1910 to Otto Wallach (1847–1931) of Germany "for his Innovative Work in the Field of Alicyclic Substances"

Wallach, educated at Göttingen, carried out his famous studies at Bonn, where he was stimulated by Kekulé's work on the nature of benzene. He was in charge of pharmacy beginning in 1879 and in this way came face to face with the challenge of "ethereal oils." Attacking the separation and structure of the components of these mixtures, which Kekulé said was impossible, he soon found them to be largely composed of substituted six-membered rings (terpenes) but with a higher hydrogen content than benzene. His efforts to understand and correlate the structures of these compounds led him to lay the foundations of alicyclic chemistry (i.e., the chemistry of nonbenzenoid rings). It was this particular chemical subject that the prize cited, but by defining the structures of the terpenes and enunciating the "isoprene rule" he had far more impact on the future course of science. Principally through his efforts it became clear that biological systems must have an isopentenoid pattern of biosynthesis. In 1889 he returned to Göttingen, working there until 1915, when he retired to devote himself to art.

2. In 1927 to Heinrich Wieland (1877–1957) of Germany "for his Research on Bile Acids and Analogous Substances"

After completing his doctorate at Munich under Thiele, Wieland remained there on the faculty. His academic career was interrupted by the First World War, during which he worked with Haber at the Kaiser Wilhelm Institute for Chemistry in Berlin-Dahlem. In 1921 he accepted a post at Freiburg and five years later succeeded to the chair recently vacated by Willstätter (Nobel Laureate, 1915) at Munich. From his earlier days at Munich he was impressed with biochemistry, having worked first on respiration and later on the structure of "natural products," notably the alkaloids morphine and strychnine, and the pigments of butterflies, the latter opening the door to pterin chemistry. In 1912 he began his work on bile acids. These investigations, spanning the next 20 years, together with those of Windaus, who was awarded the prize the following year, all but solved the mystery of steroid structure. Actually, in 1927 Wieland thought he had arrived at the correct formula and in his Nobel address he declared that "the last puzzles of our constitution problems have been solved." The structure proposed, however, was not entirely right, and it remained largely for others to resolve the problem during the next five years. Nevertheless, had it not been for Wieland's work, the structure of steroids would not have been elucidated at this time. The problem of the wrong structure only illustrates the immense complications of the molecule and the fact that both its investigation and its investigator were on the frontier of a science where the unexpected is a way of life. The talented Wieland had both talented parents and children. His father was a pharmaceutical chemist and one of his sons (Wolfgang) is a doctor of pharmaceutical chemistry. His other two sons are professors; Theodor is professor of chemistry at Frankfurt and Otto is professor of medicine at Munich. His daughter, Eva, is the wife of F. Lynen, who is himself a professor and Nobel Laureate (1964) in iso-pentenoids.

3. In 1928 to Adolf Windaus (1876–1959) of Germany "for his Studies on the Constitution of the Sterols and Their Connection with the Vitamins"

Windaus very early developed an abiding interest in living systems. At age nineteen he began the study of medicine in Freiburg and Berlin, and in 1897 he passed his preliminary examinations. By listening to lectures of Emil Fischer (Nobel Laureate, 1902) he became indelibly imprinted with the molecular approach to biology. He therefore changed from medicine to chemistry and was accepted by Kiliani as a doctoral student at Freiburg. Kiliani was interested in plant glycosides, especially those with unusual effects on man and other mammals. He had, for instance, studied the constituents of the upas tree, which natives of the Malayan archipelago used as an arrow poison. Thus it was that Windaus began his scientific career by investigating the nature of cardiotonic glycosides found in the Digitalis plant. It so happens that these glycosides are steroidal. Windaus recognized that he had only scratched the surface of the subject when he completed his degree in 1900. After a postdoctoral year with Fischer in Berlin, he returned to Freiburg and the aegis of Kiliani. In preparation for his Habilitation, he began his work on cholesterol, which he believed was the parent steroidal substance. This work ultimately won him the title of Assistant Professor in 1903, which he assumed at Innsbruck. In 1915 he succeeded Wallach as Professor of Chemistry at Göttingen, where he re-mained until his retirement in 1944. During the first quarter of the century, the work that Windaus did on the structures of cholesterol and vitamin D complemented what Wieland was doing simultaneously on the bile acids. To these two men we owe the essence of our knowledge of the steroid mole-cule. Windaus made many other contributions, however, not the least being a classic set of investigations of the imidazoles, which led him to the discovery of histamine. In addition, he spawned many discoveries through his students. One of these was Butenandt, who also won the Nobel Prize for work on isopentenoids. He is discussed in Section 6.

4. In 1937 to Paul Karrer (1889–1971) of Switzerland "for his Investigations on Carotenoids, Flavins and Vitamins A and B₂," and Walter N. Haworth (1883–1950) of England "for his Investigations on Carbohydrates and Vitamin C"

Karrer's career was from its earliest inception closely connected with the great ideas of the times. He studied chemistry with Werner (Nobel Laureate, 1913) at Zurich, working on organic arsenic complexes. Graduating in 1911, he spent an additional year there before going to Frankfurt, where he worked for six years with Ehrlich (Nobel Laureate, 1908) on the relationship of metal complexes and therapeutic effectiveness. A silver-salvarsan was developed from their collaboration. Returning to Zurich, he succeeded Werner in 1919 as Professor of Chemistry and began a study of plant pigments. His efforts were concentrated on the yellow-red pigments, the carotenoids. Only six had been described by then, and little was known about their structure. By the time Karrer gave his Nobel address, and largely through his efforts, 40 different carotenoids had been established in nature and the basic structural problems had been solved. It was also through Karrer's work that we know the structure of vitamin A and its relation to the carotenoids. Working in Karrer's laboratory, Wald (Nobel Laureate, 1967) proved the presence of large quantities of vitamin A in the retina, which contributed to Wald's later monumental investigations of the role of isopentenoids in the visual process. Karrer's mind was always inquisitive. As his carotenoid work led him to think about and study vitamin A, vitamin A led him to wonder about the relationship of vitamins to coenzyme action. He elucidated the structure of lactoflavin (riboflavin, vitamin B₂) and with Warburg (Nobel Laureate, 1931) went on to show the central significance of hydrogen transfer in the interaction of nicotinamide and lactoflavin. Karrer has also been a leader in the bringing together of vast amounts of scientific information in a digestable form. His textbook on organic chemistry has gone through 13 editions and is among the most famous in the world. He has been honored by election both to the Royal Society (London) and the National Academy of Sciences (Washington).

Since Haworth's contributions were not in the isopentenoid field, the reader is referred to such biographies as Farber (1953) (87) and to Nobel Lectures (4) for further information.

5. In 1938 to Richard Kuhn (1900–1967) of Austria and Germany "for his Work on Carotenoids and Vitamins"

Born in Vienna, Kuhn traveled to Munich to study in the laboratory of the famous Willstätter, who in 1915 had won the Nobel Prize for his work on chlorophyll. Kuhn's doctor's thesis on enzymes was completed in 1922. This, together with the fact that Willstätter had deduced the empirical formula for carotene and showed that the alkaloid pelleterine contained an eight-membered ring containing a conjugated set of double bonds, led Kuhn to an interest in polyunsaturated plant materials. His first task was to develop syntheses for polyenes. With pure materials of defined structure in hand he then began a study of their chemical, optical, dielectric, and magnetic properties. In all he synthesized more than three hundred such compounds, but as early as his sixth paper was already reporting structure determinations on naturally occurring materials. It was therefore inevitable that his work should parallel that of Karrer, and in 1931 he, Karrer, and Rosenheim simultaneously reported the successful separation of "carotene" into two isomers named α-carotene and β-carotene, distinguishable by different optical rotations and chromatographic properties. Two years later Kuhn discovered a third isomer, γ-carotene. This was followed by isolation, physical characterization, and structural analysis of many others, not the least of which were the oxygenated carotenoids (xanthophylls) such as violaxanthin and β-cryptoxanthin. Most of Kuhn's professional life was spent in Heidelberg, where he headed the Max Planck Institute for Medical Research. He was also Professor of Biochemistry at Heidelberg University. Besides his carotenoid contributions, Kuhn was associated with the discovery of vitamin B_6, and it is because of him that we know its structure. In collaboration with Szent-Gyorgi (Nobel Laureate, 1937) and Wagner-Jauregg (Nobel Laureate, 1927), he isolated lactoflavin and ultimately synthesized it. In one of his last papers he returned to the carotenoid problem with a detailed study of carotenoid-protein complexes. Despite his tremendous achievements, Kuhn was prevented from accepting the Nobel Prize by the prevailing political conditions in Germany.

6. In 1939 to Adolf Butenandt (1903–   ) of Germany "for his Work on Sex Hormones" and to Leopold Ruzicka (1887–   ) of Yugoslavia and Switzerland "for his Work on Polymethylenes and Higher Terpenes"

Butenandt won his doctorate at Göttingen under Windaus in 1927, the year before his professor won the Nobel Prize. He was thus well aware of the great story that was developing on sterols. Moreover, in the same year Aschheim and Zondek had demonstrated the presence of estrogens in the urine of pregnant women. Butenandt made good use of this information and by 1929, while still working at Göttingen, he isolated estrone, a feat independently carried out by Doisy (Nobel Laureate, 1943). The following year he confirmed Marrian's discovery of estriol, showed a relationship to estrone, and by 1932 had related them to cholesterol. By this time he had also isolated androsterone. After several interim years at Danzig, he became Professor at Berlin in 1936 and began a life-long association with the Max Planck Society, assuming Directorship of its Institute for Biochemistry at Berlin-Dahlem. The Institute was successively moved to Tubingen and finally to Munich. Butenandt moved both times, continuing his academic career at the respective universities of these cities. In 1960 he became President of the Max Planck Society. In the meantime he isolated urinary pregnanediol and converted it to progesterone. The year the Nobel Prize was awarded, he obtained this hormone from cholesterol and converted androsterone, as did Ruzicka independently, to testosterone. From these classic investigations the steroidal nature of the principal sex hormones was established, but Butenandt's scientific accomplishments encompassed even more, through, for instance, his investigations of tryptophan metabolism and the influence of genetics on it. Unfortunately, like Kuhn, he was prevented from accepting the Nobel Prize by the political climate of Germany.

Although a native of Yugoslavia by birth, Ruzicka was educated at the Technische Hochschule in Karlsruhe under Staudinger, whom he followed to the Eidgenossische Technische Hochschule (ETH) in Zurich. He has remained there to this day except for a period with friends in Geneva (1925–1926) and as a faculty member at Utrecht (1926–1929). His interest in isopentenoids stems from support he received prior to his Habilitation at the ETH from the perfume industry (Haarman and Reimer) of Germany and, after he became Privatdozent, from the Swiss pharmaceutical industry (CIBA). He very early achieved syntheses of fenchone, linalool, pinene, nerolidol, and farnesol. He coined the term "Wagner rearrangement," established the structure of jasmone, corrected Tiemann's structure of irone, and deduced the structures of the macrocyclic polymethylenes, civetone and muscone. His work on the terpenes, though, excited an interest that he has continued throughout his career. By investigating the structures of the sesqui- and higher terpenes, beginning in 1920, he extended Wallach's ideas into the more complicated realm of the polyisopentenoids. Through the "isoprene rule" he was able to postulate that the suggested formulas for phytol, abietic acid, caryophyllene, and many other substances were wrong. Probable formulas were then deduced from the "isoprene rule" and experiments designed to prove their structures. He also realized that many compounds, such as santene, with 9 C atoms, and the ionones, with 13 C atoms, were understandable in terms of an isopentenoid (or terpenoid as he called it) skeleton that had lost one or more carbon atoms. He therefore suggested that cholesterol, with 27 C atoms, might well be isopentenoid having a skeleton that had lost 3 C atoms. While he was not alone in making such a suggestion, his extensive and successful use of the "isoprene rule" gave a great weight to it. That we now know the hypothesis is correct is the result of experiments conceived in no small measure with the help of his thinking. The proof of this relationship, which he writes has been "one of my old cherished reveries," was left to others, but he did succeed in interrelating various steroids and in so doing he contributed to their structural elucidation. More recently, together with the powerful group of intellects he came to surround himself with, he developed an extensive theoretical correlation of the triterpenes with one another and with the steroids. It is based on the assumption of a fundamental precursor and the operation of reasonable chemical processes. "The biogenetic isoprene rule," as he calls it, remains today the basis of thought on the subject. Like his great intellectual predecessor Wallach, Ruzicka is devoted to art, especially Dutch and Flemish. With Switzerland isolated in 1939 by conditions in Germany, he was unable to travel to Sweden and accept his Prize, but when the war was over in 1945 he attended the ceremonies and was formally presented the Certificate and Nobel Medal.

7. In 1943 to Henrik Dam (1895–1976) of Denmark "for his Discovery of Vitamin K" and to Edward A. Doisy (1893–   ) of the United States "for his Discovery of the Chemical Nature of Vitamin K"

Dam studied chemistry at Copenhagen's Polytechnic Institute. Following graduation in 1920 he assumed the post of Instructor in Chemistry at the School of Agriculture and Veterinary Medicine. By 1928, after an interim in Pregl's laboratory in Austria, he moved to the Institute of Biochemistry at the University of Copenhagen as Assistant Professor and was named Associate Professor the following year, a post he held until 1941. Dam was always curious to find out what was happening in other laboratories, and this period at the University found him spending time in 1932–1933 as a Rockefeller Fellow with Schoenheimer in Freiburg, where he was introduced to the budding science of sterol metabolism. Three years later he went to Karrer's laboratory in Zurich. The beginning of the Second World War found him on a lecture tour in the United States. The German occupation of his native country prevented his return, but he made good use of his time by doing research at the Woods Hole Marine Biological Laboratories, the University of Rochester, and the Rockefeller Institute for Medical Research. Meanwhile, despite his absence from Denmark, he was appointed Professor of Biochemistry at Copenhagen's Polytechnic Institute. After the war he returned home and was honored in 1956 by being appointed Director of the Biochemical Division of the Danish Fat Research Institute. Dam published many papers during his career, mainly on the biochemistry of sterols, fats, and vitamins E and K. Except for the fats, all of these compounds are partly or wholly isopentenoid. In 1935 he discovered vitamin K in soybeans and other seeds and thus was among the first to contribute to our knowledge of the biological importance of the nonsteroidal isopentenoids to the biochemistry of animals and man. He was led to the discovery from studies he had made on cholesterol metabolism in chicks. Although he and others showed that animals could biosynthesize sterols, it also became evident that chicks would not thrive on diets from which sterols had been removed by extraction. In particular, they developed hemorrhages under the skin, in muscles or other organs, and blood taken for examination showed delayed coagulation. Sterols, as well as vitamins A and D, failed to solve the problem, but he finally succeeded in demonstrating that extraction of the diet was removing a substance, vitamin K, which would prevent the symptoms of disease.

Doisy's professional attainments began at the University of Illinois, his native state, where he won the A.B. (1914) and M.S. (1916) degrees. He embarked immediately on his postgraduate studies at Harvard. Although they were interrupted by service in the U.S. Army for two years, he completed his Ph.D. degree in 1920 and took up the post of Instructor at St. Louis' Washington University School of Medicine. His abilities were quickly recognized; by 1923 he was appointed full Professor and the following year Director of the Department of Biochemistry, St. Mary's Hospital. All of Doisy's work was done in St. Louis. Although he was cited in the Nobel Prize for proof of structure of vitamin K, he is at least as well known for his contributions to steroid biochemistry and physiology. As early as 1923, with E. Allen he devised a biological test for the estrogenic hormones. By making ovarian extracts and showing they induced estrus in animals, Allen and Doisy also established that the active principle is a chemical substance. Finally, simultaneously with Butenandt (Nobel Laureate, 1939), but independently, Doisy isolated pure estrone. The year 1929, less than a decade after his Ph.D. award, was not yet finished before Doisy was able to make the announcement of this great achievement. He continued work on the structure of estrone but soon found his attention, like Dam's, turning to the vitamin K problem. By establishing its structure through degradation as well as synthesis, Doisy, along with Fieser, Karrer, and Alongquist and Klose, who made similar contributions, proved the presence of an isopentenoid (phytyl) portion of the molecule.

8. In 1947 to Sir Robert Robinson (1886–   ) of England "for his Investigations on Plant Products of Biological Importance"

Robinson was born near Chesterfield, Derbyshire, England and educated at the University of Manchester, where he received the B.Sc. in 1906 and D.Sc. in 1910. He later received honorary doctorates from no less than 20 universities in England, Wales, Scotland, Ireland, India, Australia, France, Spain, and Yugoslavia. From 1912 to 1915 he was the first Professor of Pure and Applied Organic Chemistry at the University of Sydney, after which he held a variety of academic and industrial jobs in England until 1930, when he became a Fellow of Magdalen College and Waynflete Professor of Chemistry at Oxford University, a post he held until his retirement in 1955. In the latter year he published a book, *Structural Relations of Natural Products,* which in many ways crowned his career. In both it and his earlier research papers he presented structural facts and ideas which, as Wallach had done much earlier, he used to analyze probable biosynthetic pathways. His contributions dealt primarily with alkaloids, but his exploration and grasp of chemistry in general had a substantial effect in the steroid field. He had long been interested in cyclic molecules as a result of his alkaloid work, and the steroids, with their complicated stereochemistry, offered a suitable challenge to his ingenuity. In 1935 he began a series of investigations directed toward the total synthesis of estrogens. In the period 1938–1945, after encountering some difficulties with estrone, he succeeded in obtaining one (isoequilenin) with both A and B rings aromatic. In the same period he succeeded in synthesizing a degradation product of desoxycholic acid. One of the substances obtained, a tricycle composed of rings A, B, and C, possessed *cis-anti-trans-* stereochemistry, and Robinson felt this achievement also presaged the total synthesis of coprosterol. The work with the estrogens led him to still another accomplishment. Reasoning that estrogenic activity was related to structure by a phenolic group and three-dimensional characters of the rest of the molecule, with the cooperation of Professor E. C. Dodds he made the steroidal analog, stilbestrol, (also known as diethystilbestrol), which is a simple stilbene (diphenylethylene) derivative. Stilbestrol not only proved to be a potent estrogen but it retains today an important place in clinical medicine. At the end of his career, writing for his book, his attention was drawn to the origin of the "extra" alkyl group at C-24 of phytosterols. He suggested they were derived from carboxylic acids other than acetate that were inserted early in the pathway. While he was later proved to be wrong, his thoughts stimulated the first experiments actually to be done on the problem; these experiments then led to the discovery of the methyl group of *S*-adenosylmethionine as the correct precursor.

9. In 1950 to Edward Calvin Kendall (1886–1972) of the United States, Philip Showalter Hench (1896–1965) of the United States, and Tadeus Reichstein (1897–   ) of Poland, Russia, and Switzerland "for their Discoveries Concerning the Suprarenal Cortex Hormones, Their Structure and Biological Effects"

Although a New Englander by birth, Kendall received all of his college and postgraduate education in New York City, where he received his Ph.D. degree in chemistry at Columbia in 1910. During the next year he was with Parke, Davis, and Company in Detroit, then for three years with St. Luke's Hospital in New York City. In 1914 he joined the staff of the Mayo Foundation in Rochester, Minnesota, as Professor of Physiological Chemistry and Head of the Section of Biochemistry. Many years later, despite formal retirement at the age of 65, Kendall did not cease to devote himself to experimental biochemistry. Leaving Rochester he went to Princeton, New Jersey, where he continued his work at Princeton University's James Forrestal Research Institute (the former Princeton branch of the Rockefeller Institute), where another Nobel Laureate, W. H. Stanley, did his famous work on tobacco mosaic virus. Kendall very early became interested in the active constituents of endocrine glands (and even earlier with science, having connected his home to a friend's with a telephone at the age of ten). Except for a relatively brief concern with enzymes, glutathione, and oxidative metabolism, he has spent his whole professional life in endocrinology. Known to his colleagues as an indefatigable worker, he achieved the isolation of hormones from two different glands. The first, thyroxine, which he named after the thyroid gland of its origin, crystallized for him on the morning of December 25th after a feverish Christmas Eve of work when he was but 29 years old. This paved the way for effective treatment of countless patients with defects in basal metabolism. While he went on to make important contributions to its structure, success was achieved ahead of him by C. R. Harrington. Kendall therefore turned his attention to the isolation of glutathione. After accomplishing this and proving it to be a tripeptide, he tackled the adrenal cortex, "the last of the ductless glands to yield its secrets to the investigator," as he was fond of saying. Between 1934 and 1936 he succeeded in isolating eight steroidal components of the adrenal cortex, which he named "Compounds A–H." Simultaneously, Reichstein was doing much the same thing. In the same year, 1936, both isolated the famed cortisone, known to Reichstein as his Substance F_a and to Kendall as his Compound E. Through their efforts, together with those especially of O. Wintersteiner and J. J. Pfiffner, we know that the adrenocortical hormones are steroids, and steroids of particular and unique structures. While the isolations were almost superhuman in terms of hard work (Kendall processed 150 tons of beef adrenals in one period of several months), the structural elucidation took an equal amount of intellectual agility, for there existed no established prototypes and the basic steroidal structure was itself only just becoming known. Kendall added to these accomplishments an avid interest in chess, which he played by mail, and the old English game of skittles, which he played with visitors to his home. His mind and interest in science were active to the day of his sudden death at 86.

Hench was born in Pittsburgh and graduated from Lafayette College with the A.B. degree in 1916. He was awarded the M.D. degree four years later from the University of Pittsburgh, and after an internship at St. Francis Hospital in the same city he began his life-long association with the state of Minnesota. First a Fellow of the University, he soon became First Assistant in Medicine at the Mayo Clinic, Instructor in Medicine in the University-affiliated Graduate School of the Mayo Foundation, and Head of the Clinic's Section on Rheumatic Diseases. In 1947 he became full Professor. His driving force intellectually was that "within every rheumatoid patient corrective forces lie dormant, awaiting proper stimulation." What can this force be? His mind searched endlessly. "Regardless of the supposed validity of the microbic theory," he wrote, "rheumatoid arthritis can be profoundly influenced by phenomena which are primarily biochemical." He had in mind the reversibility of the disease, which can be induced by jaundice, pregnancy, surgical procedures, etc. Hans Selye had made it clearly known that the adrenal glands were related to man's reaction to stressful conditions such as surgery. Maybe the "antirheumatic substance" originated in the adrenals. Kendall agreed. In January, 1951, Hench made an entry in his notebook "Try Compound E," but seven years elapsed before enough material could be obtained for him to do so. Through cooperative efforts between L. H. Sarett and J. van de Kamp at Merck and Company and Kendall in Rochester, Hench succeeded in having enough cortisone to inject into a 29-year-old woman who had been a pathetically crippled rheumatoid patient for four and a half years. Although she was to the point where she scarcely was able to rise from bed, after cortisone treatment for less than a week she was making a shopping trip to downtown Rochester. This dramatic result was repeated later on many other patients. Subsequent work both at the Mayo Clinic and elsewhere also showed that Kendall's and Reichstein's steroids together with aldosterone (discovered in Kendall's laboratory by his associates, H. L. Mason and V. R. Mattox, after his retirement and independently by the Taits in England) do indeed have the classic functions attributed to this gland. Hench's great accomplishments were made despite a serious speech impediment, which remained with him until his death.

Reichstein was born in Poland and spent his early childhood in Kiev. After a period in Berlin the family moved to Zurich and became Swiss citizens. He graduated in chemical engineering from the Eidgenössische Technische Hochschule in 1920. After a year in industry he returned to the E.T.H. and completed his doctorate (1922) in organic chemistry. Remaining there, he worked with Karrer on the aromatic (volatile compounds with aroma) constituents of roasted coffee, a project that resulted in today's Nescafe. Then as a faculty member in his own right at the E.T.H. (Assistant Professor, 1934; Associate Professor, 1937) he spent many years teaching before being called to Basel. There he assumed Chairmanship of the University's Department of Pharmacy and of the Pharmaceutical Institute. Eight years later he was asked to head the Organic Division, a post he continues to hold. He has always loved nature. Several Alpine paths have been named for him and he has climbed the Alps' most treacherous peaks. "You're quite apt to find him," a friend once said, "face upward, floating serenely down the Rhine." His intellect was equally fixed on high places. He synthesized vitamin C and published over a hundred papers in carbohydrate chemistry. But his greatest accomplishment was, like Kendall's, the isolation and structural elucidation of the adrenal cortical hormones, which he began in 1934. He did not think they were steroidal because their solubilities were very different from those of known steroids, but in the first chemical degradations the results strongly suggested a relationship to cholesterol. He was subsequently able to prove this in several ways. By 1937 he had even succeeded in converting an oxidative product of cholesterol to one of the hormones, desoxycorticosterone, a year before it was actually isolated from the gland. Following his work in the hormones, with equal brilliance Reichstein investigated the sources and structures of plant steroids and ways in which they might be used to synthesize the hormones.

10. In 1950 to Otto Paul Hermann Diels (1876–1954) of Germany and Kurt Alder (1902–1958) of Germany "for the Development of the Diene Synthesis"

Although this award, like Wallach's, did not itself specify anything isopentenoidal in the formal citation, it was so integrally associated with the field that it deserves inclusion here. Indeed, Diels' Nobel Address was entitled "Description and Importance of the Aromatic Basic Skeleton of the Steroids." Both men were interested in the unusual properties of polyenes, and from their work comes the modern "Diels-Alder addition" to dienes, so useful in synthetic chemistry. Diels, however, had an early and abiding interest as well in dehydrogenations leading to the aromatic hydrocarbons and especially in their use to elucidate the structure of the compounds from which they were derived. As his Nobel Address shows, he was also strongly drawn to the sterol problem. By dehydrogenation of cholesterol he obtained chrysene and later (1927) the methylcyclopentanophenanthrene which bears the basic tetracyclic system of the steroids. This latter hydrocarbon, known as "Diels hydrocarbon," figured heavily in the work of Windaus, Wieland, and others which ultimately proved how the steroids are constructed. Diels studied under Emil Fischer (Nobel Laureate, 1902) at Berlin, graduating in 1899. Seven years later, after passing rapidly through the assistant and lecturer phases of his academic career, he became Professor. In 1915 he accepted a call to the University of Kiel as Professor and Director of the Institute of Chemistry, where he remained until his retirement in 1945.

Since Alder's work was not directly concerned with isopentenoids his biography is omitted.

11. In 1964 to Konrad Bloch (1912–   ) of Germany and the United States and to Feodor Lynen (1911–   ) of Germany "for their Discoveries Concerning the Mechanism and Regulation of Cholesterol and Fatty Acid Metabolism"

Born in Germany, Bloch left his native land in 1936 because of the Nazi situation and settled in the United States. He won his Ph.D. (1938) in biochemistry at Columbia in the laboratory of the famed Rudolf Schoenheimer, whose interest in the purity, stereochemistry, and origin of cholesterol had already spanned many years. In 1937, with David Rittenberg, Schoenheimer published a classic paper in which experiments with deuterium-enriched water led to the conclusion that cholesterol was derived in animals from numerous small molecules. Working further with Rittenberg, Bloch was able to show in 1942, using deuterioacetate, that the small precursor molecule is acetate. R. Sonderhoff and H. Thomas had in the meantime shown the same thing for ergosterol in yeast. Thus, a building-up principle was operating and Bloch set out to unravel it. By showing ultimately through remarkably elegant experiments that acetate led to squalene, squalene to lanosterol, and lanosterol to cholesterol, he discovered the basic elements of sterol biosynthesis which had been sought for during a period of at least a century. In 1954 he became Higgins Professor of Biochemistry at Harvard, the post he now holds, after a number of years at the University of Chicago. While much of his interest still remains in the sterol field, it is not confined to it. Early in his career, during the period of work with deuterium-labeled substrates, he was able to show that fatty acids are derived by polymerization of acetate, which opened the huge field of fatty acid metabolism to its current state of extensive investigation. Furthermore, his investigations of sterol biosynthesis in insects both showed an unusual character in not having early steps in the pathway and also led him to an important hypothesis widely used today concerning the role of sterols in biological systems. He found that but little of the sterol the insect needed was metabolized and suggested that it functions therefore as an architectural component in some way. From his and other people's efforts it now appears probable, if not yet certain, that the architectural role is in membrane structure.

Lynen, born and educated in Munich, where he studied under Wieland (Nobel Laureate, 1927), has spent his whole career in his native city. Joining the Chemistry Department of the University in 1942, he was made Professor a scant five years later, and in 1954 accepted the direction of the Max Planck Institute for Cell Chemistry. His professional life has been deeply involved with the role and mechanism of action of small acids. Searching for the nature of "active acetate," he succeeded in discovering acetyl coenzyme A. Few molecules have such a ubiquitous and multiple biochemical significance, among many other things being utilized for isopentenoid biosynthesis. Lynen's further work on fatty acid biosynthesis and on the function of biotin in the intermediate conversion of acetyl CoA to malonyl CoA brought him equal success. Then, "with the discovery of mevalonic acid in the laboratory of K. Folkers," as he wrote in 1958, "the study of the biosynthesis of terpenes and steroids from acetic acid has entered upon a new phase." It was especially because of Lynen's work that the "new phase" was placed on a sound footing, for he showed, just a step ahead of Bloch's closely similar findings, that mevalonic acid leads to the isopentenyl pyrophosphates, which in turn lead to the "terpenes and steroids." Indeed, the isopentenyl pyrophosphates so carefully identified by Lynen constitute the true C_5 unit of isopentenoid biosynthesis, which two generations earlier Wallach and later Ruzicka has foreseen conceptually if not precisely as isoprene.

12. In 1965 to Robert Burns Woodward (1917–   ) of the United States "for his Outstanding Achievements in the Art of Organic Synthesis"

Woodward's contributions to synthesis, for which his Nobel prize was awarded, have spanned most of organic chemistry. Among his most notable achievements was the synthesis of the alkaloids (quinine, reserpine, and strychnine), the antibacterial agent cephalosporin C, and the photosynthetic pigment chlorophyll. In addition, he has contributed to the structural determination of antibiotics, e.g., aureomycin and terramycin, and paved the way for their synthesis. Of special interest to the isopentenoid field, Woodward was responsible for the synthesis of cholesterol, the total synthesis of cortisone, and the synthesis of lanosterol from cholesterol (in collaboration with Barton, Nobel Laureate, 1969). In the area of structural determination by physical methods, Woodward also made important contributions. He applied his results from the investigation of the UV properties of 1,3-butadiene to polycyclic heteroannular dienes and concluded that bathochromic shifts would be produced by each alkyl group or ring residue bonded to any of the carbon atoms in the diene system or by additional exocyclic double bonds. These observations were subsequently refined by Fieser and Fieser and have become an invaluable tool for the prediction of steroidal structure on the basis of UV absorption. His mastery and understanding of the ways in which organic molecules interact intra- and intermolecularly prompted him, in collaboration with the biochemical genius of Bloch (Nobel Laureate, 1964), to propose a scheme for the cyclization of squalene to lanosterol. Their proposals, i.e., appropriate folding pattern of squalene, electrophilic attack, and subsequent Wagner-Meerwein rearrangements, have been substantiated over the years by numerous brilliant experiments carried out by Bloch and others.

Born in Boston in 1917, Woodward has spent his entire professional career there. He received his Bachelor of Science and doctorate degrees at the Massachusetts Institute of Technology and joined Harvard University in 1937 as a Postdoctoral Fellow. In 1953 he was made Morris Loeb Professor of Chemistry and in 1960 the Donner Professor of Science, a position he still holds. Not only is his reputation world-wide, but his activities extend beyond his native shores. He is director of the Woodward Research Institute in Basel, Switzerland, and is a Member of the Board of Governors of the Weizmann Institute of Science in Israel.

13. In 1969 to Derek H. R. Barton (1918–   ) of England and to Odd Hassel (1897–   ) of Norway "for their Contributions to the Development of the Concept of Conformation and Its Application in Chemistry"

In 1950, Barton published a brief paper entitled "The Conformation of the Steroid Nucleus" (88) which has had enormous impact on the structural determination of triterpenes, steroids, and other molecules. In this historic paper he described the tool of conformational analysis, which allows the chemical and physical properties of a molecule to be interpreted in terms of a preferred conformation and which allowed him to examine in considerable depth the relationship between configuration and conformation of steroids, triterpenes, etc. Among his more notable achievements was the structural elucidation of lanosterol, cycloartenol, euphol, α-onocerin, and oleanic acid, all of which are pivotal polycyclic isopentenoids.

Barton was born on September 8, 1917, and educated at the Imperial College, University of London, from where he received his undergraduate degree in 1940 and Ph.D. (Organic Chemistry) in 1942. In 1945 he again became associated with the Imperial College in various capacities, culminating with his appointment as Professor of Organic Chemistry in 1957. Barton was also appointed Regius Professor of Chemistry at the University of Glasgow in 1955.

The biography of Odd Hassel will not be discussed here since his contributions have not been directly related to the isopentenoid field. His work on the structure of cyclohexane, its derivatives, and other compounds containing six-membered rings related to cyclohexane was generalized and applied by Barton to more complicated systems, i.e., the triterpenes, culminating in conformational analysis.

14. In 1975 to John W. Cornforth (1917–   ) of England "for his Researches on the Stereochemistry of Enzyme-Catalyzed Reactions" and to Vladimir Prelog (1906–   ) of Switzerland "for his Researches on the Stereochemistry of Organic Molecules and Reactions"

Cornforth has devoted his career to the study of the stereochemistry of natural products. He received his doctorate at Oxford in 1941 under Sir Robert Robinson (Nobel Laureate, 1947) and continued working with him during the war on the structure of penicillin and on the chemical syntheses of steroids, an effort culminating in the total synthesis of epiandrosterone. While investigating squalene, Cornforth developed a novel stereospecific synthesis of olefins that is now in general use. More recently, he has synthesized the plant hormone dormin (abscisine II) of terpenoid origin as well as proved its structure. During his stay at the Mill Hill Research Laboratories of Medical Research Council (1946–1962), Cornforth's interest in the stereochemistry of enzyme processes developed. While director of the Milstead Laboratory of Chemical Enzymology of Shell Research Ltd. in Kent from 1962 to the present, Cornforth pursued detailed studies of the stereochemistry of enzyme-catalyzed reactions in the early stages of the isopentenoid pathway from mevalonate to squalene, for which his Nobel Prize was awarded. With the use of stereospecifically labeled mevalonic acid (labeled at C-2, C-4, and C-5 with deuterium or tritium), he was able to follow the fate of the label in the products of the various enzymatic reactions leading to squalene (i.e., decarboxylation, isomerization, and two types of condensation reactions). From his data on labeling patterns in the precursors and products of each step he was able to determine the stereochemical course of squalene biosynthesis and gain insight into the mechanism of the enzyme-catalyzed reactions. Thus, Cornforth was able to resolve 13 out of the 14 stereochemically defined steps leading from mevalonate to squalene. The last step involved the brilliant use of tritium and deuterium labeling in the same molecule to define the stereochemistry of H^+ addition to C-4 of isopentyl pyrophosphate during its isomerization to dimethylallyl pyrophosphate. Cornforth's wife, the former Rita H. Harradence (also an Oxford Ph.D.), has worked with him for more than 35 years. It was she who was responsible for the actual synthesis of the labeled mevalonate precursors.

Since Prelog's award was not in the terpenoid field, his biography will not be discussed here.

LITERATURE CITED

1. M. E. Chevreul, Ann. Chim. 95:5 (1815).
2. M. Berthelot, Ann. Chim. Phys. 56:51 (1859).
3. F. Reinitzer, Sitzungber. Kaiserl. Wiss. Wein, Math.-Naturwiss. Kl. Abt. I 97:167 (1888).
4. Nobel Lectures. Chemistry. Nobel Foundation, Vols. 1-4. Elsevier, New York, 1964-1972.
5. A. Strecker, Ann. Chem. Pharm. 67:1 (1848).
6. F. Mylius, Ber. Dtsch. Chem. Ges. 19:374 (1886).
7. O. Wallach, Justus Liebigs Ann. Chem. 227:283 (1884).
8. O. Wallach, Justus Liebigs Ann. Chem. 230:262 (1885).
9. O. Wallach, Justus Liebigs Ann. Chem. 239:34 (1887).
10. A. Kawalier, J. Prakt. Chem. 58:226 (1853).
11. O. Jacobsen, Ann. Chem. Pharm. 157.234 (1871).
12. W. A. Tilden and W. A. Shenstone, J. Chem. Soc. 31:554 (1877).
13. H. Wackenroder, Geigers Magazin Pharm. 33.144 (1831).
14. W. C. Zeise, Ann. Chem. Pharm. 62:380 (1847).
15. R. Willstätter and W. Mieg, Justus Liebigs Ann. Chem. 355:1 (1907).
16. R. Willstätter and H. H. Escher, Hoppe-Seyler's Z. Physiol. Chem. 64:47 (1910).
17. F. A. Hartsen, Chem. Zentralbl. 204 (1873); C. R. Hebd. Séances Acad. Sci. 76:385 (1873).
18. A. Millardet, Bull. Soc. Sci. Nancy 1.111 S.21 (1875).
19. M. Faraday, Quart. J. Sci. 21:19 (1826).
20. A. E. Souberain and H. Capitaine, Ann. Chem. Pharm. 34:323 (1840).
21. O. Wallach, Justus Liebigs Ann. Chem. 238:78 (1887).
22. J. W. Bruhl, Ber. Dtsch. Chem. Ges. 21.163 (1888).
23. A. Vesterburg, Ber. Dtsch. Chem. Ges. 18:333 (1885).
24. F. Bouchardat, Bull. Soc. Chim. Fr. 24:108 (1875).
25. C. G. Williams, Proc. Roy. Soc. 10:516 (1860).
26. W. A. Tilden, Chem. News 46:129 (1882).
27. Gladziatsky, Bull. Soc. Chim. Fr. 47:168 (1887).
28. W. A. Tilden, J. Chem. Soc. 45:410 (1884).
29. O. Wallach, Justus Liebigs Ann. Chem. 238:78 (1887).
30. F. W. Semmler and K. Bartelt, Ber. Dtsch. Chem. Ges. 40:4595 (1907).
31. F. W. Semmler and K. Bartelt, Ber. Dtsch. Chem. Ges. 41:128 (1908).

32. F. W. Semmler and K. Bartelt, Ber. Dtsch. Chem. Ges. 41:389 (1908).
33. F. W. Semmler and K. Bartelt, Ber. Dtsch. Chem. Ges. 41:867 (1908).
34. P. de Mayo, Chemistry of Natural Products. In K. W. Bentley (ed.), Mono- and Sesquiterpenoids, Vol. II. Interscience, New York 1959.
35. W. Loebisch, Ber. Dtsch. Chem. Ges. 5:510 (1872).
36. A. Windaus and C. Resau, Ber. Dtsch. Chem. Ges. 46:1246 (1913).
37. L. Ruzicka, Proc. Chem. Soc. 341 (1959).
38a. A. Eschenmoser, L. Ruzicka, O. Jeger, and D. Arigoni, Helv. Chim. Acta 38:1890 (1955).
38b. R. Robinson, The Structural Relations of Natural Products. The Clarendon Press, Oxford, 1955.
39. R. B. Woodward and K. Bloch, J. Am. Chem. Soc. 75:2023 (1953).
40. E. H. Rodd, Chemistry of Carbon Compounds, Vol. II B. Elsevier, New York, 1953.
41. L. F. Fieser and M. Fieser, Natural Products Related to Phenanthrene. 3rd Ed. Reinhold, New York, 1949.
42. L. F. Fieser and M. Fieser, Steroids. Reinhold, New York, 1959.
43. F. Kindt, Tromms J. Pharm. 11:132 (1802).
44. M. Berthelot, Ann. Chem. Pharm. 110:367 (1859).
45. M. Berthelot, C. R. Hebd. Séances Acad. Sci. 55:496 (1862).
46. J. Riban, Ann. Chim. 6:363 (1875).
47. G. Wagner, J. Russ. Phys. Chem. Soc. 31:680 (1899).
48. H. Meerwein, Justus Liebigs Ann. Chem. 376:152 (1910).
49. H. Meerwein, Justus Liebigs Ann. Chem. 405:129 (1914).
50. H. Meerwein, Justus Liebigs Ann. Chem. 417:255 (1918).
51. F. W. Semmler, Ber. Dtsch. Chem. Ges. 23:2965 (1890).
52. F. Tiemann and F. W. Semmler, Ber. Dtsch. Chem. Ges. 28:2132 (1895).
53. L. Ruzicka and V. Fornasir, Helv. Chim. Acta 2:182 (1919).
54. W. H. Perkin, J. Chem. Soc. 85:416 (1904).
55. G. Vavon, C. R. Hebd. Séances Acad. Sci. 150:1127 (1910).
56. G. Vavon, C. R. Hebd. Séances Acad. Sci. 150:1428 (1910).
57. F. Richter and W. Wolff, Ber. Dtsch. Chem. Ges. 59:1733 (1926).
58. A. von Baeyer, Ber. Dtsch. Chem. Ges. 29:25 (1896).
59. M. Kerschbaum, Ber. Dtsch. Chem. Ges. 46:1732 (1913).
60. C. Harries and R. Haarmann, Ber. Dtsch. Chem. Ges. 46:1737 (1913).
61. L. Ruzicka and J. Meyer, Helv. Chim. Acta 4:505 (1921).
62. L. Ruzicka and C. F. Seidel, Helv. Chim. Acta 5:369 (1922).
63. W. F. Campbell and M. D. Soffer, J. Am. Chem. Soc. 64:417 (1942).
64. R. Willstätter and F. Hocheder, Justus Liebigs Ann. Chem. 354:205 (1907).
65. R. Willstätter, F. Hocheder, and E. Hug, Justus Liebigs Ann. Chem. 371:1 (1909).
66. R. Willstätter and A. Oppe, Justus Liebigs Ann. Chem. 378:1 (1911).
67. R. Willstätter, E. W. Mayer, and E. Huni, Justus Liebigs Ann. Chem. 378:73 (1911).
68. R. Willstätter, O. Schuppli, and E. W. Mayer, Justus Liebigs Ann. Chem. 418:121 (1918).
69. F. G. Fischer, Justus Liebigs Ann. Chem. 464:69 (1928).
70. A. Vesterberg, Ber. Dtsch. Chem. Ges. 36:4200 (1903).
71. A. C. Chapman, J. Chem. Soc. 111:56 (1917).
72. M. Tsujimoto, J. Ind. Eng. Chem. 8:889 (1916); see also Chem. Z. I:638, 1048.
73. I. M. Heilbron, E. D. Kamm, and W. M. Owens, J. Chem. Soc. 1630 (1926).
74. I. M. Heilbron, W. M. Owens, and I. A. Simpson, J. Chem. Soc. 873 (1929).
75. I. M. Heilbron and A. Thompson, J. Chem. Soc. 883 (1929).

76. P. Karrer and A. Helfenstein, Helv. Chim. Acta 14:78 (1931).
77. N. Nicolaides and F. Laves, J. Am. Chem. Soc. 76:2596 (1954).
78. W. E. Bachmann, W. Cole, and A. L. Wilds, J. Am. Chem. Soc. 61:974 (1939).
79. W. E. Bachmann, W. Cole, and A. L. Wilds, J. Am. Chem. Soc. 62:824 (1940).
80. R. Robinson, J. Chem. Soc. 1390 (1938).
81. A. Koebner and R. Robinson, J. Chem. Soc. 1994 (1938).
82. A. J. Birch, R. Jaeger, and R. Robinson, J. Chem. Soc. 582 (1945).
83. O. Diels and W. Gadke, Ber. Dtsch. Chem. Ges. 60:140 (1927).
84. O. Diels, W. Gadke, and P. Kording, Justus Liebigs Ann. Chem. 459:1 (1927).
85. P. de Mayo, The Higher Terpenoids. Interscience, New York, 1959.
86. G. Ourisson, P. Crabbe, O. R. Rodig, Tetracyclic Triterpenes. Holden-Day, San Francisco, 1964.
87. E. Farber, Nobel Prize Winners in Chemistry, 1901-1950. H. Schuman, New York, 1953.
88. D. H. R. Barton, Experientia 6:316 (1950).

Chapter
2

Structure
and
Nomenclature

A. Chemical Classification of Steroids.................................... 37
    1. *Steroidal Character* 37
    2. *Sterols* 44
    3. *Ring System* 44
    4. *Numbering of Carbons* 45
    5. *Stereochemistry* 46
    6. *Naming of Steroids* 57
B. Biological Classification of Steroids 71
    1. *General* 71
    2. *Progestogens* 71
    3. *Corticoids* 71
    4. *Androgens* 72
    5. *Estrogens* 72
    6. *Cardiac-Active Steroids* 73
    7. *Bile Acids and Alcohols* 74
    8. *Vitamin D* 75
C. Other Classifications of Steroids....................................... 76
    1. *Sapogenins* 76
    2. *Steroidal Alkaloids (Azasteroids)* 77
D. I Classification 80
    1. *Introduction* 80
    2. *I_1 Stage* 82
    3. *Higher Acylic I Stages* 82
Literature Cited.. 83

A. CHEMICAL CLASSIFICATION OF STEROIDS

1. Steroidal Character

   a. Early and Current Usage Louis and Mary Fieser were the first to struggle with the problem of what a steroid is. The name itself is derived from the term "sterol," which in turn comes from that part of "cholesterol" that originated in the Greek "stereos," meaning solid, since cholesterol is a solid substance. From the use of the suffix "oid," "steroid" thus means something that is like cholesterol, and the implication is a structural similarity. Exactly in what way, however, there is a structural similarity is not so simple to arrive at, and the current literature is anything but consistent. Workers in medicine and endocrinology frequently use "steroid" to mean only hormones (or hormone metabolites) such as cortisol, testosterone, etc., and distinguish cholesterol by referring to it as a "sterol." On the other hand, structural chemists refer to the closely related cycloartenol as a "triterpenoid." The compound lanosterol has an even more ambiguous history. Its name implies steroidal character, while it most often is referred to as a triterpenoid and has at times been called a "C_{30} steroid" to distinguish it from, as well as to relate it to, cholesterol, which has 27 carbon atoms. These inconsistencies have crept into the literature despite the fact that all of the compounds mentioned fall under the term "steroid" as defined by Fieser and Fieser (1, 2). Why should this be? The principal problem lies in the fact that no really unique definition of "steroid" has been proposed. In fact, it was only in 1959 that Fieser and Fieser came to use the word in a book title (1). Previously their famous steroid books, in three editions, were entitled *Natural Products Related to Phenanthrene*, and in the last edition (1949) (2) morphine was included.

While steroidal uniqueness, if there is such a thing, was not apparent 20 years ago, Fieser and Fieser's efforts at that time (1) succeeded in giving us an extremely useful working definition, as follows: *The term steroid is employed to indicate all those substances that are structurally related to the sterols and bile acids to the extent of possessing the characteristic perhydro-1,2-cyclopentanophenanthrene ring system* ("perhydro" meaning fully hydrogenated). This definition places the essence of steroidal character on the tetracyclic system (Scheme 2.1) present in the sterols (which, as Fieser and Fieser (1949) (2) recognized, embraces both saturated and unsaturated members) and in the bile acids. Examples of sterols used by Fieser and Fieser are cholesterol, cholestanol, and coprostanol, cholic acid being one of their bile acid examples. This definition is therefore clear in one regard, that steroids have in common the partly or wholly hydrogenated skeleton of 1,2-cyclopentanophenanthrene. What it does not define is the stereochemistry, since cholestanol and coprostanol, for instance, are diastereoisomers; nor does it define the presence or absence or character of any substituents, especially of methyl groups. Recent knowledge has made these two questions of very considerable importance, because: (1) there are naturally occurring compounds, e.g., euphoids, which have the common skeleton, if stereochemistry is ignored, but which do not appear to have a common polycyclic biosynthetic precursor with cholesterol, cholestanol, etc.; (2) there are natural compounds that have from one to five additional carbon atoms on the

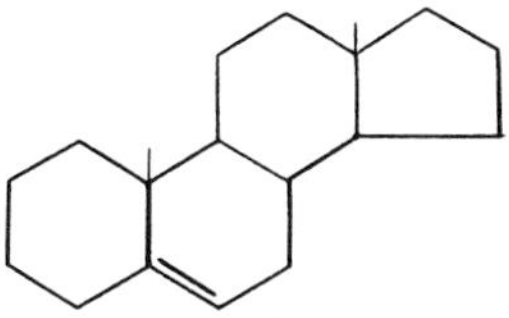

(Cholesterol)

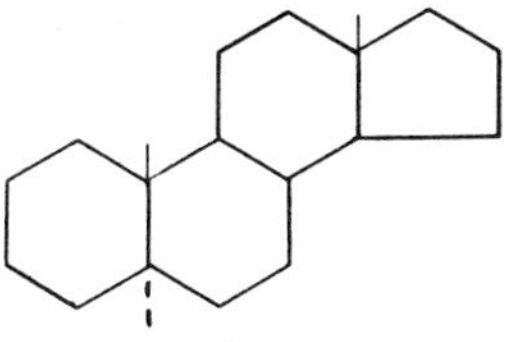

H   (Cholestanol)

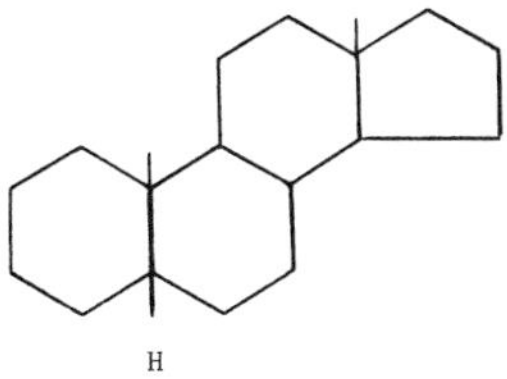

H

(Coprostanol, Cholic Acid)

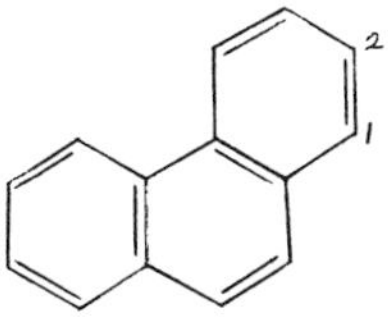

Phenanthrene

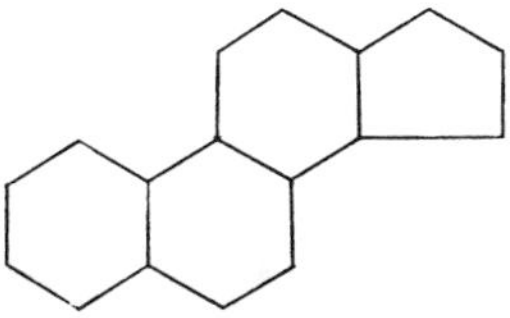

Common Saturated Steroid Tetracycle
1,2-Cyclopentanoperhydrophenanthrene

Scheme 2.1. *Polycyclic systems employed by Fieser and Fieser in defining steroidal character.*
(Names given in parentheses are for common molecules bearing the polycycle shown.)

common skeleton; and (3) there are natural compounds with substituents that are not even methyl groups. Examples of these differences are: (1) euphol, with five methyl substituents compared to the common skeleton but, more importantly, with three more than in cholesterol, and an inverted stereochemistry compared to cholestanol at three positions (between the five- and six-membered rings and at the juncture of the C_8 side chain); (2) lanosterol with the same stereochemistry as cholesterol but three additional carbon atoms; and (3) cycloartenol, with, among other things, an additional methylene substituent forming a cyclopropyl ring (Scheme 2.2).

Fieser and Fieser's definition of a steroid would, strictly speaking, encompass all of these compounds. However, in common usage among investigators of the field this has not been the case. As already briefly mentioned, euphol and cycloartenol are regarded as belonging to the distinct triterpenoid class of C_{30} compounds, while the problem is begged with lanosterol by usually classifying it as a triterpenoid and naming it as a sterol. The problem lies in the following facts. Historically, the majority of known subtances in nature with the 1,2-cyclopentanophenanthrene skeleton had the stereo-

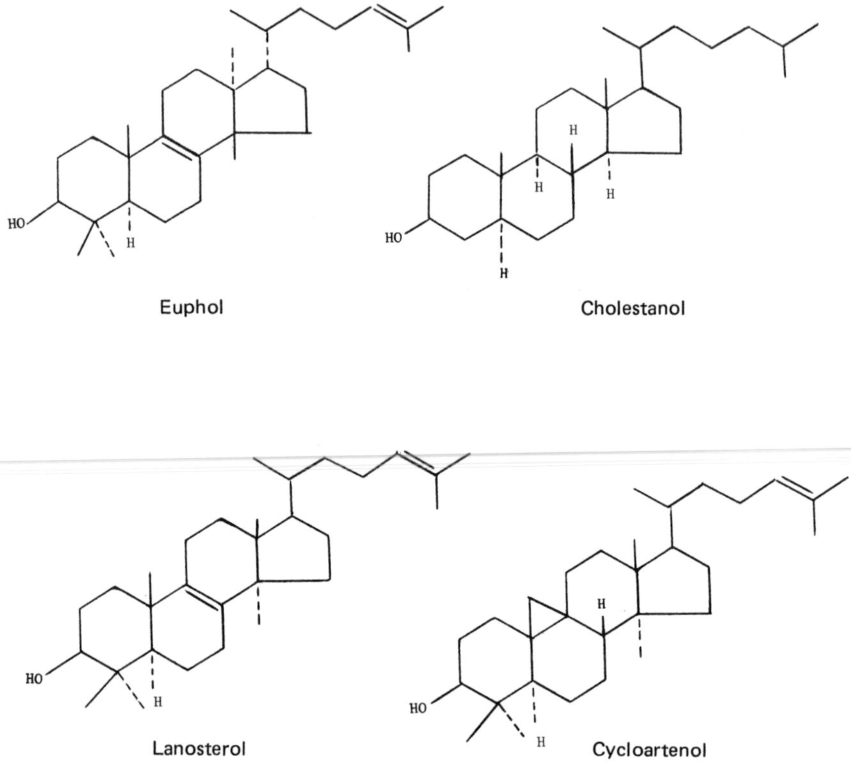

Euphol   Cholestanol

Lanosterol   Cycloartenol

Scheme 2.2. Some different tetracycles.

chemistry either of cholestanol or coprostanol, possessed no more than two C_1 groups on the tetracyclic skeleton, and possessed in entirety no more than 29 carbon atoms, and usually 27 or less. Furthermore, the biological origin of these "steroids" was obscure. On the other hand, the historically fewer tetracyclic C_{30} compounds, such as euphol and cycloartenol, more or less following the isoprene rule, clearly were triterpenoid. Man's sense of simplicity and order, therefore, put them in a class with other C_{30} compounds that were already known to vary from acyclic to pentacyclic. With the development of the biogenetic isoprene rule this classification became eminently reasonable, because it became clear that the various C_{30} compounds all had a common biosynthetic precursor (squalene).

The problem has become further complicated by the fact that a number of "C_{30} compounds" actually have more or less than 30 carbon atoms. An example is eburicoic acid, with an extra carbon atom (methylene group) on the side chain (Scheme 2.3). This we now know to be added to the primary C_{30} skeleton, and by defining a triterpenoid in a biosynthetic sense as one being derived from an isopentenoid C_{30} precursor we would have the

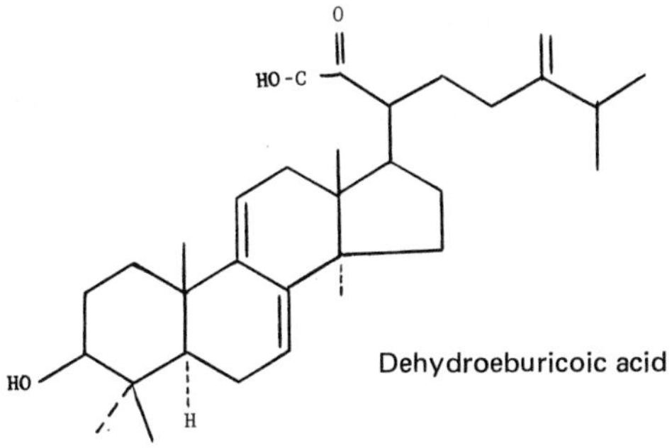

Dehydroeburicoic acid

Scheme 2.3. A C$_{31}$-tetracycle.

problem resolved. The C$_{31}$ compounds would become triterpenoid by virtue of having been derived biosynthetically from a "true" triterpenoid. If carbon additions are allowed biochemically, why not carbon subtractions? In fact, macdougallin (Scheme 2.4), with only 28 carbon atoms, is clearly a tri-

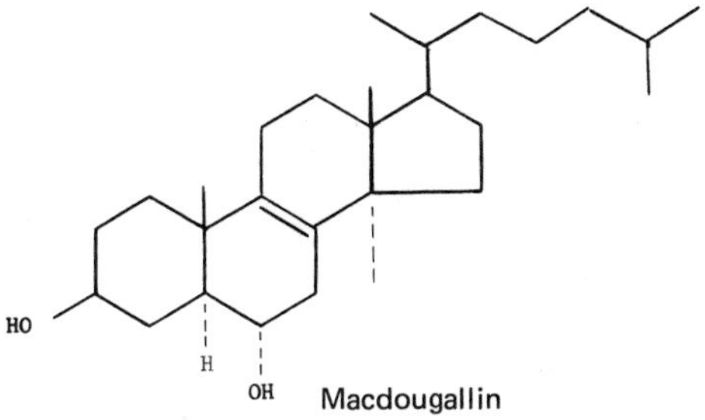

Macdougallin

Scheme 2.4. A C$_{28}$-tetracycle.

terpenoid in this view, representing a hydroxydihydrolanosterol from which two carbon atoms have been removed. What then about the mammalian equilenin and estrone (Scheme 2.5)? They have only 18 carbon atoms. In

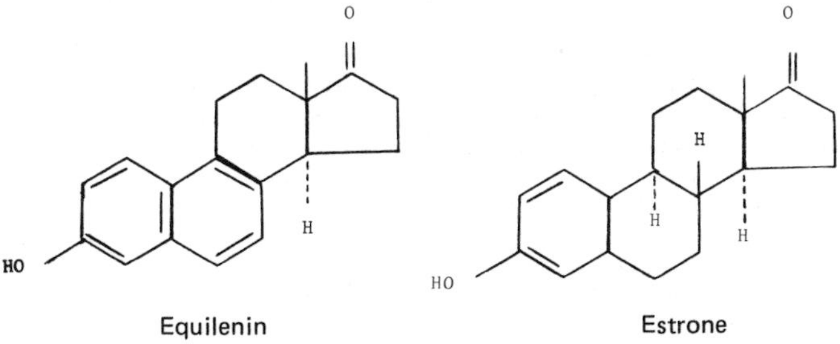

Equilenin

Estrone

Scheme 2.5. C$_{18}$-tetracycles.

chemical, physical, and biological properties they are much more closely related to simple phenolic compounds than they are to either cholesterol or lanosterol; yet we know that estrone is a physiologic metabolite of lanosterol through cholesterol by oxidative removal of carbon and hydrogen, and equilenin almost certainly is, too. Are they then triterpenoids, as macdougallin could be called, or are all of these compounds steroids? We believe an answer to this problem can be given.

b. Definitions of Steroid and Triterpenoid   For the reasons brought out in the foregoing section, current usage is ambiguous. It should also be evident that whatever system is used a certain amount of arbitrariness must be present to prevent an unmanageable continuum. The authors therefore recommend and will use in this book the definitions that are explained in what follows. When one views the manner in which the polycyclic C_{30} compounds are formed in nature, it becomes evident that the folding or cyclization pattern leading from squalene to lanosterol and its stereochemical analogs is unique. Squalene is also the known precursor of a variety of other polycyclic types. Despite considerable differences in structure among these various compounds, the transitions from the acyclic to the cyclic states are basically of only two kinds (Scheme 2.6). One is what we shall call the *triterpenoid transition*, in which a condition (probably bonded to the cyclase at C-20) is reached having *trans-anti-trans-anti-trans-anti* stereochemistry.[1] This is thermodynamically the most stable of the stereochemical possibilities. The other and obviously less stable is the *trans-syn-trans-anti-trans-anti* stereochemistry, which we shall call the *steroid transition*. Through the latter arise lanosterol and cycloartenol, while most of the other C_{30} types arise through the former. This difference is the basis for our definition of steroidal character.

We shall define a *steroid as a compound with the 1,2,-cyclopentanophenthrene skeleton, which either in its own biosynthesis or in the biosynthesis of one of its precursors has passed through a state possessing stereochemistry similar to the trans-syn-trans-anti-trans-anti configuration.* Because the common steroids, such as cholesterol, result from several different kinds of metabolism ensuing after formation of the "steroid transition" (also known as the "protosteroid cation"), a full appreciation of what a

---

[1] The terms *cis* and *trans* refer, respectively, to similar and opposite configurations at a ring junction where two carbons atoms are common to the two rings. The terms *syn* and *anti* refer, respectively, to similar and opposite configurations when there are no common atoms. The series of terms, e.g., *trans-anti*, is taken to refer to the stereochemical condition as one encounters the junctures from left to right in the structure.

trans-anti-trans   *cis-syn-cis*

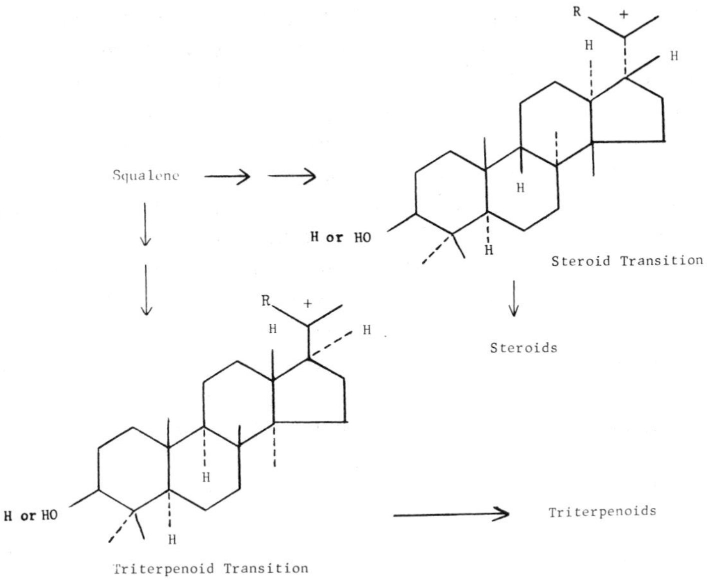

Scheme 2.6. Biosynthetic basis for steroid and triterpenoid classification. (The cations shown probably are not really charged entities but are bonded to the cyclase at C-20 with the enzyme in front in the steroid transition and in the back in the triterpenoid transition.)

steroid is requires an understanding of these processes, which are described in subsequent chapters. It will be found by examining what happens that the "transition definition" proposed here encompasses all the compounds, e.g., cholesterol, sitosterol, bile acids, corticoids, and estrogens, that fall under the "structural definition" of Fieser and Fieser (1), but that the "transition definition" specifically excludes euphol and its relatives, which would be tetracyclic triterpenoids (not by virtue of having 30 carbon atoms but as a result of having passed through the triterpenoid transition). Furthermore, the "transition definition" classifies the two C_{30} compounds, lanosterol with four rings and cycloartenol with five, as well as all of their metabolites as steroids and not as triterpenoids. This has great merit, since both are precursors to the common steroids. It therefore becomes possible to say that steroids and triterpenoids are distinct biosynthetic classes and that neither group has a defined number of rings nor a defined number of carbon atoms. It is, however, necessary to subdivide the steroid category according to the extent of methyl migration, methyl elimination, and methyl or other carbon addition. Steroids bearing the carbon skeleton of the "steroid transition" are already known as *"protosteroids"* or *"protosterols"* (3), a practice we subscribe to. Steroids that have a methyl group at C-13 (lacking in protosteroids) could then be distinquished for emphasis where the occasion requires by borrowing from taxonomic use in biology of the prefix "eu" (Greek, "well"; commonly used to imply "true") and calling them *eusteroids*. Steroids lacking one or more methyl groups are frequently described, as we also recommend, by the term "desmethyl." Thus, we speak of "4β-desmethyllanosterol," usually shortened to "4-desmethyllanosterol" since the remaining methyl group nearly always has the α-configuration, making the β-designation for the one that is missing superfluous. When a methyl group is added, one simply so designates, as in the description "24α-ethylcholesterol" for sitosterol. Because we define a steroid without reference to the exact number of carbon atoms, "4,4-dimethylsteroid" is a perfectly acceptable and common term to imply that the two methyl groups at C-4 of ring A have not been removed. Contrariwise, "4,4-desmethylsteroid" implies that both methyl groups are missing.

A triterpenoid is then any molecule which passed through the all-*trans-anti*-state ("triterpenoid transition") in its biosynthesis or in the biosynthesis of its precursor. Not only the tetracyclic euphol but the pentacyclic amyrins and many other compounds can be accounted for in this way.

2. Sterols

The term "sterol" has never been formally defined to the authors' knowledge, although it is one of the commonest biochemical words. It is usually taken to mean a steroidal alcohol with lipid properties. Historically, the first example was cholesterol, followed by its simple derivatives (sitosterol, 7-dehydrocholesterol, etc.). Derivatives of cholesterol bearing an additional hydroxy group have more recently come to be recognized in nature, but they pose no real problem to the tacit definition and can be called sterols. On the other hand, we now know that higher animals in particular degrade cholesterol to C_{21}-steroidal alcohols, which no longer are lipid-like in their solubilities. What grouping they are to belong to has never been agreed to. Some of them, especially those with ketonic groups, have endocrinologic properties and are classified as "hormones," but this leaves the others, which fail to give a defined biological response, in a sort of limbo. The authors see no real resolution to this problem nor can they propose a better definition of "sterols." However, just for the sake of clarity we will use the term *sterol* to mean *any hydroxylated steroid that retains some or all of the carbon atoms of squalene in its side chain and partitions nearly completely into the ether layer when it is shaken with equal volumes of water and ether*. This is only a more precise definition of common usage. Although it suffers from inclusion of detailed solubility, this characteristic is probably very important in determining the biological role of cholesterol and other classic sterols (Chapter 11).

3. Ring System

The four rings characteristic of steroids are denoted by the capital letters of the alphabet, A-D, as shown in Scheme 2.7. If, as in the case with certain steroids, substitution by heteroatoms (X and Y) with formation of two

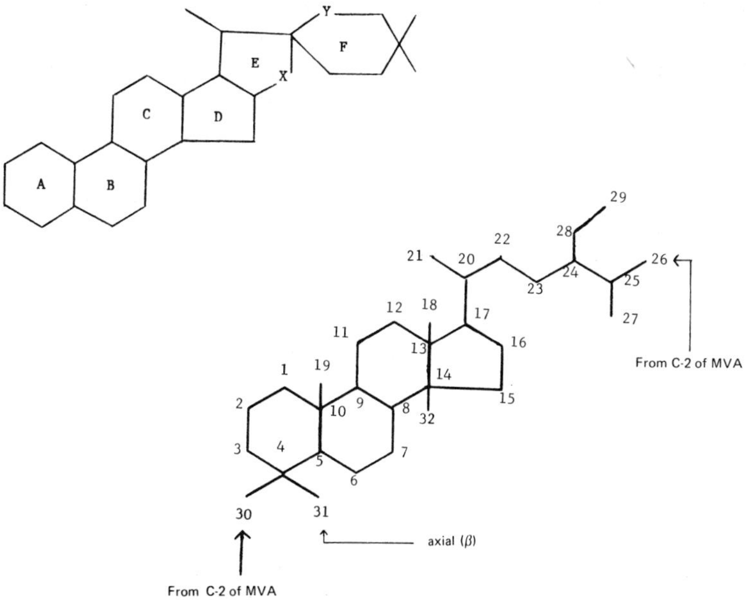

Scheme 2.7. Designations of carbon atoms and rings. Stereochemistry is ignored.

additional rings occurs in the side chain, the latter are designated E and F. The letter designation of rings also applies to triterpenoids.

4. Numbering of Carbons

The accompanying formula (Scheme 2.7, which ignores stereochemistry) shows the maximum number of carbon atoms that a steroid was known to bear until recently. The conventional numbering system is also shown. The numbering system appears haphazard and is the result of the chronology of structural elucidation. Steroids with additional methyl groups attached to C-23 and C-29 as well as with a cyclopropyl bridge between C-22 and C-23 are now known. Again with deference to chronology, we propose that the methyl group on C-29 be accorded the C-33 designation, that the group at C-23 be called C-34, and that the methylene bridge be referred to as C-35. We also will use the numbering system of Fieser and Fieser (1) as shown so that the methyls on C-4 and C-14 are designated 30, 31, and 32. This is different from, but the authors believe preferable to, the system used by Boiteau et al. (4). Neither the two methyls on C-4 nor those on C-25 are biosynthetically equivalent. This was not envisioned in the original numbering, but in order to accommodate the newer information the authors propose and will use in this book a system in which the lower numbered of the two atoms is derived from C-2 of mevalonic acid which is equivalent to the *trans*-methyl group at the terminus of squalene. Insofar as C-30 and

C-31 are concerned, this also has gross stereochemical significance, since one of the two is equatorial (C-30) and the other is axial. At the other end of the molecule the same convention (Scheme 2.7) will apply to C-26 and C-27. It is unfortunate that in a steroid, such as lanosterol, bearing no substituent at C-24, there will be a break (no C-28 or C-29) in the consecutive numbering. However, the alternative, to change the numbering of C-28 and C-29, destroys simple comparison with well-established usage in the literature. This is not to say the history of nomenclature is consistent. In the older literature (before about 1950) the numbered description of C-18 and C-19 is reversed.

When a name is used as a parent and the parent bears a carbon that is not present in the compound under consideration, the prefix "nor" is used, preceded by the number of the absent atom. If two or three atoms are missing, the prefix "bisnor" or "trisnor," respectively, is used. For instance, the cholestane skeleton is also the 30,31,32-trisnorlanostane skeleton.

5. Stereochemistry

a. Tetracyclic Skeleton   The tetracyclic skeleton of steroids in the *trans-anti-trans-anti-trans* configuration is like a table top, in that it is solid with two coplanar surfaces (or planes). Where a double bond (Δ^5, Δ^8, etc.) is present at a ring juncture, the stereochemistry is similar to that of the *trans*-fusion. All of the carbon atoms lie approximately in the two surfaces. If the molecule is viewed on its edge (Scheme 2.8) so that ring A is to the

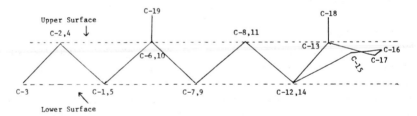

Scheme 2.8. Steroid skeleton viewed from an edge, illustrating table top quality.

left and C-2 is away and C-4 toward the observer, then C-1, C-3, C-5, C-7, C-9, C-12, and C-14 lie in the bottom surface and C-2, C-4, C-6, C-8, C-10, C-11, and C-13 lie in the upper surface. C-15, C-16, and C-17 are a bit different, because they are in a five-membered ring, but they conform approximately by being closer to the upper than to the lower surface. Because of this stereochemistry, in which the steroid is extended or spread out, the molecule is frequently said to be "flat." It should be noted, however, that the "flat" character is three dimensional and not like that of benzene, in which all 12 atoms lie in a single plane.

If one of the carbons at a ring juncture is inverted from the foregoing condition, the molecule loses its flatness. There are several results, depending on which carbon or carbons are inverted, but a common one is inversion of C-5 yielding the *cis-anti-trans-anti-trans* configuration (A/B-*cis* configuration). In this case the molecule approximates the shape of an L in which the angle is at the A/B-juncture.

The flat condition of the steroid skeleton is dependent on all rings being in the chair conformation. This is normally achieved. However, if a boat form is present, interesting phenomena result from the proximity of otherwise distant atoms. For instance, in the A/B-*cis* configuration it is not impossible for ring A to assume the boat conformation, and, when it does, C-3 and C-9 are sufficiently close to bond to a common atom. Thus, the 3,9 epoxide of the A/B-*cis* (but not of the A/B-*trans*) series can be prepared synthetically.

Studies of the x-ray diffraction pattern of more than 80 steroids by Bernal, Crowfoot, and their collaborators (5) [see Turner, 1949 (6) for a key to the literature and a more extensive discussion] during the 1930s and 1940s demonstrated the stereochemical nature of the skeleton and in addition made possible calculation of its average dimensions. An observed 4-Å thickness represents both the separation of the "table top surfaces" as well as of the bond distances for the protruding atoms on either side. It will be seen to be in excess of the value (3.08 Å) for two covalent bonds placed linearly adjacent to one another (protruding atoms). The difference (measured to be 0.8 Å) represents the distance between the two surfaces holding the carbon atoms of the rings. See Chapter 11 for additional information derived from x-ray patterns.

b. Angular Methyl Groups   Extensive chemical and x-ray crystallographic work has established that both C-18 and C-19 are on the same side of the molecule and arranged vertically when the molecule is viewed on edge, as described in Section A.5a. When the molecule is viewed on its side in the usual manner (with ring A down and to the left and ring D up and to the right) the methyls project toward the observer. The C-10—C-19 and the C-13—C-18 bonds lie approximately at 90° to the upper surface of the "table top." The C-18 and C-19 groups are, therefore, frequently spoken of as "angular methyl groups," and the side they are on is known as the "front side."

c. Effect of Double Bonds   When double bonds are introduced into a six-membered ring, the stereochemistry is significantly but not greatly altered. Of particular importance, the stereochemistry of a ring junction approximates the *trans* or *anti* condition when a double bond is present at the junction. Thus, cholesterol (with a double bond between C-5 and C-6), lanosterol (with a double bond between C-8 and C-9), and cholestanol (with no double bonds) all have essentially the same stereochemistry.

d. Conformations, Configurations, and Stereochemical Nomenclature for Tetracyclic Nucleus   The conformation and configuration of steroids are known to play an enormously large role in their biochemistry. Inversion of a single configuration can abolish a given biologic effect. We have already seen something about the gross stereochemistry of the ring system in Sections A.5a–A.5c. The purpose of the present section is to refine this and to consider substituents other than C-18 and C-19.

The word "conformation" refers to spatial orientation when any two atoms joined by a single bond are rotated with respect to each other. *Conformational isomers* (or *conformers*) are therefore *rotational isomers*. This is to be contrasted with *configurational isomerism*, which can only be induced by breaking two bonds and remaking them in an opposite fashion (placing X where Y was). In a conformational analysis of steroids, bonds that are at 90° to the two "table top" planes (Section A.5a) of the steroid skeleton are designated as "axial," while those that lie in planes approximately coplanar with the "table top" are termed "equatorial."

In Scheme 2.9 it will be seen that substituents on the tetracyclic skeleton

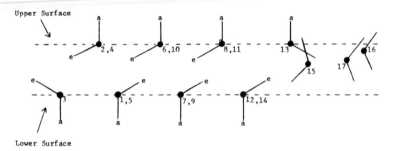

Scheme 2.9. Steroid skeleton viewed on edge showing spatial orientation of substituents. a, axial; e, equatorial.

(viewed on edge) project above and below the "table top" as well as more or less coplanar with it. It will also be seen that on adjacent carbons, e.g., C-2 and C-3, the axial substituent of each one is on the side opposite from the other. Furthermore, none of the substituents on C-15, C-16, and C-17 are clearly axial or equatorial, except the downward substituent (H in natural steroids) at C-17, which is more nearly axial than equatorial. The other five substituents in ring D have both axial and equatorial characteristics. True equatorial substituents are to be found in each of the other three rings at all positions not at a ring junc-ture. Because the tetrahedral angle is 109° instead of 90°, the equatorial bonds point slightly up or down and away from the rings (Scheme 2.10). If a deeper in-sight is to be had into these steric phenomena, the reader should study an ac-tual molecular model. See also Chapter 11.

As in all cyclohexane stereochemistry, of which steroidal stereochemistry is a part, rotational isomerism from the chair form (assumed in the foregoing) to the boat form inverts the conformation of substituents, but it does not invert the configuration (since no bonds are broken). For this reason, conformational integrity is dependent on rotational integrity. In so far as rings B, C, and D are

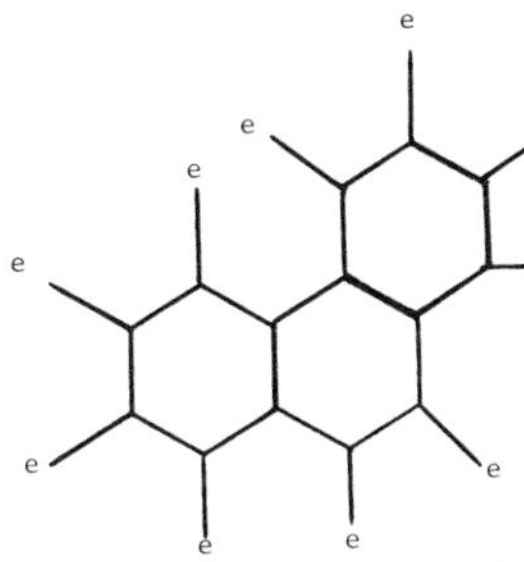

Scheme 2.10. Steroid skeleton viewed on its side. e, equatorial.

concerned, diaxial interactions appear to be large enough in the boat form to ensure that these rings are in the chair form. Ring A is also usually in the chair form, although it is easier for it to "flip" into the boat conformation.

The two possible configurations of substituents on the steroid skeleton are designated α and β. At any given carbon, there are two valences involved in ring formation and two available for substituents. For any given substituent, then, there are two possible valences to use. These valences are not stereochemically equivalent, because on each carbon atom the other two valences (used for ring formation) are not equivalent. This is another way of saying that each carbon atom in the steroid ring system is essentially asymmetric. It becomes formally asymmetric when the two substituents are different, and there are two configurations, α and β. It was known quite early that the angular methyl groups are both on the same side of the molecule. They were arbitrarily assigned the β-configuration. Since they are axial, there is no ambiguity about what the word "side" means. It follows that all other substituents that are axial and on the same side as the angular methyls are given the β-designation, while axial substituents on the opposite side are α-oriented.

What about equatorial substituents? Unfortunately, at the time the original framers of the α, β-designation worked, conformational analysis was unknown. They thought "side" would always be clear and did not envision that there would be (equatorial) substituents projecting strongly on neither side. Nor did conformational analysis actually help, because it only made clear that at C-3, for instance, the change from the chair form to the boat form places both α- and β-substituents on the same side of the molecule as C-18 and C-19. Furthermore, C-16 does not have true axial and equatorial substituents. In fact, the situation in ring D approximates the assumptions of the framers of both this and the sugar stereochemical designation, namely, that all rings are completely flat, with a substituent above and one below the plane. If this were true, there would be no ambiguity and a simple and accurate convention could be established. Although it is not true, it is possible to force the molecule into this shape without breaking bonds. This imaginary process is what one does to establish configurational relationships. *Assume that the angles of the bonds involved in ring formation are bent so that all carbons in the rings lie in a single plane. A substituent on the same side of this plane as C-18 and C-19 is designated β, while one on the opposite side is designated α (Scheme 2.11).*

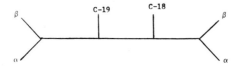

Scheme 2.11. Edge view of steroid in which bonds are distorted so that ring carbon atoms are all in a plane. Only four positions other than C-18 and C-19 are shown.

If one studies an undistorted molecular model, it becomes evident in and due to the chair puckering of the six-membered rings that there will be an alternation of configuration and conformation as one proceeds from one carbon atom to another. Thus, at C-1 the α-substituent is axial. On C-2 the α-substituent is equatorial. On C-3 the α-substituent is axial again, and so on. Similarly, on adjacent carbon atoms β-substituents will be axial on one and equatorial on the other.

Since the configuration of a substituent controls and fixes its conformation in a given chair-boat situation, the substituent is given only a configurational assignment in nomenclature. This is done by placing the Greek letter immediately after the position number followed by a dash and the description of the substituent, e.g., 2β-hydroxy. In order to deduce the conformation of a substituent, it is useful to memorize the configurational-conformational relationship of a substituent in two different parts of the molecule. In the usual chair condition, for example, the 3β-position is equatorial while the 11β-position is axial. With these in mind one can rapidly deduce, for instance, that the 5α- and 12α-substituents are axial.

In steroid drawings, an α-substituent is shown by an interrupted line (Scheme 2.12). A β-substituent is shown by a solid line. This specialized *con-*

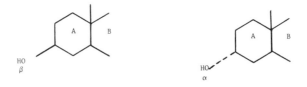

Scheme 2.12. Configurational conventions.

figurational convention for steroids is related to the more generalized spatial convention of solid and interrupted lines described in the next section. In most cases the two conventions have overlapping meanings. However, there are special cases involving chair-boat conformations when they do not. For the sake of uniformity, unless otherwise mentioned, solid and interrupted lines connected to the *steroid nucleus* (annular carbon atoms) in this book will always be in the configurational rather than the spatial convention. In all other cases, except where mentioned, they will be used in the spatial convention, e.g., when attached to the side chain. This distinction is important, because stereochemical nomenclature in the side chain is different from that in the nucleus.

e. Absolute Configuration of Steroids There are always two possible configurations of an asymmetric system. In a molecule such as a steroid containing more than one asymmetric center, *inversion of all the centers* leads to the *enantiomer* or *optical antipode* or *mirror image*, all three terms being equivalent. *Inversion of less than all the asymmetric centers* yields a *diastereoisomer* or *epimer*. Thus, the 3α- and 3β-hydroxy steroids are epimers. If, however, simultaneously with inversion at C-3 we inverted all the other asymmetric carbon atoms, the enantiomer, not the epimer, would be produced. Now, these considerations have only to do with the configurations of the asymmetric centers relative to each other in the same molecule. At the same time we could also relate them, say, to one of the carbons in the dextro-rotating enantiomer of glucose. We might determine experimentally, for instance, that the 3β-hydroxyl group of cholesterol had the same or the opposite configuration as the hydroxyl group at C-2 of (+)-glucose. *By relating one configuration to another we establish* what is known as *relative configuration*. However, while one can build up in this way a completely correct relative system both within and between molecules, one is left with an ambiguity about whether the whole system is one or the other of the two possible mirror-image situations. This can be settled by examination of any asymmetric carbon atom (in any of the molecules) in such a way that one can associate a particular configuration with the (+)- or (−)-rotating isomer of that carbon atom. Knowing this, then from the relative configurations we know the particular configuration of every other atom in the system. X-ray crystallography offers a method by which this can be done, and several asymmetric compounds have been so examined.

To depict a three-dimensional condition in two dimensions, *a solid line joining two atoms is taken to mean that the atom or group considered the substituent is directed toward the observer, while an interrupted line means the substituent points away from the observer.* This is the *spatial convention of solid and interrupted lines*. If the configuration is unknown, a wavy line (or the symbol ξ) is used. From x-ray information on, for instance, an enantiomer of tartaric acid and determination of the relative configurations we know that the dextro-rotating or (+)-isomer of glyceraldehyde has its H and OH groups directed, respectively, to the left and right of the observer and the CHO and CH₂OH groups directed, respectively, upwards and downwards with respect to the observer, when the molecule is viewed, as is conventional, with the largest carbon substituents (CHO and CH₂OH) directed vertically and away from the observer (Scheme 2.13). It follows that, with this view, the (−)-isomer will have the OH on the left. Glyceraldehyde is taken as a standard for nomenclature.

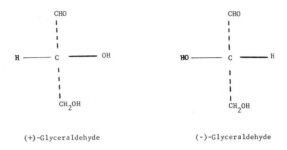

(+)-Glyceraldehyde   (-)-Glyceraldehyde

Scheme 2.13. Absolute configuration of glyceraldehyde.

With agreement on how the substituents A, B, C, and D on a given carbon atom shall relate to the H, CHO, and OH, and CH₂OH of glyceraldehyde, we can say the configuration of the carbon under consideration is the same as (D) or opposite to (L) that of (+)-glyceraldehyde. We use the term *absolute configuration* of a molecule (as opposed to the ambiguous relative configuration). Thus, the absolute configuration of (+)-glyceraldehyde is shown in Scheme 2.13.

By degradatively removing a carbon atom from a steroid and determining its configuration relative to glyceraldehyde, stereochemical investigators have been able to show, for instance, that C-3 of 3β-hydroxy steroids has the D-configuration when C-2 and C-4, respectively, are taken to correspond to the CHO and CH₂OH groups of glyceraldehyde (Scheme 2.14). From stereochemical

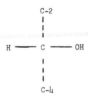

Scheme 2.14. Absolute configuration at C-3 of cholesterol.

work of this and related sorts carried out by Bergstron (*7*), Lardon and Reichstein (*8, 9*), Prelog et al. (*10*), Prelog and Meier (*11*), Dauben et al. (*12*), Cram and Elhafez (*13*), Prelog and Tsatas (*14*), Riniker, Arigoni, and Jeger (*15*), Cornforth, Youhotsky, and Popjak (*16*), Viscontini et al. (*17*, *18*), Brenneisen, Tamm, and Reichstein (*19*) and others and from still more extensive work on relative configuration, we know that the absolute configuration of steroids is as shown in Scheme 2.15. Very recently it has also been shown by Nes, Varkey, and Krevitz (*20*) that sterols from algae, fungi, higher plants (Tracheophytes), and animals all have a configuration at C-20 with the H-atom projecting toward the observer when C-22 is to the right (*trans*-oriented with respect to C-13). Moreover, in this configuration, the right-handed conformer is the stable one (Scheme 2.15). In the opposite configuration the left-handed conformation is skew and preferred (Scheme 2.15). For a more detailed analysis, see Chapter 7, Section B.11.

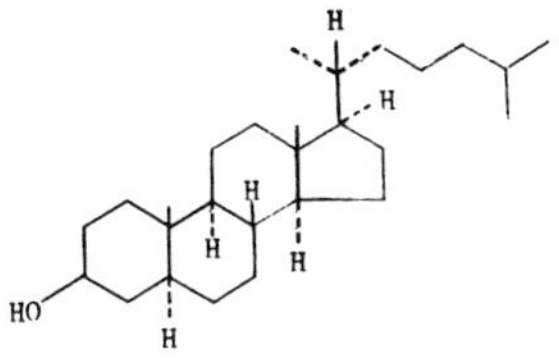

5α-Cholestanol
(Natural enantiomer and
preferred skew 17,20-
conformer)

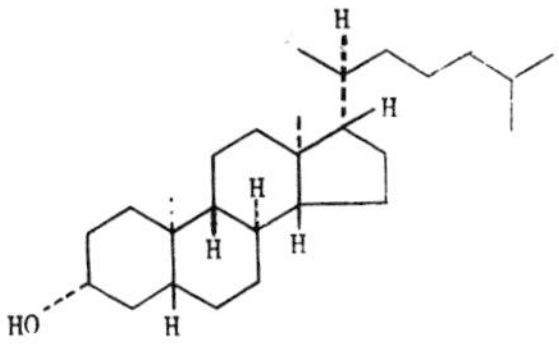

Enantiomer of 5α-Cholestanol
(Unnatural)

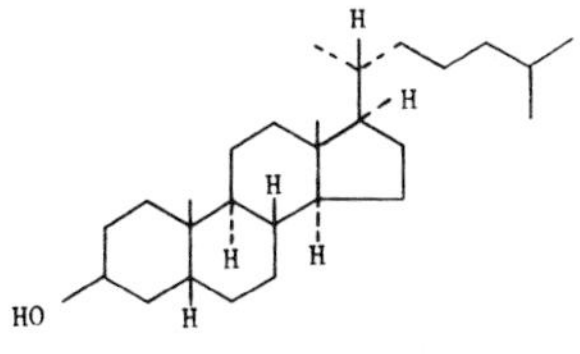

5β-Cholestanol

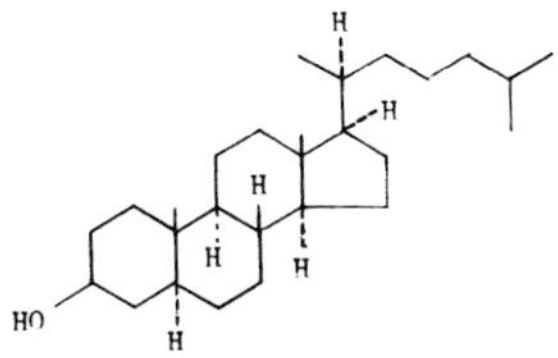

20-Epi-5α-cholestanol in unstable
eclipsed conformation

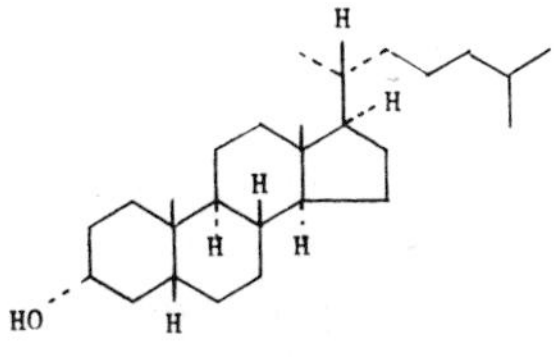

3-Epi-5β-cholestanol

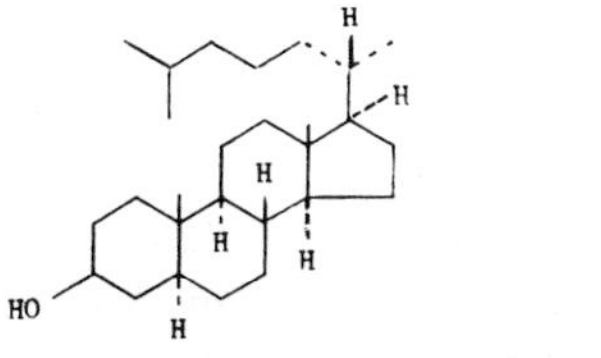

20-Epi-5α-cholestanol in preferred
skew conformation

Scheme 2.15. Configuration and conformation of steroids.

The *R, S notation* (*21, 22*), also known as the Sequence Rule, will at times be used in this book. It states that if, after assigning priorities to the groups on an asymmetric atom and after viewing the atom with the group of lowest priority (highest number) away from him, the observer finds the groups are in a clockwise order of ascending priority, then the asymmetric atom is assigned the *R* configuration (*R* for *rectus*). If they are in a counterclockwise order, then the assignment is the *S* configuration (*S* for *sinister*). Higher priority is given to higher atomic number; for isotopes it is given to higher atomic weight; for different carbon substituents, the larger the group the higher the priority; for —C—X versus —C—Y the order depends on the atomic number of X and Y; and for saturation versus unsaturation the higher priority is for the higher unsaturation. Thus we have the decreasing order of priority: F, O, N, C, NH_2—CH_2, CH_3—$C\equiv C$, CH_3—$CH=CH$, CH_3—CH_2—CH_2, CH_3—CH_2, CH_3, H^3, H^2, H. For a carbon with substituents ^1H, ^2H, CH_3—CH_2, NH_2—CH_2, the molecule would be viewed with the H pointing away as shown in Scheme 2.16 with the numbers indicating priorities. H would have priority 4, the lowest, indicating that it be below the plane observed.

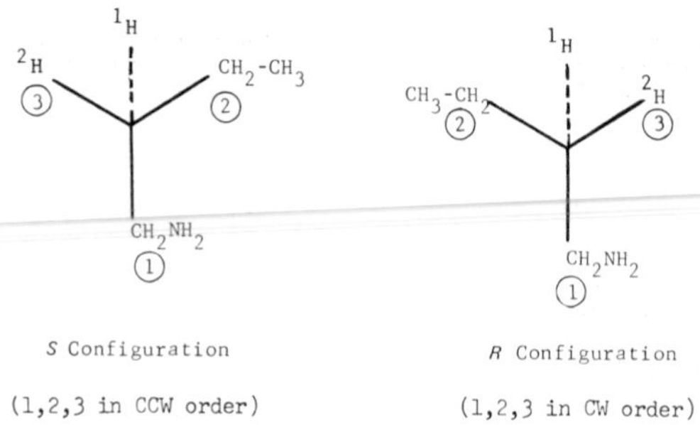

S Configuration

(1,2,3 in CCW order)

R Configuration

(1,2,3 in CW order)

Scheme 2.16. The R,S notation (example with 2-deutero-n-butylamine).

f. Configurational Nomenclature for Side Chain   The spatial orientation of the various carbon atoms of the side chain was not thought to be very precise by the early workers, and they were unable to relate it and consequently its configurational nomenclature to the front or back of the tetracyclic nucleus. Nevertheless, it has been known for decades that two asymmetric centers (at C-20 and C-24) commonly are present, e.g., in sitosterol. Fieser and Fieser (*1*), modifying a suggestion of Plattner, made a proposal which has been widely used to deal with this problem. The Fieser convention is as follows. The side chain is first imagined to be twisted about the 17 (20)-bond as well as about all succeeding bonds along the longest or most highly substituted chain so that at every carbon atom the next one projects downwards in an eclipsed conformation. The entire chain, which has now described something similar to a circle at right angles to the observer, is next stretched and distorted upwards (in the usual front-side view of the molecule) so that the side chain forms a linear array of C atoms. Now, those substituents to the left are designated β and those to the right α. This is illustrated in Scheme 2.17 for C-20 of cholesterol (and other common sterols) and compared with the $R.S$ notation. Natural sterols have a 20β_F-methyl group and a 20α_F-H atom in this notation (often but not always shown by the subscript F). In the R, S notation, C-20 has the R configuration. Unfortunately, both of these conventions are so dependent on arbitrary choices that important cases arise where two steroids have the same configuration

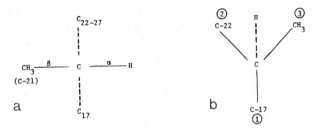

Scheme 2.17 (a) Absolute configuration of C-20 in cholesterol using the spatial convention of solid and interrupted lines and the Fieser notation. (b) Absolute configuration of C-20 of cholesterol showing *R,S* priorities leading to an *R* designation in the *R,S* notation.

with opposite notations. Thus, at C-24 sitosterol has the *R* configuration but its Δ^{22}-derivative, stigmasterol, with the same absolute configuration has the *S* notation as a result of the way priorities concerning saturated and unsaturated groups are established in the Sequence Rule. In the Fieser notation, shortening the sterol side chain has an analogous effect. For steroids with only a C_2-side chain, C-21 becomes the end of the longest chain replacing C-22 in the way the side chain is viewed (cf. Scheme 2.17). The result is that 20-hydroxysteroids with different configurations can have the same notation depending on the presence of two or more C atoms in the chain (Scheme 2.18).

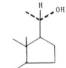

20α$_F$-Hydroxysteroid
with a C_2-side chain

20α$_F$-Hydroxysteroid
with a side chain
longer than C_2

Steroid with *R*-Designation
at C-24

Steroid with *S*-Designation
at C-24

Scheme 2.18. Anomalies of the Fieser and *R, S* notations.

These problems can be resolved in the following way as suggested by Nes (*23*). Let us simply agree to view the molecule perpendicularly to the 17(20)-bond as shown in Scheme 2.18 with the side chain in the staggered conformation, C-21 to the left, and carbon atoms, numbers 17, 20, and 22 lying in a plane, e.g., the plane of the paper. Carbon atoms, numbers 20-26 inclusive, will then lie in this plane, and all substituents in the front will be designated as α-oriented and those in back as β-oriented. The choice of α and β is made so that most of the designations will agree with the Fieser notation. With a cholesterol backbone, only C-23 will have inverted notation in the two conventions. If we further agree that with a C_2-side chain C-21 will remain on the left but rotated into the plane, we have a simple set of rules for nomenclature that obviate the previous difficulties. Cholesterol has as before a 20α-H-atom and 20β-methyl group, and sitosterol has a 24α-ethyl group, as does stigmasterol. Furthermore, 20α-hydroxysteroids, regardless of side chain length, will have a consistent designation. The α-orientation, for instance, will always imply that the designated substituent, C-20, and the third substituent (C-22, H, or whatever) are to be found in a clockwise order when viewed from the top and that the substituent designated is in front when C-21 is placed to the left. When the side chain extends at least to C-23, the proposal and the Fieser convention agree, but reverse notation in the two conventions will be found when only a C_2 side chain is present. In this book we will use the new convention (Scheme 2.19) unless otherwise indicated by R, S, or an F subscript.

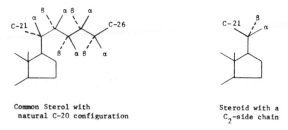

Common Sterol with
natural C-20 configuration

Steroid with a
C_2-side chain

Scheme 2.19. Proposed stereochemical nomenclature for the side chain.

It should be noted that, when the side chain is cyclized, a rigid relationship to the stereochemistry of the nucleus is established. We will use the α,β convention of the steroid nucleus except in the case of spirostanes. In the spirostanes, ring F is perpendicular to ring E with the oxygen atom in the back. Ring F is believed to have the chair conformation placing C-20 in an equatorial relationship, which means that the terminal methyl group (C-26 or C-27) is either axial (up) or equatorial (down) depending on its configuration. An arbitrary convention has arisen for the configuration of this terminal methyl of spirostanes. It assigns α or β to C-25, as shown in the next section, and no attempt will be made to alter this situation.

6. Naming of Steroids

a. Parent Systems   There are three widely used ways in which a steroid can be named. 1) A compound can be given a *trivial name,* by which we mean a nonsystematic name. They are entirely arbitrary, are coined usually by the discoverer, and more often than not memorialize some aspect of the origin of the substance (cholesterol, cortisol, testosterone, stigmasterol, etc.); less commonly they memorialize a structural feature (aldosterone), another investigator (Marrianolic acid, Marker-Lawson acid), a biological activity (androsterone, estrone), etc. 2) Naming can be part systematic and part trivial. This is usually done by adding a prefix to a trivial name, e.g., 7α-hydroxycholesterol, 24-dihydrolanosterol, 24-ketocholesterol, etc. 3) Systematic nomenclature, which follows rules (see Section A-6e) established under the auspices of the International Union of Pure and Applied Chemistry and other assemblies of scientists, may be used. The main aspects of systematic nomenclature are discussed in what follows.

Parent substances, usually hydrocarbons, are used as a base for nomenclature. Prefixes and suffixes are added to these in a systematic way in order to describe the functionality and in part the stereochemistry. Insofar as the carbon skeleton is concerned, the parent name fixes most or sometimes all of its stereochemistry. The principal parent substances are shown in Scheme 2.20. In all structural formulas a *line ending in nothing signifies a methyl group.* The names given in parentheses in Scheme 2.20 are alternatives either for the name or for some aspect of it. Stereoisomerism at C-5 is frequently encountered. It was first observed in the reduction product of cholesterol, viz., a sterol (coprosterol, Greek "kopro," feces) found in feces (produced by metabolism of intestinal flora). Consequently, the parent hydrocarbons, cholestane and coprostane, came into use for the C-5 epimers. With recognition of a wider occurrence of C-5 epimerism, the prefix "copro" was added to other stem names (coproergostane, etc.) for the 5β-H isomer. An analogous system arose in the pregnanes, except that the prefix "allo" (Greek, other) came into use (allopregnane). "Allo" and "copro," however, have reverse meanings, viz., 5α-H and 5β-H, respectively. It is therefore preferable not to use them, and simply to add 5α or 5β to the historically most common parent name, e.g., 5α-cholestane and 5β-cholestane, 5α-androstane and 5β-androstane, etc. The Greek letter refers to the configuration of the H atom. Such a configurational system could be used in the side chain, but parent hydrocarbons have not been named for all the known substituents at C-22, C-23, and C-24. We recommend the use of 5α- and 5β-cholestane as basic parents from which we can then derive 24α-methylcholestane, 23β-methylcholestane, etc., as working parents. This would give campesterol the systematic name 24α-methylcholest-5-en-3β-ol, and chondrillasterol would be 24β-ethylcholesta-7,22-*trans*-dien-3β-ol. The α,β-designation refers to the substituent carbon atom, not to the H atom. The use of the designation for the H atom is peculiar to ring junc-

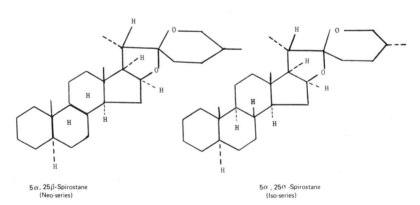

5β-Cholestane
(Coprostane)

Scheme 2.20. Parent hydrocarbon for nomenclature purposes.

R = H, 5α-Cholestane

R = CH₃, 5α,24α-methylcholestane

R = C₂H₅, 5α, 24α-ethylcholestane

R = H, 5α-Cholestane

R = CH₃, 5α, 24β-methylcholestane

R = C₂H₅, 5α, 24β- ethylcholestane

5α, 25β-Spirostane
(Neo-series)

(Terminal methyl up
and axial)

5α, 25α-Spirostane
(Iso-series)

(Terminal methyl down
and equatorial)

Scheme 2.20. *Continued.*

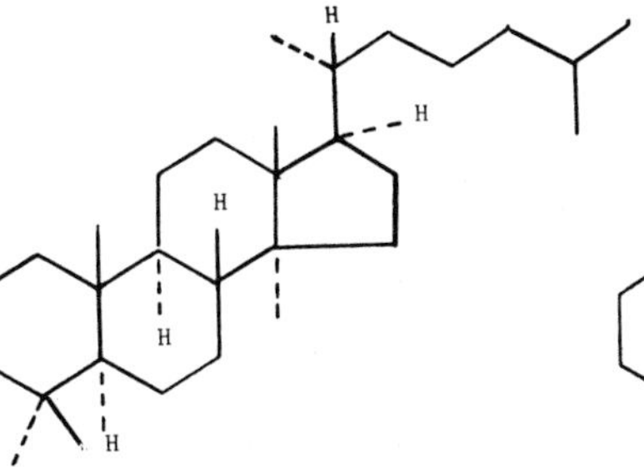

Lanostane

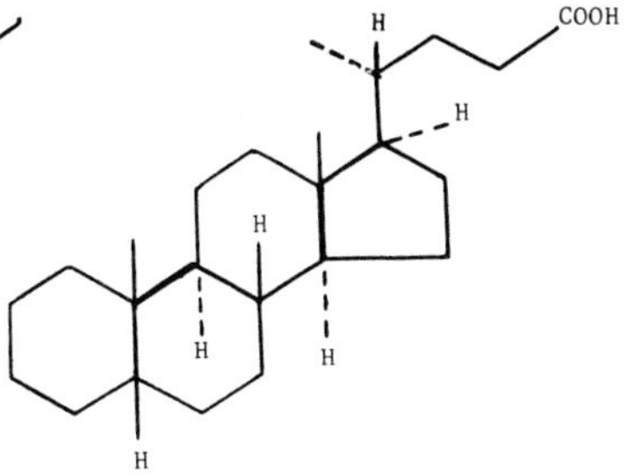

5 β -Cholanic acid
(Cholanic acid)
(the hydrocarbon is
5 β -Cholane)

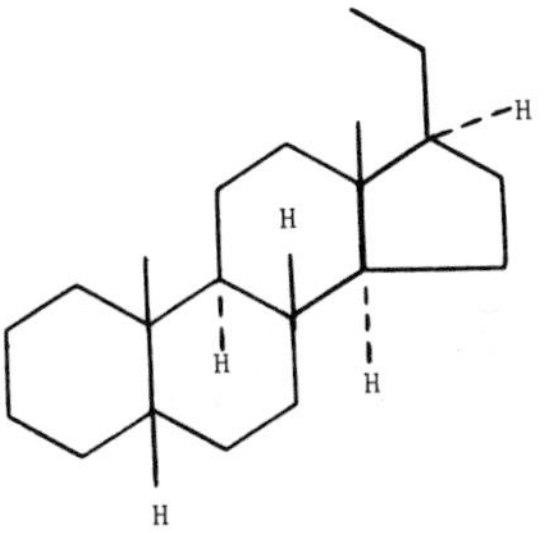

5 β -Pregnane
(Pregnane)

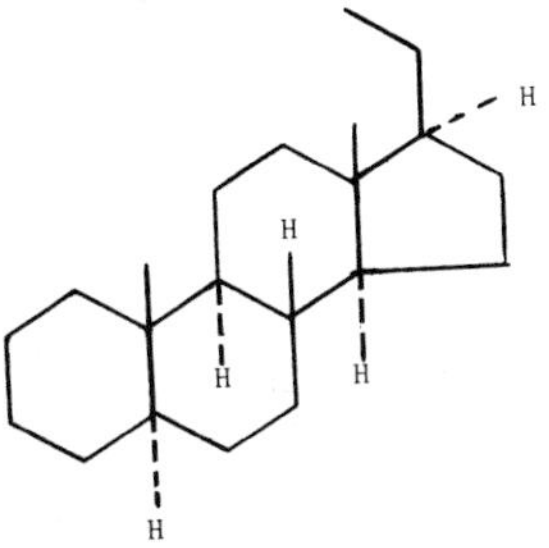

5 α -Pregnane
(Allopregnane)

Scheme 2.20. *Continued.*

tions, especially at C-5. Alternatives for the side chain case are to use 24α- and 24β-ergostane (or campestane and ergostane) for the epimeric 24-methyl hydrocarbons and 24α- and 24β-stigmastane (or stigmastane and poriferastane) for the 24-ethyl epimers. However, it is not as simple as using 24-alkylcholestanes as parents and becomes more arbitrary. Why, for instance, choose the names stigmastane and poriferastane over sitostane and clionastane, respectively? The respective pairs, in fact, are identical compounds.

The terms "neo" and "iso" for the C-25 epimers of sapogenins (spirostanes) have been used. Again, since these prefixes also have other meanings (e.g., "neoergosterol" signifies a compound with an aromatic ring B), it is preferable to indicate the configurations at C-25 by a number. The system that has come into use, unfortunately, is the opposite of that for C-5. Unless otherwise noted, at C-25 the configuration given refers to the methyl group (rather than the hydrogen atom), and the convention for α and β is in the Fieser system and assumes that the CH$_2$O group [or CH$_2$-N group in spirosolanes (tomatanines)] is directed upwards and C-24 downwards. Under these circumstances 25β implies that the methyl is on the

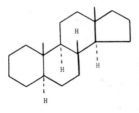

5 α -Androstane
(Androstane)

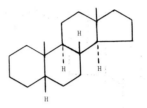

5 β -Androstane
(Testane, Etiocholane)

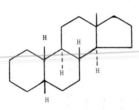

5 β-Estrane
(Estrane)

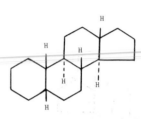

5 β -Gonane
(Gonane, Sterane, 18-Norestrane)

Scheme 2.20. *Continued.*

D-Homo-5 β -androstane

3,5-Cycloandrostane

3,4-Seco-5 α -androstane

Scheme 2.20. *Continued.*

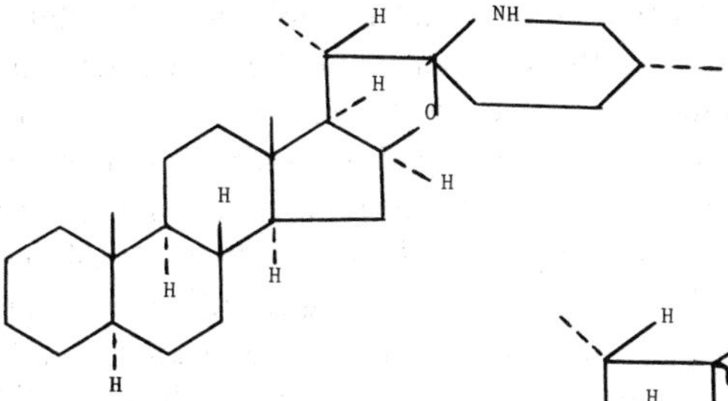

5α,25α-Tomatanine
(25R-series)

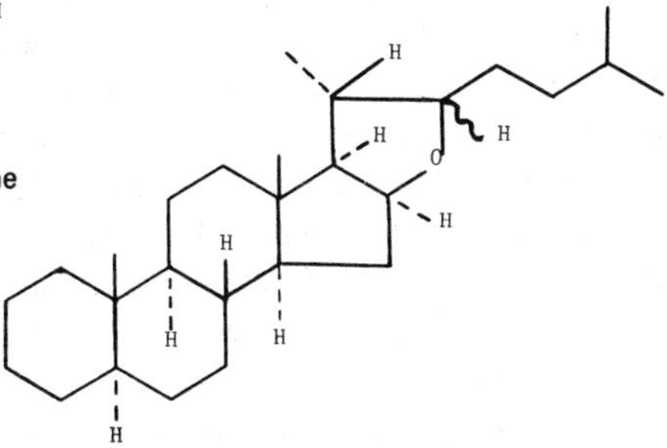

5α-Furostane

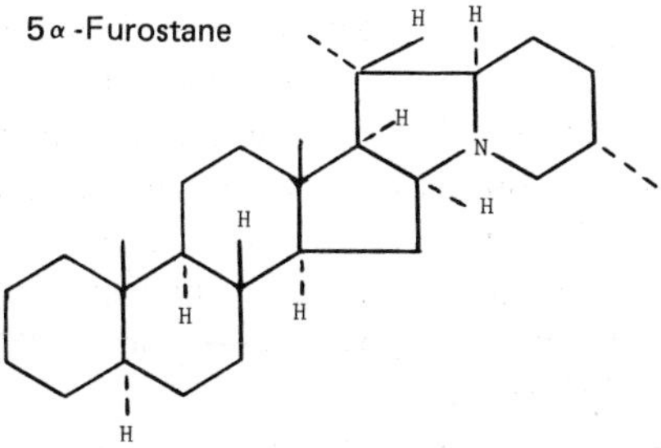

5α,22α,25α-Solanidanine
(Solanidane)

Scheme 2.20. *Continued.*

left. Moreover, it should be noted that ring F in the spirostanes is turned approximately 90° to the planes of rings A, B, and C. Therefore the question of "side" for the substituent on C-25 is meaningless relative to the nucleus. The same thing applies to the spirosolanes. The α configuration at C-25 is the same as the R configuration.

The prefix "3,5-cyclo" indicates the presence of an α-oriented bond between C-3 and C-5. The prefix "seco" indicates the bond between two carbon atoms has been severed. The prefix "homo" indicates a carbon atom has been added to a ring enlarging it. The prefix "nor" indicates a carbon atom has been eliminated.

   b. *Suffixes*   It is preferable not to have more than two suffixes on a name. These are generally taken from the following: "ol" for hydroxy, "one" for ketonic oxygen, "oic" for oxidation to the carboxylic acid stage, "ene" for olefinic unsaturation, "yne" for acetylenic unsaturations, or the "ane" in the parent signifying "saturated." If more than one of a kind is present it is indicated by "di," "tri," etc., and does not count as one of the allowed suffixes. The suffixes are placed in alphabetical order of the first letter of the suffix stem. If the first letter of the entire first suffix (other than "ane" but including "di," etc.) is a consonant, the vowel at the end of the parent is retained, but it is dropped if the first letter is a vowel. This is also done between the suffixes. If multiple unsaturation occurs, only the "a" of "ane" is retained for euphony. Thus, we have "cholestadienol" or "pregnatrienol," but "cholestene" and "pregnene." The position of the functionality is indicated by insertion of the position number and configuration between the stem and suffix, e.g., "cholestan-3β-ol-11-one," "cholest-5-en-3β-ol," "cholesta-5,7-dien-3β-ol," and "24α-ethylcholest-7-en-3β-ol."

c. *Double and Triple Bonds*   The position of a double or triple bond is frequently indicated by the Greek letter Δ as a prefix, to which the unsaturated carbons are added as a superscript. If the unsaturation occurs at two consecutively numbered atoms, it is common only to use the lower numbered one unless emphasis is desired. If they are not consecutive, the higher numbered one is placed in parentheses. Thus, we arrive at "Δ^5-cholestene" for the carbon system of cholesterol, but "$\Delta^{5,8(14)}$-cholestadiene" for its 8(14)-dehydro derivative. "Δ^5-Cholestene" could also be written "$\Delta^{5(6)}$-cholestene" for emphasis, if, for instance, one wanted to distinguish carefully from "$\Delta^{5(10)}$-cholestene." Some authors do not use the Δ symbol and simply add the position numbers as prefixes, e.g., "5-cholestene." In fully systematic literature, the position number is added between the stem and suffix, e.g., "cholest-5-ene."

d. *Prefixes*   Two kinds of prefixes have been discussed in the foregoing sections, viz., for configurations at ring junctions and for double bonds. In addition, when more than two kinds of functionality are present, all but one are indicated by prefixes. The suffix chosen is usually, in order of preference, "ene" (or "yne"), "ol," or "one" with the appropriate "di," "tri," etc. Prefixes are generally placed in alphabetical order with "di," etc., and the position number and configuration preceding it, e.g., 3β,11α-dihydroxy-6-keto-Δ^8-5β-cholestene. In some of the literature "oxo" is used for "keto," and "oxy" is used for "hydroxy."

e. *Sources of Further Information*   More detailed accounts of the conventions for nomenclature may be found in the International Union of Pure and Applied Chemistry Revised Tentative Rules for Nomenclature of Steroids (24).

f. *Absence of Stereochemical Notation or Knowledge*   When no stereochemical notation is given, it is implied that it is the same as in cholesterol. An unknown or ambiguous configuration is designated by the Greek letter xi (ξ) and a wavy line.

g. *Common Naturally Occurring Sterols*   The sterols that comprise approximately 95% or more of the mixture in a given biological system have been called the "dominant sterols" (25). They usually represent the end product of the biosynthetic pathway. In the great majority of plants and animals these dominant sterols lack C-30 through C-32 and are 4,4,14-trisdesmethyl compounds. The common ones have been given trivial names, and their structures are shown in Schemes 2.21 to 2.27. A more complete

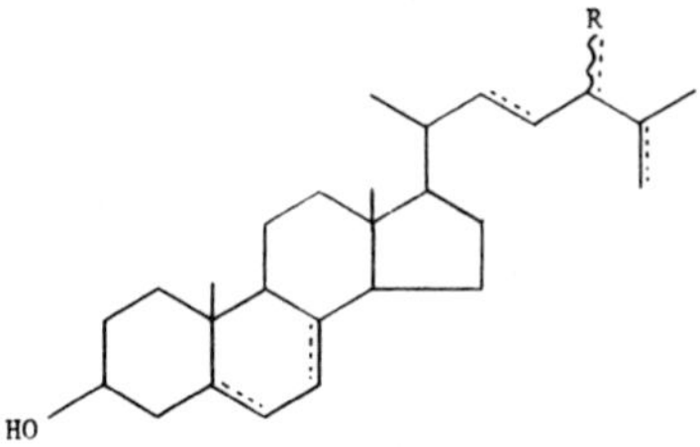

Scheme 2.21. Common dominant sterols. The interrupted lines mean a double bond may or may not be present, and the wavy line at C-24 implies that saturated R groups of either configuration may occur. R may vary from H to CH_3 to C_2H_5. In some cases there is a $\Delta^{24(28)}$-bond indicated by the interrupted line to R. Variations beyond what is shown here are found, but not commonly.

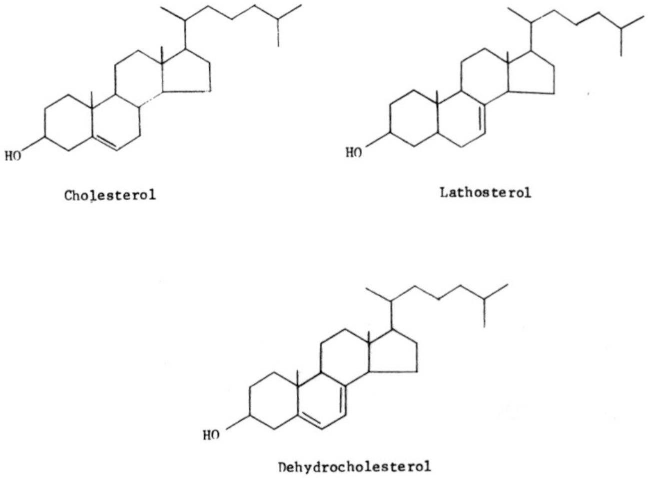

Cholesterol

Lathosterol

Dehydrocholesterol

Scheme 2.22. Principal 24-desalkylsterols lacking C-30 to C-32.

listing is given in Table 2.1. Cholesterol (cholest-5-en-3β-ol), lathosterol (5α-cholest-7-en-3β-ol), and their common diene, cholesta-5,7-dien-3β-ol, are the sterols most often encountered lacking a substituent at C-24. We will use these as semisystematic parents in many cases. Cholesta-5,7-dien-3β-ol, for instance, is well known as 7-dehydrocholesterol, where cholesterol is taken as the semisystematic parent. In this and a few other cases we will drop the numbered prefix and reduce the semisystematic name to the status

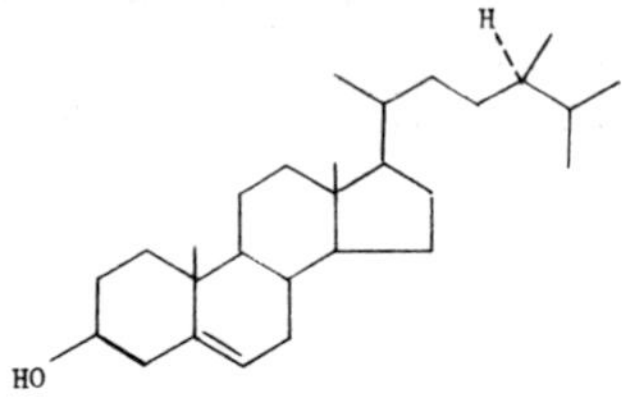

Campesterol

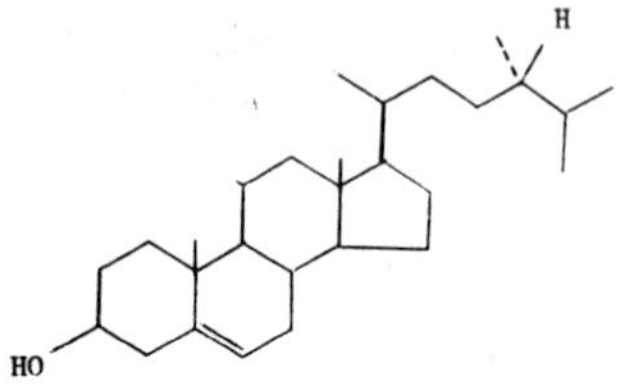

Dihydrobrassicasterol

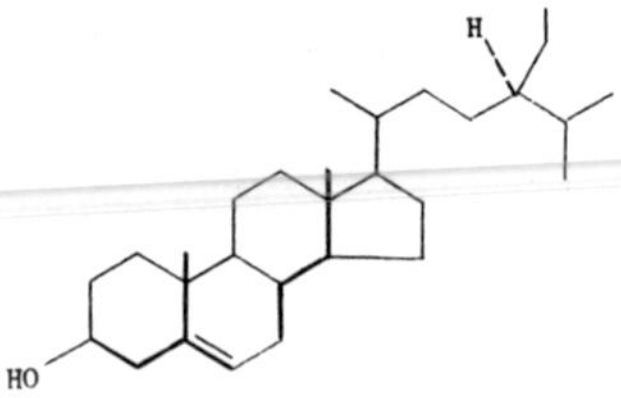

Sitosterol

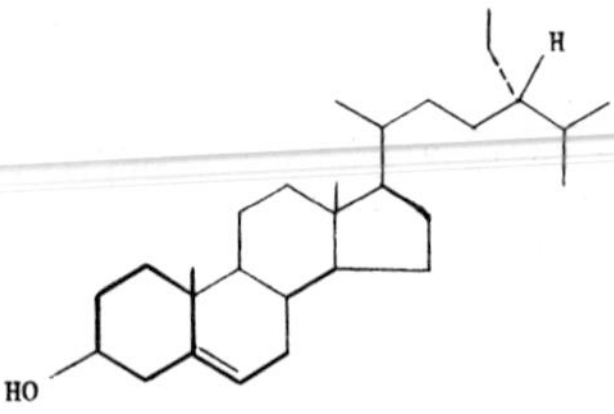

Clionasterol

Scheme 2.23. The 24-methyl- and 24-ethylcholesterols.

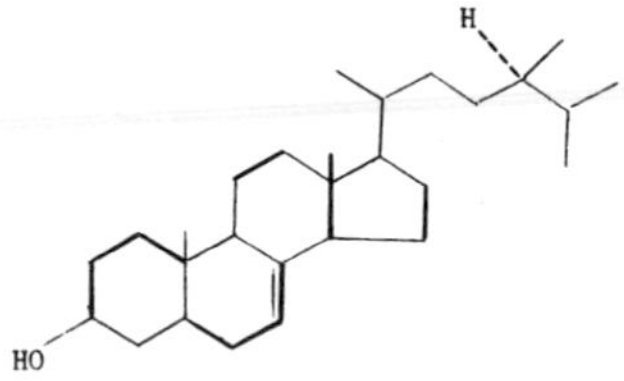

Epifungisterol

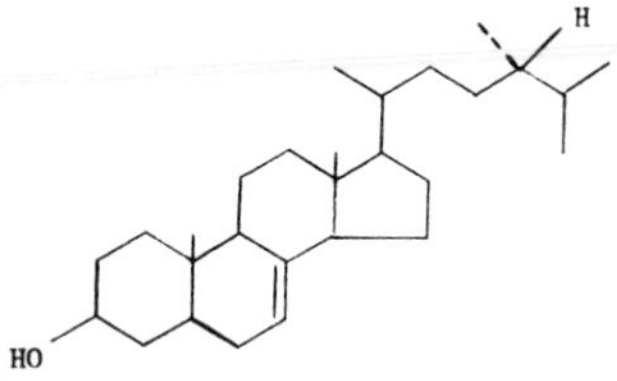

Fungisterol

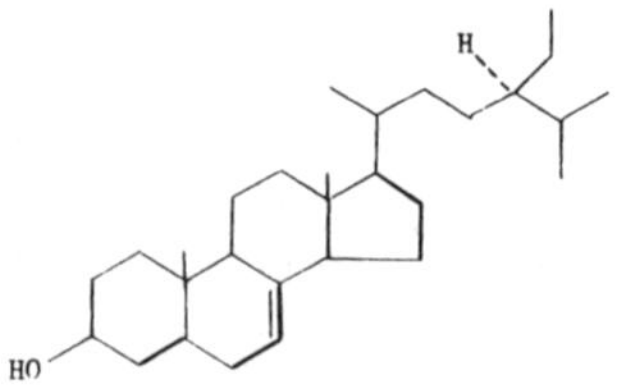

Schottenol

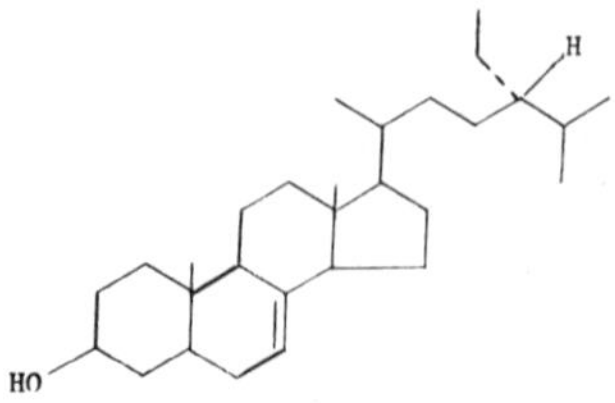

Dihydrochondrillasterol

Scheme 2.24. The 24-methyl- and 24-ethyllathosterols.

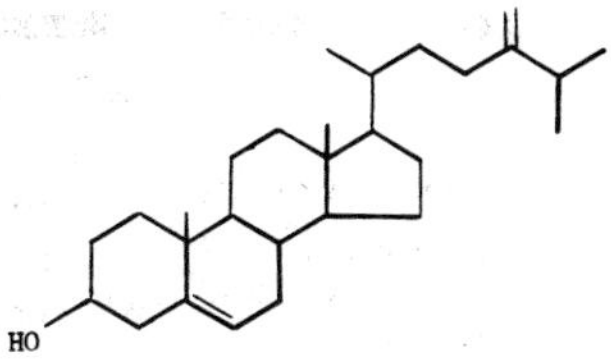

Ostreasterol

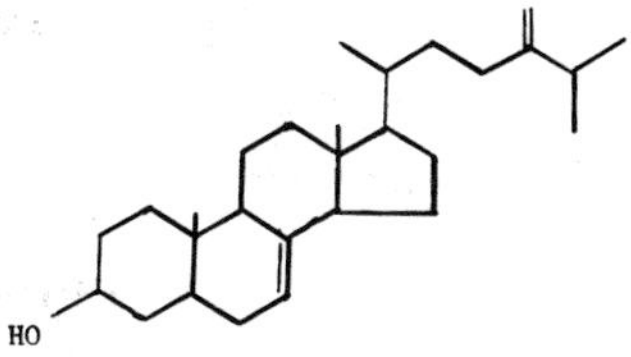

Epialterol

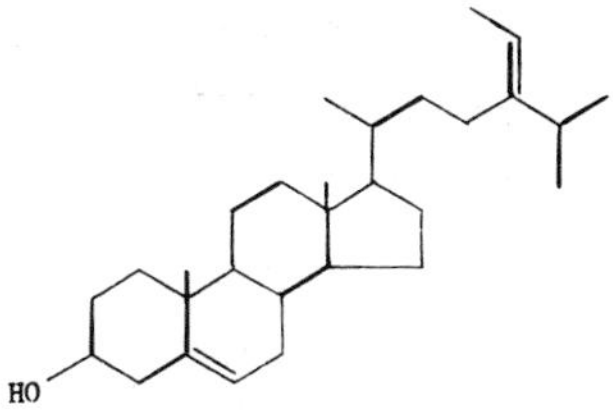

Fucosterol

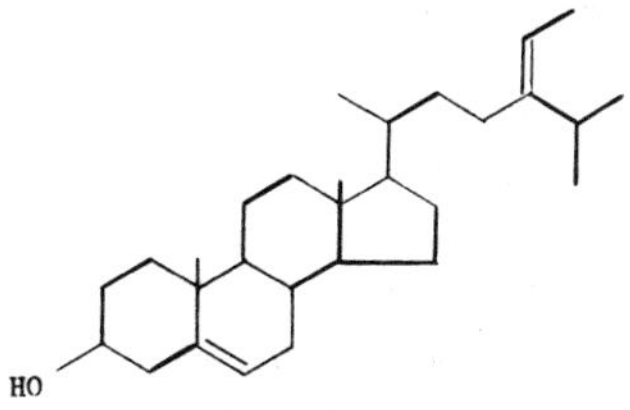

Isofucosterol

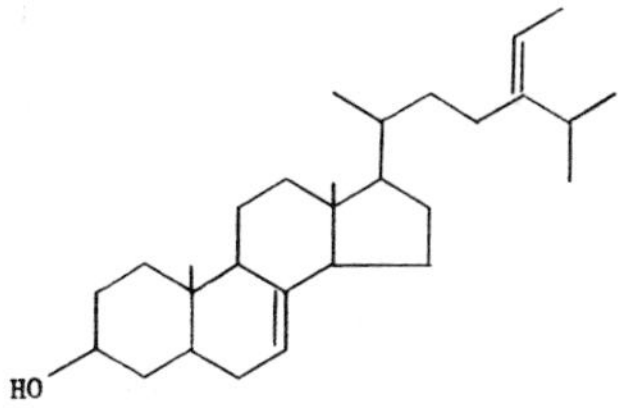

Avenasterol

Scheme 2.25. Principal 24-alkylidenesterols lacking C-30 to C-32.

of a trivial name. In some cases we will drop a number from the prefix "epi," "iso," and "methylene" thereby also developing a trivial name. A well-established example is dehydroepiandrosterone (DHEA, also known as dehydroisoandrosterone) for the 17-ketone derived from cholesterol by oxidative cleavage of the 17(20)-bond. The latter name comes from androsterone (5α-androstan-3α-ol-17-one) and semisystematically is 5-dehydro-3-epiandrosterone. Illustrations to be found in the schemes and table include dehydrocholesterol for 7-dehydrocholesterol, dihydrobrassicasterol for 22-dihydrobrassicasterol, dihydrolanosterol for 24-dihydrolanosterol, epiergosterol for 24-epiergosterol, isofucosterol for 28-isofucosterol, and methylenecycloartanol for 24-methylenecycloartanol. In Scheme 2.27 and Table 2.1 will also be found the names and structures of some of the more important sterols bearing one or more methyl groups at C-4 and C-14. Only very rarely do

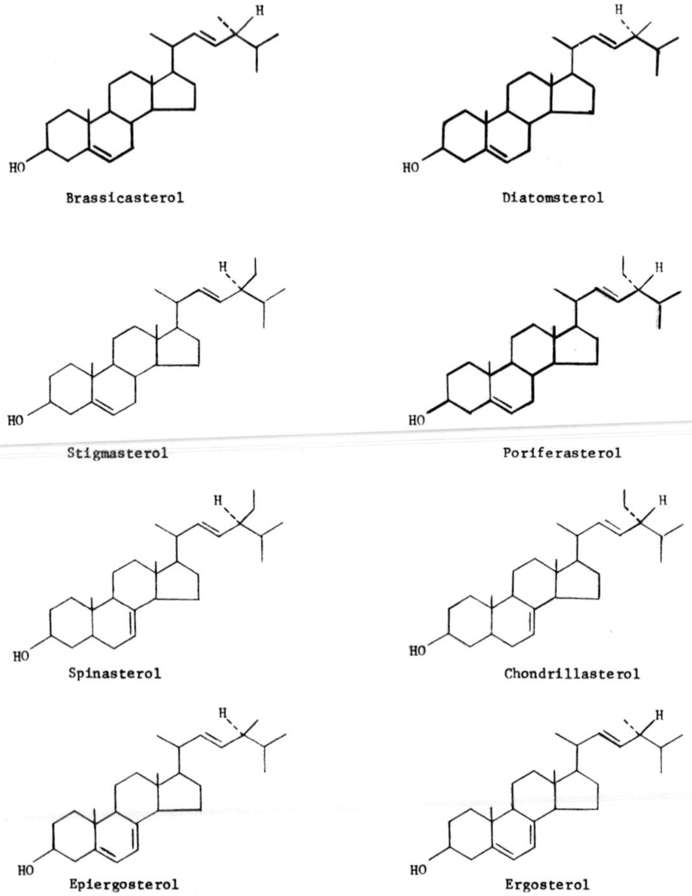
H
HO
Brassicasterol
H
HO
Diatomsterol
H
HO
Stigmasterol
H
HO
Poriferasterol
H
HO
Spinasterol
H
HO
Chondrillasterol
H
HO
Epiergosterol
H
HO
Ergosterol

Scheme 2.26. Some sterols with a Δ^{22}-bond.

these compounds comprise part of the dominant sterols. Many of them, as well as many other intermediates to the dominant sterols, do not possess trivial names. It is necessary in these cases to use either systematic or semi-systematic nomenclature. Cholesta-8,14-dien-3β-ol, for instance, is present in and converted to cholesterol by mammalian liver but lacks a trivial name.

Since use of fully systematic names or of many trivial names requires thought of the reader, making comparisons more time-consuming and difficult, we will use as often as possible only a few such names. Cholesterol and lathosterol assume special importance in this regard, since they are the Δ^5-and Δ^7-cholesten-3β-ols, respectively. Most dominant sterols have either the Δ^5-, Δ^7, or $\Delta^{5,7}$-bonds, with or without a *trans*-oriented Δ^{22}-bond, $\Delta^{25(27)}$-bond, $\Delta^{24(28)}$-bond, or (rarely) a $\Delta^{24(25)}$-bond and are in the homol-

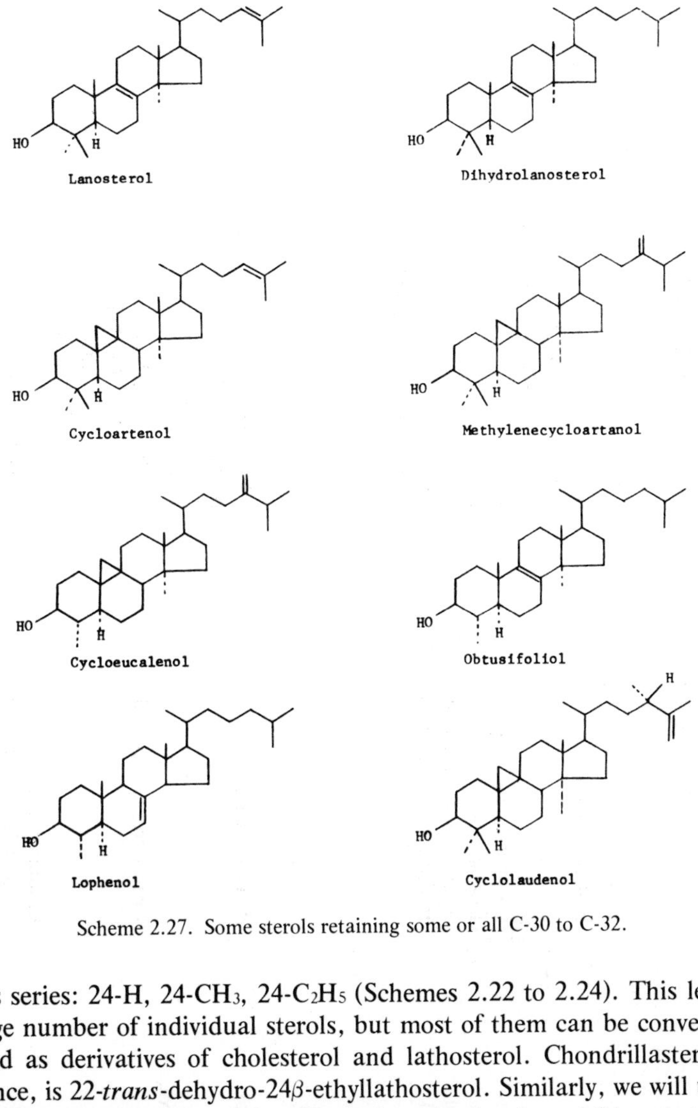

Lanosterol

Dihydrolanosterol

Cycloartenol

Methylenecycloartanol

Cycloeucalenol

Obtusifoliol

Lophenol

Cyclolaudenol

Scheme 2.27. Some sterols retaining some or all C-30 to C-32.

ogous series: 24-H, 24-CH₃, 24-C₂H₅ (Schemes 2.22 to 2.24). This leads to a large number of individual sterols, but most of them can be conveniently named as derivatives of cholesterol and lathosterol. Chondrillasterol, for instance, is 22-*trans*-dehydro-24β-ethyllathosterol. Similarly, we will use the term 24β-methylcholesterol for dihydrobrassicasterol, and 24α-ethylcholesterol for sitosterol. This allows immediate recognition, without our resorting to mental gymnastics about the detailed meaning of the trivial names, that these two sterols differ both in configuration and size of the substituent at C-24, that the substituents are CH₃ and C₂H₅, respectively, and that these are the only differences. It is worth noting in passing that trivial names are very precise and imply skeleton, configuration, functionality, and in nearly all cases also conformation as a derived fact from configuration. They are often used more loosely, which is unfortunate. Sitosterol, for instance, is

Table 2.1. Trivial names of sterols

Name	Alternate names	Structure based on changes or additions to 5α-cholestan-3β-ol
Δ⁰-Sterols		
Cholestanol	5α-Cholestanol	5αH
Coprostanol	5β-Cholestanol	5βH
Lanostanol		4,4,14α-Trimethyl
Cycloartanol		9β,19-Cyclo-4,4,14α-trimethyl
24α-Methylcholestanol	Campestanol	24α-Methyl
24β-Methylcholestanol	Ergostanol	24β-Methyl
24α-Ethylcholestanol	Stigmastanol, sitostanol	24α-Ethyl
24β-Ethylcholestanol	Poriferastanol, clionastanol	24β-Ethyl
Pollinastanol		9β,19-Cyclo-14α-methyl
Δ⁵-Sterols		
Cholesterol		Δ^5
Desmosterol		$\Delta^{5,24}$
Campesterol		Δ^5-24α-Methyl
Dihydrobrassicasterol		Δ^5-24β-Methyl
Sitosterol		Δ^5-24α-Ethyl
Clionasterol		Δ^5-24β-Ethyl
22-Dehydrocholesterol	Δ⁵-Ergostenol	$\Delta^{5,trans-22}$
Diatomsterol	Crinosterol, pinesterol	$\Delta^{5,trans-22}$-24α-Methyl
Brassicasterol		$\Delta^{5,trans-22}$-24β-Methyl
Stigmasterol		$\Delta^{5,trans-22}$-24α-Ethyl
Poriferasterol		$\Delta^{5,trans-22}$-24β-Ethyl
Ostreasterol	Chalinasterol, methylenecholesterol	Δ^5-24-Methylene
Fucosterol		Δ^5-cis-24-Ethylidene
Isofucosterol	Δ⁵-Avenasterol	Δ^5-trans-24-Ethylidene
Codisterol		$\Delta^{5,25(27)}$-24β-Methyl

Clerosterol	$\Delta^{5,25(27)}$-24β-Ethyl
Haliclonasterol	Δ^5-20-epi-24α-Methyl (probably not natural)
Sargasterol	Δ^5-20-epi-cis-24-Ethylidene (probably not natural)
22-Hydroxycholesterol	Δ^5-(22S)-22-Hydroxy
Saringasterol	Δ^5-24-Hydroxy-24-vinyl (probably not natural)
Celsianol	$\Delta^{5,9(11)}$-24α-Ethyl
Δ^7-Sterols	
Lathosterol	Δ^7
Lophenol	Δ^7-4α-Methyl
Epifungisterol	Δ^7-24α-Methyl
Fungisterol	Δ^7-24β-Methyl
Avenasterol (Δ^7-Ergostenol)	Δ^7-trans-24-Ethylidene
Citrostadienol (Δ^7-Avenasterol)	Δ^7-4α-Methyl-trans-24-ethylidene
Dihydrospinasterol	Δ^7-24α-Ethyl
Dihydrochondrillasterol (Schottenol, Δ^7-stigmastenol)	Δ^7-24β-Ethyl
Dehydrolathosterol	$\Delta^{7,trans-22}$
Episterol	Δ^7-24-Methylene
Gramisterol	Δ^7-4α-Methyl-24-methylene
Epidehydrofungisterol	$\Delta^{7,trans-22}$-24α-Methyl
Dehydrofungisterol	$\Delta^{7,trans-22}$-24β-Methyl
Spinasterol	$\Delta^{7,trans-22}$-24α-Ethyl
Chondrillasterol	$\Delta^{7,trans-22}$-24β-Ethyl
Elasterol	$\Delta^{7,16,25}$-24α-Ethyl
Carpesterol	Δ^7-6-Keto-22α-hydroxy-4α-methyl-24α-ethyl
$\Delta^{5,7}$-Sterols	
Dehydrocholesterol	$\Delta^{5,7}$
Dehydroepisterol	$\Delta^{5,7}$-24-Methylene
Dehydrocampesterol	$\Delta^{5,7}$-24α-Methyl

Table 2.1. (continued)

Name	Alternate names	Structure based on changes or additions to 5α-Cholestan-3β-ol
Dihydroergosterol	7-Dehydro-Δ⁵-ergostenol, 7-dehydrodihydrobrassicasterol	$\Delta^{5,7}$-24β-Methyl
Dehydrositosterol		$\Delta^{5,7}$-24α-Ethyl
Dehydroclionasterol		$\Delta^{5,7}$-24β-Ethyl
Dehydrostigmasterol		$\Delta^{5,7,trans\text{-}22}-24\alpha$-Ethyl
Dehydroporiferasterol		$\Delta^{5,7,trans\text{-}22}-24\beta$-Ethyl
Epiergosterol		$\Delta^{5,7,trans\text{-}22}-24\alpha$-Methyl
Ergosterol		$\Delta^{5,7,trans\text{-}22}-24\beta$-Methyl
Δ^8-Sterols		
Ascosterol		$\Delta^{8,23}$
Zymosterol		$\Delta^{8,24}$
Fecosterol		Δ^8-24-Methylene
Vernosterol		$\Delta^{8,14}$-trans-24-Ethylidene
Peniocerol		Δ^8-6α-Hydroxy
Macdougallin		Δ^8-6α-Hydroxy-14α-methyl
Lanosterol		$\Delta^{8,24}$-4,4,14α-Trimethyl
Obtusifoliol		Δ^8-4α,14α-Dimethyl-24-methylene
$\Delta^{9(11)}$, and Other Sterols		
Indosterol		$\Delta^{9(11),22}$-24α-Ethyl
Parkeol		$\Delta^{9(11),24}$-4,4,14α-Trimethyl
Agnosterol		$\Delta^{7,9(11),24}$-4,4,14α-Trimethyl
Cycloartenol		Δ^{24}-9β,19-Cyclo-4,4,14α-trimethyl
Cycloeucalenol		9β,19-Cyclo-4α,14α-dimethyl-24-methylene
Cyclobranol		Δ^{24}-9β,19-Cyclo-4,4,14α,24ξ-tetramethyl
Cyclosadol		Δ^{23}-9β,19-Cyclo-4,4,14α,24-tetramethyl
Cyclolaudenol		$\Delta^{25(27)}$-9β,19-Cyclo-4,4,14α,24β-tetramethyl

not an acceptable term for 24ξ-ethylcholesterol. The latter term should be used when the configuration is unknown.

B. BIOLOGICAL CLASSIFICATION OF STEROIDS

1. General

It is very common to group steroids together according to their biological activity even though there may not be a simple structural similarity between them. One of the reasons for this is the need to have names in cases where the exact structures are not known. Therefore it should be noted that biological classifications do not unequivocally imply steroidal character.

2. Progestogens

Progestational activity is associated with a variety of effects related especially but not exclusively to the luteal phase of the menstrual cycle. The only well-characterized natural steroid with physiological activity of this sort is progesterone (Scheme 2.28). It is produced in several kinds of tissue, most

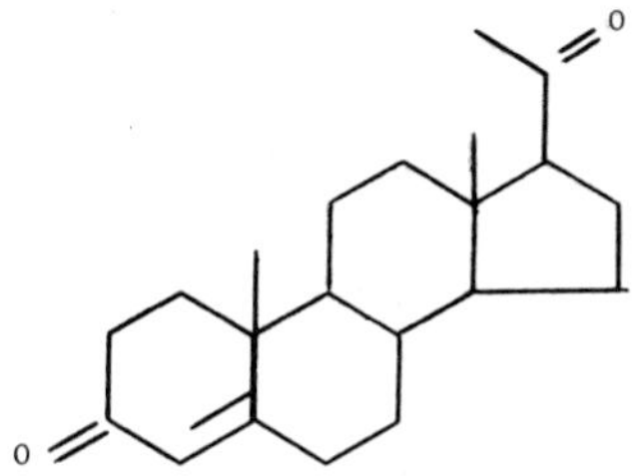

Progesterone

Scheme 2.28. A natural progestogen (progesterone).

notably the corpus luteum and placenta. Its most important activities are as an inducer of proliferation of the uterine endometrium and as a messenger to the pituitary gland (perhaps via the hypothalamus), which controls production of polypeptide hormones controlling ovarian function. A fuller account of physiological and pharmacological behavior is to be found in Chapter 11. Several unnatural steroids mimic one or another activity of progesterone and are considered to be progestogens. They are used, *inter alia*, as oral contraceptives and are discussed in Chapter 11.

3. Corticoids

The cortex of the adrenal gland biosynthesizes two major groups of steroids, the behavior of which constitutes the physiologic function of the cortical tissue. These steroids are therefore known variously as *adrenal corticoids*, *adrenocorticoids*, *adrenocortical steroids*, or more simply as *corticoids*. The two major functions have been found to be (1) control of carbohydrate metabolism by the *glucocorticoids*, and (2) control of the concentrations of sodium and potassium ions by the *mineralocorticoids*. There are a number of such compounds. They generally possess a C_2 side chain at C-17 and often are referred to as "C_{21} steroids." This term, however, preferably should and will be used in this book exclusively with its chemical rather than biological meaning, since not all C_{21} steroids are corticoids and not all C_{21} steroids of the adrenal cortex are biologically active. Cortisol and aldosterone (Scheme 2.29) are most important to human physiology. A fuller account of assays and physiological and pharmacological aspects is to be found in Chapters 3 and 11.

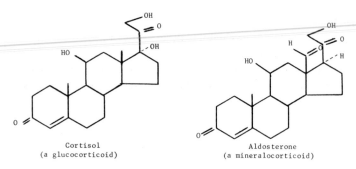

Cortisol
(a glucocorticoid)

Aldosterone
(a mineralocorticoid)

Scheme 2.29.

4. Androgens

The androgens (Greek, *andros*, man) have biological activity associated with male sexual characteristics and behavior. Examples include stimulation of the growth of the penis and other secondary sex tissue, induction of the growth of pubic hair, and production of at least a part of libido. Steroids with this sort of biological activity usually possess no side chain at C-17 and therefore are often referred to as "C_{19} steroids." However, not all C_{19} steroids are androgenic, and the term is used preferably and in this book will be used only in a chemical sense. The most important steroidal androgens in human physiology are testosterone (Scheme 2.30), formed in the testes and one of its dihydro derivatives. A fuller account of assays and of physiologic and pharmacologic behavior is to be found in Chapters 3 and 11.

5. Estrogens

The word "estrogen" is derived from and is associated with estrus in animals and its counterpart, the menstrual cycle, in the human female. Estrogens play their role especially but not exclusively in the early phase of the cycle. In ways only poorly understood they help regulate ovarian function and appear to be interrelated with the maturation of the corpus luteum. In

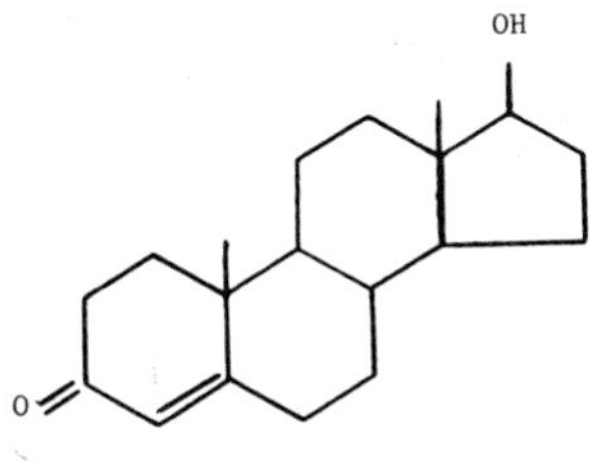

Testosterone

Scheme 2.30.

addition, they stimulate the growth of certain female secondary sex tissue. All known estrogens are aromatic in their active state. The steroidal ones have either a benzenoid ring A or a naphthalenic ring A/B. Examples are estrone and equilenin (Scheme 2.31). Estrogens are sometimes referred to

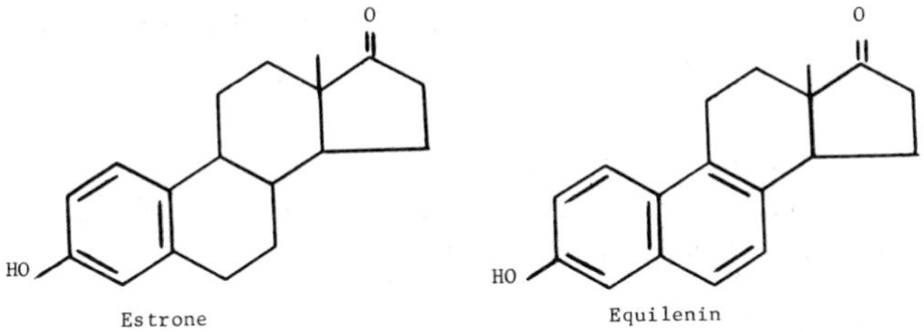

Estrone   Equilenin

Scheme 2.31.

as "C_{18} steroids," but the term should and will be used in this book exclusively in a chemical sense, since not all C_{18} steroids are estrogenic. A fuller account of the biology of estrogens is to be found in Chapter 11.

6. Cardiac-Active Steroids

Steroids that have marked effect on the cardiovascular system have been isolated from both plants (especially of the orders *Apocynaceae*, *Scrophulariaceae*, *Liliaceae*, and *Ranunculaceae*) and animals (especially the toad, *Bufo*). This has been the subject of a great deal of pharmacologic study, and primitive men have used them for arrow poison. Earlier civilized cultures (Egyptian, etc.) have used them medicinally. The steroidal aglycones are principally lactones of two types, those with a six-membered and those with a five-membered lactone ring as a side chain at C-17. Examples are digitoxigenin from the purple foxglove (*Digitalis purpurea*) and bufalin from the skin secretions of the toad (*Bufo vulgaris*) (Scheme 2.32). The term "genin" is given to the aglycone. Digitoxigenin, as other cardiac-active genins, occurs naturally as several different conjugates (glycosides), e.g., as digitoxin and digilamide A. Bufalin exists naturally both as the free genin and as the

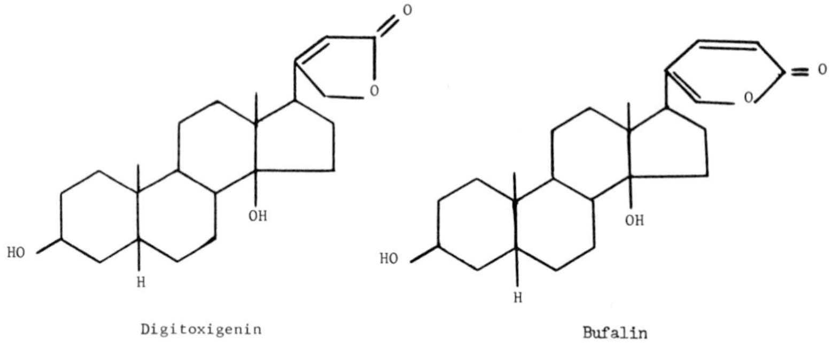

Digitoxigenin   Bufalin

Scheme 2.32.

suberylarginine ester $(C(NH_2)(NH)-NH-CH_2-(CH_2)_2-CH(COOH)-$ $NH-CO-CH_2(CH_2)_4-CH_2-COO-)$. The six-membered lactone ring is found in plants as well as animals. An example of a bufalin analog found in the plant kingdom is scillirosidin (the 6β-acetoxy-8-hydroxy-Δ^4-derivative of bufalin) present as a glycoside in the red variety of *Scilla maritima* (the red squill).

The term *cardenolide* refers to the steroids with a five-membered lactone ring at C-17, while *bufenolide* refers to those with a six-membered lactone ring. The latter usually also possess a 14β-hydroxyl group.

7. Bile Acids and Alcohols

In the animal kingdom, at least among the *Vertebrata*, the digestive tract contains a series of steroids that are derived biosynthetically from sterols by oxidation of the side chain and other nuclear changes. In higher animals they are found in the bile and are formed in the liver. If the carbon skeleton is intact and hydroxylated in the side chain, the substance is called a *bile alcohol*. If it has been converted to the carboxyl stage, the steroid is a *bile acid*. In some cases, especially mammals, the side chain is found degraded to the C-24 acid. The acids generally occur as the amides with glycine (*glyco* being used as a prefix to the bile acid name) or taurine (*tauro* being used as a prefix). Taurine (CH_2NH_2- CH_2-SO_3H) is the sulfonic acid corresponding to glycine. When only a hydroxyl group is present (the bile alcohols), an ester is frequently formed formally with sulfuric acid and the hydroxyl group of the side chain. Typical examples of these steroids are cholic acid from mammals and man and scymnol from sharks and other elasmobranchs (Scheme 2.33). It will be seen that there is an α-OH at C-3 and that rings A and B are *cis*-fused. This is usually found for both the alcohols and the acids in their final functional states from at least fish to man. There are about two dozen natural representatives of bile acids, differing in the number and position of the nuclear hydroxyl groups

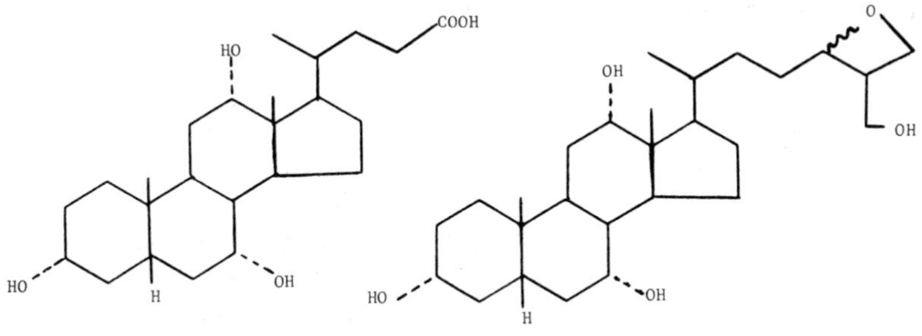

Cholic acid   Scymnol

Scheme 2.33.

and in the extent of oxidation and degradation of the side chain. Chapter 11 should be consulted for a fuller discussion.

8. Vitamin D

Vitamin D is a steroidal metabolite in which ring B has been opened between C-9 and C-10. It prevents rickets in man and other animals. Vitamin D_3 (Scheme 2.34) has the side chain of cholesterol, while vitamin D_2 has the side chain of ergosterol. Vitamin D_1 is not a pure entity. The stereochemistry of the vitamins is the same as in the sterols. In the crystalline state the 4-iodo-5-nitro derivative assumes the conformation in which the H atoms on C-6 and C-7 are *trans*-oriented (rather than *cis*-oriented as shown in Scheme 2.34). The term *provitamin D* is given to the $\Delta^{5,7}$-steroids, because upon

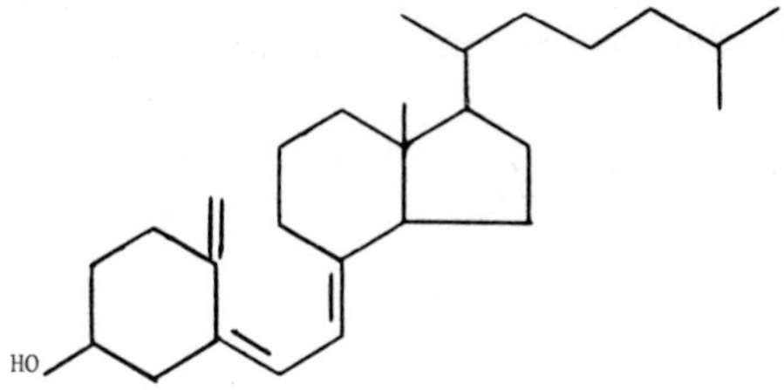

Vitamin D_3

Scheme 2.34.

irradiation they yield the vitamin. An intermediate is *previtamin D*, which is the initial product of irradiation. It possesses the $\Delta^{5(10),6,8}$-triene system, which isomerizes to the more stable $\Delta^{5,7,10(19)}$-triene system characteristic of the vitamin. A thorough discussion is given in Chapter 11.

C. OTHER CLASSIFICATIONS OF STEROIDS

1. Sapogenins

There are various kinds of classifications of steroids that are not clearly chemical or biological. An important example is the sapogenins. These are steroids found in plants, e.g., the *Liliaceae*, *Dioscoreaceae*, and *Scrophulariaceae*, which, as the natural glycosides (saponins), have the property of forming a soapy lather when added to water. Mexicans and others beat clothes against such plants during washing to take advantage of this. In addition, the saponins have the ability to effect the hemolysis of red blood cells. Digitonin (not to be confused with digitoxin), which is isolable from *Digitalis purpurea*, causes destruction of erythrocytes and liberation of hemoglobin in defibrinated blood at a concentration of one part in 10^5.

The aglycones (genins) are structurally derived from the sterols by oxidation in the side chain and at C-16. They are formally 16,26-dihydroxy-22-ketones which have undergone internal ketal formation leading to the formation of two new rings (E and F). Since the two rings are joined at a single carbon atom (C-22), the two rings are of the spirane type and lie at approximately 90° to one another. For these reasons they are called *spiroketals* and the parent system is called *spirostane*. Stereoisomerism exists at C-25 in the natural representatives (see Section A.6a), but apparently not at other centers in the side chain. The oxygen in ring F is believed to be α-oriented and is usually written at the top rather than the bottom of the ring. Typical examples of sapogenins are diosgenin isolable, for instance, from *Dioscorea mexicana* and digitogenin from *Digitalis purpurea* (Scheme 2.35). It will be seen that they differ at C-5 and in the extent of hydroxylation. These are typical but not the exclusive natural differences. There are more than 50 individual sapogenins in nature. Little or nothing is known

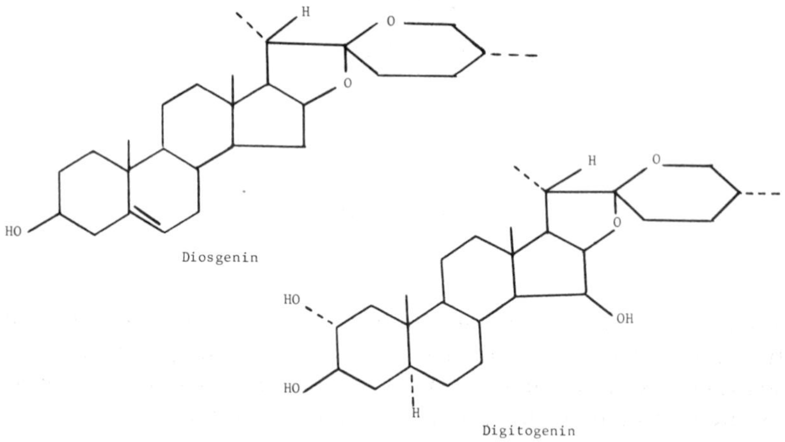

Diosgenin

Digitogenin

Scheme 2.35.

about their biological role or biosynthesis. The prefix *pseudo* in the sapogenin field refers to the product derived from eliminating O and H, respectively, from C-22 and C-20 yielding a $\Delta^{20(22)}$, 26-hydroxy compound retaining the five-membered ring E. The parent name of this compound with an O-containing ring E, no ring F, no 3-hydroxyl or 26-hydroxyl group, and no $\Delta^{20(22)}$-bond but retaining all carbons of the side chain, is *furostane*.

2. Steroidal Alkaloids (*Azasteroids*)

The plant kingdom has yielded many nitrogen-containing steroids. They are frequently grouped for historical reasons with the alkaloids, although they do not share with such classic alkaloids as morphine an amino acid origin of their skeletal carbon atoms. For this reason the term "azasteroid," used by many authors, is probably preferable and will be used in this book. Nitrogen occurs at quite a variety of positions, both with and without changes in the number and kind of rings. They have been found principally in the *Solanaceae*, the *Veratraeae*, the *Liliceae*, and among *Holarrhena* species. In addition, the salamander has yielded C_{19}-A-homosteroids in which one of the atoms in the seven-membered ring A is nitrogen.

There are several different structural kinds of azasteroids (Scheme 2.36). The simplest (represented by jurubidine, a 3β-aminospirostane) contains a nitrogen atom in place of the 3β-hydroxyl group. Conessine is both of this general kind as well as representative of the introduction of a nitrogen atom followed by ring closure. It possesses a 3β-dimethylamino group and a nitrogen atom attached to both C-19 and C-20, forming a five-membered ring. In tomatillidine the latter kind of effect with the nitrogen attached to C-22 and C-26 produces a six-membered ring, as is also true for solasodine, in which the oxygen atom in ring F of a sapogenin is replaced by nitrogen. The nitrogen atom may also be attached to three positions. An important example is solanidine, in which the attachment is at C-16, C-22, and C-26, forming fused five- and six-membered rings E and F. In addition to these, there is a large group of substances that are clearly related to the steroids but that nevertheless are not strict steroids (Section A.1b) in that ring C is five-membered and ring D is six-membered. An important representative is veratramine.

Similarly, the compounds isolated from salamanders, e.g., samandarine, are not strict steroids, since ring A is not intact. It remains to be seen whether they are steroidal metabolites, as seems likely, or whether they represent, as the veratramine type very probably does represent, an alternative cyclization biosynthetically.

Stereochemically, the spirosolane azasteroids all have the same skeletal configurations except at C-22 and C-25. The solasodanes, e.g., solasodine and soladulcidine, are believed to possess (26) the 22R configuration, while the tomatidanes, e.g., tomatidine, are thought to possess (26) the 22S configuration. The former is designated $22\alpha N$ and in this book are written as

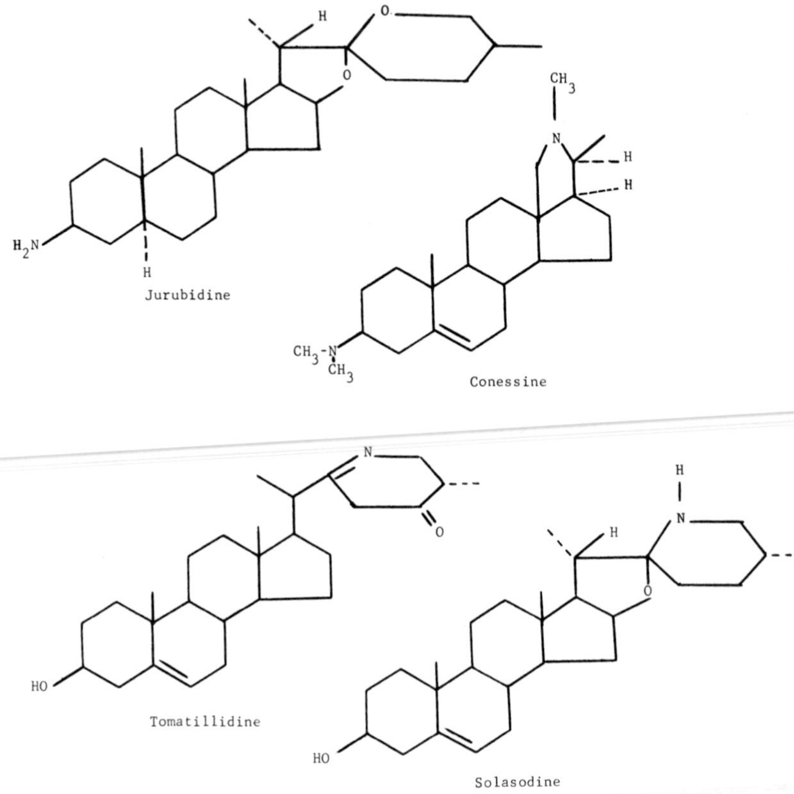

Scheme 2.36. Examples of azasteroid structural types.

with the sapogenins with the N at the top. The 22*S* configuration is designated 22βN and is written down. At C-25 both configurations also are known,
and in Scheme 2.36 the methyl group is shown according to the convention
for noncyclic side chains as for the sapogenins, since ring F is at 90° to the
rest of the molecule. For purposes of correlation, it may be noted that in
solasodine C-25 has the *R* configuration and is designated α, while in tomatidine it is the *S* configuration and is designated β. At the other asymmetric centers, the configurations are as in cholestanol.

In veratramine C-25 has the *S* configuration and is shown in Scheme
2.36 in the stereochemical convention for sapogenins where N replaces O.
The methyl group in the chair form is axial. On the assumption that C-20
(being the largest group on the heterocyclic ring) is equatorial and that the
heterocyclic ring is in the chair form, there is evidence to indicate that the
OH-group at C-23 also is equatorial and therefore α-oriented (in the noncyclic side chain convention). Shown as it is in Scheme 2.36 with the hetero-

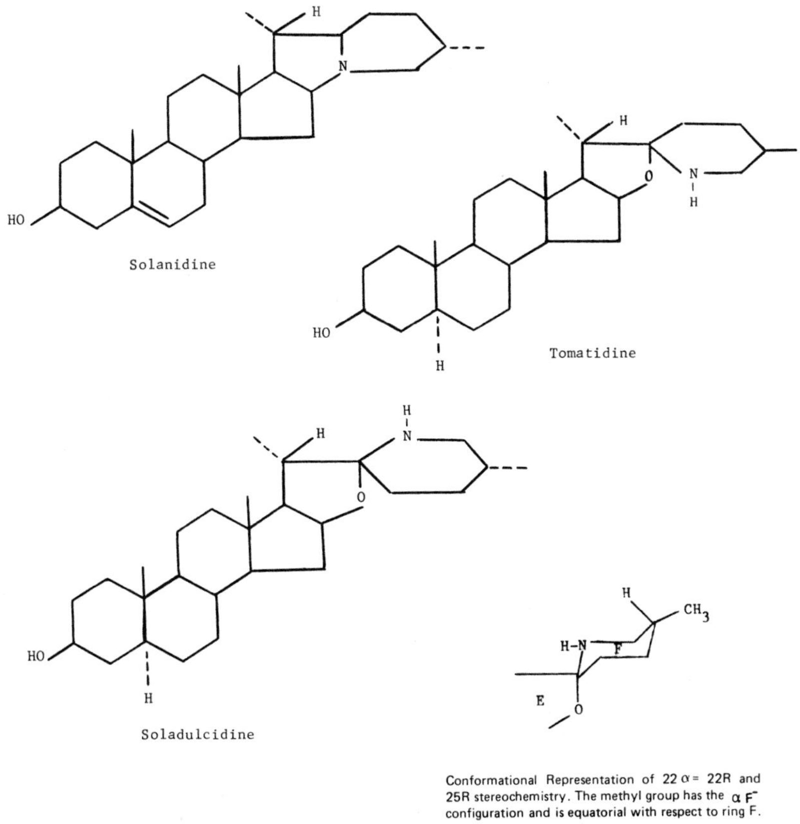

Solanidine

Tomatidine

Soladulcidine

Conformational Representation of 22 α = 22R and 25R stereochemistry. The methyl group has the α F⁻ configuration and is equatorial with respect to ring F.

Scheme 2.36. *Continued.*

cyclic ring viewed from above with the N at the top in the chair form, the noncyclic side chain rotation is equivalent to the more generalized convention of solid and interrupted lines and the substituents with solid lines point toward the observer and those with interrupted lines point away from him. The remaining asymmetric centers are as in cholesterol. A number of analogs of veratramine are known in nature in which there are varying substituents and in which ring D is not benzenoid. In addition, more extensive cyclization is found, especially between the nitrogen atom and C-18, yielding a hexacyclic compound, and between the oxygen at C-23 and C-17, which also yields a hexacyclic compound. The latter is represented by jervine. Zygacine represents the former as well as further ring closure through oxygen between C-4 and C-9. Zygacine is also of the A/B-*cis* type. Since the entire system in zygacine is rigid and no spiro atoms exist, the stereochemical notations are as for the tetracyclic steroid system.

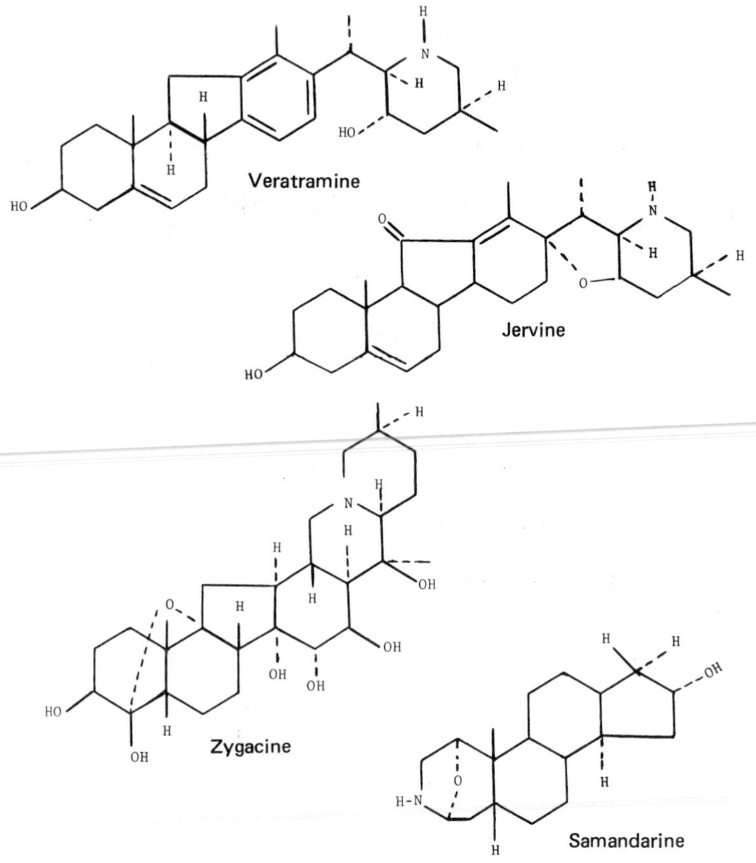

Scheme 2.36. *Continued.*

D. I CLASSIFICATION

1. Introduction

The classification of isopentenoids has historically followed a tortuous course. Terms like "terpene," "triterpene," "isoprenoid," "vitamin," "hormone," etc., have been and continue to be very useful and cannot be abandoned, but they do not lend themselves to an overall system of biochemical inter-relationships. Difficulties in defining the term "steroid" have already been dealt with in Section A-1. Since most of the sophisticated conventions in the isopentenoid field have their origins in steroids and since the steroids are the most well-investigated group, they have been discussed under the heading "steroid." However, before proceeding to the other groups, an attempt will be made here to define a classification, based on biosynthetic principles, that tends to unify all the compounds with which we shall be dealing.

So far as we know, all isopentenoids are biosynthetically derived from a derivative of isopentenol that has the carbon skeleton C—C(C)—C—C. Let us therefore regard any such C_5 compound as an I_1 compound, where the capital letter I stands for the isopentenoid unit and the subscript denotes the number of these units. Compounds that have dissimilar ends of the I unit linked together (called "head-to-tail" linking) would then be I_2 compounds. If a third unit were added, we would have an I_3 compound, etc. If, on the other hand, the units are linked at the same end of each (head-to-head) let us denote this by separating the I units, e.g., I—I, or I_3—I_3, etc. Scheme 2.37 illustrates several types of I compounds. Steroids are thus I_3—I_3 com-

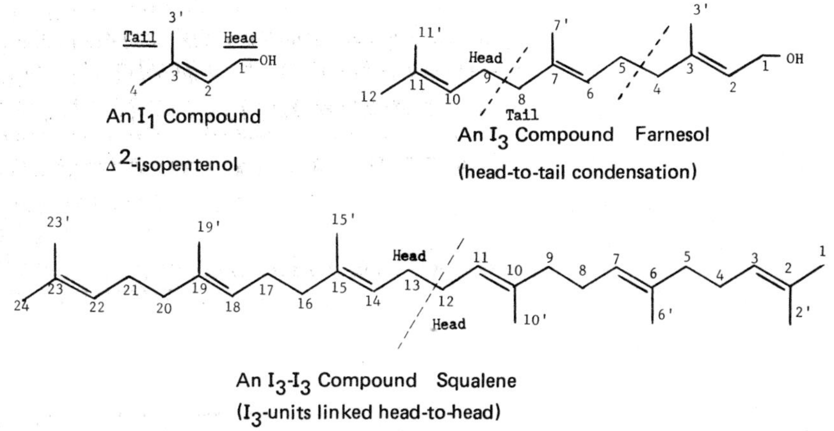

An I_1 Compound

Δ^2-isopentenol

An I_3 Compound   Farnesol

(head-to-tail condensation)

An I_3-I_3 Compound   Squalene

(I_3-units linked head-to-head)

Scheme 2.37.

pounds without (lanosterol, cycloartenol, etc.) or with (cholesterol, cortisone, etc.) removal of carbon atoms. Pentacyclic triterpenoids, e.g., β-amyrin, and the acyclic triterpenoid squalene are also I_3—I_3 compounds. The merit of the I classification is that these very different chemical substances fall into a single biosynthetic group depending upon the degree of polymerization and condensation of the I unit. This is, of course, the true condition. The terms steroid, etc., then can be used to distinguish the precise kind of cyclization or other metabolism at any given I stage of biosynthesis. We shall also employ a numbering system in the head-to-tail case such that C-1 is at the end of the chain that possesses or originally (in a biosynthetic sense) possessed at the C_5 stage a primary alcoholic function. The carbon atoms in the chain will be numbered consecutively, with the methyl groups given a primed number corresponding to the carbon in the chain to which they are attached. In the case of head-to-head condensation, the chain will be numbered in a reverse fashion such that the terminal methyl group that is *trans*-oriented to the rest of the longest head-to-tail chain is taken as No.1. The entire chain will then be numbered consecutively, with the methyl groups given primed numbers. These numbering systems will be called the I system of numbering as opposed to the steroid system described in Section A-4. The latter will be used for polycyclic systems (steroids, pentacyclic triterpenoids, etc.) when they are well established in the literature. The I system will be used in other cases.

2. I$_1$ Stage

The term *isopentane* will be used to denote what in Geneva nomenclature would be 2-methylbutane, and the term *isopentanol* without any numbering for the hydroxyl group will be used for 3-methyl-butan-1-ol. At the I$_1$ stage of polymerization there are three possible olefinic isomers, the Δ^2-, the $\Delta^{3(3')}$-, and the $\Delta^{3(4)}$-compounds. The latter two of these are formally but not biochemically equivalent. In view of simplicity and clarity of the use of the Δ symbol, it will always be used where appropriate.

3. Higher Acylic I Stages

In the last few years, acyclic I compounds with many I units have been found in nature. No systematic nomenclature has been developed for these. Moreover, at the I$_2$ stage, stereoisomerism at the double bonds is already not only possible but present in nature. Thus, geraniol, first isolated from the geranium, and nerol, first isolated from *Neroli* species, are *cis-trans* isomers. The use of trivial names, however, at, say, the I$_{10}$ stage with all the possibilities of *cis-trans*-isomerism, etc., becomes prohibitively complicated. Furthermore, trivial names for all the known cases have not even evolved. Consequently, parent I hydrocarbons will be given names depending systematically on the degree of polymerization using the common prefixes derived from Latin added to the monomeric unit isopentane. Thus, we have diisopentane, triisopentane, tetraisopentane, etc., respectively for the I$_2$-, I$_3$-, and I$_4$-hydrocarbons, etc. For a compound of unknown chain length, the prefix "poly" will be used instead of the Latin specification of degree of polymerization. For simplicity, in certain cases the letter "a" meaning "all" will be added as a superscript to Δ, that is, every fourth numbered carbon atom beginning with No. 2 carries a double bond. Thus, $\Delta^{2,6,10,14,18,22(trans)}$-hexaisopentahexenol could be written $\Delta^{a(trans)}$-hexaisopentahexenol, or a large rubber hydrocarbon could be called $\Delta^{a(cis)}$-polyisopentapolyene. We may also describe, for instance, farnesol as a "$\Delta^{a(trans)}$-isopentenoid at the I$_3$ stage," or we may write "Δ^a-diisopentenoid" to describe the geraniol and nerol structures and various of their derivatives without specifying the stereochemistry of the double bonds or the nature of any other groups. The term "Δ^a-isopentenol," on the other hand, would refer only to geraniol or nerol. The I nomenclature is extended in Chapter 5.

LITERATURE CITED

1. L. F. Fieser and M. Fieser, Steroids. Reinhold, New York, 1959.
2. L. F. Fieser and M. Fieser, Natural Products Related to Phenanthrene. 3rd Ed. Reinhold, New York, 1949.
3. E. J. Corey, P. R. Ortiz de Montellano, and H. Yamamoto, J. Am. Chem. Soc. 90:6254 (1968).
4. P. Boiteau, B. Pasich, and A. R. Ratsimamanga, Les Triterpenoides en Physiologie Végétale et Animale. Gauthier-Villars, Paris, 1964.
5. J. D. Bernal, D. Crowfoot, and I. Fankuchen, Trans. Roy. Soc. London A 239:135 (1940).
6. R. B. Turner, in L. F. Fieser and M. Fieser (eds.), Natural Products Related to Phenanthrene. 3rd. Ed. Reinhold, New York, 1949. pp. 620-670.
7. S. Bergstrom, Helv. Chim. Acta 32:3 (1949).
8. A. Lardon and T. Reichstein, Helv. Chim. Acta 32:1613 (1949).
9. A. Lardon and T. Reichstein, Helv. Chim. Acta 32:2003 (1949).
10. V. Prelog, A. Furlenmeier, D. F. Dickel, and W. Keller, Helv. Chim. Acta 36:308 (1953).
11. V. Prelog and H. L. Meier, Helv. Chim. Acta 36:320 (1953).
12. W. G. Dauben, D. F. Dickel, O. Jeger, and V. Prelog, Helv. Chim. Acta 36:325 (1953).
13. D. J. Cram and F. A. A. Elhafez, J. Am. Chem. Soc. 74:5828 (1952).
14. V. Prelog and G. Tsatas, Helv. Chim. Acta 36:1178 (1953).
15. B. Riniker, D. Arigoni, and O. Jeger, Helv. Chim. Acta 37:546 (1954).
16. J. W. Cornforth, I. Youhotsky, and G. Popjak, Nature (London) 173:536 (1954).
17. M. Viscontini and H. Kohler, Helv. Chim. Acta 37:41 (1954).
18. M. Viscontini and P. Miglioretto, Helv. Chim. Acta 38:930 (1955).
19. K. Brenneisen, C. Tamm, and T. Reichstein, Helv. Chim. Acta 39:1233 (1956).
20. W. R. Nes, T. E. Varkey, and K. Krevitz, J. Am. Chem. Soc. 99:260 (1977).
21. R. S. Cahn, J. Chem. Ed. 41:116 (1964).
22. R. S. Cahn, C. K. Ingold, and V. Prelog, Angew. Chem., Int. Ed. Engl. 5:385 (1966).
23. W. R. Nes, in R. Paoletti and D. Kritchevsky (eds.), Advances in Lipid Research. Vol. 15. Academic Press, New York, 1977.
24. IUPAC-IUB Revised Tentative Rules for Steroid Nomenclature, Steroids, 13:277 (1969); Biochemistry, 8: 2227 (1969); ibid., 10: 4994 (1971).
25. W. R. Nes, Lipids 9:596 (1974).
26. H. Ripperger, K. Schreiber, and G. Snatzke, Tetrahedron 21:727 (1965).

Chapter
3

Analytical
Procedures

A. **Chemical Methods** 85
    1. *General Comments* 85
    2. *Acylable Hydroxyl Groups* 86
    3. *Ketones* 88
    4. *Double Bonds* 92
    5. *Aromatic Systems* 92
    6. *Aldehydes* 93
    7. *Tests for Other Steroids* 93
    8. *Summary of Chemical Selectivity* 94
B. **Physical Methods** 97
    1. *General Comments* 97
    2. *Ultraviolet and Visible Spectroscopy* 100
    3. *Infrared Spectroscopy* 104
    4. *Nuclear Magnetic Resonance Spectroscopy* 108
    5. *Mass Spectroscopy* 114
    6. *Polarimetry* 122
    7. *Methods Using Radioactivity* 123
    8. *Enzyme Assays* 123
C. **Chromatographic Methods** 124
    1. *Fundamental Principles* 124
    2. *Liquid-Liquid and Liquid-Solid Chromatography* 127
    3. *Gas-Liquid Chromatography* 131
D. **Methods Using Protein-Steroid Interactions** 137
    1. *Radioimmunoassay* 137
    2. *Competitive Protein Binding* 140
Literature Cited 140

A. CHEMICAL METHODS

1. General Comments

With the exception of protein binding (see Section D) and other interactions with polymers, chemical reactions generally occur not with an entire molecule but rather with a given type of functional group, the precise reactivity of which depends on its environment. Consequently, although there are no reactions that are really distinctive for a steroid, there are those that will show 1) what and how many functional groups are present, and 2) the environment and therefore the position of the group. To the extent that one can eliminate (by other procedures) the presence of nonsteroidal materials, these procedures are useful for structural and analytical purposes. Whether a compound is or is not a steroid can be ascertained from a combination of the various chemical, physical, and biological techniques. The information obtainable from each of these is discussed in what follows.

2. Acylable Hydroxyl Groups

With but a few exceptions, all naturally occurring steroids possess at least one hydroxyl and/or keto group. They are consequently of tremendous analytical value. Several ways by which the hydroxyl group can be measured are available.

a. Digitonin Precipitation   Windaus (1) discovered that the highly oxygenated steroidal glycoside, digitonin (Scheme 3.1), a sapogenin, formed

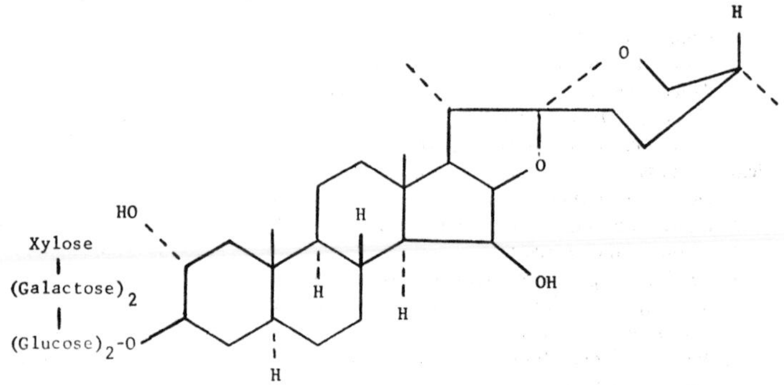

Scheme 3.1. Digitonin ($C_{56}H_{92}O_{29}$).

an insoluble 1:1 complex with cholesterol, only 14 mg in 100 ml of 95% ethanol being soluble. Such complexes are called *digitonides*. It has since been found that this complex formation is nearly restricted to unesterified 3β-hydroxy steroids in either the 5α- or the 5β-series, for reasons that are not clear. The 3α-hydroxy steroids are not precipitated, and the addition of digitonin in a 1% solution of 95% ethanol to a steroid mixture thus affords an easy way to separate the epimers. The solid digitonide may be weighed for quantitative estimation. Dissociation of the complex is accomplished in pyridine (2, 3), and the digitonin is then selectively precipitable with ether. Similar complexes of 3β-hydroxy steroids are also formed with other sapogenins, e.g., tigonin, the 2,15-bisdesoxy derivative of digitonin. Complex formation occurs without much regard for the nature of the side chain in the sterol. Even 3β-hydroxy-17-keto steroids form digitonides. In view of the usefulness of the method over the years, it is unfortunate that a thorough systematic study of structural effects has not been made, and a note of caution must be injected into its use. It is known, for instance, that the introduction of an acyloxy group at C-4 or C-7 prevents complex formation, as does inversion at C-10. A further drawback of the method is that milligram rather than microgram quantities are necessary.

b. Acylation With the advent of radioactive techniques, it has become possible to determine the presence of acylable hydroxyl groups in samples weighing far less than a milligram. After the addition of labeled acetic anhydride to the steroid in question (dissolved in pyridine) and reisolation of the steroid, the extent of radioactivity is measured. A positive response indicates an acylable hydroxyl group. If the number of molecules can be measured, e.g., by spectroscopy or gas-liquid chromatography, the number of hydroxyl groups can be calculated from the molar specific activities of the acetic anhydride and acetate. Thus, if the specific activity of the acetate in d.p.m./μM were the same as that of the acetic anhydride (labeled with ^{14}C in both acyl halves), the steroid would contain two acylable hydroxyl groups (since only half the ^{14}C from each anhydride molecule is incorporated into the acetate).

Similar use can be made of ultraviolet spectroscopy by the preparation of benzoates [λ_{max} 230 (ϵ 14,000)] and other esters in which the acyl moiety has a chromophore. If one knows the number of molecules as described above for the labeled case, measurement of the absorbance and comparison with the molar extinction coefficient of monoesters of the same class yields the number of acylable hydroxyl groups. Qualitatively, of course, just the presence of the appropriate absorption indicates an OH group. The method is applicable on a scale of about 50 μg, which is less than necessary for the digitonin method but more than is required by the labeling technique.

Ether formation with labeled or UV-absorbing reagents can be used in much the same way as acylation, but experimentally it is not as feasible.

Acylable hydroxyl groups are sterically unhindered. They include most of the primary and secondary hydroxyl groups of the usual steroids, e.g., at C-21 and C-3, respectively. However, the secondary hydroxyl group at C-11 with the β configuration is not acetylated under the usual conditions. Corticosterone, for instance, gives only monoacetate (at C-21). Tertiary hydroxyl groups, of which the one at C-17 is of the most importance, are not acylable under the usual conditions. Thus, cortisol yields only a monoacetate. In the hindered cases, recourse must be had to acylating reagents such as isopropenyl acetate which are more reactive (of higher energy in the biochemical sense).

3. Ketones

a. Imino Derivatives   The formation of light-absorbing imino derivatives of ketones is an easy chemical step quite diagnostic for the presence of a keto group. Moreover, these derivatives are readily used for quantitation. Of special importance are the semicarbazones and 2,4-dinitrophenylhydrazones. The former absorb near 228 nm (ϵ 12,900) and the latter near 370 nm (ϵ 24,400). A bathochromic shift occurs for α, β-unsaturation, and other detailed structural features about the environment of the carbonyl group can also be ascertained from the precise nature of the spectrum. Of special importance are the derivatives of the Δ^4-3-keto system, the semicarbazone absorbing at 270 nm (ϵ 30,000) and the 2,4-dinitrophenylhydrazone absorbing at 392 nm (ϵ 31,200). The 2,4-dinitrophenylhydrazones also exhibit a peak of lower intensity about 25 nm toward shorter wavelengths, but it is the peak closer to 400 nm which is responsible for the visually observed color that is useful qualitatively and for chromatographic identification. A thorough discussion is to be found elsewhere (4). As a first approximation, the decreasing order of reactivity is saturated 3-ketones, Δ^4-3-ketones, 17- or 20-ketones, 21-hydroxy-20-ketones, and 17α,21-dihydroxy-20-ketones. 11-Carbonyls usually do not form such derivatives.

b. 17α,21-Dihydroxy-20-Keto System   Since this type of side chain is characteristic of cortisol and other glucocorticoids, many methods for quantitative and selective analysis of it have been reported. Probably the most useful has been a reaction devised by Porter and Silber (5, 6) in which a 2,4-dinitrophenylhydrazone is formed under acid conditions (Scheme 3.2). The importance of the procedure is that the hydrazone formed is not

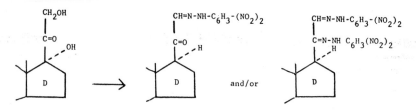

Scheme 3.2. Chemistry of the Porter-Silber reaction.

the simple derivative of the original 20-keto compound but rather the hydrazone of a rearranged substance. Consequently the ability to give the test is highly restricted to compounds bearing the 17α,21-dihydroxy-20-keto moiety and very closely related structures involved in or capable of undergoing the rearrangement. This rearrangement was discovered by Mattox (7) and involves simultaneous reduction at C-17 and oxidation at C-21 such that C-21 bears an aldehyde grouping. The end product thus appears to be a 2,4-dinitrophenylhydrazone of the 20-keto-21-aldehyde and it possesses a very distinctive spectrum with an absorption peak near 410 nm. The bathochromic shift in the peak from the position of unconjugated ketones is due to the presence of π-electrons at the positions adjacent to the C=N group. As expected from this, 20-keto-21-aldehydes also produce the same type of end product. Similar results are also obtained when the 17α-hydroxyl group is replaced by unsaturation at C-16, C-17. The methodology was discussed in detail by Silber and Porter (8) in 1957, and more recently the Taits and their associates (9) have added certain advantages to the experimental procedure as applied to blood and urine samples.

Oxidation with sodium bismuthate, developed by Norymberski (10, 11), is also useful for quantitative and qualitative analysis. This procedure cleaves the molecule at the C-17, C-20-bond and the C-20, C-21-bond, yielding formaldehyde and 17-ketosteroids, which can be analyzed colorimetrically. In the absence of the 17α-hydroxyl group, formaldehyde is obtained with no 17-ketosteroid formed. Sodium bismuthate cleaves various 1,2-glycols, 1,2-ketols, and α-hydroxyacids, and any compound with these groupings may also yield formaldehyde.

Table 3.1 summarizes the use of these reagents, and the literature has been reviewed more extensively by Peron (12) and by Eik-Nes (13). In these reviews can also be found a discussion of other methods, which tend to be more empirical. Of these the formation of light-absorbing products by dehydration and rearrangement in the presence of sulfuric acid ("sulfuric acid chromogens") has been widely used.

  c. 20,21-Ketol System   Compounds containing an α-ketol system are readily oxidized by a variety of reagents, probably the oldest known being silver ion, which yields easily visible (black) silver metal. The most important steroids with an α-ketol system possess a 21-hydroxyl and a 20-keto group. In the presence of alkaline silver nitrate they readily give a black deposit. However, the metallic silver is not easily measured. Better reagents are cupric ion (14), originally used by Folin and Wu for carbohydrates, and the yellow 2,3,5-triphenyltetrazolium chloride (15) better known as "blue test tetrazolium reagent." In the former case the resultant cuprous ion is measured colorimetrically as a blue complex formed on addition of phosphomolybdic acid. With blue tetrazolium, the reduced product, diformazan, possesses its own distinctive absorption spectrum (also a blue color, from which the name of the reagent is derived) measurable directly. 21-Hydroxy-20-ketosteroids with and without the 17α-hydroxy group give a positive, quantitative test.

These and other methods, e.g., the formation of chromogens on treatment with sulfuric acid, have been reviewed (12, 13) more extensively elsewhere.

  d. The 17-Ketones   17-Ketosteroids are common metabolites found in mammalian blood and urine. Although they produce reactions with

Table 3.1. Identification of Cortical-type Side Chains

Steroid	Type of Test					
	CH_2O with HIO_4	CH_2O with $NaBiO_3$	17-KS[a] with HIO_4	17-KS[a] with $NaBiO_3$	P.S.[b]	BT[c]
CH_2OH—C=O— ... D	+	+	–	–	–	+
CH_2OH—C=O—OH ... D / CH_2OH—CHOH	+	+	–	+	+	+

Structures (steroid D-ring fragments):

- D — CH_3 — $C{=}O$, OH
- D — CH_2OH, OH
- D — $C{-}HOH$, OH

−	−	−
−	−	−
−	+	+
−	−	+
+	−	+
+	−	+

[a] 17-Ketosteroids
[b] Porter-Silber Chromogen
[c] Reducing with Blue Tetrazolium Reagent

reagents such as 2,4-dinitrophenylhydrazine with about the same ease as 20-ketosteroids, a more specific reaction was discovered by Zimmermann (16) with m-dinitrobenzene in alkali. This reagent produces a blue complex with an absorption maximum near 500 nm that can be quantitated spectrophotometrically. Wilson (17) and others studied the influence of steroidal structure on chromogenicity. Certain other aromatic compounds yield similar complexes, notably m-dinitrobenzoic acid and benzyltrimethylammonium hydroxide. The formation of the typical blue complex seems to depend on the presence of a CH_2 or CH_3 group adjacent to a carbonyl group. Thus, acetone yields a positive test, as do 3-ketosteroids, but the intensity and precise spectrophotometric character of the color produced with 17-ketosteroids tend to be unique.

4. Double Bonds

Double bonds yield complexes with various reagents. Among these is tetranitromethane, which Heilbronner (18) showed could be used spectrophotometrically to distinguish the extent of substitutions. Osmium tetroxide, which adds to double bonds to form osmate esters, has also been used (19) to show the presence of a double bond in the side chain of sterols, and a micromethod using metaperiodate has been developed (20). However, the most widely used tests of both the qualitative and quantitative levels are the formation of chromogens with acids. In 1885 Liebermann (21) found that cholesterol produced a series of transient colors (from red to blue to green) when a few drops of sulfuric acid are added to the sterol in cold acetic anhydride. The saturated stanols give no color. The precise nature of the color and the speed with which it is developed depend on the kind of unsaturation present. $\Delta^{5,7}$-Steroids, for instance, develop colors much faster than Δ^5-steroids. The method has been used widely for the determination of cholesterol in tissues and fluids following modifications of Schoenheimer. A more complete discussion is to be found elsewhere (22). The Liebermann reaction is the forerunner of the assays of corticoids using sulfuric acid chromogens (12, 13). In the latter case, sulfuric acid is usually used without dilution and the products depend more on oxygenated substituents than on positions of double bonds. The application of o-phthalaldehyde to the formation of usable colored complexes of Δ^5-steroids with or without a long side chain has been reported (23).

5. Aromatic Systems

Most of the aromatic steroids known are estrogens or their metabolites. A great deal of effort has been expended on their analysis. Unfortunately, they have not lent themselves readily to precise and usable chemical reactions on the aromatic nucleus, and nearly all the chemical processes used are empirical. Of the colorimetric procedures, the most widely employed devices are from the work of Kober (24) in 1931, who found that a pink color develops when phenolsulfonic acid and sulfuric acid are added to estrogens followed by addition of water. The color is produced with estrone, estradiol, and estriol. Modifications by Ittrich (25, 26) and by Salokangas and Bulbrook (27) are widely used. As little as 0.2 μg of estrogen is measurable.

The conversion of estrogens to fluorescing polyunsaturated materials by reaction with phosphoric or sulfuric acids has been found more recently to be the method of choice. By measurement of the fluorescent spectrum it is possible to quantitate 0.005 μg of estrone (28), which is a remarkable sensitivity, but the method suffers from lack of selectivity, especially when sulfuric acid is the reagent. The Ittrich modification (25) of the Kober reaction is also applicable to fluorescence techniques and appears to be more selective. A review is available (29). More recently, Touchstone et al. (30) reported that diazotization of estrogens with "fast violet B salt" (the diazonium salt of 6-benzoyl-4-methoxy-5-toluidine) produces stable yellow compounds which are chromatographically separable and directly quantitated at 412 nm. The method allows 0.02 μg to be detected. The 3-methyl ethers do not react and neither equilenin nor non-estrogenic steroids behave similarly to estrone, etc. The site of diazotization appears to be at C-2, since neither 2-hydroxy- nor 2-methoxyestrone formed the yellow product.

6. Aldehydes

Aldosterone is the only steroidal aldehyde that has attracted enough attention for extensive analytical study. Although the reactions with 2,4-dinitrophenylhydrazine, with the blue tetrazolium reagent, and other procedures for corticoids have been modified for use with aldosterone, they suffer from lack of selectivity. In fact, no completely specific assay for aldosterone has been developed, and more or less rigid purification is necessary before assay. Purification is made either with the compound itself or with the etiolactone formed by oxidatively removing C-21. The Taits and their associates (31) have developed procedures for purification via the etiolactone followed by an assay depending on fluorescence induced by alkalicatalyzed reactions with sodium hydroxide (soda fluorescence). Fluorescence induced by potassium t-butoxide is also currently used (32). Brodie and Tait (33) have reviewed the literature on these and other methods.

7. Tests for Other Steroids

Analytical procedures for other types of steroids have not been extensively investigated, especially with regard to quantitations and careful correlations with structure. Nevertheless, it is known that many of the saponins, e.g., digitonin, will cause hemolysis of blood, and that cardenolides, e.g., strophantidin but not dihydrostrophantidin, produce a deep red color when sodium nitroprusside is added to a pyridine solution of the steroid followed by a little alkali (Legal test). This test is characteristic of the strophanthus-digitalis group. The double bond in the lactone ring must be β,γ-oriented to the carbonyl group. The steroidal alkaloids give typical alkaloidal reactions. The bile acids, however, which have received considerable analytical attention recently, are usually examined by chromatographic procedures.

8. Summary of Chemical Selectivity

Together with the accompanying collection of structural formulas (Schemes 3.3 to 3.9) is given a list of the tests in which each of the compounds gives

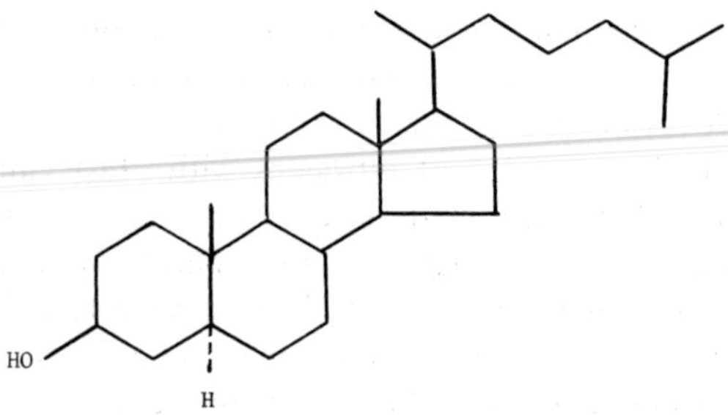

Cholestanol

Digitonin
Labeled Ac$_2$O (1)

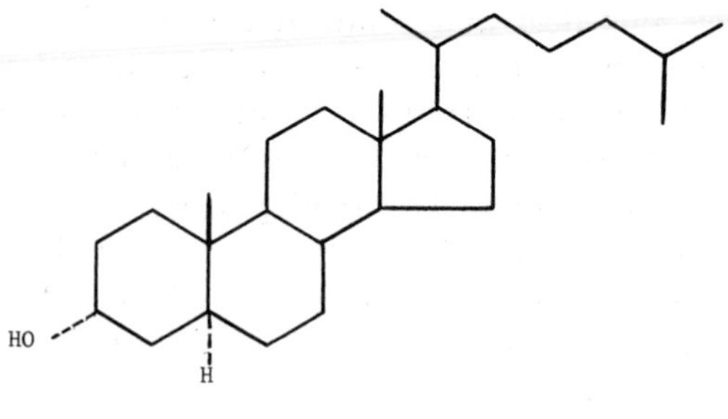

3-Epicholestanol

Labeled Ac$_2$O (1)

Scheme 3.3.

a positive result. If no test is mentioned, the test is negative. The tests included are: precipitation with digitonin; assay for acylable hydroxyl groups with radioactive acetic anhydride, in which the number in parentheses indicates the number of acyl groups introduced; the Liebermann test for unsaturation; the Zlatkis-Zak test for unsaturation; the formation of

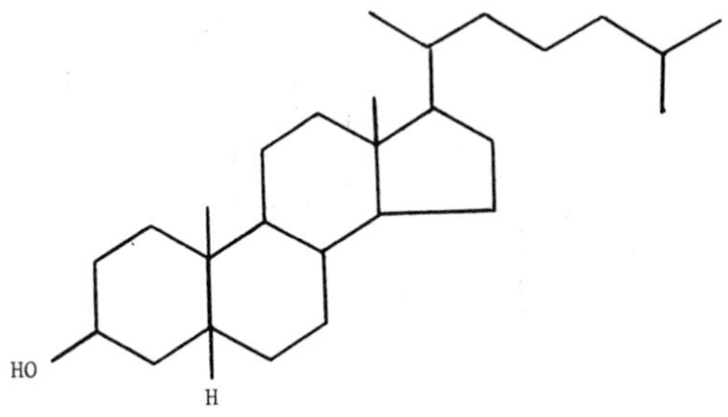

Coprostanol

Digitonin
Labeled Ac$_2$0 (1)

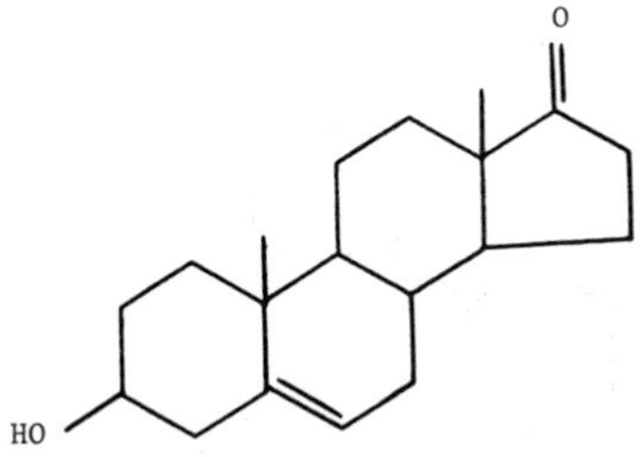

Dehydroepiandrosterone

Digitonin
Labeled Ac$_2$0 (1)
Lieberman
Zlatkis-Zak
Zimmerman
2,4-DNPH

Scheme 3.4.

2,4-dinitrophenylhydrazones as a test of keto groups; the formation of a typical Zimmermann color for 17-keto groups; the periodate test of Mallory et al. for the Δ^{22} group; the development of appropriate fluorescence under strong alkaline conditions, with NaOH or t-C$_4$H$_{10}$O as an indication of the Δ^4-3-keto group; the formation of formaldehyde from periodate or bismuthate oxidation which is indicative of a 21-hydroxy-20-keto system; the formation of 17-ketosteroids from such oxidations when a 17α-hydroxy-20-keto system is present; the capacity to reduce cupric and silver ions as well as the blue tetrazolium reagent characteristic of α-ketols; the formation of a colored product on diazotization, as described by Touchstone, proving the presence of an aromatic ring; and finally the development of appropriate fluorescence by Ittrich's modification of the Kober reaction or the production of a pink color in the Kober reaction proper, both of which indicate phenolic steroids.

It will be seen that the use of these reactions can lead to a great deal

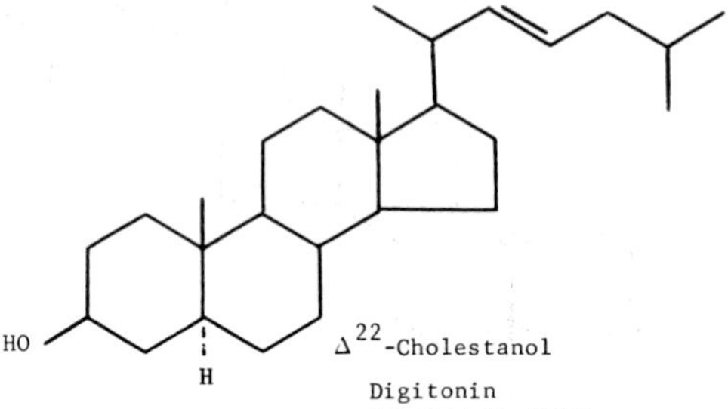

Δ^{22}-Cholestanol

Digitonin
Labeled Ac_2O (1)
Mallory et al. Periodate

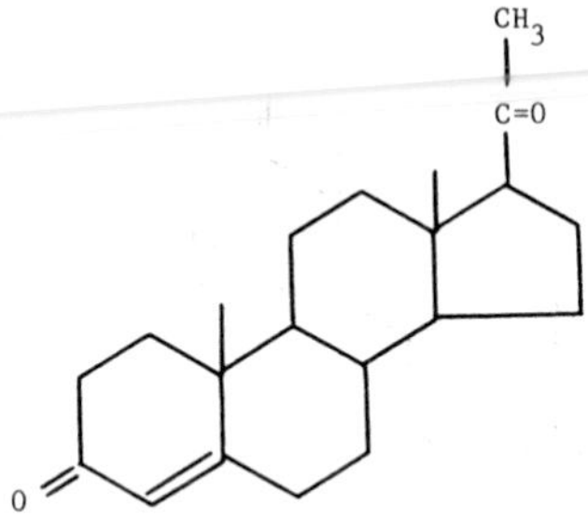

Progesterone

2,4-DPNH
Soda fluorescence
t-Butoxide fluorescence

Scheme 3.5.

of structural information. Since all the methods mentioned here have also been developed to some degree of quantitative sophistication and frequently are applicable on a scale of micrograms (or even less in some cases), qualitative and quantitative analyses have been possible with very small amounts of tissues and fluids (thin tissue slices, milliliter quantities of blood, etc.). Extensive information, summarized in subsequent chapters, on the distribution, biosynthetic pathways, and dynamic physiology of these and related substances has thus been obtained.

However, these methods are not entirely sufficient. This is especially so when the compound is a new one. Restricted conditions (time, nature or amount of tissues, etc.) under which an assay must be carried out also often make a given test useless. Furthermore, most cells contain mixtures of two or more, often as many as thirty, steroids. For these and other reasons it has been necessary to utilize equally sophisticated procedures of separation, many of which allow numbers to be assigned to the extent of separation and thereby function in their own right as methods of functional group identification. Each of these procedures yields different but frequently overlapping information. Aldosterone is a case in point. It is not easily

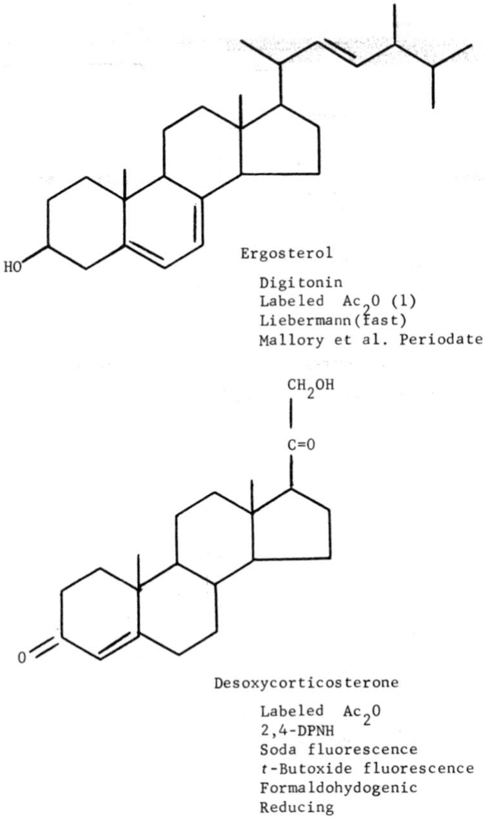

Ergosterol

Digitonin
Labeled Ac$_2$O (1)
Liebermann(fast)
Mallory et al. Periodate

CH$_2$OH
|
C=O

Desoxycorticosterone

Labeled Ac$_2$O
2,4-DPNH
Soda fluorescence
t-Butoxide fluorescence
Formaldohydogenic
Reducing

Scheme 3.6.

differentiated from certain other corticoids by chemical methods, so it is identified chromatographically and then quantitated chemically and fluorimetrically.

B. PHYSICAL METHODS

1. General Comments

Physical methods of analysis described in this section are restricted to measurements of the steroids themselves. The results therefore are directly referable to the molecule and do not depend on interpretations about intervening chemical reactions. The information derived is obviously of immense value, but, since many of the methods require as much as milligram quantities of material, their use is limited. It should also be pointed out that each of the methods described yields only certain kinds of information. As a first approximation, spectroscopy in the ultraviolet and

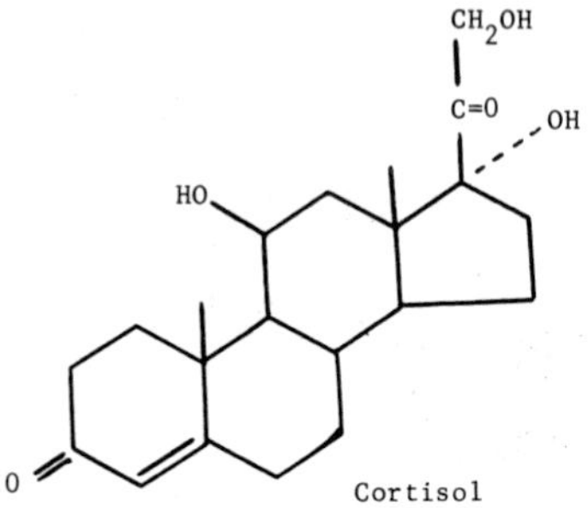

CH$_2$OH

C=0   OH

HO

0

Cortisol

Labeled   Ac$_2$0 (1)
2,4-DPNH
Alkali fluorescence
Porter-Silber
Formaldohydogenic
17-Ketogenic
Reducing

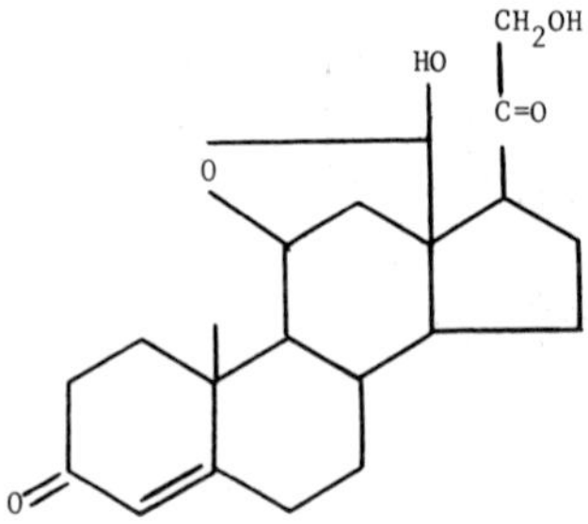

CH$_2$OH

HO

C=0

0

0

Aldosterone
(Internal hemiacetal)

Labeled   Ac$_2$0 (2)
Alkali fluorescence
2,4-DPNH
Formaldohydogenic
Reducing

Scheme 3.7.

visible regions is particularly useful for interpretations about the position
and number of double bonds and is frequently amenable to precise quantitation. Infrared spectroscopy is also useful for interpretations about the
presence of double bonds; it also yields information about hydroxyl and
carbonyl groups. Nuclear magnetic resonance spectroscopy reflects the
number and environment of hydrogen nuclei, and is of special usefulness in
determining the presence and position of methyl groups. It can be used to
deduce the number of hydrogen atoms on a double bond or the number
adjacent to various groups. Mass spectroscopy is the method *par excellence*
for the determination of molecular weights. This feature alone makes the
method important, but it yields a tremendous amount of additional information, particularly about the presence and nature of a steroidal ring

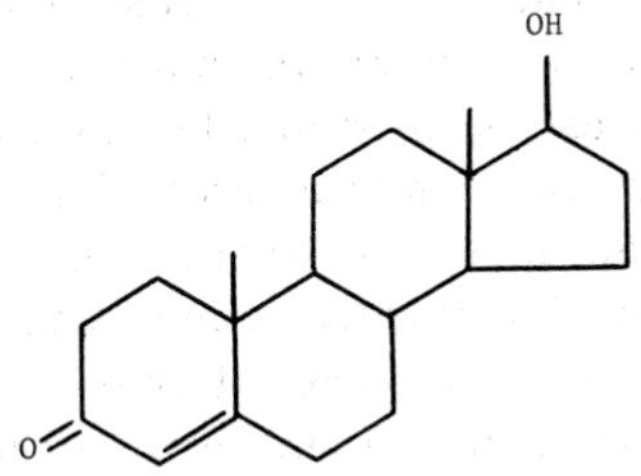

OH

Testosterone

Labeled   Ac$_2$0 (1)
Alkali fluorescence
2,4-DPNH

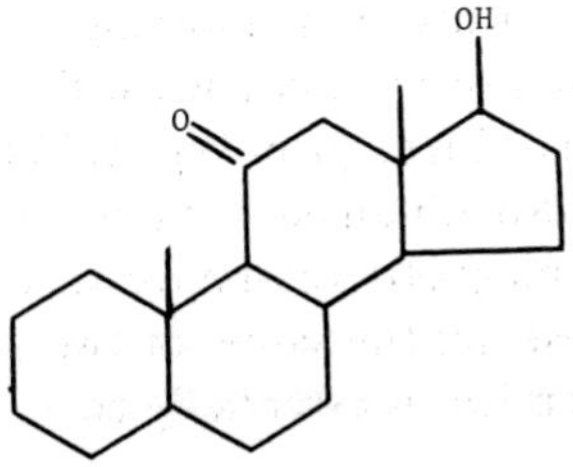

OH

11-Keto-androstan-17 β -ol

Labeled   Ac$_2$0 (1)

Scheme 3.8.

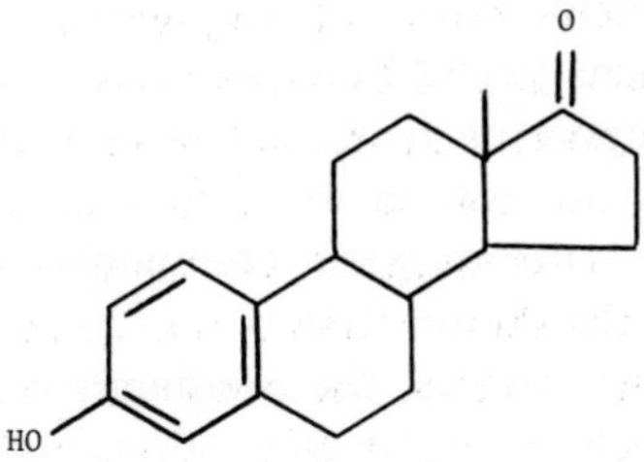

O

Estrone

Labeled   Ac$_2$0
DPNH
Zimmermann
Diazotization
Ittrich fluorescence
Kober

Scheme 3.9.

system. Measurements of optical rotations at single or especially at multiple (optical rotatory dispersion) wavelengths allow deductions to be made about the asymmetry of the molecule. Since steroids and related substances are highly asymmetric at various centers, the positioning of certain groups, of which carbonyls are the easiest to study, becomes possible. In the reverse sense, if one knows the position of a carbonyl group, optical rotatory dispersion yields information about the adjacent positions. Finally, x-ray diffraction, when applied to its fullest extent, can and has yielded nearly complete structural elucidation, as in the case of vitamin D. However, it has not been developed as a laboratory tool and requires the interest, extensive time, and special equipment of the rare expert in the field. For this reason it deserves only mention at this point. While it was used with signal success in the early studies of steroidal structure, the current interests of workers in the field tends toward protein structure (myoglobin, etc.).

As described in the foregoing paragraphs, these methods yield precise structural information. It is worth remembering that they can also be used empirically for identification of an unknown with a standard sample. This was first achieved with the "finger print region" of the infrared spectrum. A distinctive pattern is also obtained with mass spectroscopy and to a great extent with nuclear magnetic resonance spectroscopy. If the spectral patterns in all three of these are the same for two samples, the chance that the compounds are not identical is essentially zero.

2. Ultraviolet and Visible Spectroscopy

a. Fundamental Principles   The energy of photons in the visible and experimentally usable ultraviolet regions of the electromagnetic spectrum raises the electrons in double (but not single) bonds to higher levels. Since the process is quantized, only certain transitions are allowed and they are dependent on the environment, extent of conjugation, degree of substitution, and nature of the atoms joined by π-electrons. The C=C and C=O bonds are the ones most important in steroids of natural origin. The C=N group also plays an important role in derivatives used for analysis. The absorption peaks for the unconjugated chromophores (light-absorbing groups) appear at wavelengths shorter than is readily measured. Because of the presence of air and other factors, the commonly measurable region is from 210 to 800 nm, of which the region from 400 to 800 nm is regarded as the visible and lower wavelengths as the near ultraviolet region. Although some of the unconjugated chromophores absorb outside of the usable region, the peaks are frequently so close to 210 nm that the long-wavelength side of the band is observed between 210 and 225 nm. This is known as "end-absorption." When used carefully, it is of great value. Its very presence indicates unsaturation (or, of course, contamination). Pure cholestanol, for instance, has no significant absorption from 210 to 800 nm, and when wavelength (λ) is plotted against intensity of absorption (A

for *absorbance*, or, in the older literature, O.D. for optical density), an essentially straight line at $A = 0$ is obtained. On the other hand, 5,6-dehydrocholestanol (cholesterol) exhibits end-absorption because of a peak for the Δ^5-bond near 200 nm.

The intensity of absorption is measured usually as the logarithm of the ratio of the intensity of the light incident on the sample (I_0) to that of the light transmitted by the sample (I). The reciprocal of the latter ratio is "percent transmittance" $(\%T)$. When the absorbance (A) is divided by the molarity (M) multiplied by the length $(l$, in centimeters) of solution through which the light travels, the result is the *molar extinction coefficient* (ϵ). When absorbance is plotted against molar concentration, a straight line is obtained, the slope of which depends on ϵ, if there are no intermolecular interactions. In such cases, which correspond to the behavior of most steroids in dilute solution, the absorbance is said to obey Beer's law, and quantitation is easily possible. For most instruments and for steroidal samples with ϵ = 10,000 or greater, one can quantitatively measure 0.1 mg. Absorption is denoted by the symbol λ_{max} for the position of maximal absorption followed by the value of ϵ in parentheses. Some important relationships are;

$$\%T = \frac{I}{I_0}$$

$$A = \text{O.D.} = \log \frac{I_0}{I}$$

$$\epsilon = \frac{A}{M \times l}$$

Two valuable reviews (*4, 34*) of steroidal absorption are available.

b. Unconjugated Carbonyl Group Unconjugated carbonyl groups exhibit a low intensity (ϵ 30-100) maximum in the 280-294-nm range. No important generalizations are possible about the relationship of structure to this absorption despite the availability (*4*) of some detailed information. The low extinction coefficient of this group makes it of very limited value.

c. Unconjugated Double Bonds Woodward (*35*) showed that, as one increases the substitution on a double bond, there is shift in the absorption peak toward longer wavelengths (*bathochromic shift*). This explains the observations of Bladon et al. (*36*) that the intensity of end-absorption depends on the position of a double bond. As the peak is shifted toward longer wavelengths, a greater share of it will appear in the measurable spectrum. Consequently, at a given wavelength the intensity will increase. This is illustrated for actual cases by Table 3.2.

d. Conjugated Double Bonds When two C=C groups are placed adjacent to each other (conjugation), a bathochromic shift occurs. For

Table 3.2. UV absorption by isolated double bonds

Position of Double Bond	Number of Substituents	ϵ at λ (nm)		
		210	215	220
Δ^2	2	200		
Δ^6	2	750	225	100
Δ^{11}	2	900	275	75
Δ^4	3	3,000	1,500	850
Δ^5	3	1,950	780	410
Δ^7	3	4,300	3,100	1,600
$\Delta^{9(11)}$	3	2,650	1,450	500
Δ^{14}	3	2,600	900	200
Δ^8	4	4,470	3,970	3,470
$\Delta^{8(14)}$	4	9,900	8,350	6,100
Δ^9	4	7,450	4,900	2,600

each double bond added the shift amounts to approximately 40 nm. Thus, the $\Delta^{3,5}$-, $\Delta^{4,6}$-, $\Delta^{6,8(14)}$-, $\Delta^{7,9(11)}$-, $\Delta^{8,14}$-, and $\Delta^{16,20}$- systems all yield absorption peaks in the region between 235 and 255 nm, with most appearing near 240 nm. This represents a displacement of about 40 nm from the position of the unconjugated double bonds. If, in addition, two of the double bonds lie in a single ring (*homoannular*) instead of being in different rings (*heteroannular*), a further shift of about 40 nm occurs. The biosynthetically important $\Delta^{5,7}$-system appears, for instance, at 282 nm.

The trienes follow the foregoing rules just as the dienes do. The heteroannular $\Delta^{4,6,8,(14)}$-system absorbs at 283 nm, which is about 40 nm beyond the $\Delta^{4,6}$-system. Similarly, the homoannular $\Delta^{5,7,14}$-triene system is found at 319 nm, which is about 40 nm beyond the position for the $\Delta^{5,7}$-system.

A more precise calculation of the position of absorption comes from Woodward's rules (*35*), which have been extended by Fieser (*37*) and discussed fully by Dorfman (*4*). In brief, one adds to a basic diene value 5 nm for each alkyl substituent, plus 30 nm for each double bond added to the diene system, plus 5 nm for the special case when a double bond is *exocyclic*, i.e., when a double is attached to the outside of a ring as in methylenecyclohexane. The basic values are 214 nm for a heteroannular diene and 253 nm for a homoannular diene. An example is with the $\Delta^{4,6,8(14)}$-system. One adds to 214 nm $4 \times 5 = 20$ nm for the four substituents (C-3, C-10, C-9 and C-13) plus $1 \times 30 = 30$ nm for the third double bond plus $2 \times 5 = 10$ nm for the doubly exocyclic character of the $\Delta^{8(14)}$-bond. The calculated value ($214 + 20 + 30 + 20 = 284$ nm) is within 1 nm of the experimental value (283 nm, ϵ 33,000). Nearly all the known polyene systems are well within 5 nm of the calculated value.

The extinction coefficients for the conjugated dienes generally lie in the 12,000–24,000 range. As double bonds are added ϵ increases. The increase is variable but is of the order of magnitude of 5,000–10,000. Polyene systems in which all the the double bonds are *trans*-oriented about the intervening single bond generally have higher extinction coefficients than do those with *cis*-oriented single bonds. This means, for instance, that heteroannular systems usually have higher extinction coefficients than homoannular ones, as in the cases, respectively, of $\Delta^{4,6}$-systems (ϵ 23,000) and $\Delta^{5,7}$-systems (ϵ 12,000).

   e. Conjugated Carbonyl Groups   The foregoing discussion of the polyene systems applies to the conjugated carbonyl systems (*4*) with but a little modification. The ethylenic band near 200 nm is again shifted bathochromically about 40 nm by conjugation with a carbonyl group, and an additional double bond adds another 40 nm. The Δ^4-3-ketones, for instance, absorb at 241 nm (ϵ 16,600) and the band for $\Delta^{4,6}$-3-ketones is found at 284 nm (ϵ 26,400). The influence of homoannularity and heteroannularity is similar to the polyene situation. Thus, the $\Delta^{3,5}$-7-ketones absorb at 279 nm (ϵ 26,000) while the $\Delta^{1,3}$-6-ketones absorb at 315 nm (ϵ 7,600). However, the precise calculations of the positions of maximal absorption are not quite as simple as for the polyenes themselves, since there is greater variability in the contribution of substituents and in other effects. Dorfman (*4*) has discussed the Fiesers' method of calculation, which assumes an absorption of 215 nm for a basic α, β -unsaturated steroidal ketone to which is added 10–18 nm (depending on its position) for each alkyl substituent, plus 5 nm for each exocyclic double bond, plus 30 nm for each double bond extending the system, plus 38 nm if the system is homoannular. The calculation for the hormonally important Δ^4-3-ketone system is: 215 + 24 + 5 + 0 + 0 = 244 nm, in which an increment of 12 is used for each of the two β-substituents (C-6 and C-10). The substituent (C-2) on the side of the carbonyl group that is away from the ethylenic linkage is never counted. The experimental value is 241 nm.

   Many steroidal α-diketones also show absorption characteristic of ethylenic and carbonyl groups in conjugation. This results from enolization. The peaks usually occur near 270–280 nm.

   The five-membered α,β-unsaturated lactone ring of the cardenolides, e.g., strophanthidin, possesses an absorption peak near 217 nm (ϵ 15,000), while the six-membered α, β, γ, δ-diunsaturated lactone rings of the bufadienolides, e.g., bufotalin, have maximal absorption near 300 (ϵ 6,000).

   f. Benzenoid Systems   The 3-hydroxy benzenoid steroids have absorption typical of similarly substituted derivatives of benzene. They show a strong absorption band near 210 nm and a weaker one near 280 nm. The latter one shows occasional fine structure and in certain cases (*38*) is of diagnostic value. It can be used, for instance, to distinguish steroids with an aromatic ring B from steroids with this ring aromatic but which have a rearranged ring A (*38*). The 3-hydroxy steroids with ring A aromatic have a higher extinction coefficient (ϵ 2,000–7,000) for the band near 280 nm than do those with ring B aromatic (ϵ 400–700). When a double bond extends the conjugation (4, 34, 38) dramatic changes take place in the spectrum. These include a shift in the shortest wavelength maximum to the measurable region near 224 nm with ϵ about 25,000. In addition, a tremendous increase in the extinction coefficient of the longer-wavelength band occurs. The latter is found in this instance near 270 nm with ϵ from 10^3 to 10^4 depending on detailed structural features. Bands also appear in the 300-nm region with ϵ of the order of magnitude of 10^3. The effect of substituents and of introducing aromaticity into other rings has recently been reviewed (34). If rings A and B are both aromatic, typical naphthalenic spectra arise with a very strong band near 230 nm (ϵ 50,000) and a series of characteristic peaks near 270, 280, 290, 330, and 340 nm with extinction coefficients of several thousand.

   g. Fluorescence and Sulfuric Acid Spectra   The spectra of steroids derived from treatment with various reagents frequently are highly specific and can be quantitated. Of these, the formation of fluorescing materials by a variety of techniques has been the best exploited. It has been reviewed by Goldzieher (39). The formation of ultraviolet absorbing chromogens has also been reviewed recently (40). In neither case is the methodology sufficiently well understood theoretically to allow generalizations here. The results depend highly on experimental details that have been established more or less empirically and that vary from laboratory to laboratory. However, they have been of great value in the hormone field. In the case of sapogenins, analysis of their sulfuric acid chromogens (41) constitutes about the only established micro method of identification.

   h. Visible Spectra   Almost no steroids per se have absorption in the visible region. Of the isopentenoids, the best-investigated ones with color are the carotenoids.

3. Infrared Spectroscopy

   a. Fundamental Principles   When electromagnetic radiation with wavelengths in the 2–15-μ region (the infrared region of the spectrum) impinge on a molecule, they can be absorbed. Their energies then excite the atoms to increase in vibrational modes of movement. Only certain frequencies of vibration are allowed, i.e., the system is quantized. Consequently, only certain wavelengths of light are absorbed, and the precise values correspond to precise energies of vibration. These in turn depend on the precise nature of atoms involved, on the kind of electronic bonding, and on the intramolecular environment of the atoms vibrating. There are two major kinds of vibration, stretching and bending:

$$W—X \leftrightarrow Y \qquad\qquad W—X \updownarrow Y$$

Stretching motion of   Bending motion of Y
X relative to Y relative to the W-X axis

These motions are so numerous that they produce an overlapping series of absorption bands in the 7-15-μ region that are nearly unique for a given compound. Hence the name "finger print region" is used. In addition, various peaks of absorption can be associated with particular atomic arrangements.

Instead of wavelength [measured in microns (μ), which are millionths of a meter] its reciprocal is more generally used. This reciprocal is called *wave number* and given the symbol ν. It generally is multiplied by 10^4 and therefore is expressed in cm^{-1}.

The stronger the bonding cement between two atoms, the more energetic (shorter wavelength) is the photon absorbed. This is exemplified by hydrogen bonding. The absorption bands for the H—O bond and for the C=O bond are moved to longer wavelengths when the group is H-bonded. Carboxyl compounds, for instance, can readily dimerize, but the extent of dimerization is concentration dependent. A single absorption peak is found

$$
\begin{array}{c}
\text{O---H---O} \\
R-C \overset{//}{\underset{\backslash\backslash}{}} \quad \overset{\backslash\backslash}{\underset{//}{}} C-R \\
\text{O---H---O}
\end{array}
$$

Carboxyl Dimer

in the 6-μ region for the carbonyl portion of the carboxyl group in either very dilute or very concentrated solutions. However, in the latter case it is at somewhat longer wavelengths (1,710 cm^{-1}) than in the former (1,760 cm^{-1}). At intermediate concentrations, both peaks are found corresponding to the dimeric and monomeric forms, respectively.

Infrared spectroscopy has been studied extensively. A general discussion of the method is to be found in the book by Nakanishi (*42*), and specific application to steroids has been discussed by Fieser and Fieser (*43*). A large catalog of steroidal spectra has been collected by Jones and his associates (*44*) and by Neudert and Röpke (*45*). Some examples of the more useful correlations are discussed in what follows.

b. O—H and C—H Stretching Absorption   The H—O stretching frequency is to be found near 3,630 cm^{-1}, and a band in this region is diagnostic for the presence of alcoholic hydroxyl groups. Phenolic hydroxyl groups tend to appear closer to 3,610 cm^{-1}. With hydrogen bonding, broadening of the band frequently occurs with a shift to the 3,500-3,600-cm^{-1} region. In the 2,900-cm^{-1} region the absorption for C-H stretching vibrations occurs. This is very strong in steroids, because of the numerous C-H bonds. In fact, a large ratio for the intensities of the C-H stretching to O-H stretching frequencies is a strong suggestion of steroidal or at least of polyisopentenoidal character. Very few other natural products exhibit this kind of ratio.

c. C=O Stretching Absorption   Carbonyl groups absorb near 1,700 cm^{-1} with an intensity similar to the intensity of the C-H stretching band of sterols. The exact position of the band depends on the environment of the carbonyl group and is exceedingly important diagnostically. Keto groups in the side chain and in six-membered B-, C-, and D-rings absorb near 1,710 cm^{-1}. The band is shifted to shorter wavelengths (1,745 cm^{-1}) because of ring strain in the five-membered D-ring. Thus, 17-ketosteroids are easily distinguished from steroids with keto groups either in the side chain or other rings. The carbonyl group of esters also appears at the shorter wavelengths (1,745 cm^{-1}) but is distinguishable from 17-ketones by the presence of C-O-C stretching vibrations that appear strongly near 1,240 cm^{-1}. As already mentioned, the carbonyl of carboxylic acids is distinguishable by two bands, the intensities of which are strongly concentration dependent; this dependence is much stronger than is the case for H-bonding of other carbonyls, which usually do not dimerize. The carbonyl group of aldehydes appears at 1,725 cm^{-1}, and the CHO grouping is readily identified by its C-H stretching frequency at 2,820 cm^{-1}. Very few other groups absorb at this latter frequency. The most widely known aldehydic steroid, aldosterone, however, does not show such absorption, because of internal hemiacetal formation.

The intramolecular ester (lactone) system of the cardenolides bearing the α,β-unsaturation exhibits a carbonyl peak near 1,750 cm^{-1} with a subsidiary peak near 1,785 cm^{-1}. The six-membered doubly unsaturated lactone system of the bufadienolides absorbs near 1,740 cm^{-1}, sometimes as a doublet.

Conjugation of carbonyl groups with an ethylenic bond, e.g., the Δ^4-3-ketone, usually shifts the peak to a longer wavelength (1,679 cm^{-1}).

d. C=C Stretching Absorption   The carbon-carbon double bond absorbs in the 1,650-cm^{-1} region, but not strongly. The influence of structure on this absorption is also not very great. For these reasons the region has not been exploited much in the steroid field. The bending vibrations generally are diagnostically more useful (see next section). The presence of absorption in this region is perhaps most helpful in ascertaining whether or not a carbonyl group is conjugated, e.g., a band at 1,617 cm^{-1} for Δ^4-3-ketones, but this can be determined more precisely by ultraviolet spectroscopy. Aromatic systems show typical absorption in the 1,600-cm^{-1} region and they have been studied carefully (*38, 44*). The steroidal benzenoid phenols show a peak at 1,610 cm^{-1}, often with a subsidiary maxima near 1,590 cm^{-1}. The naphthalenic and aromatic ring B steroids are similar to this but different in detail (*38*).

e. C—H Bending Absorption   Many steroids differ only in the number and position of double bonds. The C—H bending vibration can be of great value in obtaining structural information.

A very common double bond occurs at the 22-position. In most natural cases it is *trans*-oriented and shows a very strong band near 967 cm^{-1}. This so-called "out-of-plane" vibration originating from the 22-H and the 23-H vibrating in opposite directions is characteristic (*42*) of 1,2-disubstituted, *trans*-oriented carbon-carbon double bonds and is not exhibited by the *cis*-isomers. In the usual spectrum of steroids with and without the Δ^{22} bond, e.g., stigmasterol versus sitosterol, the band at 967 cm^{-1} is the only observable spectroscopic difference. A similar vibration (the two H atoms vibrating in opposite directions) is exhibited by the biosynthetically important CH$_2$ group, found, for instance, in 24-methylenecholesterol, but it appears at 890 cm^{-1}. It is of moderate intensity and easily distinguished. Generally, nothing else absorbs as strongly at that frequency.

The bending vibrations of the trisubstituted double bonds appear in the 790–850-cm^{-1} range. They generally are much weaker than the bending vibrations for the disubstituted cases already described and consequently are subject to overlap with other absorptions. However, when used carefully they are of important diagnostic value. Among the more useful correlations is a very distinct doublet of moderate intensity near 805 and 840 cm^{-1} found in the biosynthetically important $\Delta^{5,7}$-compounds. The peak at 840 cm^{-1} is the stronger. The Δ^{5}- and Δ^{7}-compounds containing only one of these double bonds yield triplets in the same region. In the Δ^{5} case, two peaks of nearly the same intensity are found at 802 and 845 cm^{-1} with a very weak peak in between at 830 cm^{-1}. With Δ^{7}-compounds the middle peak (830 cm^{-1}) is stronger and becomes nearly as intense as the one at 845 cm^{-1}, and the longest wavelength maximum is shifted to 795 cm^{-1}. The $\Delta^{24(25)}$-bond exhibits a peak at 822 cm^{-1} with a much weaker subsidiary one at 805 cm^{-1}. The pattern remains essentially the same for 24-deuterocompounds. In the $\Delta^{5,24(25)}$-diene, the maximum at 822 cm^{-1} becomes superimposed on the Δ^{5}-triplet to give a very characteristic multiplet that reverts to the Δ^{5}-type in the Δ^{5}-24-ketone. The introduction of a trisubstituted *cis*-$\Delta^{24(28)}$-bond (for instance, by a 24-ethylidene group) into Δ^{5}-steroids yields an effect similar to introduction of a $\Delta^{24(28)}$-bond in that marked absorption appears between the peaks at 802 and 845 cm^{-1}. The new band (825 cm^{-1}) becomes the strongest and in this way is distinguishable from the $\Delta^{5,24(25)}$-steroids in which it is of slightly less intensity compared to the other two. In the *trans*-$\Delta^{5,24(28)}$-compounds the middle peak is shifted to 812 cm^{-1} but remains dominant.

Since the tetrasubstituted ethylenic linkage fails to have attached hydrogen atoms, such bonds ($\Delta^{8(9)}$, $\Delta^{8(14)}$, etc.) do not possess significant absorption in the 800–850-cm^{-1} region.

f. C—O Stretching Absorption   The C—O stretching vibration appears in the 1,000–1,100-cm^{-1} region as a strong band. It is diagnostic for the presence of the hydroxyl group and its derivatives. Changes of various sorts in rings A and B produce subtle differences in the exact character of this absorption. In the Δ^{5}-3β-alcohols, for instance, a broad single peak is usually obtained at 1,040–1,050 cm^{-1}, but in the $\Delta^{5,7}$-3β-alcohols the band is split into two distinct peaks separated by 25 cm^{-1}. In the Δ^7-3β-alcohols it tends to be split with a smaller separation factor and displaced closer to 1,033 cm^{-1}. The effect of the double bond is presumably mediated in a conformational way. It has been shown that equatorial hydroxyl groups of steroids lacking a 4,4-dimethyl group absorb about 40 cm^{-1} toward larger frequencies than do the axial substituents (46). The situation is reversed if the 4,4-dimethyl group is present (47). An analogous effect is found in the C—O—C stretching absorption of acetate esters at 1,240 cm^{-1}. The equatorial acetoxy group gives rise to a singlet, while the axial groups yield a multiplet (46).

4. Nuclear Magnetic Resonance Spectroscopy

a. *Fundamental Principles* The nucleus of a hydrogen atom (the proton) has, in addition to vibratory motion associated with infrared spectra, a rotational motion or spin around an axis. Being a charged body in motion, it can interact with an applied magnetic field. This interaction is related to the precession of the axis of rotation around the north-south axis at the field. Protons that have a spin quantum number of 1/2 are allowed to orient their own magnetic fields either with or against the external field. If a proton is placed in an external field and an oscillating force with a frequency equivalent to the angular momentum of precession is applied from an alternating current, the proton undergoes transitions between the two orientations. The precise frequency producing this effect is the *resonance frequency*. All protons would yield the same results if they could interact similarly with the applied field. However, because of differing electronic environments, the proton is shielded to greater or lesser extents from the applied field. The variations in the shielding result in altered positions of absorption (*chemical shift*) and can be measured. They allow deductions to be made about the electronic environment and therefore about the position of a proton in the steroidal molecule.

The angular momentum (ω), applied magnetic field (H_o), and irradiation frequency (ν) are related as shown in the accompanying equation where γ and σ are, respectively, a constant (the *magnetogyric ratio* of the nucleus) and the *screening parameter:*

$$\nu = \frac{\omega}{2\pi} = \frac{\gamma H_o (1-\sigma)}{2\pi}$$

The screening parameter depends on the environment of the proton and is in essence what one measures. In practice, one places the substance under the influence of a given alternating current with a frequency usually of 60, 100, or 220 megacycles per second and then varies the magnetic field. Since the frequency and field strength are interrelated it will be found that, at certain values for the field strength, energy is absorbed corresponding to the excitation (*resonance*) of the proton. The experimental values are usually now given as displacements of the field strength in parts per million (δ) from the value at which tetramethylsilane absorbs. This is expressed more precisely by

$$\delta \text{ in ppm} = \frac{H_{\text{TMS}} - H}{H_{\text{TMS}}} \times 10^6$$

where H_{TMS} is the value for the 12 equivalent hydrogens in tetramethylsilane and H the value for the proton(s) in question. The results are also sometimes expressed in cycles per second (cps). These are obtained by multiplying ppm by the operating frequency in megacycles, i.e., by 60, 100, 220, etc. The terms "downfield" or "lower field" strength refer to larger δ values.

As a first approximation, the absorption peak will be a singlet only if there are no hydrogen atoms adjacent to the carbon atom to which the proton in question is attached. If there is one adjacent, a doublet is produced; if two, a triplet, etc.; i.e., the number of peaks in an absorption band equals $n + 1$ where n is the number of adjacent hydrogen atoms. The multiplet position is given as the center of the whole band. The distance between peaks in a given multiplet is usually expressed in c.p.s. and is called the *coupling constant* (J). The intensity (area under the band) of absorption is directly related to the number of absorbing protons. Hence, important quantitative information on the number of a given type of proton in a molecule can be obtained. In principle, therefore, the method could also be used to determine the number of molecules, but because of the rather large amounts of material necessary (5-50 mg) the method is usually not of practical use in this way.

There are several important types of information about steroids obtained from nuclear magnetic resonance spectroscopy. To start with, strong singlets are obtained from the angular methyl groups, the 4,4-dimethyl group, and the 14α-methyl group, since there are no adjacent hydrogen atoms; a series of doublets arise from C-21, C-26, C-27, and C-28 (when present as a methyl group); and a triplet is seen from C-29. There is no other method that so elegantly shows the presence and environmental characteristics of these groups. Similarly, methyl groups attached to carbon atoms bearing π-electrons (C=C or C=O) or to atoms with lone electrons, notably oxygen as in the methoxyl group, give rise to such a chemical shift that they are easily distinguished. Hydrogen atoms directly on double bonds also show distinctive chemical shifts, as do hydrogen atoms attached to carbon-bearing hydroxyl groups. Of special importance are the cases in which the multiplicity of the absorption band is small, because the peak height is then large and the group responsible for it is readily apparent. In steroids the multiplicity for most of the hydrogen atoms on saturated carbons is actually large, and only a few major and unequivocal peaks are observed above the general absorption. It is these peaks that are useful and are discussed in what follows. Our understanding of them stems from work

by Shoolery and Rogers (*48*) and of Bishop, Cox, and Richards (*49*). Neudert and Röpke (*45*) and especially Bhacca and Williams (*50*) have collected and reviewed most of the data on the subject that have accumulated
in the meantime. Smith (*51*a) has reported a great deal of data on hormonal
and other highly oxygenated steroids.

b. Methyl Groups From the work of Shoolery and others, information on several hundred steroids has been obtained with reference to the
methyl groups. Of particular interest are C-18 and C-19. Not only are they
clearly discernible, but the exact position of absorption depends greatly
on a number of other structural features. The stereochemistry of the skeleton paricularly influences the peaks. For instance, in the *trans-anti-trans-
anti-trans* system ($5\alpha,14\alpha$-androstane) the C-19 protons appear at 0.792
ppm, while in the C-5 epimer they appear at 0.925 ppm. The C-18 protons,
appearing at 0.692 ppm., are unchanged. There is essentially no effect
on the C-19 protons if one inverts C-14, but the latter inversion produces
a large effect on the C-18 protons, which are found in $5\alpha,14\beta$-androstane
at 0.992 ppm. Similarly, introduction of a Δ^5-bond or a 3-keto group influences the absorption of the C-19 protons but not that of the C-18 protons. These and other correlations are apparent from the data of Tables
3.3 to 3.5. It will be seen that *the shifts produced by various structural features are essentially additive,* which is of great value in structural elucidation when carefully used.

It should be evident from the tabular information that there are two
kinds of structural information one can get, i.e., *direct information* that
a group is present and *indirect information* from the chemical shift about
its environment. Thus, the presence of a strong singlet near 2.14 ppm
not only directly proves the presence of a methyl group, but it also indirectly shows that adjacent to it is a carbonyl function. Since in non-acety-
lated steroids the $CO\text{-}CH_3$ grouping is almost entirely limited to C-20 and
C-21, respectively, the absorption can be used still more precisely to identify
the nature of both of these atoms. The values for the methyl groups in a
variety of natural sterols have recently been determined at 220 MHz (*51*b, c).
Among the more important aspects of the measurements is that it pro-
vides detailed information which allows discrimination of Δ^0-, Δ^5-, Δ^7-, and
$\Delta^{5,7}$-sterols from each other as well as determination of the size and configuration of substituents at C-24. For instance, with regard to the latter,
24β-alkyl groups move the signal from C-21 downfield by 0.01 ppm compared to the 24α-epimers. The experimental values for progesterone and
cholesterol are identified in Scheme 3.10. They agree well with the values
expected from the information in Table 3.3.

c. Protons on Double Bonds When a proton is attached to a double
bond a strong shift downfield occurs, and they are usually found in the
5–6-ppm region. The exact position, multiplicity, and *J* value depend
heavily not only on the number of adjacent protons but also on the stereo-

Table 3.3. Effect of changes in steroid structure on PMR spectra

Steroid	C-18 δ (ppm)	C-19 δ (ppm)
5α-Cholestane	0.64	0.78
5α-Cholestanol	0.67	0.82
5α-Androstane	0.692	0.792
5β-Androstane	0.692	0.925
12-Ketocholanic Acid Acetate	1.01	1.01
Cortisone	0.66	0.40
3-Ketones	0.042	0.242
Δ⁴-3-Ketones	0.075	0.417

Grouping	Downfield Shift (ppm) from 5α-Sterol	
5β-H	0.00	0.13
Δ⁴	0.04	0.25
Δ⁵	0.04	0.23
Δ⁵,⁷	−0.06	0.17
Δ⁷	−0.15	0.02
Δ⁸	−0.01	0.21
3-Keto	0.04	0.24
11-Keto	−0.03	0.22
12-Keto	0.38	0.10
Δ⁴-3-Keto	0.08	0.42
3β-OH	0.02	0.03
Δ⁵-3β-OH	0.00	0.23
3α-OH	0.01	0.00
3β-OAc	0.01	0.05

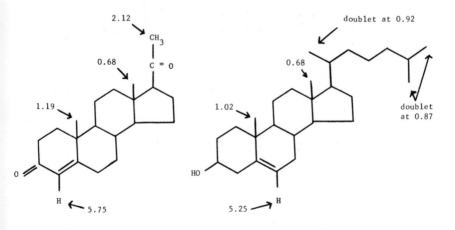

Progesterone   Cholesterol

Scheme 3.10. NMR absorption of various protons (in ppm).

Table 3.4. PMR spectra of common sterols[a]

Side Chain Character at C-24 and C-22	Chemical Shift in ppm from TMS at 220 MHz for Δ^5- and (Δ^7)-sterols								
	H	α-CH$_3$	β-CH$_3$	α-C$_2$H$_5$	β-C$_2$H$_5$	α-CH$_3$-Δ^{22}	β-CH$_3$-Δ^{22}	α-C$_2$H$_5$-Δ^{22}	β-C$_2$H$_5$-Δ^{22}
Proton Position									
C-18	0.68 (0.53)	0.68	0.68 (0.54)	0.68 (0.54)	0.68 (0.54)	0.69	0.70 (0.54)	0.70 (0.55)	0.70 (0.55)
C-19	1.01 (0.80)	1.01	1.01 (0.80)	1.01 (0.80)	1.01	1.02	1.01 (0.80)	1.01 (0.80)	1.01 (0.80)
C-21	0.91 (0.92)	0.91	0.92 (0.91)	0.92 (0.93)	0.93 (0.93)	1.00	1.01 (1.01)	1.02 (1.02)	1.03 (1.03)
C-26,27	0.87 (0.86) (0.87)	0.77 0.85	0.77 (0.77) 0.86 (0.85)	0.81 (0.82) 0.84 (0.84)	0.81 (0.82) 0.83 (0.84)	0.82 0.83	0.82 (0.82) 0.83 (0.83)	0.80 (0.80) 0.85 (0.85)	0.79 (0.79) 0.85 (0.85)
C-28	—	0.80	0.78 (0.78)	—	—	0.91	0.91 (0.91)	—	—
C-29	—	—	—	0.85 (0.85)	0.86 (0.86)	—	—	0.80 (0.80)	0.81 (0.82)

[a] Adapted from Ref. 51b, c, and d. Values have been rounded to nearest hundredth.

Table 3.5.   PMR absorption of various steroidal methyl protons

Group	Multiplicity	Coupling Constant, (cps)	Absorption Band (ppm)
C-18($5\alpha,14\alpha$)	1	0	0.69
C-19($5\alpha,14\alpha$)	1	0	0.79
C-21 protons	2	6-7	0.93
C-26 protons	2	6-7	0.88
C-27 protons	2	6-7	0.88
C-28 protons	2	6-7	0.78
C-21 protons in 20-ketones	1	0	2.14
N—CH$_3$	1	0	2.25
O—CH$_3$	1	0	3.36
$\overset{\overset{\text{O}}{\|\|}}{\text{C-OCH}_3}$	1	0	3.66
$\overset{\overset{\text{O}}{\|\|}}{\text{CH}_3\text{-C-O}}$	1	0	2.05
6α-CH$_3$ (Δ^4-3-Keto)	2	7	1.08
6β-CH$_3$ (Δ^4-3-Keto)	2	7	1.26
=CH-CH$_3$ (C-28,C-29)	2	7	1.57
=C-(CH$_3$)$_2$ (C-25,C-26,C-27)	1	0	1.60
CH$_3$ on C-14	1	0	0.88
CH$_3$ on C-4	1	0	0.88
CH$_2$-CH$_3$(C-28,C-29)	3	8-9	0.85

chemical relationship between them. In addition, in many cases *both* protons on the two olefinic carbon atoms may couple with an adjacent proton. Thus, in Δ^{11}-steroids the C-11 and C-12 protons are themselves coupled yielding two doublets at 5.55 and 6.22 ppm with J values of 10 cps each, but the two peaks in each doublet are further split into two with J values of 2–3 cps by coupling with the adjacent proton (on C-9). This phenomenon of coupling with protons on the allylic carbon atom is known as *allylic coupling*. On the other hand, the C-16 and C-17 protons of Δ^{16}-steroids lacking a substituent at C-17 are coupled such that a doublet appears at 6.16 ppm with $J = 5.5$ cps and no further splitting occurs (no allylic coupling). Both the splitting and the J value are stereochemically determined. As a first approximation, *as the value of the angle between two protons increases from 90° to 180° or decreases from 90° to 0°, the larger is the value of J*. At 0° or 180° J is found to be 9–16 cps, while at 60° J is only 1–7 cps. This means that, for instance, diaxial coupling or coupling of the two protons on ethylenic carbon atoms in a six-membered ring will yield the larger values, while equatorial coupling or coupling of the protons on a double bond in a five-membered ring will result in the lower J values. See Karplus (52) for a more detailed discussion.

Allylic coupling often perturbs the absorption without yielding a clear multiplet. This is found for the proton on C-4 of Δ^4-3-ketones, which is neither a clear singlet, as the simple $n + 1$ rule would predict, nor is it a well-resolved multiplet, but rather a broad band (centered at 5.7 ppm) with an inflection. Allylic coupling to the 6β-H causes this effect. The proton at C-5 in Δ^5-steroids also gives rise to a very poorly resolved multiplet centered at 5.3 ppm, but the proton on C-28 of steroids bearing a *trans*-ethylidene group at C-24, e.g., isofucosterol, shows a very clearly resolved quartet as predicted by the $n + 1$ rule. Although it is separated well from the Δ^5-band in the *trans*-case, in the *cis*-isomer the Δ^5- and $\Delta^{24(28)}$-absorptions overlap.

d. Protons on Carbon Atoms Bearing a Hydroxyl Group   Protons on carbon atoms bearing hydroxyl groups give rise to absorption in the 3.5–4.5-ppm region. The 17α-proton of 17β-hydroxy steroids appears as a well resolved triplet with $J = 8$ cps at 3.67 ppm. The 3α-proton exhibits a broad band near 3.5 ppm. When inversion occurs either at C-3 or at C-5, the absorption is shifted downfield to the 4-5 ppm region. The 12β-proton is found at 5.2 ppm.

e. Configuration and Conformation at C-20   As a result of changing the environment of C-21, inversion of C-20 produces an upfield shift of 0.10 ppm in the signal from C-21, as is discussed in some detail in Chapter 2.

5. Mass Spectroscopy

a. Fundamental Principles   In mass spectroscopy a sample is vaporized, usually at elevated temperature in a vacuum, and bombarded with electrons. Positively charged ions are produced which are accelerated toward the negative pole of an electrostatic field. The ions are thereby focused into a beam which then passes perpendicularly through a magnetic field. The path that any given ion follows through the magnetic field depends on its momentum and charge, which can be expressed as its velocity and the ratio of its mass to charge (m/e). If a collector is placed so that the point of impact of the ions can be measured, it will be found that the greater the value of m/e the smaller the deflection of the ion from the center of the original beam. Since most of the ions will have a charge of one, the deflection becomes a measure of mass. This method in turn becomes a way of measuring molecular weight, if, as is true in most cases, a measurable percentage of the molecules lose just one electron and the resultant *molecular ion* has a period of existence sufficiently long to be accelerated through the electrostatic and magnetic fields and be collected.

The half-life of the molecular ion is obviously a function of its structure. Consequently, the percentage of molecules which are not further changed is immediately of interpretive value. For instance, the molecular ion of cholesterol is much more stable than that of its acetate, which loses acetic acid much more readily than the free alcohol loses water. Thus, the intensity of the response from the molecular ion of cholesterol is relatively greater than that from cholesteryl acetate. Moreover, the fragment formed after removal of acetic acid or water will retain a charge and appear on the final collecting device. This means that cholesteryl acetate will give two ionic responses, the molecular ion (M) *and* the deacetylated fragment (M-60, where 60 is the molecular weight of acetic acid). Cholesterol will result in its own molecular ion but will also yield an M-18 fragment identical with the M-60 one from the acetate. The relative intensities, however, of the molecular ion responses and the fragment responses will be markedly different in the two cases. Much more deep-seated eliminations and/or rearrangements followed by eliminations can and do take place, all highly dependent on the original structure. Many of them can be correlated with distinct structural features, and the complete pattern is much like the "finger print" produced in the infrared, although the mass spectrum tends to be even more characteristic. There are consequently three major values to mass spectroscopy: (1) determination of molecular weight, (2) empirical identification with a standard, and (3) elucidation of structural features.

While it is not used widely in steroid biochemistry, a fourth application can sometimes be of importance. This is the determination of empirical formulas by "high-resolution" techniques. By this is implied the ability to detect much less than integral values of a mass unit. Most mass spectroscopists adhere to the IUPAC scale in which the mass of ^{12}C is taken as 12.0000 and other atomic weights are then related to it. Oxygen becomes 15.9949, hydrogen 1.0078, and nitrogen 14.0031. Combinations of these numbers give different precise values even when the nominal value is an integer. Consider $M = 28$. It might represent either CO ($M = 27.9949$) or H_2CN ($M = 28.0187$), and by measuring the exact mass with a high-resolution spectrometer a discrimination is possible.

Our general knowledge of the fragmentation processes has been greatly enhanced by McLafferty and others, and in the steroid and related fields the work of Djerassi, who has coauthored excellent books on the subject (*53, 54*), has been especially important. High-resolution mass spectroscopy was pioneered independently by Beynon and by Biemann. Several reviews are available (e.g., *54, 55*). Material for the calculation of empirical formulas has been brought together in tabular form by Lederberg (56).

   b. Process of Fragmentation   The molecular ion is generally formed by extraction of an electron from an oxygen (or nitrogen, if present) rather than a carbon atom. There then ensue electronic shifts. The molecular ion has an odd number of electrons (a *radical ion*) and is denoted by a positive sign and a dot. When a single electron shifts, it is symbolized by a "fishhook" (⇀) instead of an "arrow" (→), which is reserved for shifts of an electronic pair. These points are simply illustrated by the fragmentation of the ethylene ketal of androstan-3-one shown in Scheme 3.11. The ketal

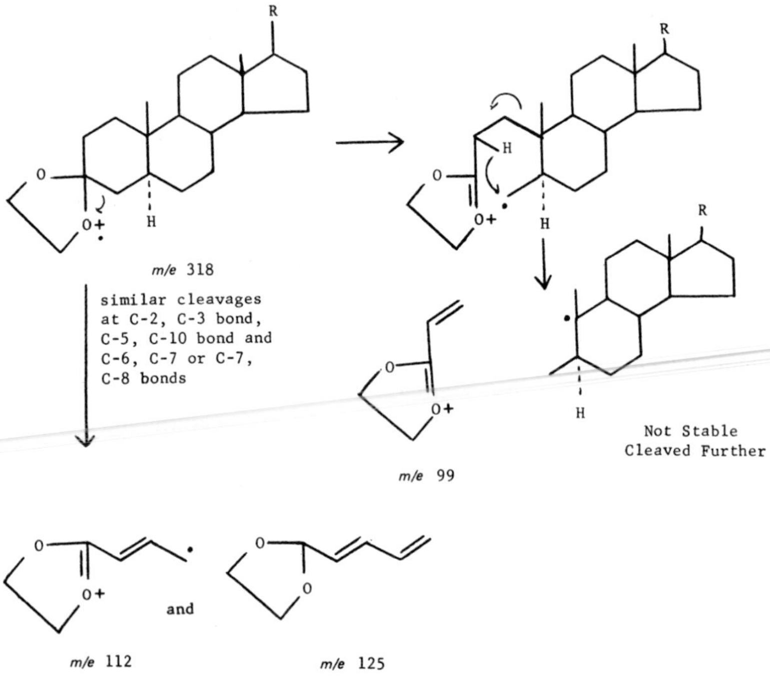

m/e 318

similar cleavages
at C-2, C-3 bond,
C-5, C-10 bond and
C-6, C-7 or C-7,
C-8 bonds

m/e 99

Not Stable
Cleaved Further

m/e 112   m/e 125

Scheme 3.11. Principal fragmentations of ethylene ketals at C-3, illustrating one-electron movements during mass spectral fragmentation.

exhibits a weak peak for the molecular ion at m/e 318 and two strong peaks at m/e 99 and 125. The latter two represent elimination, respectively, of the ketal ring with C-3, C-2, and C-1 and the ketal ring with C-3, C-4, C-5, C-6, and C-7. A fragment (m/e 112) containing the ketal ring with C-3, C-4, C-5, and C-6 also appears in the spectrum. The peak at m/e 99 is the dominant one in all saturated or Δ^5-containing 3-ethylene ketals studied demonstrating the importance of the charged oxygen atom. This is also illustrated by elimination of H_2O or HOAc from alcohols and acetates. That the removal of 18 or 60 mass units is indeed due to H_2O and HOAc, respectively, has been shown by deuterium labeling. When the 2,2,4,4-tetradeutero compound is examined, CH_3—COOD is eliminated and the peak is observed at M-61 (Scheme 3.12). By the use of labeling experiments of this kind, Djerassi has been able to elucidate the process of fragmentation in many more complicated cases (54).

c. *Sterols*   Sterols have been examined by several workers (54, 56–63) who have shown that there are important characteristics of the group as well as of the individual members. Some of the most important fragmentations are shown in Scheme 3.13. They include dehydration or its equivalent (M—H_2O, M—HOAc, etc.), loss of the side chain (M-SC), and in many

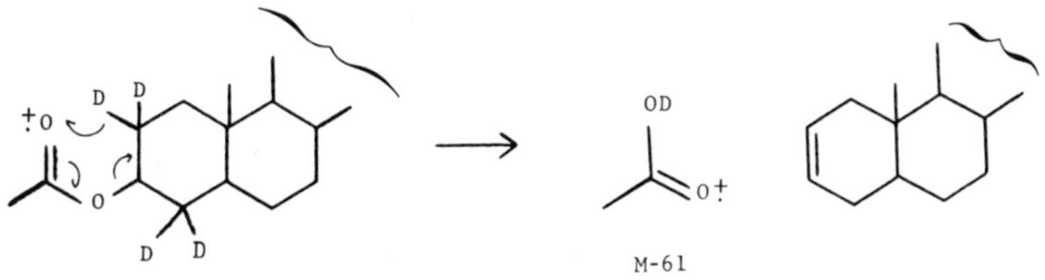

Scheme 3.12. Fragmentation of deuterosteryl acetate, demonstrating loss of acetic acid.

cases loss of the side chain plus C-15, C-16, and C-17 together with their hydrogen atoms plus one more (M-SC-42). The latter fragmentation is quite complex (60). In addition, combinations of these fragmentations occur. In the absence of a double bond in rings A or B, the dehydrated fragment (or its equivalent) undergoes a retro-Diels-Alder reaction with the elimination of C-1, C-2, C-3, and C-4 as butadiene (m/e 54) yielding an M-ROH-54 fragment. When a Δ^5-bond is present, dehydration apparently yields a $\Delta^{3,5}$-diene in which the elimination of butadiene is no longer chemically feasible. Evidence for this is that the spectrum of $\Delta^{3,5}$-cholestadiene is the same as that of cholesteryl acetate.

The fragmentations which yield ions retaining C-4 and C-14 (M-SC, M-SC-42, etc.) are of immense value in diagnosing the presence or absence of methyl groups at this position. Thus, while the M-HOAc-SC-42 fragment of Δ^7-cholestenyl acetate appears at m/e 213, it is found at 227 for the 4-methyl derivative and at 241 in the 4,4-dimethyl derivative (61). The latter two peaks are 14 and 28 mass units higher corresponding to the inclusion of the equivalent of one and two CH_2-groups in the fragment.

The character of the side chain can also be inferred in several cases (Scheme 3.14). The saturated cholesteryl-type side chain loses the terminal isopropyl group (m/e 43), which is stable enough to appear as a strong peak. Similarly, Δ^{24}-compounds yield an isoprene peak at m/e 69 by an allylic extension of the isopropyl loss. 24-Ethylidene compounds also lose C-23, C-24, C-25, C-26, C-27, C-28, and C-29 plus one hydrogen atom (m/e 98) by an allylic cleavage at the C-22, C-23 bond, but in this case further fragmentation occurs and the peak at m/e 98 is not prominent. However, the M-98 peak is very strong. In a similar fashion, allylic cleavage of the side chain of Δ^{22}-sterols occurs at the C-17, C-20 bond, yielding an unusually intense peak for M-SC with or without dehydration or its equivalent (59, 64).

The relative proportion of the various fragmentations depends on a number of factors. One of them is the temperature of the sterol at the place where it is introduced into the mass spectrometer (the *inlet temperature*). Dehydration and loss of acetic acid, for instance, are quite sensitive to this temperature, so that it is not easy to make exact comparisons from one

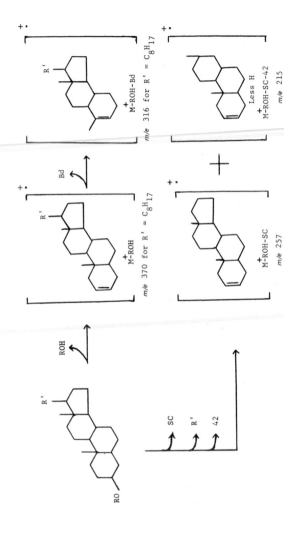

Scheme 3.13. Fragmentation of stanols. Bd, butadiene from C-1, C-2, C-3, and C-4. SC, side chain. The loss of 42 mass units is principally from C-15, C-16, and C-17. When R = H, fragments as shown also are found with HOH except for the one, M-ROH-Bd, which is sequential from the M-ROH fragment.

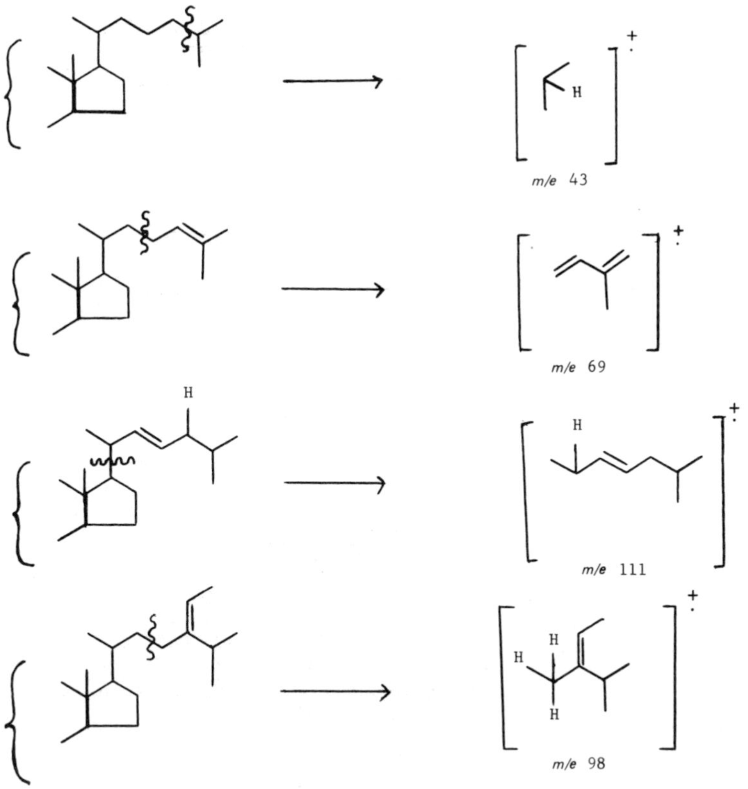

Scheme 3.14. Fragmentations of the side chain.

laboratory to another. However, when the temperature and other instrumental factors are kept constant, it is found that significant differences in the spectra arise from small changes in the sterol structure. Thus, it has been reported (61) that the parent molecular ion (M) is found in much greater proportion in Δ^7- than in Δ^5- or $\Delta^{5,7}$-steroids. Presumably, this results from the lack of stabilization of the (dehydrated) diene by conjugation in the Δ^7-case. In Table 3.6 is a list of the major peaks for the common Δ^5- and Δ^7-sterols. Of the nuclear double bonds the system which is most distinctive is $\Delta^{5,7}$-unsaturation (61). Such dienes show two strong peaks at m/e 143 and 158, probably corresponding to fragments containing rings A and B as shown in Scheme 3.15. They differ by 15 mass units, presumably representing C-19. Δ^5-Sterols are believed (61) to be characterized by peaks at m/e 120, 245, and 247, and Δ^7-sterols by peaks at m/e 94, 108, and 122. As a key to a much more detailed analysis of fragmentations the literature (51d,e, 59, 60, and 63) should be consulted.

d. *Hormones*   Estrogen spectra are dominated by cleavages derived

Table 3.6. Mass spectra of Δ^5 and Δ^7-sterols

| | | Cholesterol Series | | | | Lathosterol Series | |
Side Chain	24-H	24-CH_3	24-C_2H_5	24-C_2H_5-Δ^{22}	24-H	24-C_2H_5	24-C_2H_5-Δ^{22}
Fragmentation							
M^+	386 (100)	400 (100)	414 (100)	412 (66)	386 (100	414 (100)	412 (28)
M^+—CH_3	371 (32)	385 (29)	399 (29)	397 (9)	371 (29)	399 (26)	397 (10)
M^+—H_2O	368 (47)	382 (42)	396 (44)	394 (11)	368 (2)	369 (2)	394 (1)
M^+—CH_3—H_2O	353 (33)	367 (30)	381 (28)	379 (13)	353 (5)	381 (4)	379 (1)
M^+—C_3H_7	—	—	—	369 (22)	—	—	369, (13)
M^+—85	301 (43)	315 (41)	329 (39)	327 (5)	—	—	—
M^+—$C_7H_{11 \text{ or } 12}$	275 (56)	289 (47)	303 (44)	300 (42)	—	—	—
M^+—(SC = Side Chain)	273 (26)	273 (24)	273 (25)	273 (23)	273 (21)	273 (21)	273 (31)
M^+—SC—2H	271 (15)	271 (2)	271 (2)	271 (59)	—	—	271 (100)
M^+—SC—H_2O	255 (36)	255 (29)	255 (28)	255 (100)	255 (75)	255 (67)	255 (40)
M^+—SC—H_2O—2H	253 (6)	253 (1)	—	—	—	—	—
M^+—SC—C_3H_6	231 (30)	231 (27)	231 (24)	231 (18)	231 (31)	231 (25)	231 (18)
M^+—SC—C_3H_8	229 (18)	229 (12)	229 (11)	229 (21)	229 (24)	229 (20)	229 (21)
M^+—SC—C_3H_6—H_2O	213 (43)	213 (39)	213 (39)	213 (45)	213 (33)	213 (24)	213 (20)
M^+—SC—C_3H_8—H_2O	211 (9)	211 (2)	211 (1)	—	211 (2)	211 (1)	211 (3)

m/e (%)

Adapted from Nes et al. (51d).

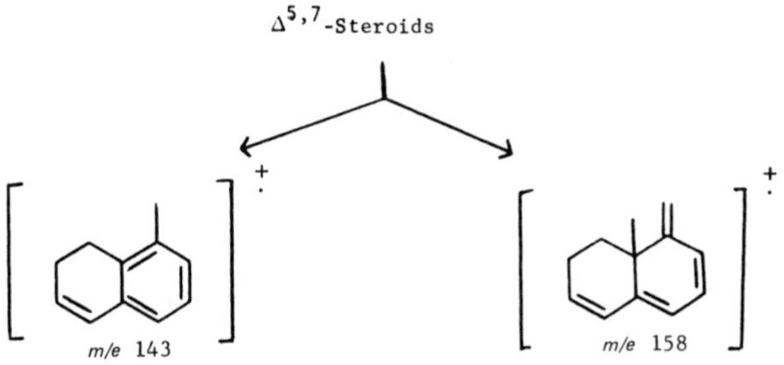

$\Delta^{5,7}$-Steroids

Scheme 3.15. Fragmentation of $\Delta^{5,7}$-sterols.

from elimination of an electron from the benzenoid ring and, if present, oxygen atoms in rings other than ring A, as shown in Scheme 3.16.

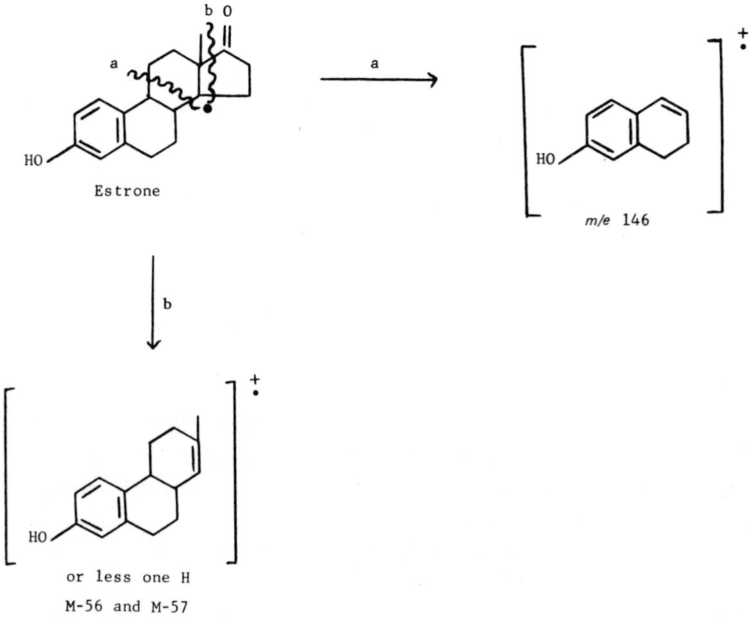

Scheme 3.16. Fragmentation of estrogens.

The nonaromatic hormones and their relatives being highly oxygenated undergo extensive H migrations, dehydrations, and rearrangements. This leads to very unique spectra for identification but also makes group analysis difficult. However, the α,β-unsaturated system present in the hormones themselves does have a characteristic fragmentation (Scheme 3.17). The largest peak greater than m/e 100 usually is derived from a cleavage

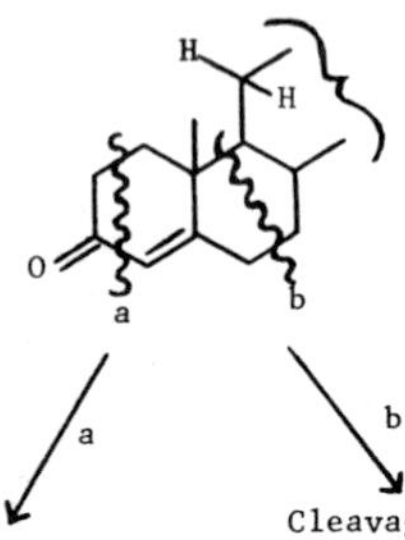

Loss of C_2H_2O
yielding M-42

Cleavage yielding
Rings A and B, C-19, and C-6
plus two H-atoms with *m/e* 124

Scheme 3.17. Fragmentation of Δ^4-3-ketones.

allylic to the Δ^4-bond producing an ion containing ring A, C-19 and C-6 plus two hydrogen atoms. The H-transfer occurs from C-8 and C-11, and, when C-11 is ketonic preventing the transfer, the fragment appears at two mass units lower. Δ^4-Cholestenone, progesterone, and testosterone all show a peak at *m/e* 124, while in cortisone and Δ^4-androsten-3,11-dione the peak is shifted to *m/e* 122. In the 19-nor-series the peak is 14 mass units lower as expected. The next largest peak results from elimination of C-2 and C-3 with the attached oxygen atom yielding an M-42 fragment.

e. Bile Acids In the spectra of the acetates of the bile acid methyl esters, the principal peaks result from loss of HOAc and the side chain in various combinations. The methyl ester of cholic acid triacetate, for instance, shows strong peaks in decreasing order at *m/e* 253, 368, and 313 corresponding to M-SC-3HOAc, M-3HOAc, and M-SC-2HOAc.

6. Polarimetry

Measurement of the rotation of the plane of polarized light when it passes through an asymmetric system is known as polarimetry. Barton (65) was the first to show that there were rotational increments which could be as-sociated with distinct steroidal features, and in the early work on struc-ture it was of very great value. α-Oriented 3-OH groups, for instance, pro-duce a positive increment on acetylation, while β-ones yield a negative movement. The method has been well reviewed (66, 67). Unfortunately, in common practice several milligrams or preferably more of the substance is needed. In addition, at a single wavelength the changes in the rotational value are small (approximately 30°) in all but a few specialized cases. Consequently, the method is of only limited value today. On the other hand, measurements at many wave lengths (*optical rotary dispersion*) can still produce important information. When plane polarized light possessing a wavelength near the wavelength at which a group absorbs is passed through a steroid, a very pronounced effect is produced. For instrumental reasons the long-wavelength part of the ultraviolet region has been the most useful, and only chromophores, largely the saturated keto group, absorbing in this region have been carefully examined. If one plots the optical rotation of a ketone against wavelength, a pronounced peak in the rotation is observed at a wavelength slightly higher than the absorption peak and another peak (a so-called *trough*) of opposite sign is observed on the other side of the absorption maximum. At maximal absorption the rotation is zero. Such behavior is known as the *Cotton effect*. Since the asymmetric environment of the different steroidal positions is different, the details (position and intensity of peaks and troughs) of the Cotton effect differ from one ketonic position to another. This allows location of the carbonyl group, or, if this is known, it allows deductions about adjacent positions. 3-Keto and 4-keto systems show opposite effects in that the peaks on the long-wavelength side of the absorption maxima have, respectively, positive and negative values. A third extreme effect is shown by 2-keto steroids in which the rotation does not cross the zero value and only a single positive peak is observed. In view of the large rotations (ca. 1000°) involved in the Cotton effect, quantitative microanalytical use of polarimetry could be devised, but it has not been exploited. Excellent reviews of optical rotatory dispersion are available (*68, 69*).

7. Methods Using Radioactivity

The use of a labeled reagent to determine the number of functional groups, e.g., hydroxyl groups, in a steroid has already been mentioned (see Section A.2.b). A much wider use has been given to labeling for quantitative assay. In principle, if a steroid of known structure has been separated from blood, etc., and can be considered pure, the amount can be determined from the disintegrations per minute (dpm) of its derivative after reaction with a reagent of known specific activity (dpm/mM). ^{14}C, ^{3}H, ^{131}I, and ^{35}S have been used for this purpose via acetyl, pipsyl, and tosyl derivatives. In so-called *double isotope dilution,* a derivative containing a different label is added as a carrier during any further processes of separation. If the ratio of the two radioactive atoms remains constant, it can be concluded that the labeled unknown has the same structure as that of the carrier. The precise and successful use of this procedure coupled with appropriate chromatographic methodology has been extensively examined especially in the case of aldosterone (*70–72*). In this way blood levels as little as 1–10 ng/100 ml have been determined.

8. Enzyme Assays

Although very few enzymes in the steroid and related pathways have been purified, methods are now available even with the relatively impure proteins for determination of enzyme levels as well as for steroid assays. Some of the more important enzymatic systems that have been studied for these purposes are the epoxysqualene cyclases, Δ^5-3-ketosteroid isomerase, hydroxylases, hydroxysteroid dehydrogenases, the cholesterol side chain cleaving enzyme, mevalonic acid kinases, geranylgeranyl pyrophosphate synthetase, and certain of the carotenoid enzymes involved in synthesis and conversion to retinal. For a key to the literature, see Ref. 73a. Of special importance is the enzymatic determination of cholesterol (73b–g). An intracellular oxidase of the actinomycete, *Nocardia*, which converts Δ^0-or Δ^5-3β-hydroxysterols to Δ^0-3-keto- or Δ^4-3-ketosterols, can be obtained by treatment with Triton X-100. Hydrogen peroxide, formed in the reaction, is converted to oxygen with peroxidase and used to couple 4-aminoantipyrine and phenol in an oxidative reaction yielding a pigment which is measured colorimetrically. Other end products have also been used. An extracellular oxidase from *Brevibacterium* has been reported (73h).

C. CHROMATOGRAPHIC METHODS

1. Fundamental Principles

All chromatographic procedures in essence depend upon the *phenomenon of partition,* which is the equilibration of a substance between two (or rarely more) phases that are not mutually miscible. In practice, the biphasic systems liquid-liquid, liquid-solid, and gas-liquid are used. If 1) after equilibration the two phases are mechanically slipped past each other so that a fresh amount of each phase is presented to the point of original equilibration on the other phase, and 2) if equilibration is then achieved again, a *chromatographic system* is said to be in operation. The ratio between the amounts of substance that distribute into the two phases at equilibrium is called the *partition coefficient* (K). Let us assume K to be 1.00. By reference to Scheme 3.18 it will be seen that, while the initial distribution will place equal amounts of substance in the two phases at a given point on each, as the phases move, i.e., as the substance is chromatographed, two things happen: 1) the region on each phase where the substance is found changes; and 2) the distribution in each phase widens with a consequent drop in the concentration at any point. This behavior in an ideal system is described by the binomial expansion:

$$\left(\frac{1}{K+1} + \frac{K}{K+1} \right)^n$$

where n is the number of equilibrations with "slippage." It is possible to construct an experimental system with discrete numbers of equilibrations and "slippage" with liquid-liquid phases in a series of separatory funnels. By successive equilibrations (shaking) and transfer of lower phase to the next funnel containing fresh upper phase and the addition of fresh lower phase to the first funnel (*counter current distribution*), it has been demonstrated that the binomial expansion holds very precisely if the concen-

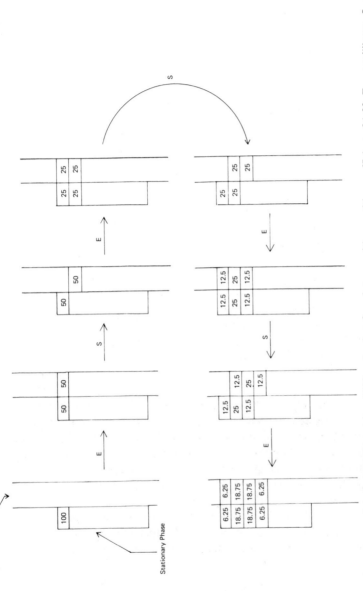

Scheme 3.18. Schematic representation of chromatography of 100 molecules of a substance with a partition coefficient of 1.00. E = equilibrate. S = slip, and means the two phases have been allowed to slip past each other. In the drawing the mobile phase is moving downwards at each "slip" by an amount equal to one box containing the number of molecules at the side of the box. The stationary phase remains at its original position relative to the observer during the entire process and can be imagined as a column of Al₂O₃, etc.

tration of solute is low. If each equilibration and transfer of lower phase is called a *transfer*, then from binominal theory:

$$r_{max} = \frac{Kn}{K+1}$$

where K is the ratio of concentrations in lower to upper phases, r_{max} is the funnel containing the maximal concentration, and n is the number of transfers. It will be seen 1) that the larger the number of transfers the more the solute moves through the series of funnels, and 2) that the larger the value of K the faster the movement will be. Thus, for 100 transfers and $K = 1.0$, r_{max} is 50, while for the same number of transfers with $K = 0.10$, r_{max} becomes 9. Obviously if two substances, one with $K = 1.0$ and one with $K = 0.10$, were mixed, after this procedure they would once again be separated. Herein lies the utility of chromatographic systems: if a bi-phasic system can be found for a series of compounds such that each has a distinct partition coefficient, then the individual compounds can be separated from each other. Since the value of K depends on structure, structural information is also obtained.

If the phases are arranged so that one of them does not move relative to the observer, it is called the *stationary phase*. The other is the *mobile phase*. The term *chromatography* is usually applied to systems in which the stationary and mobile phases move past one another in a continuous fashion rather than in the discontinuous fashion of counter-current distribution. The continuous mode of operation increases the efficiency of separation. Names for chromatographic systems are frequently derived from the manner in which the phases are manipulated. The more important ones are: 1) *column chromatography*, in which a liquid (mobile phase) is passed through a column filled with a stationary phase of pulverized solid or filled with liquid adsorbed to particles of solid; 2) *paper chromatography*, in which a mobile phase of liquid is passed (by gravitation down or sometimes by surface tension up) over a second liquid phase held stationary by impregnation in paper; and 3) *thin-layer chromatography*, in which a liquid (mobile phase) is allowed to move by phenomena of surface tension through and along a thin layer of solid. Another category of nomenclature depends on the nature of the forces binding the substance to one of the phases, viz., *adsorption chromatography*, in which the substance equilibrates between a liquid or a gas and a solid surface. Names also are derived, e.g., *gas-liquid chromatography* or *vapor-phase chromatography*, from the physical state of the phases. Finally, the name *reversed-phase chromatography* is a combination of these categories. It depends upon the fact that in ordinary chromatography the stationary phase itself is the more polar of the two phases or is capable of adsorption of a polar phase, i.e., it acts as a support for the polar phase such as water or ethyleneglycol. In order to preserve two phases, the mobile phase is then of less polar character. In reversed-phase chromatography the situation is reversed. The stationary phase itself is either less polar, as in the case of lipophilic Sephadex, or the support is changed chemically to cellulose acetate, glass fiber, etc., and a nonpolar stationary phase is held to it by surface tension. The word *polar* refers to any effect (H bonding, coulombic attraction, etc.) which strongly attracts a substance to a chromatographic phase. Thus, the more polar phase of ordinary paper chromatography is the stationary one, while in the reversed-phase system it is the mobile one. The rates of movement of two compounds are reversed when they are chromatographed first in the one system and then in the other.

As a first approximation, in liquid-liquid systems the distribution coefficients for steroids do not depend on concentration at the usual levels employed. This means that symmetrical peaks or spots are produced, although with increasing concentrations it is possible to "overload" the system and to obtain asymmetric distributions. In liquid-solid chromatography, however, an asymmetric distribution is nearly always obtained. This is brought about by the fact that distribution of the steroid into the solid phase is favored by dilute solution. Consequently, as the band moves forward the substance at the rear with a smaller concentration is adsorbed more strongly and moves relatively slower than the leading edge. The result is a tail of material following the major substance, and the phenomenon is therefore called *tailing*. It can be remedied at least partly by gradually increasing the polarity of the eluent (*gradient elution*).

2. Liquid-Liquid and Liquid-Solid Chromatography

Liquid-liquid chromatography, in which the mobile phase is the more polar, is generally carried out as a paper system, although occasionally it is accomplished in a column with diatomaceous earth, shredded paper, etc. as a support for the stationary phase. It has been most useful for separation and identification of hormones and their metabolites in microgram quantities. The method, which was pioneered by Zaffaroni and by Bush, has been the subject of numerous papers and reviews. A variant, countercurrent distribution has also been useful. A key to the literature and extensive tabulations are to be found in the recent reviews by Engel and Carter (74); by Neher (75), and by Heftmann (76).

Two major kinds of solvent systems are in use, the *Bush systems* containing water (77) and the *Zaffaroni systems* containing no water (78). The rates of movement (R) are expressed either relative to the advancing front of the mobile phase (R_F) or relative to a standard (R_S). It is common practice to express the biphasic system in terms of amount of solvents mixed together. They are then equilibrated, separated into two phases, and used, but the concentrations of the components in each of the phases are not usually known. For instance, a typical Bush system contains ligroin, benzene, methanol, and water in the ratio by volume of 33:17:40:10. This will have two phases principally but not exclusively composed of ligroin-benzene and of methanol-water. The polar characteristics of Bush and Zaffaroni systems are quite different. Thus, in the Zaffaroni system of propyleneglycol and ligroin, progesterone has an R_F of 0.17 and its 21-hydroxyderivative one of 0.03. In the Bush system, ligroin-methanol-water (100:80:20), not only do both compounds move faster (progesterone, R_F = 0.67; 21-hydroxyprogesterone, R_F = 0.15) but the relative rates of movement are different. This sort of behavior is of great value for identification.

The rates of movement of hundreds of steroids have been measured and perhaps fifty solvent systems have been used. Ten or twenty systems are in common use today. In Table 3.7 are given some representative values

Table 3.7. R_s values for different steroids[a]

(s = 21-Hydroxy-Δ^4-pregnen-3,20-dione)

Steroid	Solvent System[b]	
	P/Tol	B$_3$
Δ^4-Androstene-3,17-dione	1.26	—
Δ^4-Pregnene-3,20-dione	1.28	1.70
Δ^4-Pregnene-3,11,20-trione	1.22	1.15
Δ^4-Androstene-3,11,17-trione	1.07	—
3β-Hydroxy-Δ^5-pregnen-20-one	1.04	—
21-Hydroxy-Δ^4-pregnene-3,20-dione	1.00	1.00
20β-Hydroxy-Δ^4-pregnene-3,20-dione	0.99	1.35
20α-Hydroxy-Δ^4-pregnene-3,20-dione	.88	1.25
17α-Hydroxy-Δ^4-pregnene-3,20-dione	.86	0.93
11β-Hydroxy-Δ^4-pregnene-3,20-dione	.81	0.80
18-Hydroxy-Δ^4-pregnene-3,20-dione	0.73	1.78
17β-Hydroxy-Δ^4-androsten-3-one	0.70	—
6β-Hydroxy-Δ^4-pregnene-3,20-dione	0.59	0.60
11β-Hydroxy-Δ^4-androstene-3,17-dione	0.56	—
3β,21-Dihydroxy-Δ^5-pregnen-20-one	0.47	—
11β,21-Dihydroxy-Δ^4-pregnen-3,20-dione	0.32	—

[a]From Neher (75).
[b]P/Tol is propyleneglycol-toluene. B$_3$ is ligroin-benzene-methanol-water (33:17:40:10) at 38°.

for the polyoxygenated nonaromatic steroids. It will be seen that the Zaffaroni system with large polar differences between the two phases separates the compounds largely according to the number and kind of oxygen functions. Of the ones shown, the least polar (largest R_s) are the diketones. Next are the triketones, followed by the monohydroxymonoketones and monohydroxydiketones. The most polar are the dihydroxydiketones. While small differences in R_s are found for the position of the group, very much larger differences of this sort will be observed with the more complicated Bush system, in which structural subtleties become manifest at the expense of group categorization. Thus, the shift in the hydroxyl group from C-11β to C-18 doubles the R_F in the Bush system but causes only a 10% change in the Zaffaroni system. By a judicious choice of the many systems at hand, it is now possible to separate almost any pair of steroids.

Estrogens are separable in the same systems used for nonaromatic steroids, although some special ones have been devised. In the propylene-glycol-toluene system estrone moves 41% as fast as progesterone while estradiol moves only 13% as fast, and estriol barely moves from the origin. When compared with 21-hydroxy-Δ^4-pregnen-3,20-dione (R_F = 0.73), estrone (R_F = 0.38) moves much slower even though both compounds are dihydroxy steroids. The high polarity in the estrogen case is due to phenolic character not present in the alcohols.

The steroidal hormones and related compounds can also be chromatographed in liquid-solid systems. Usually alumina, silica gel, or silicic acid act as the adsorbent. In the thin-layer technique the hormonal types of lower polarity are usually chromatographed with $CHCl_3$-MeOH (95:5) or $CHCl_3$-ether (80:20), as the eluent, while for steroids with higher polarity $CHCl_3$-MeOH (90:10) and ether-MeOH (99:1) are used. A system in which both groups have been studied is butyl acetate-MeOH (99:1) and the R_F values of representative hormones and related steroids are given in Table 3.8.

Table 3.8. Thin-layer chromatography of the hormones
and related steroids[a]

Steroid	R_F in Butyl Acetate-MeOH (99:1)
Aldosterone	0.17
Corticosterone	0.32
Cortisol	0.48
Cortisone	0.49
Cortexone	0.50
Testosterone	0.57
Pregnanediol	0.60
Androstenedione	0.60
Progesterone	0.67
Pregnenolone	0.69
Estradiol	0.71
Estrone	0.78

[a] From Neher (75).

Sterols have been examined in liquid-solid systems in a thin layer by several groups of investigators (79–90). The thin-layer technique yields separations similar to the column method except that, with the former, smaller amounts can be used, the separations are generally better, and the time required is shorter. Liquid-solid chromatography on alumina or silica gel by either the column or thin-layer technique separates sterols readily into groups. Major examples in increasing order of polarity are: hydrocarbons, ketones, monohydroxy-4,4-dimethylsterols, monohydroxy-4-methylsterols, monohydroxysterols lacking substitution at C-4, and polyhydroxysteroids of various types. This sort of chromatography usually does not differentiate the number or position of double bonds, the extent of alkylation at C-14 or C-24, or the presence or absence of the 9,19-ring (e.g., cycloartenol versus lanosterol). However, exceptions exist. Polyenes, notably the $\Delta^{5,7}$-sterols, and certain monoenes, especially the Δ^{7}-sterols, move slower than the corresponding Δ^{5}-sterols. When silicic acid is used as the adsorbent (*91*), the subtle structural differences become more clearly manifest. Two types of reversed-phase systems are now available. They both have the advantage of separating sterols according to the number of carbon atoms and number of double bonds. Thus, a homologous series (cholesterol and its 24-methyl and ethyl derivatives) as well as mono-, di-, and trienes are separable. The technique can be used either as a thin layer of equilibrated paraffin oil (stationary phase) and acetone-water (mobile phase) on kieselguhr as the support (*92*) or as a column of lipophilic Sephadex (stationary phase) and 5% hexane in methanol (mobile phase) (*93a-e*). Sephadex itself is a cross-linked polysaccharide. It is rendered lipophilic by conversion of some of the hydroxyl groups to ether linkages with a long chain of carbon atoms. The latter then bind, by Van der Walls' attraction, to alkyl moieties of the sterol, retarding their movement. The paraffin oil in the thin layer system plays the same role. Thus, sitosterol moves slower than campesterol, which moves slower than cholesterol, and cholesterol moves slower than 7-dehydrocholesterol. Rates of movement of some sterols in the thin layer system are shown in Table 3.9. In a given series (of numbers of double bonds or alkyl groups), a straight line is produced when log $(1/R_F - 1)$ is plotted against the number of carbon atoms or against the number of double bonds. This is true, for instance, for the Δ^{5}-series: cholesterol, 24-methylcholesterol, and 24-ethylcholesterol, and for the C_{27}-series: cholestanol, cholesterol, and 7-dehydrocholesterol. Separations can be carried out on a column of the modified Sephadex on a 100-mg scale and on a 1-mg scale in the thin-layer method. Reversed phase chromatography is the technique of choice for the separation of sterols differing in the number of carbon atoms in the side chain or at C-14 and for certain differences, e.g., $\Delta^{5,7}$ versus Δ^{5} or $\Delta^{5,22}$ versus Δ^{5}, in double bond structure. The separation of Δ^{5}- from Δ^{7}-sterols is best achieved by ordinary thin-layer means, while differences in the extent of methylation at C-4 induce separation by all the techniques. Examples of lipophilic Sephadex are Sephadex LH-20 (a hydroxypropyl derivative of Sephadex G-25) and its alkoxy derivatives, Lipidex-1000 and Lipidex-5000. Lipidex-1000 is approximately 10% sub-

Table 3.9.   Chromatographic behavior of sterols in a reversed-phase system[a]

Sterol	Paraffin Oil/Acetone-H_2O (4:1)		
	$R_s{}^b$	R_F	$R_m{}^c$
5,7,22-Ergostatrien-3β-ol (ergosterol)	1.26	0.65	-0.260
5,24-Cholestadien-3β-ol (desmosterol)	1.24	0.64	-0.25
5,7-Cholestadien-3β-ol (7-dehydrocholesterol)	1.22	0.63	-0.23
24-Methylene-5-cholestene-3β-ol	1.12	0.58	-0.14
5,24(28)-Stigmastadien-3β-ol (fucosterol)	1.01	0.53	-0.052
5-Cholesten-3β-ol (cholesterol)	1.00	0.52	-0.035
7-Cholesten-3β-ol (lathosterol)	0.99	0.51	-0.017
7,22-Stigmastadien-3β-ol (spinasterol)	0.94	0.49	0.017
5,22-Stigmastadien-3β-ol (stigmasterol)	0.92	0.48	0.035
5-Ergosten-3β-ol (campesterol)	0.90	0.47	0.052
5-Stigmasten-3β-ol (β-sitosterol)	0.78	0.41	0.158
8,24-Lanostadien-3β-ol (lanosterol)	0.68	0.35	0.269
Cholestan-3β-ol	0.66	0.34	0.288
24-Methylene-8-lanosten-3β-ol	0.58	0.30	0.368
24-Ethylidine-7-lanosten-3β-ol	0.47	0.25	0.477
8-Lanosten-3β-ol (dihydrolanosterol)	0.47	0.25	0.477

[a] From deSouza and Nes (92).
[b] s = Cholesterol.
[c] $R_m = \log(1/R_F - 1)$.

stituted, while Lipidex-5000 is approximately 50% substituted. In both, the alkoxy group chain length is 15 C-atoms.

Argentation chromatography (silica gel or other adsorbent impregnated with silver nitrate) is an effective way to separate steroids as a function of the number and position of double bonds. Complex formation between the silver ion and a double bond retards the movement of the steroid so that saturated compounds move faster than monoenes, which move faster than dienes, etc. (*80–88*). Significant differences in R_F are also found for the nature of the double bond. Thus, a mixture of 24-methylene-, *cis*-24-ethylidene-, and *trans*-24-ethylidenecholesterol can be resolved (*94*), as can 24-methylene- and Δ^{24}-sterols (*95*). The argentation technique also separates certain pentacyclic from tetracyclic triterpenes [e.g., β-amyrin versus lanosterol (*96*)]. While the Δ^8- and 9,19-cyclosterols (e.g., lanosterol and cycloartenol) have not been separated by any thin-layer chromatographic techniques, a pair of Δ^7- and 14α-methyl 9,19-cyclosterols (24-methylenelophenol and cycloeucalenol) are separable by the argentation method (*97*).

3. Gas-Liquid Chromatography

a. General Comments   The chromatographically useful partition of a substance between a gas and a liquid was first achieved by James and

Martin (98) in 1952, following earlier considerations of its possibility by Martin and Synge (99). In 1960 Vandenheuvel, Sweeley, and Horning (100) succeeded in applying the technique to steroids using a thermally stable, nonpolar liquid phase (SE-30) without decomposition of the steroids. This was followed shortly by the work of Clayton (101), who introduced polar phases (e.g., polydiethyleneglycol succinate). Clayton also demonstrated that, when the logarithm of the retention time is plotted against the number of carbon atoms in a defined series, e.g., of 3β-methoxy-5α-stanols differing only in the size of the side chain, a straight line is produced. These observations, together with evidence that the introduction of double bonds, hydroxyl groups, etc., produces definite and in part qualitatively understandable effects, placed the method on a sound footing in the steroid field. It has been extensively examined in the intervening years, especially in Horning's laboratory. Two excellent reviews (102, 103) have been published in the hormone field.

Since many parameters (rate of gas flow, temperature, size of column, amount of liquid phase, etc.) influence the rate of movement of the substance chromatographed, it is common to express the rate of movement in terms of the ratio of the time required for the substance to move through the column (retention time) to the time required for a standard substance, usually either cholestane or cholesterol. This ratio is known as the relative retention time.

b. **Nature and Effect of Liquid Phases**   The nature and, to a lesser extent, amount of liquid phase used have a profound effect on the rates of movement of steroids. Liquid phases are usually deposited in films on a support consisting of diatomaceous earth of mesh size about 100. The amount of liquid phase is given as a percentage relative to the amount of support. In most cases the support is first deactivated toward adsorption by reacting it with dimethyldichlorosilane. This procedure "coats" the surface with dimethylsiloxy groups. The liquid phases that have been employed most successfully for steroids are either substituted siloxanes (silicones) or polyesters of succinic acid, e.g., "neopentylglycol succinate" shown in Scheme 3.19. The siloxanes differ from one another by the nature of the substituents on the silicon (R groups in the accompanying formula) and are named accordingly. Thus, in dimethylsiloxanes R = CH_3. Several preparations of the latter are available under the trade names SE-30, SE-52, JXR, and OV-1. The p-chlorophenylmethylsiloxane is called F-60, the methylphenylsiloxane OV-17, the fluoroalkylsiloxane QF-1, and the cyanoethylmethylsiloxane XE-60. The neopentylglycol succinate is known as NGS, and, when the neopentylglycol portion is replaced by cyclohexanedimethanol, the designation for the polyester is CHDMS. The alkylsiloxanes, e.g., SE-30, tend to be the least polar. Introduction of unsaturation, as the XE-60, or fluoro atoms, as in QF-1, increases the polarity and the succinates tend to be the most polar of all. The less polar the liquid phase, the

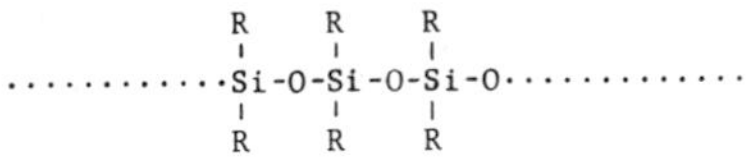

$$\cdots\cdots\cdots Si-O-Si-O-Si-O\cdots\cdots\cdots$$

with R groups above and below each Si.

Siloxane Structure

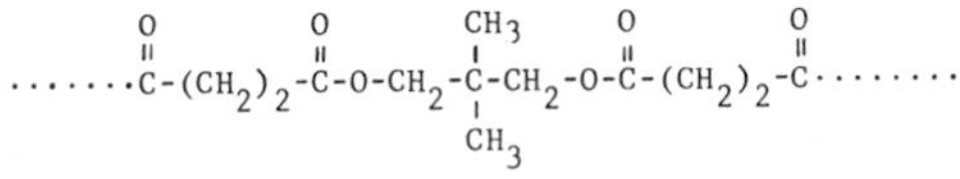

$$\cdots\cdots C-(CH_2)_2-C-O-CH_2-\overset{CH_3}{\underset{CH_3}{C}}-CH_2-O-C-(CH_2)_2-C\cdots\cdots$$

Neopentylglycol Succinate

Scheme 3.19. Structure of some liquid phases for gas-liquid chromatography.

more the rate of movement of a steroid will depend on its moleular weight and intrinsic volatility. As the polarity of the liquid phase is increased, increasing interaction with the steroid occurs. This frequently produces greater selectivity [but also may retard the movement of a polar (hydroxylated, etc.) steroid]. Thus, 7-cholesten-3β-ol and 5,7-cholestadien-3β-ol are separable on each of the four liquid phases; SE-52, QF-1, XE-60 and NGS, and the separation factors (respectively, 0.93, 0.86, 0.83 and 0.74, for rate of movement of the Δ^5-sterol divided by that of the $\Delta^{5,7}$-sterol) increase with increase in polarity of the liquid phase (*64, 101, 104*). The retardation of the movement of a steroid by increasing polarity of the liquid phase is best seen in ketones versus hydrocarbons. The 5α- and 5β-pregnane-3,20-diones, for instance, move (*105*) 1.6 times as fast as does cholestane on SE-30, reflecting a smaller molecular weight of the ketones, but on QF-1 or XE-60 they move only 0.18 times as fast, because of the carbonyl interactions with the liquid phase. Such differential behavior is immensely useful in separation and identification. Thus, on SE-52 the Δ^5- and $\Delta^{5,7,22}$-sterols are not separable, but on NGS they are (*64*).

   c. Separation of Sterols   Sterols have been converted to various derivatives in order to reduce polarity, increase the rate of movement, and decrease decomposition during gas-liquid chromatography. Early reports by Clayton (*101*) and by Tsuda, Sakai, and Ikekawa (*106*), for instance, dealt with methyl ethers, but more recent work has shown that for the common monohydroxy or monohydroxy-monoketo sterols the free compound suffices quite well. Formation of the derivative only adds an additional step to the procedure. In certain cases derivative formation could conceivably enhance a separation factor, by reducing the strong H-bonding effect of the hydroxyl group and allowing other features, e.g., double bonds, to manifest themselves more clearly. Systematic studies of this problem unfortunately are not available, but what little data have been published suggest that derivative formation does *not* significantly enhance separations. Thus, the separation factor for the Δ^5- versus $\Delta^{5,7}$-sterols is substantially the same on polysuccinates whether or not the free sterols or methyl ethers are used. The value $(\Delta^5/\Delta^{5,7})$ for the free sterols is 0.74 on NGS (*64*) and 0.71 for the methyl ethers on polydiethyleneglycol succinate (*101*). More important than ethers are acetates, since they are frequently prepared for other reasons. Again, however, no significant differences (above the 2% level) have been found between the separation factors for two acetates versus two alcohols (for sterols lacking a substituent at C-4). The data of Conner et al. (*64*) are especially useful in examining this problem. Their work also shows that on SE-52 the separation factor for alcohols/ acetates is 0.72; on QF-1, 0.65; and on NGS, 1.2. In the authors' laboratory the factor on XE-60 was found to be 0.93. Presumably, these values can be translated to other laboratories, since reasonable coincidence of retention times from one laboratory to another is found. For instance, on QF-1, Conner et al. (*64*) find the retention time (relative to cholestane) for cholesteryl acetate, 7-dehydrocholestryl acetate, and lathosteryl acetate to be 4.73, 5.42, and 5.35, respectively, while the values from Schroepfer's laboratory (*107*) are 4.69, 5.33, and 5.14. The validity of the alcohol/acetate factors is also demonstrated with values from these two laboratories. Schroepfer and his associates find cholesteryl acetate moves 4.93% as fast as cholestane on QF-1. The data of Conner's group shows a separation factor (alcohol/acetate) of 0.65 for six pairs of sterols. Correcting the Schroepfer value with this factor (4.93 × 0.65), we obtain 3.05 for the alcohol. Conner et al. report 3.06.

In Table 3.10 are compiled the retention times (relative to cholestane) of a variety of biochemically important sterols on several liquid phases. The data illustrate that very small changes in structure can be detected. Because, as first carefully illustrated by Clayton (*101*), the contributions of structural features to the retention times are additive, or more precisely multiplicative, gas-liquid chromatographic information constitutes a way of analyzing the structure of an unknown. The constancy of this contribution (on a given liquid phase) is illustrated by the separation factors for alcohols versus acetates previously discussed.

Stereochemical and isomeric differences frequently are also manifest in retention times. Examples, respectively, are the difference (*104, 108*) in retention times of the C-9 and C-10 isomers of 5,7,22-ergostatrien-3β-ol, the values (*109*) relative to cholesterol on XE-60 being 1.36 for the 9α-H, 10β-CH₃ derivative (ergosterol), 1.10 for its 9β-epimer (isopyrocalciferol), and 0.80 for the 9β,10α-epimer (pyrocalciferol), and the separation (*95,109a*) of α- and β-amyrin (Table 3.11), which differ only in the position of a methyl group. The important biosynthetic intermediates, lanosterol and

Table 3.10. Influence of carbonyl groups and double bonds on retention time
of sterols[a]

Position of Double Bonds in Derivatives of 5α-Cholestan-3β-ol		Retention Times Relative to Cholestane			
		SE-52	XE-60	QF-1	NGS
H at C-24	None	—	4.00	3.20	—
	5	2.00	4.00	3.06	6.0
	7	2.34	4.60	3.41	8.4
	8	—	—	3.07	—
	8(14)	—	—	2.92	—
	14	—	—	2.87	—
	5,7	2.15	4.80	3.50	8.1
	5,22	1.79	4.60	2.81	5.7
	8,14	—	—	2.95	—
	5,7,22	1.99	—	3.16	7.6
	5 plus 24-Oxo	—	12.04	—	—
	5 plus 3-Oxo	—	7.96	—	—
C₁ at C-24	5	—	5.12	—	—
	5,22	—	4.32	—	—
	5,24(28)	—	5.52	—	—
	5,7,22	2.46	5.44	3.84	9.0
	5,7,22,24(28)	—	6.04	—	—
	5,7,9(11)	—	4.96	—	—
C₂ at C-24	5	—	6.40	—	—
	5,22	—	5.28	—	—
	7,22	—	6.40	—	—
	5,cis-24(28)	—	6.52	—	—
	5, trans-24(28)	—	6.68	—	—
	5,7 cis-24(28)	—	7.24	—	—
	5,7,22, trans-24(28)	—	7.12	—	—

[a] From Refs. 64, 94, 104, 107, and (for XE-60) unpublished observations of the authors and their associates. Some of the values for QF-1 originally reported (107) for the acetates have been corrected by the factor 0.65 (64) for conversion to alcohols. Where more than one value was reported in the literature, an average is given here.

cycloartenol, are also resolved on XE-60 and other liquid phases, and the C_{27}-, C_{28}-, and C_{29}-sterols, differing only in substitution at C-24, move at markedly different rates. Similarly, 4α-methylsterols are separable from each other and from other sterols (97). An important example of the *lack* of separation is with 24-epimers (106), e.g., 24α- and 24β-methyl-cholesten-3β-ol. 24-Epimers, especially in the Δ^5-series, exist naturally. A lack of resolution also occurs when two groups of opposite contribution are added simultaneously, e.g., Δ^7 and Δ^{22} to a Δ^5-sterol (see Table 3.11). Patterson (109b) has published data on the rates of movement of a hundred sterols on SE-30, QF-1, Hi-Eff 8BP, and PMPE. Although cholestane used to be reported as a standard by many authors, it is now common practice to use

Table 3.11. Behavior of C_{30}-isopentenoids in a gas-liquid chromatography[a]

C_{30}-Isopentenoid	Retention Time Relative To Cholestane on XE-60
Squalene	0.84
Lanosterol	5.88
24,25-Dihydrolanosterol	5.04
Cycloartenol	6.84
24-Methylenelanosterol	6.88
24-Methylenecycloartanol	8.24
24-Ethylidenelanosterol	8.60
β-Amyrin	6.32
α-Amyrin	7.04
Tetrahymanol	11.00

[a] Unpublished observations of the authors and their associates.

cholesterol in its place. The abbreviation RRT (for relative retention time) also is frequently employed. Thus, with cholesterol as the standard, the RRTs for cholesterol, 24α-methylcholesterol, and 24α-ethylcholesterol are 1.00, 1.30, and 1.63, respectively, on SE-30 (*109b*), or we may say that ergosterol, with RRT 1.22, moves faster on SE-30 than clionasterol, with RRT 1.63. Groups added to a sterol make a definite contribution to the RRT as a percent. The introduction of the *trans*-Δ^{22}-group, for instance, lowers the RRT by 12% on XE-60. Its contribution is, therefore, 0.88, while that of a 24β-methyl group is 1.31. Brassicasterol, then, has an RRT of 1.00 × 0.88 × 1.31 or 1.15.

d. Separation of Hormonal Steroids The hormonal steroids tend to be highly oxygenated and hence subject to long retention times and ready decomposition. Their importance to clinical medicine, however, has spurred extensive and successful work with many of them. The problem of decomposition and artifact formation has largely been circumvented by the use of glass columns. In addition derivative formation has retarded such processes as dehydration and in addition rendered the compounds more volatile. The trimethylsilyl ethers have been especially useful. The book by Eik-Nes and Horning (*102*) should be consulted for a detailed discussion of this problem. Horning et al. (*110*) have described in detail how to prepare such derivatives. Methoximes ($R_2C\!=\!N\!-\!O\!-\!CH_3$) are frequently used to protect the keto group in other reactions, e.g., ether formation, and to decrease its chromatographic polarity. With the less polar liquid phases the trimethylsilyl ethers usually move faster than the free alcohols, but with more polar phases the reverse is often true. The 11β- and 17α-hydroxyl groups usually do not form ethers due to steric hindrance. Steric hindrance at C-11 also decreases the effect of OH versus C$=$O at this position.

In most cases a ketone moves substantially more slowly than an alcohol, but the 11-keto and 11β-hydroxy groups have approximately the same effect on retention time. This and other effects can be seen from Tables 3.12 and 3.13. Other data (*102*) indicate the alcohol/acetate separation

Table 3.12.   Behavior of trimethylsilyl ethers of C_{19}-steroids in gas-liquid chromatography[a]

Steroidal Ether	Retention Time Relative to Cholestane Liquid Phase			
	1-2% SE-30	1-2% XE-60	1-2% QF-1	1% NGS
3α-Hydroxy-5α-androstan-17-one	0.38	1.56	1.25	1.09
3α-Hydroxy-5β-androstan-17-one	0.39	1.81	1.25	1.34
3α,11β-Dihyroxy-5α-androstan-17-one	—	4.53	—	—
3α-Hydroxy-5β-androstan-11,17-dione	—	4.10	2.14	—
3β-Hydroxy-5-androsten-17-one	0.46	2.20	1.30	1.57
3-Hydroxy-1,3,5-estratrien-17-one	—	1.15	1.51	3.25
3,17β-Dihydroxy-1,3,5-estratriene	—	0.83	0.81	—
3,16α,17β-Trihydroxy-1,3,5-estratriene	—	1.41	1.43	1.77
2,3-Dihydroxy-1,3,5-estratrien-17-one	—	1.84	2.03	3.28
2-Methoxy-3-hydroxy-1,3,5-estratrien-17-one	—	2.06	2.29	—

[a] From Eik-Nes and Horning (*102*).

factor for oxygenated pregnanes is 0.7 on SE-30, 0.9 on XE-60, and 0.6 on QF-1. These values are in reasonable agreement with values found for sterols. Exact comparisons from one laboratory to another, however, are made difficult by temperature variations and the inexactness of measuring temperatures in the ovens of many instruments. While the influence of temperature on retention times depends on steroidal structure, at 200-240°, which is the region usually employed, temperature effects can be of the order of magnitude of 1% per degree, higher temperatures decreasing retention time by increasing the vapor pressure.

D. METHODS USING PROTEIN-STEROID INTERACTIONS

1. Radioimmunoassay

Berson et al. (*111*) were the first to describe a novel radioimmunoassay (RIA) technique for the polypeptide hormone, insulin. It was not until

Table 3.13.   Behavior of some free hormonal steroids in gas-liquid chromatography[a]

	Retention Time Relative to Cholestane Liquid Phase		
Steroid	1–2% SE-30	XE-60	1–3% QF-1
5α-Androstan-17-one	0.19	—	0.64
3α-Hydroxy-5α-androstan-17-one	0.34	—	1.96
5α-Androstan-3,17-dione	0.42	—	4.06
3α-Hydroxy-5β-androstan-17-one	0.32	—	2.05
3β-Hydroxy-5-androstan-17-one	0.34	—	1.99
4-Androstene-3,17-dione	0.57	—	—
17β-Hydroxy-4-androstene-3-one	0.65	—	—
4-Pregnene-3,17-dione	0.80	9.7	9.9
3α-Hydroxy-5α-pregnan-20-one	0.65	3.78	2.74
3β-Hydroxy-5α-pregnan-20-one	0.66	4.26	3.06
3α-Hydroxy-4-pregnen-20-one	0.65	4.7	3.7
3α,20α-Dihydroxy-5α-pregnane	0.71	—	—

[a] From Eik-Nes and Horning (102).

about 10 years later that the usefulness of the assay technique was realized and it was applied to the assay of other polypeptide hormones. RIAs are typically sensitive to as little as nanograms or picograms of sample per milliliter of plasma, urine, etc. The actual assay can often be carried out in crude samples without prior extraction or partial purification. RIA has allowed for the first time the easy and simple quantitation of minute amounts of biologically active compounds at physiologic levels in small volumes of sample.

In RIA the compound being assayed acts as an antigen that competes with a small amount of purified, radioactive antigen for binding sites on the antibody (Scheme 3.20). The amount of radioactive antigen bound by antibody varies inversely with the concentration of unlabeled antigen. Measurement of the amount of antibody-bound radioactive antigen separated from the milieu yields the amount of unlabeled antigen after comparison with a standard curve (Scheme 3.20). Various RIAs differ in the method of antiserum preparation and in the mode of separation of free from antibody-bound antigen. RIAs have been described for a variety of protein or protein-derived substances, including, for example, the gonadotropins (112–117), growth hormone (118, 119), corticotropin (120), thyroid-stimulating hormone (121), prolactin (122), β-melanocyte-stimulating hormone (123), LH-releasing hormone (124–126), fibrinopeptide B (127), clostridial toxin (128), mescaline (129), prostaglandin $F_{2\alpha}$ (130), triiodothyronine (131), and somatomedin B (132).

Steroid hormones can also be quantitated in plasma, etc. (133–135).

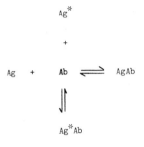

Ag = Antigen

Ag* = Radioactive Antigen

Ab = Antibody

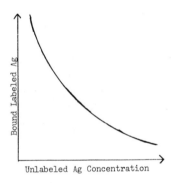

Scheme 3.20. Binding of radioactive and nonradioactive antigen by antibody and an RIA standard curve.

A major problem in the development of sensitive steroid (and small poly-peptides or amino acid derivatives) RIAs has been the production of anti-sera. Small molecules below 1,000 molecular weight, such as steroids, are not antigenic. Steroids are rendered antigenic by conjugation to large pro-teins, frequently bovine serum albumin. Hemisuccinate or chlorocarbonate derivatives of the alcohols or oxime derivatives of the ketone are prepared; these are conjugated to the albumin via a mixed anhydride reaction, the Schotten-Baumann reaction, or carbodiimide. The extent of conjugation can be monitored by UV or the addition of trace amounts of radioactive steroids before derivative preparation. Conjugated proteins with a steroid/protein ratio 20 or greater appear to produce more useful antisera. For the production of antisera in rabbits or sheep, the conjugated steroid is suspended in complete Freund's adjuvant and injected at intervals of 6-12 days for four to six series of injections followed by bimonthly or monthly boosters. Many antisteroid antisera are most specific for the portion of the steroid molecule protruding the farthest from the conjugated protein and least specific for the portion of the steroid adjacent to the site of conjugation (*136*, *137*); i.e., when a steroid is conjugated at C-17 the antibodies to the conjugate are least specific for ring D and most specific for ring A. Antibodies which are specific for both rings A and D, the sites of greatest structural variability in the steroids, can be produced from conjugates at C-6, -7, or -11.

Some purification of steroid RIA samples is often necessary before measurement, especially when the steroid is present in low concentrations. Many steroid antibodies are not completely specific and could react with other structurally related steroids in the sample. Selective solvent extraction of the steroid followed by any one of several forms of chromatographic purification are the most frequently used methods of steroid purification (*136*).

Several methods of separating antibody-bound from free antigen are commonly used after incubation of the mixture containing antiserum, sample, and radioactive steroid. Antibody-bound steroids can be precipitated by antibody to the antisteroid gamma globulin (*137*) or by ammonium sulfate (*138*). Free steroid can be adsorbed by dextran-coated charcoal which is removed by centrifugation, leaving antibody-bound steroid in the supernatent (*139*). In solid-phase RIAs the incubation medium containing free steroid is merely rinsed from the surface containing preadsorbed antiserum and bound antigen (*140*).

RIAs have been reported in the literature for a large number of the steroid hormones, for example, aldosterone (*138*), estrone and estradiol (*141*), progesterone (*142*), testosterone (*143*), and cortisol (*144*). The digitalis glycosides are also assayed by RIA (*145*). Many of the reagents for these and other steroid assays are available commercially in many instances in the form of kits. Whether a literature or a commercial method is followed, only 1 ml of plasma or urine is required for many assays. Most assays are sensitive to 5–50 pg of steroid with a between assay variance of 10 to 20% (usually 10–15%).

2. Competitive Protein Binding

The binding of steroids to blood constituents was perhaps first well documented in the case of cortisol and the protein called corticosteroid-binding globulin (CBG) or transcortin (*146*, *147*). Shortly thereafter, sulfates, e.g., that of dehydroepiandrosterone, were found to bind to serum albumin (*148*, *149*). Binding of the unconjugated steroids has now been utilized as a very sensitive quantitative method (*150*, *151*) for C_{21}-steroid assay. The idea was first conceived by Murphy (*152*). Progesterone, for instance, will compete with corticosterone for binding sites of protein(s) (presumably transcortin, with which it binds better than does cortisol) in dog serum, and when unlabeled progesterone is mixed with tritiated corticosterone, a lowering of the bound radioactivity is found to be precisely dependent on the amount of progesterone added (*153*). Millimicrograms of hormone have been measured in this way.

LITERATURE CITED

1. A. Windaus, Ber. 42:238 (1909).
2. R. Schoenheimer and H. Dam, Z. Physiol. 215:59 (1933).
3. W. Bergmann, J. Biol. Chem. 132:471 (1940).
4. L. Dorfman, Chem. Rev. 53:47 (1953).
5. C. C. Porter and R. H. Silber, J. Biol. Chem. 185:201 (1950).
6. C. C. Porter and R. H. Silber, J. Biol. Chem. 210:923 (1954).
7. V. R. Mattox, J. Am. Chem. Soc. 74:4340 (1952).
8. R. H. Silber and C. C. Porter, *in* D. Glick (ed.), Methods in Biochemical Analysis, Vol. 4. Wiley, New York, 1957. p. 139.
9. C. Flood, D. S. Layne, S. Ramcharan, E. Rossipal, J. F. Tait, and S. A. S. Tait, Acta Endocrinol. 36:237 (1961).
10. J. K. Norymberski, Nature 170:1074 (1952).
11. C. Brooks and J. K. Norymberski, Biochem. J. 55:371 (1953).
12. F. G. Peron, *in* R. I. Dorfman (ed.), Methods in Hormone Research. 1st Ed., Vol. I. Academic Press, New York, 1962. p. 199.
13. K. B. Eik-Nes, *in* R. I. Dorfman (ed.), Methods in Hormone Research. 2nd Ed., Vol. I. Academic Press, New York, 1968. p. 304.
14. R. D. H. Heard and H. Sobel, J. Biol. Chem. 165:687 (1946).
15. R. B. A. Burton, A. Zaffaroni, and E. H. Keutmann, J. Biol. Chem. 188:763 (1951).
16. W. Zimmermann, Z. Physiol. Chem. 233:257 (1935).
17. H. Wilson, Arch. Biochem. Biophys. 52:217 (1954).
18. E. Heilbronner, H. Chim. Acta 36:1121 (1953).
19. P. T. Russell, R. T. van Aller, and W. R. Nes, J. Biol. Chem. 242:5802 (1967).
20. F. B. Mallory, K. A. Ferguson, and R. L. Conner, Anal. Biochem. 33:230 (1970).
21. C. Liebermann, Ber. 18:1803 (1885).
22. B. L. Oser (ed.), Hawks Physiological Chemistry. 14th Ed. McGraw-Hill, New York, 1965. p. 1062.
23. A. Zlatkis and B. Zak, Anal. Biochem. 29:143 (1969).
24. S. Kober, Biochem. Z. 239:209 (1931).
25. G. Ittrich, Z. Physiol. Chem. 312:1 (1958).
26. G. Ittrich, Z. Physiol. Chem. 320:103 (1960).
27. R. A. A. Salokangas and R. D. Bulbrook, J. Endocrinol. 22:47 (1961).
28. J. R. K. Preedy, *in* C. A. Paulsen (ed.), Estrogen Assays in Clinical Medicine. Univ. of Washington Press, Seattle, 1965. p. 162.
29. J. R. K. Preedy, *in* R. I. Dorfman (ed.), Methods in Hormone Research. 2nd Ed., Vol. I. Academic Press, New York, 1968. p. 23.
30. J. Touchstone, A. K. Balin, and P. Knapstein, Steroids 13:199 (1969).
31. S. A. S. Tait, J. F. Tait, M. Okamoto, and C. Flood, Endocrinology 81:1213 (1967).
32. W. Siegenthaler, A. Dowdy, and J. A. Leutscher, J. Clin. Endocrinol. Metab. 22:172 (1962).
33. A. H. Brodie and J. F. Tait, *in* R. I. Dorfman (ed.), Methods in Hormone Research. 2nd Ed., Vol. I. Academic Press, New York, 1968. p. 334.

34. J. P. Dusza, M. Heller, and S. Burstein, *in* L. Engel (ed.), Physical Properties of the Steroid Hormones. Pergamon Press, London, 1963. p. 69.
35. R. B. Woodward, J. Am. Chem. Soc. 64:72 (1942).
36. P. Bladon, H. B. Henbest, and G. W. Wood, J. Chem. Soc. 2737 (1952).
37. L. F. Fieser, J. Org. Chem. 15:930 (1950).
38. I. Scheer, W. R. Nes, and P. Smeltzer, J. Am. Chem. Soc. 77:3300 (1955).
39. J. W. Goldzieher, *in* L. Engel (ed.), Physical Properties of the Steroid Hormones. Pergamon Press, London, 1963. p. 288.
40. L. L. Smith and S. Bernstein, *in* L. Engel (ed.), Physical Properties of the Steroid Hormones. Pergamon Press, London, 1963. p. 321.
41. H. A. Walens, A. Turner, and M. Wall, Anal. Chem. 26:325 (1954).
42. K. Nakanishi, Infrared Absorption Spectroscopy. Holden-Day, San Francisco. 1962.
43. L. F. Fieser and M. Fieser, Steroids. Reinhold, New York, 1959. pp. 169-175.
44. G. Roberts, B. S. Gallagher, and R. N. Jones, Infrared Absorption Spectra of Steroids. Vols. I and II. Interscience, New York, 1958.
45. W. Neudert and H. Röpke, Atlas of Steroid Spectra. Springer-Verlag, New York, 1965.
46. R. N. Jones and G. Roberts, J. Am. Chem. Soc. 80:6121 (1958).
47. I. L. Allsop, R. H. Cole, D. E. White, and R. L. S. Willix, J. Chem. Soc. 4868 (1956).
48. J. N. Shoolery and M. T. Rogers, J. Am. Chem. Soc. 80:5121 (1958).
49. E. O. Bishop, J. S. G. Cox, and R. E. Richards, J. Chem. Soc. 5118 (1960).
50. N. S. Bhacca and D. H. Williams, Applications of NMR Spectroscopy in Organic Chemistry, Illustrations from the Steroid Field. Holden-Day, San Francisco, 1964.
51a. L. L. Smith, Steroids 4:395 (1964).
  b. I. Rubinstein, L. J. Goad, A. D. H. Clague, and L. J. Mulheirn, Phytochem. 15:195 (1976).
  c. W. R. Nes, K. Krevitz, and S. Behzadan, Lipids 11:118 (1976).
  d. W. R. Nes, K. Krevitz, J. M. Joseph, W. D. Nes, B. Harris, G. F. Gibbons, and G. W. Patterson, Lipids, in press (1977).
  e. L. J. Mulheirn and G. Ryback, J. Chem. Soc. Chem. Commun. 886 (1974).
52. M. Karplus, J. Am. Chem. Soc. 85:2870 (1963).
53. H. Budzikiewicz, C. Djerassi, and D. H. Williams, Interpretation of Mass Spectra of Organic Compounds. Holden-Day, San Francisco, 1964.
54. H. Budzikiewicz, C. Djerassi, and D. H. Williams, Structure Elucidation of Natural Products by Mass Spectroscopy. Vol. II, Steroids, Terpenoids, Sugars, and Miscellaneous Classes. Holden-Day, San Francisco, 1964.
55. K. Biemann, Special Lecture Presented at the Third International Symposium on the Chemistry of Natural Products. Butterworths, London, 1964. p. 95.
56. J. Lederberg, Computation of Molecular Formulas for Mass Spectrometry. Holden-Day, San Francisco, 1964.
57. S. S. Friedland, G. H. Lane, Jr., R. T. Longman, K. E. Train, and M. J. O'Neal, Jr., Anal. Chem. 31:169 (1959).
58. B. A. Knights, J. Gas Chromatog. 5:273 (1967).
59. S. G. Wyllie and C. Djerassi, J. Org. Chem. 33:305 (1968).
60. L. Tokes, G. Jones, and C. Djerassi, J. Am. Chem. Soc. 90:5465 (1968).
61. G. Galli and S. Maroni, Steroids 10:189 (1967).
62. G. J. Gibbons, L. J. Goad, and T. W. Goodwin, Phytochemistry 7:983 (1968).

63. B. A. Knights and C. J. W. Brooks, Phytochemistry 8:463 (1969).
64. R. L. Conner, F. B. Mallory, J. R. Landrey, and C. W. L. Iyengar, J. Biol. Chem. 244:2325 (1969).
65. D. H. R. Barton, J. Chem. Soc. 813 (1945).
66. L. Fieser and M. Fieser, Steroids. Reinhold, New York, 1959. p. 177.
67. D. H. R. Barton and W. Klyne, Chem. Ind. 755 (1948).
68. C. Djerassi, Optical Rotatory Dispersion, McGraw-Hill, New York. 1960.
69. P. Crabbé, Optical Rotatory Dispersion and Circular Dichrosim in Organic Chemistry. Holden-Day, San Francisco, 1965.
70. P. J. O. Ayers, S. A. Simpson, and J. F. Tait, Biochem. J. 65:639 (1957).
71. B. Kliman and R. E. Peterson, J. Biol. Chem. 235:1639 (1960).
72. J. P. Coghlan and J. R. Blair-West, in C. H. Gray and A. L. Bacharach (eds.), Hormones in Blood. Vol. 2. Academic Press, New York, 1967. p. 420.
73a. R. B. Clayton (ed.), Steroids and Terpenoids, Vol. 15 of S. P. Colowick and N. O. Kaplan, (eds.), Methods in Enzymology. Academic Press, New York, 1969.
  b. W. Richmond, Clin. Chem. 19:1350 (1973).
  c. H. M. Flegg, Ann. Clin. Biochem. 10:79 (1973).
  d. P. N. Tarbutton and C. R. Gunter, Clin. Chem. 20:724 (1974).
  e. C. C. Allain, L. S. Poon, C. S. G. Chan, W. Richmond, and P. C. Fu, Clin. Chem. 20:470 (1974).
  f. V. P. Röschlau, E. Bernt, and W. Gruber, Z. Klin. Chem. Klin. Biochem. 12:403 (1974).
  g. D. L. White, D. A. Barrett II, and D. A. Wycoff, Clin. Chem. 20:1282 (1974).
  h. T. Uwajima, H. Yagi, and O. Terada, Agr. Biol. Chem. 38:1149 (1974).
74. L. L. Engel and P. Carter, in L. L. Engel (ed.), Physical Properties of the Steroid Hormones, Macmillan, New York, 1963. p. 1.
75. R. Neher in L. L. Engel (ed.), Physical Properties of the Steroid Hormones, Macmillan, New York, 1963. p. 37.
76. E. Heftmann, Chromatography. A laboratory handbook of Chromatographic and Electrophoretic methods, Van Nostrand Reinhold Co., New York, 1975.
77. I. E. Bush, Recent Prog. Hormone Res. 9:321 (1954).
78. A. Zaffaroni, Recent Prog. Hormone Res. 8:51 (1953).
79. R. D. Bennett and E. Heftmann, J. Chromatog. 9:359 (1962).
80. J. Avigan, DeW. S. Goodman, and D. Steinberg, J. Lipid Res. 4:100 (1963).
81. R. Ikan, S. Harel, J. Kashman, and E. D. Bergmann, J. Chromatog. 14: 504 (1964).
82. R. Ikan and M. Cudzinovski, J. Chromatog. 18:422 (1965).
83. N. Ditullio, C. S. Jacobs, Jr., and W. L. Holmes, J. Chromatog. 20:354 (1965).
84. A. S. Truswell and W. D. Mitchell, J. Lipid Res. 6:438 (1965).
85. J. R. Claude, J. Chromatog. 17:596 (1965).
86. R. Kammereck, W. H. Lee, A. Paliokas, and G. J. Schroepfer, Jr., J. Lipid Res. 8:282 (1967).
87. L. J. Morris, J. Lipid Res. 7:717 (1966).
88. J. W. Copius-Peereboom and H. W. Beekes, J. Chromatog. 17:99 (1965).
89. J. W. Copius-Peereboom in C. B. Marini-Bettolo (ed.), Thin-Layer Chromatography, Elsevier, Amsterdam, 1964. pp. 197-204.
90. J. W. Copius-Peereboom and H. W. Beekes, J. Chromatog. 9:316 (1962).

91. G. A. Blondin, J. L. Scott, J. K. Hummer, B. D. Kulkarni, and W. R. Nes, Comp. Biochem. Physiol. 17:391 (1966).
92. N. J. de Souza and W. R. Nes, J. Lipid Res. 10:240 (1969).
93a. J. Ellingboe, E. Nyström, and J. Sjövall, Biochem. Biophys. Acta 152:803 (1968).
  b. J. Ellingboe, E. Nyström, and J. Sjovall, J. Lipid Res. 11:266 (1970).
  c. P. M. Hyde and W. H. Elliott, J. Chromat. 67:170 (1972).
  d. R. A. Anderson, C. J. W. Brooks, and B. A. Knights, J. Chromat. 75:247 (1973).
  e. G. W. Patterson, M. W. Khalil, and D. R. Idler, J. Chromat. 115:153 (1975).
94. R. T. van Aller, H. Chikamatsu, N. J. de Souza, J. P. John, and W. R. Nes, J. Biol. Chem. 244:6645 (1969).
95. L. J. Goad and T. W. Goodwin, Biochem. J. 99:735 (1966).
96. H. H. Rees, E. I. Mercer, T. W. Goodwin, Biochem. J. 99:726 (1966).
97. B. L. Williams, L. J. Goad, and T. W. Goodwin, Phytochem. 6:1137 (1967).
98. A. T. James and A. J. P. Martin, Biochem. J. 50:679 (1952).
99. A. J. P. Martin and R. L. M. Synge, Biochem. J. 35:1358 (1941).
100. W. J. A. Vandenheuvel, C. C. Sweeley, and E. C. Horning, J. Am. Chem. Soc. 82:3481 (1960).
101. R. B. Clayton, Biochemistry 1:357 (1962).
102. K. B. Eik-Nes and E. C. Horning (eds.), Gas Phase Chromatography of Steroids. Springer-Verlag, New York, 1968.
103. R. I. Dorfman (ed.), Methods in Hormone Research. Vol. I. Academic Press, New York, 1968.
104. G. A. Blondin, B. D. Kulkarni, J. P. John, R. T. van Aller, P. T. Russell, and W. R. Nes, Anal. Chem. 39:36 (1967).
105. H. J. van der Molen, in K. B. Eik-Nes and E. C. Horning (eds.), Gas Phase Chromatography of Steroids. Springer-Verlag, New York, 1968. p. 164.
106. K. Tsuda, K. Sakai, and N. Ikekawa, Chem. Pharm. Bull. (Tokyo) 9:835 (1961).
107. W. H. Lee, B. N. Lutsky, and G. J. Schroepfer, Jr. J. Biol. Chem. 244: 5440 (1969).
108. H. Ziffer, W. J. A. Vandenheuvel, E. O. A. Haahti, and E. C. Horning, J. Am. Chem. Soc. 82:6411 (1960).
109a. M. Castle, G. A. Blondin, and W. R. Nes, J. Biol. Chem. 242:5796 (1967).
  b. G. W. Patterson, Anal. Chem. 43:1165 (1971).
110. E. C. Horning, M. C. Horning, N. Ikekawa, E. M. Chambaz, P. I. Jaakonmaki, and C. J. W. Brooks, J. Gas Chromatog. 5:283 (1967).
111. S. A. Berson, R. S. Yalow, A. Bauman, M. A. Rothschild, and K. Newerly, J. Clin. Invest. 35:170 (1956).
112. M. L. McKean and W. R. Nes, Anal. Biochem. 73:397 (1976).
113. B. B. Sazena, H. Demura, H. M. Gandy, and R. E. Peterson, J. Clin. Endocrinol. Metab. 28:519 (1968).
114. R. A. Levine, R. K. Donabedian, and L. G. Sobrinho, Clin. Chem. (Winston Salem, N.C.) 17:931 (1971).
115. K. Catt and G. W. Tregear, Science 158:1570 (1967).
116. C. Faiman and R. J. Ryan, J. Clin. Endocrinol. Metab. 27:444 (1967).
117. A. R. Midgley, Jr., Endocrinology 79:10 (1966).
118. D. S. Schaloh and M. L. Parker, Nature (London) 203:1141 (1964).
119. W. M. Hunter and F. C. Greenwood, Biochem. J. 85:39P (1962).
120. A. Galskov, Radioimmunochemical Corticotropin Determination. Bogtrykkeriert Forum, Copenhagen, 1972.

121. W. D. Odell, P. L. Rayford, and G. T. Ross, J. Lab. Clin. Med. 70:973 (1967).
122. G. D. Bryant and F. C. Greenwood, Biochem. J. 109:831 (1968).
123. J. J. H. Gilkes, G. A. Bloomfield, A. P. Scott, P. J. Lowry, J. G. Ratcliffe, J. Landon, and L. H. Rees, J. Clin. Endocrinol. Metab. 40:450 (1975).
124. T. M. Nett, A. M. Akbar, G. D. Niswender, M. T. Hedlund, and W. F. White, J. Clin. Endocrinol. Metab. 36:880 (1973).
125. W. R. Keye, Jr., R. P. Kelch, G. D. Niswender, and R. B. Jaffe, J. Clin. Endocrinol. Metab. 36:1263 (1973).
126. A. Arimura, H. Soto, J. Kumasaka, R. B. Worobec, L. Debeljuk, J. Dunn, and A. V. Schally, Endocrinology 93:1092 (1973).
127. S. B. Bilezikian, H. L. Nossel, V. P. Butler, Jr., and R. E. Canfield, J. Clin. Invest. 56:438 (1975).
128. M. Lieberman, Anal. Biochem. 67:115 (1975).
129. L. J. Riceberg, H. van Vunakis, and L. Levine, Anal. Biochem. 60:551 (1974).
130. L. Levine and H. van Vanukis, Biochem. Biophys. Res. Commun. 41:1171 (1970).
131. I. Nejad, J. Bollinger, M. A. Mitnick, P. Sullivan, and S. Reichlin, Endocrinology 96:773 (1975).
132. R. S. Yalow, K. Hall, and R. Luft, J. Clin. Invest. 55:127 (1975).
133. B. F. Erlanger, S. M. Beiser, F. Borek, F. Edel, and S. Lieberman, in C. A. Williams and M. C. Chase (eds.), Methods in Immunology and Immunochemistry. Vol. 1. Academic Press, New York, 1967. p. 144.
134. I. H. Thorneycroft, S. A. Tillson, G. E. Abraham, R. J. Scaramuzzi, and B. V. Caldwell, in F. G. Peron and B. V. Caldwell (eds.), Immunologic Methods in Steroid Determination. Appleton-Century-Crofts, New York, 1970. p. 63.
135. L. Goodfriend and A. Schon, in F. G. Peron and B. V. Caldwell (eds.), Immunologic Methods in Steroid Determination. Appleton-Century-Crofts, New York, 1970. p. 15.
136. G. E. Abraham, Acta Endocrinol. (Copenhagen) Suppl., 183:7 (1974).
137. A. R. Midgley, Jr., and G. D. Niswender, Acta Endocrinol. (Copenhagen) Suppl. 147:320 (1970).
138. D. Mayes, S. Furuyama, D. C. Kem, and C. A. Nugent, J. Clin. Endocrinol. Metab. 30:682 (1970).
139. D. Tulchinsky and G. E. Abraham, J. Clin. Endocrinol. Metab. 33:775 (1971).
140. G. E. Abraham, J. Clin. Endocrinol. Metab. 29:866 (1969).
141. G. Mikhail, C. H. Wu, M. Ferin, and R. L. Vande Wiele, Acta Endocrinol. (Copenhagen) Suppl. 147:347 (1970).
142. G. E. Abraham, R. Swerdloff, D. Tulchinsky, and W. D. Odell, J. Clin. Endocrinol. Metab. 32:619 (1971).
143. S. Furuyama, D. M. Mayes, and C. A. Nugent, Steroids 16:415 (1970).
144. G. E. Abraham, J. E. Buster, and R. C. Teller, Anal. Lett. 5:757 (1972).
145. T. W. Smith, V. P. Butler, and E. Haber, N. Engl. J. Med. 281:1212 (1969).
146. W. H. Daughaday, J. Clin. Invest. 37:519 (1958).
147. W. R. Slaunwhite and A. A. Sandberg, J. Clin. Invest. 38:384 (1959).
148. R. C. Puche and W. R. Nes, Endocrinology 70:857 (1962).
149. J. E. Plager, J. Clin. Invest. 44:1234 (1965).
150. B. E. P. Murphy, J. Clin. Endocrinol. 27:973 (1967).
151. P. F. Dixon, M. Booth, and J. Butler, in C. H. Gray and A. L. Bacharach (eds.), Hormones in Blood. Vol. 2. Academic Press, New York, 1967. pp. 325–338.
152. B. E. P. Murphy, Nature 201:679 (1964).
153. J. D. Neill, E. D. B. Johansson, J. K. Datta, and E. Knobil, J. Clin. Endocrinol. 27:1167 (1967).

Chapter 4

Formation of the Isopentenoid Unit

A. General and Historical Comments 147
   1. *Biosynthetic Relationship of Steroids to Other Isopentenoids* 147
   2. *Role of Acetoacetate and β-Hydroxy-β-Methylglutarate* 150
   3. *Discovery of Mevalonic Acid* 151
   4. *Structure and Properties of Mevalonic Acid* 151
   5. *Role of Mevalonic Acid* 153
B. Biosynthesis of Mevalonic Acid 155
   1. *Development of Cell-Free Systems* 155
   2. *Roles of Coenzyme A and Acyl Carrier Protein* 155
   3. *Formation of Hydroxymethylglutarate* 156
   4. *Reduction of Hydroxymethylglutarate to Mevalonic Acid* 157
C. Structure and Biosynthesis of the C_5 Unit 159
   1. *Conversion of Mevalonate to Δ^3-Isopentenyl Pyrophosphate* 159
   2. *Interconversion of Δ^3- and Δ^2-Isopentenyl Pyrophosphate* 161
D. Stereochemistry 161
   1. *Absolute Configuration of C_6 Compounds* 161
   2. *Stereochemistry of Elimination to Form C_5 Units* 162
   3. *Stereochemistry of the Isomerization of the C_5 Units* 162
Literature Cited 166

A. GENERAL AND HISTORICAL COMMENTS

1. Biosynthetic Relationship of Steroids to Other Isopentenoids

The existence of an isopentenoid unit and its role as a biosynthetic precursor of natural products were first envisioned by Wallach in the 1880s. A discussion of his ideas and of their extension by Ruzicka into "the isoprene rule" is to be found in Chapter 1. In summary, the presence of a repeating "isoprenoid" or, now more properly, isopentenoid unit in the structures of rubber, terpenes, and carotenoids clearly indicated to the early workers that a biochemical polymerization must be operating in which an isopentenoid unit functions as the reacting monomer. They thought that isoprene might represent the monomer from which the term "isoprenoid" is derived. That the same C_5 monomer is involved in steroid biosynthesis was somewhat less clear. It was strongly indicated by the structures of the side chain and a part of ring D of cholesterol (Scheme 4.1), which were strictly composed of such units, but the remainder of the molecule was not. In particular, there was an insufficient number of carbon atoms, especially of methyl groups. Cholesterol has only 27 carbon atoms. Nevertheless, as early as 1926, Channon (1) and Heilbron et al. (2) raised the possibility that cholesterol might be derived from an otherwise obscure C_{30}-hydrocarbon called squalene, which was shown to follow the "isoprene rule." Squalene had been isolated and named just after the turn of the century by Tsujimoto (3-5) and later by Chapman (6), who called it spinacene, from shark and other fish livers, and Channon (1) actually observed an increase in rat liver cholesterol when animals were fed the substance. Its fully isopentenoid structure (Scheme 4.1)

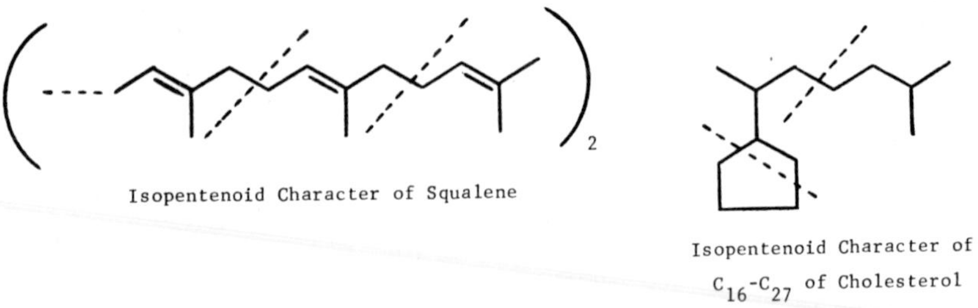

Isopentenoid Character of Squalene

Isopentenoid Character of
$C_{16}-C_{27}$ of Cholesterol

Scheme 4.1. Isopentenoid units in squalene and sterols.

was established in the laboratories of Heilbron and Karrer in 1929–1931 by degradation (7, 8) and synthesis (9), and a few years later Robinson (10) proposed a particular mode of cyclization that, followed by removal of three carbon atoms, would yield the skeleton of cholesterol. Thus, by the mid-1930s there was a theoretical framework that not only related steroids to classic "isoprenoids" such as squalene but also in consequence predicted the existence of a particular kind of biosynthetic sequence, viz., the formation of a C_5 unit, its polymerization, cyclization, and further metabolism. This was a remarkable achievement, since, as Bloch (11) has remarked, "Unlike most high molecular cell constituents (proteins, polysaccharides, fatty acids, alkaloids), the steroids display little structural information from which an a priori reasonable reaction path or the nature of the biogenetic subunits could have been deduced."

The first direct evidence that steroids and "isoprenoids" are in fact derived through a common pathway came ultimately from the discovery that acetate is the precursor both of sterols and of rubber. In 1937 Sonderhoff and Thomas (*12*) showed that trideuteroacetate is incorporated into the sterol fraction of yeast. In agreement with acetate as a sterol precursor, the same year Rittenberg and Schoenheimer (*13*) found deuterium in the cholesterol of mice fed deuterated water; 5 years later Bloch and Rittenberg (*14, 15*) demonstrated clearly that acetate serves as a precursor of cholesterol in rats. Then in the period 1949–1951, Bonner and Arrequin (*16–19*) achieved experimental biosynthesis of rubber, finding not only that acetate but also the C₅ compound, β,β-dimethylacrylate (DMA, sometimes known as β-methylcrotonate), increases its formation in guayule plants (*Parthenium argentatum*). They suggested that three molecules of acetate might condense with the loss of one carboxyl group to give the C₅ monomer. The possibility of β,β-dimethylacrylate's functioning in this capacity was tantalizing but not experimentally verifiable. Nevertheless, if acetate did lead to the monomer, the monomer would be expected to have the labeling pattern shown in Scheme 4.2 (see Section A.2 for details). The advent of radioactive carbon made it

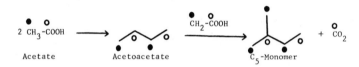

Scheme 4.2. Expected labeling pattern of C₅ monomer from acetate.

possible to explore this readily, and in 1952, through the work of Wuersch, Huang, and Bloch (*20*), exactly the expected labeling pattern was shown to arise from acetate in the side chain of cholesterol. Furthermore, at essentially the same time Grob et al. (*21*) obtained β-carotene using acetate as a source of carbon, and Langdon and Bloch (*22*) obtained squalene from this same small acid. The availability of biosynthetically labeled [¹⁴C]squalene immediately allowed the critical test: try to obtain cholesterol using it as precursor. Langdon and Bloch (*23*) did the experiment with positive and far-reaching results. By obtaining [¹⁴C]cholesterol from similarly labeled squalene, they presented final and unequivocal proof that steroids are derived from a common pathway with the classic "isoprenoids."

Subsequent extensive work by Cornforth and Popjak (*24–28*) on the labeling pattern in the ring system of cholesterol after biosynthesis from labeled acetate has substantiated that the entire molecule is derived from a C₅ monomer. The labeling pattern is shown in Scheme 4.3. As will be seen, not only is each carbon atom derived from one or the other of the carbon atoms of acetate, but the distribution of the methyl and carboxyl carbons, e.g., at C-1, C-10, C-19, C-5, and C-6, is for the most part the same

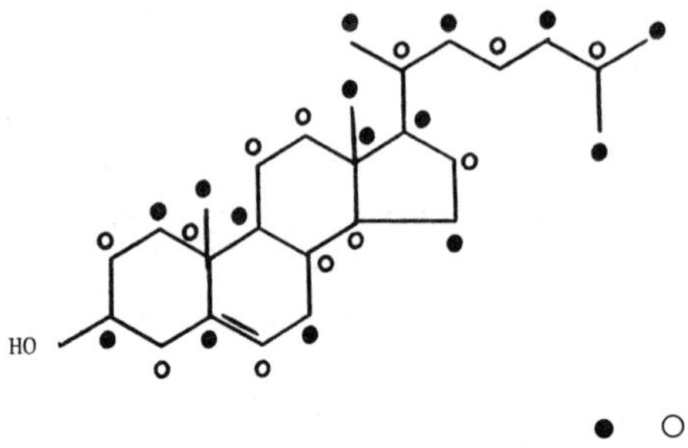

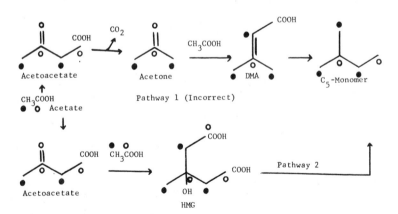

Scheme 4.3. Labeling pattern of cholesterol from CH₃-COOH.

as in the side chain, e.g., at C-26, C-27, C-25, C-24, and C-23, as predicted by the utilization of three molecules of acetate which condense and decarboxylate to the isopentenoid monomer (cf. Scheme 4.2). The fact that a regular alternation of methyl and carboxyl carbons does not fully exist, e.g., at C-13 and C-18 where both are derived from the methyl group of acetate, was ultimately explained and verified experimentally by rearrangements during cyclization (see Chapter 7).

2. Role of Acetoacetate and β-Hydroxy-β-Methylglutarate

Concurrently with the work on acetate, various investigators were studying the incorporation of label from other small molecules, e.g., isovalerate (29). Of particular significance, Brady and Gurin (30) succeeded in developing evidence for the direct utilization of all four carbon atoms of acetoacetate. This meant that a suggested (18) route from acetate via acetoacetate, decarboxylation to acetone, and a second condensation with acetate to give DMA could not precisely account for C₅ formation (see pathway 1 in Scheme 4.4).

Scheme 4.4. Possible origins of the C₅ monomer.

Acetone would contain only three of the four carbon atoms. The alternative possibility, pathway 2, that acetoacetate reacts with acetate in the manner that it does with oxaloacetate in the Krebs cycle, was quickly appreciated in several laboratories and has been reviewed by Rudney (*31*). Rabinowitz and Gurin (*32*) were able to show in 1954 that the expected product, β-hydroxy-β-methylglutarate (HMG), serves as a precursor of cholesterol, and Kloster-man and Smith (*33*) and Adams and Van Duuren (*34*) proved its natural occurrence. HMG, however, also is found on other pathways, e.g., between leucine and acetoacetate (*35*), and for this and other reasons (cf. Sections E.2 and E.4) the yield of cholesterol is experimentally poor. This made the use of HMG as a substrate for further biosynthesis quite difficult and uncertain. Therefore, all the work so far accomplished still shed but little light on the actual nature of the C_5 unit. Whatever it was, it was derived from acetate via acetoacetate and probably via HMG. β,β-Dimethylacylate might be the next step. At least the labeling patterns (Schemes 4.2 and 4.4) from acetate in both DMA and HMG in liver preparations (*36, 37*) were in accord with such a pathway. It remained for serendipity to bridge the gap between probability and certainty.

3. Discovery of Mevalonic Acid

As chance would have it, during this same period Novak and Hague (*38*) had been studying the promotion of growth in chicks and rats by "concentrates" of "dried distillers' solubles." They felt they had a new vitamin and named it vitamin B_{13}. A large group at Merck, Sharp and Dohme under Folkers (*39*) became interested in the "vitamin" and devised an assay procedure in which the growth response of the bacterium, *Lactobacillus acidophilus* ATCC 4963, was measured in a medium devoid of acetate. While they were unable to obtain a promotion of growth in chicks under certain dietary conditions (*40*), they did obtain marked response of the bacterium to preparations from the "distillers' solubles" (*41*). This still suggested the presence of an interesting material warranting continued study. On the assumption that it might be lipoic acid, they began fractionation of the "solubles" by counter current distribution using ether-water as the partition system. Evidence for lipoic acid was actually obtained, but, much more importantly, the fractionation yielded another material, which appeared to be a new one (*42, 43*). Its growth-promoting effects in the bacterial assay were remarkable, approximating the response to acetate, and it was accordingly regarded as a new "acetate-replacing factor." Being an apparently new physiologically active substance it might, the Merck group thought (*39*), have value beyond growth promotion in *Lactobacillus*. What? They had no idea, but their active pursuit of the unknown was fortunate. The "acetate-replacing factor" was soon shown to be the first specific precursor of cholesterol. Furthermore, while it was not the sought-after C_5 unit, experiments with MVA led directly to the discovery of this important unit.

4. Structure and Properties of Mevalonic Acid

Subsequent fractionations yielded the "acetate-replacing factor" as a color-less oil, unrelated to lipoic acid, with infrared absorption typical of hydroxy lactones. Hydrolysis yielded an acid with the formula $C_6H_{12}O_4$. It was con-vertible to a solid amide with benzhydrylamine showing optical activity with $[\alpha]_D - 2.0°$. The amide formed an optically active acetate, $[\alpha]_D + 1.6°$, and possessed one C-methyl group. From this and other data the free acid was shown (44) to have the structure of 3,5-dihydroxy-3-methylpentanoic acid. Since a methylpentanoic acid is, in systematic nomenclature, a methyl-valeric acid, the trivial name *mevalonic acid* (MVA) was coined (39). A solid, stable, nontoxic, and water-soluble derivative was found in the N,N'-di-benzylethylenediammonium salt, m.p. 124–125°. Known as the DBED salt, it is widely used experimentally. The numbering system for mevalonate it-self and the structure of the entire DBED salt are shown in Scheme 4.5. It will be seen that MVA possesses an isopentenoid moiety at C-2, C-3, C-3', C-4, and C-5.

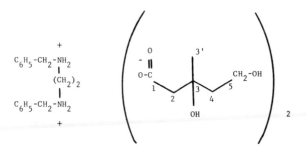

Scheme 4.5. DBED salt of mevalonic acid.

Mevalonic acid is asymmetric at position—3. Its racemate was obtained by two synthetic routes (44, 45) and resolved (46) by fractional crystallization of the α-phenyl-1-naphthalenemethylamine amides. The dextrorotatory enantiomer upon hydrolysis produced exactly the same response with *L. acidophilus* as had the material isolated from "distillers' solubles."

Curiously enough, at the same time in Japan, Tamura (47) was studying the spoilage of sake by "Hiochi" bacteria, *L. homohiochi* and *L. heterohiochi*. Evidence had accumulated that sake and broths of several microorganisms contain a growth-promoting factor for the bacteria. Tamura succeeded in isolating the substance as the quinine salt from *Aspergillus oryzae*. It was named "hiochic acid." Preliminary work on its structure proved it to be a dihydroxy-C_6-acid, and an exchange of samples with the Merck group soon showed it was identical with MVA (39).

5. Role of Mevalonic Acid

The Merck group (*39*), working on the isolation and structure of MVA, was split into two parts, one in West Point, Pa., and the other in Rahway, N.J. In West Point, just a few doors away from the laboratory where some of the MVA work was being done, Tavormina, Gibbs, and Huff were independently studying, among other things, the origin of cholesterol. They were, therefore, well aware of the implication of HMG and DMA in isopentenoid biosynthesis. When the structure of MVA became evident, it was obvious to them that MVA might also be on the pathway. Racemic [2-^{14}C]mevalonate was prepared and incubated with a rat liver homogenate. The results (*48, 49*) were a 43% incorporation of the label into sterol. On the assumption that only one enantiomer is active (which has since been verified), the yield from the active material was 86%. By contrast, [3′-^{14}C]HMG and [4-^{14}C]DMA gave only 0.16% and 3.8% incorporations, respectively. Mevalonic acid must then be truly on the pathway. Moreover, by labeling C-1 (the COOH group) with ^{14}C and incubating it with a cell-free system from rat liver, they found cholesterol to be unlabeled. The radioactivity appeared instead in CO_2. This proved that C-2, C-3, C-3′, C-4, and C-5 must ultimately constitute the C_5 unit.

During the next few years, [2-^{14}C]mevalonate became generally available, and it was enthusiastically examined in several laboratories as a precursor to a variety of isopentenoids. Squalene was soon found to be specifically derived from it both in animals (*50-52*) and in yeast (*53*) and photosynthetic plants (*54-56*). The typical plant sterol, sitosterol (*56-64*), various terpenes (*54,59, 65-69*), rubber (*70*), carotenoids (*70-73*), and the isopentenoid portion of ubiquinone (*74-76*) all were found to incorporate radioactivity readily from MVA. Furthermore, in several cases the labeling pattern was determined by degradation. Squalene is an especially important example. Both in the animal (*50, 52*) and plant (*77*) kingdoms the data are in accord with the pattern shown in Scheme 4.6. The discrimination (*77*) between the *cis*- and

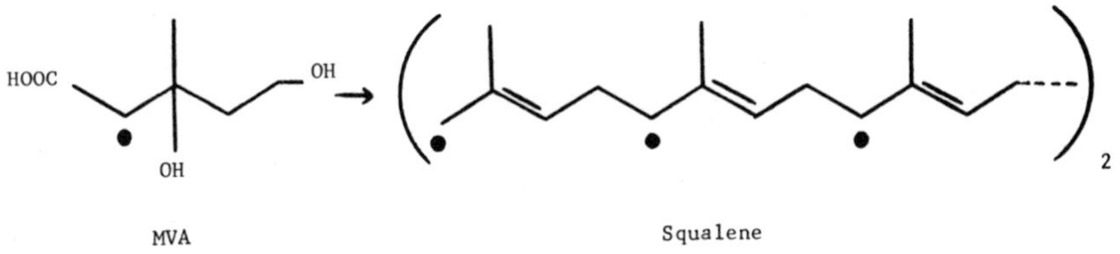

HOOC　　　　　OH　→

MVA　　　　　　　　Squalene

Scheme 4.6. Labeling pattern of squalene from [2-^{14}C]MVA.

trans-methyl groups at the terminus is, however, indirect. It is discussed in Section D.3, and relates to the details of the polymerization of the C_5 monomer. Cholesterol derived from [2-^{14}C]MVA has likewise been degraded, with results in keeping with expectation (78). Furthermore, when unlabeled squalene was incubated with [2-^{14}C]MVA, label appeared mostly in squalene, which acted as a trapping agent, but in the absence of squalene the label appeared primarily in sterol (50). This demonstrates clearly that the squalene to cholesterol pathway is operating with MVA as the source of carbon. The degradation of β-carotene (71, 79) after biosynthesis from [2-^{14}C]mevalonate also has yielded the same labeling pattern in the C$_5$ units as is indicated in Scheme 4.6 for squalene.

There were early reports that some steroids, viz., sapogenins (80) and adrenal corticosteroids (81), were not experimentally derivable from MVA in plant homogenates or tissue slices, respectively, despite incorporation of label from acetate. While the reasons for the difficulties are not entirely clear, the particular steroids in question almost certainly are derived from MVA in the usual way. Caspi and his associates (82) have obtained cortisol in vitro from [1-^{14}C]acetate with bovine adrenals and removed carbon atoms Nos. 1, 2, 3, 4, 5, 6, 7, 20, and 24. The labeling pattern is in accord with expectation (cf. Scheme 4.3). Furthermore, Eik-Nes and co-workers (83) actually achieved biosythesis of corticosteroids from mevalonate by prolonged incubation with pig adrenal slices, although the yields were not good, and other endocrine tissue of mammals, such as ovaries (84), have also yielded steroid hormones from MVA. The problem in yield appears to lie in such things as enzyme activities, transport, and compartmentation. Acetate rapidly penetrates adrenal cells but mevalonate does not (85), and broken cells release a microsomal adenosine triphosphatase (85), which reduces the availability of ATP. This behavior is much more severe than with liver tissue, but similar to chloroplasts, which have been reported not to be permeable to MVA (86). The sapogenin problem probably has its origins in similar phenomena, because in vivo conversion of mevalonate into sapogenins with either the 25α- or 25β-configuration has been achieved with Dioscorea spiculifora (62).

While experiments such as those described in Sections A.1 and A.2 had raised the possibility that DMA might be on the pathway, and while it is theoretically conceivable to place it there either after or independent of mevalonate (87), Jacobsohn and Corley (88) have clearly excluded it from the mammalian route to cholesterol. They found that in biotin-deficient animals the utilization of DMA was abolished without affecting incorporation of acetate. The reason for this is that DMA requires conversion by CO_2 fixation and hydration to HMG before its conversion to cholesterol. In biotin-deficient animals, CO_2 fixation is inhibited. Rudney and Farkas (89) in fact showed that, with liver preparations in which the incorporation of CO_2 into HMG had been abolished, the formation of HMG from acetate was not impaired. Similarly, the incorporation of [1-^{14}C]acetate into nonsaponifiable materials in biotin-deficient yeast was not depressed but in fact enhanced over levels of incorporation normally observed (90). Baisted and Nes (87) have also found that in vivo MVA is a better precursor to sterols and pent-acyclic triterpenes in plants than is DMA by a factor of 10^3 to 10^4, which mitigates heavily against the latter's direct involvement in isopentenoid bio-synthesis. In fact, evidence was obtained by Baisted and Nes (*87*) for the conversion of DMA to HMG in the plant studied (peas). As discussed in detail in Section B.3, HMG is the precursor to MVA. This, together with the facts that MVA is the first specific compound on the isopentenoid path-way and that quantitative control of the amount of isopentenoid biosynthesis resides at the mevalonate stage, explains why there is incorporation of label from DMA as well as why it happens only at a low level.

In view of all of the evidence, it is essentially certain that mevalonate is the ubiquitous precursor of the C_5 unit in all cases of de novo isopentenoid biosynthesis regardless of the tissue in which it occurs or of the structure of the final product.

B. BIOSYNTHESIS OF MEVALONIC ACID

1. Development of Cell-Free Systems

The elucidation of the details of the biosynthesis and further metabolism of mevalonic acid has depended on some very sophisticated experimentation, which would have been quite impossible had it not been for the development of cell-free systems capable of carrying out the reactions. This was first achieved in the early 1950s for animal tissue by Bucher (*91*), Bucher and McGarrahan (*92*), and Rabinowitz and Gurin (*93*). Similar preparations from yeast were subsequently found (*53, 94*). The procedures allow disrup-tion of the cell as a physiologic entity while maintaining the biosynthetic integrity of the mitochondria and microsomes, which have subsequently been shown to be the sites of a great deal of the metabolic capacity. The principal advantage of cell-free systems is that they can be treated in much the same way as a simple chemical system in that cofactors, inhibitors, etc., can be added. The input or loss of chemicals from the biosynthetic site is minimal, and clear deductions about the reactions occurring can be made.

2. Roles of Coenzyme A and Acyl Carrier Protein

Rudney (*31, 95*) found that an extract from microsomes that could synthe-size HMG from acetate required ATP and CoA, but acetyl-CoA served equally well in the absence of these cofactors. These experiments made it unequivocal that, as in other enolate condensations involving acetate such as the formation of fatty acids, the thiol ester bond is required. Although more work is required, it appears from preliminary evidence (*96, 97*) that the thiol utilized is primarily but not necessarily only CoA in both yeast and rats. The alternative is the use of acyl carrier protein (*96*) or conceivably enzyme or other protein (*98, 99*). Thus, in the presence of the yeast con-densing enzyme for the reaction of acetate and acetoacetate to give HMG, acetoacetyl-CoA reacts six times as quickly as does acetoacetyl-ACP, and the former does not undergo a transacylation with ACP to give the latter (*96*).

There are reasons for believing from investigations of fatty acid biosynthesis that the utilization of acyl carrier protein might also involve malonate. In the simplest case, acetyl-ACP condenses with malonyl-ACP, eliminating CO_2, to give acetoacetyl-ACP. In further elongation of the chain, the C_2 units are derived from malonyl-ACP. However, the utilization of malonate in mevalonate biosynthesis (*98, 99*) appears not to be an absolute requirement (*96*), although the question remains unsettled (*100–102*). The final analysis of this problem may have to contend with species and/or tissue differences as well as with other factors that regulate fatty acid biosynthesis. In subsequent sections we shall ignore the problem and employ CoA for purposes of general discussion, although literature citations will of course imply that it was actually used.

3. Formation of Hydroxymethylglutarate

Extensive work, especially by Rudney and his associates (*95, 96, 103–105*), has shown that 2 moles of acetyl-CoA condense to give acetoacetyl-CoA. The latter, by further condensation at the keto group with a third molecule of acetyl-CoA, which undergoes hydrolytic loss of CoA, yields hydroxymethyl-glutarate CoA (HMG-CoA) (Scheme 4.7). The loss of CoA (*103, 104*) from

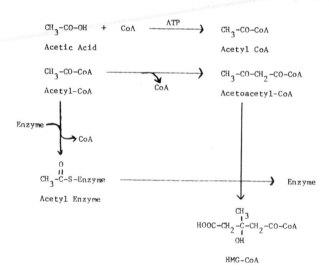

Scheme 4.7. Biosynthesis of hydroxymethylglutarate.

the last acetyl-CoA molecule to condense was demonstrated (*105*) by the alternative labeling of the carbonyl carbon atom of the acetate portion and one of the carbon atoms in the CoA portion of the molecule with ^{14}C. In the former case, radioactive HMG-CoA was obtained, while in the latter case unlabeled HMG-CoA resulted, and free radioactive CoA was identified. It has been demonstrated that the free CoA is derived from the intermediate formation of an acetyl-enzyme intermediate (94, 106), the final formation of the HMG-CoA being the resultant of the condensation of the protein bound acetyl group with the acetoacetyl-CoA and concomitant or probably (106) subsequent hydrolytic cleavage of the thioester bond between the acetyl portion of the HMG-CoA and the enzyme. The thiol ester linkage of the acetoacetyl-CoA remains intact (but see Section B.2 for the alternative use of acetoacetyl-ACP), because acetoacetyl-CoA labeled with tritium in the CoA portion leads to radioactive HMG-CoA upon incubation with unlabeled acetyl-CoA and the condensing enzyme (106).

The purification and assay of the condensing enzyme from bakers' yeast have been described in detail by Stewart and Rudney (94), who also compared it with thiolase, the enzyme that catalyzes an equilibrium between acetoacetyl-CoA, CoA, and 2 moles of acetyl-CoA. Thiolase is strongly inhibited by treatment with trypsin, while the HMG-CoA condensing enzyme is more resistant to it. Trypsin treatment has been used very effectively to free the condensing enzyme of thiolase activity, thereby preventing contamination of added acetyl-CoA with any acetyl-CoA from retrocondensation of acetoacetyl-CoA.

4. Reduction of Hydroxymethylglutarate to Mevalonic Acid

The conversion of HMG to MVA requires in principle a two-stage reduction, in which a C_6 compound at the aldehyde stage of oxidation is an intermediate. This aldehyde, named mevaldic acid by the Merck group (39), was synthesized (46) and shown to depress the incorporation of label from [1-^{14}C] acetate into cholesterol in rats (46). Since acetate labeled in this way also leads in the same animal to mevalonic acid (108), the depression in cholesterol biosynthesis is consistent with the intermediacy of mevaldate. A ^{14}C-labeled sample of the latter was also shown to lead to [^{14}C]cholesterol with rat liver homogenates (39) and to squalene and sterols in yeast (109). Partial purification of the yeast HMG-CoA reductase that catalyzes the conversion of HMG-CoA to mevalonate was soon achieved (109–112), from which it was shown that two moles of NADPH are specifically required. Mevaldic acid, however, has presented some difficulties of interpretation. While the theoretical and experimental aspects just discussed are incontrovertible, there have been problems in showing that mevaldic acid per se is involved as a free intermediate (110–111). The suggestion (113) has been made that it is present in a bound form in which the aldehyde group has been converted to an acetal-like structure by reaction with a sulfhydryl group. The addition product of mevaldate and coenzyme A actually is reduced by HMG-CoA reductase from yeast at a faster rate than is mevaldate itself (114). Kirtley and Rudney (*112*) have also examined the kinetics and other properties of a highly purified preparation of the reductase (MW 150,000–200,000), and they find that the results are compatible with a mechanism in which an enzyme-mevaldate complex exists. The reduction of HMG-CoA to mevalonic acid is strongly displaced toward the latter (*110–112*), and the enzyme is inhibited by sulfhydryl reagents (*110–112*). The structure of mevaldic acid together with a simplified version of the route from HMG-CoA to MVA is shown in Scheme 4.8. The reaction is believed to occur by a so-called "ping-

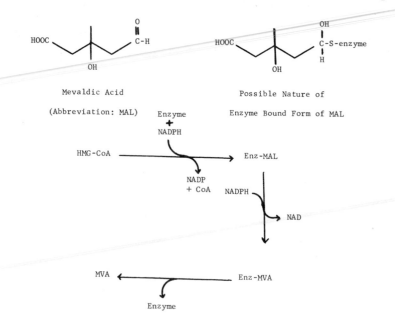

Scheme 4.8. Mevaldic acid and its role in the conversion of hydroxymethylglutarate-CoA to mevalonic acid.

pong mechanism" in which the enzyme has the alternative of being bound either to mevaldate or to mevalonate (*112*). Such a mechanism operates in other systems, such as with transaminase, which is bound alternately to pyridoxal or to pyridoxamine (*115–116*). In the "ping-pong mechanism," mevaldic acid does not occur as a true intermediate, which is released from the enzyme on which it was formed. This means that no simple pool of the free intermediate exists and that trapping experiments are necessarily doomed to failure or at best to quantitative inexactness. The capacity of added mevaldic acid to enter the enzymatic system at all depends on the more subtle point of the extent to which the enzyme will accept preformed compound in contrast to having it already available through formation at the active site. The full enzymological details have yet to be elucidated.

C. STRUCTURE AND BIOSYNTHESIS OF THE C_5 UNIT

1. Conversion of Mevalonate to Δ^3-Isopentenyl Pyrophosphate

The discovery of mevalonic acid and of the utilization of five of its six carbon atoms in high yield for isopentenoid biosynthesis (Section A.5) made it clear that the isopentenoid monomer for polymerization must be an MVA metabolite. The true nature of the unit was elucidated shortly afterwards through the use of labeled MVA as a substrate in incubations with cell-free systems. Work in Lynen's laboratory (53, 109, 117) was especially productive with these systems prepared from yeast. Squalene was readily produced, but there was little accumulation of intermediates to allow isolation and identification. The key to the problem finally lay in inhibitors and in cofactor requirements.

Popjak and Bloch and their associates (118, 119) found for both liver and yeast systems a requirement for ATP, reduced pyridine nucleotide, and a divalent cation in order to convert MVA to squalene. The requirement for pyridine nucleotide was not associated with the formation of the C_5 unit, because in its absence a C_{10} metabolite was formed (Chapter 5), but the ATP requirement was found by Tchen (120, 121) to involve an initial conversion of MVA to its primary, i.e., at C-5, phosphate ester. Bloch and his associates (122–126) then found a second and third ATP molecule to be involved in the next two steps. The second ATP molecule produces mevalonic acid 5-pyrophosphate. In the succeeding step ATP induces elimination of CO_2 and the elements of water, yielding a C_5 compound identified as Δ^3-isopentenyl pyrophosphate (122, 123). Chemical synthesis (126) provided a sample that had the same properties as the biosynthetic product and yielded squalene upon incubation with yeast extracts (126). At the same time, Lynen and his group (53) discovered that [2-^{14}C]MVA 5-phosphate, Mg^{++}, and ATP, when incubated with a cell-free yeast system in the presence of two-hundredth molar iodoacetamide, produced an acidic (collidine-extractable) radioactive compound. The same compound was formed from MVA 5-phosphate labeled with ^{32}P instead of with ^{14}C, but no label from [1-^{14}C]MVA 5-phosphate was incorporated. Thus, the product must have lost CO_2 and been converted to the same C_5 unit obtained by Bloch. Further work, including degradation and synthesis, demonstrated (53) the compound to be Δ^3-isopentenyl pyrophosphate (3-methyl-Δ^3-butenyl pyrophosphate). Reincubation of this intermediate with Mg^{++} and NADPH with the yeast system yielded squalene, and with a *Hevea brasiliensis* system it yielded rubber. The C_5-pyrophosphate was 10 times more efficient than MVA. A few years later Chichester and his associates (127, 128) found that Δ^3-isopentenyl pyrophosphate also yielded β-carotene and lycopene in appropriate plant systems and that iodoacetamide inhibited carotenoid biosynthesis from MVA. The data therefore demonstrated that for steroids, as well as for other isopentenoids, there is a common C_5 unit that, while it is not Wallach's isoprene, is a closely related hydrated ester. Corroboration of the absence of isoprene in the pathway was independently provided (50).

The formation of Δ^3-isopentenyl pyrophosphate was shown in Bloch's laboratory (124) to involve the attack of ATP on MVA 5-pyrophosphate at the tertiary alcohol group. When the MVA was labeled with ^{18}O in the latter group, ^{18}O-labeled phosphate ion could be isolated. Their stoichiometric measurements indicated one mole of ATP and one mole of MVA 5-pyrophosphate as reactants, and one mole of ADP, one mole of phosphate ion, one mole of Δ^3-isopentenyl pyrophosphate, and one mole of CO_2 as products. An intermediate tertiary phosphate ester could not be isolated and is tentatively presumed not to exist as such. The data can be interpreted at the moment to mean that a concerted elimination of CO_2 and the elements of water (as H^+ and phosphate ion) occurs as shown in Scheme 4.9. The con-

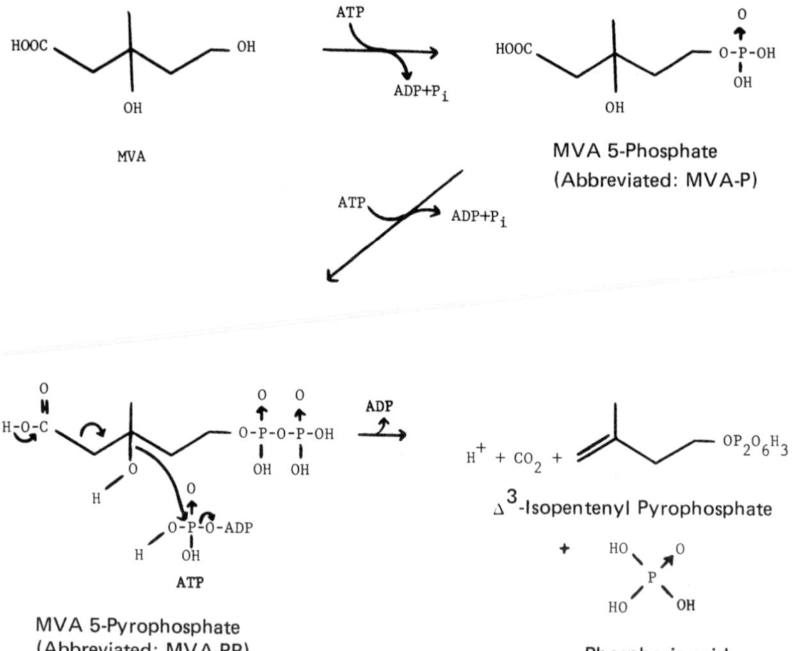

Scheme 4.9. Conversion of mevalonic acid to Δ^3-isopentenyl pyrophosphate.

certed nature of these elimination reactions to form a C_5 unit from MVA had previously been predicted by Bloch and his associates (129). Variations of the mechanism have been discussed (124). The enzyme catalyzing the formation of MVA 5-phosphate is known as mevalonic kinase (120, 121, 130, 131), that for the second phosphorylation is phosphomevalonic kinase

($122-124$, 132), and the enzyme for the final step is pyrophosphomevalonic anhydrodecarboxylase (53, 124).

2. Interconversion of Δ^3- and Δ^2-Isopentenyl Pyrophosphate

It was soon appreciated that a *pair* of C_5 units are probably involved in isopentenoid biosynthesis rather than just the one found to be Δ^3-isopentenyl pyrophosphate. More particularly, if the Δ^3-compound were to isomerize to the Δ^2-isomer, a reasonable coupling mechanism (53) for polymerization was apparent (Chapter 5). Lynen's group (117, 133) provided unequivocal proof of such an isomerization by purifying the yeast isomerase and demonstrating the formation of Δ^2-isopentenyl pyrophosphate (dimethylallyl pyrophosphate) and its equilibration with the Δ^3-compound. The equilibrium was found to lie strongly (93%) toward the Δ^2-isomer. The enzyme possesses an active SH group and is inhibited by iodoacetamide. More recently, it has been purified from mammalian liver (134, 135). It is known as isopentenyl pyrophosphate isomerase (EC 5.3.3.2) or sometimes as prenyl isomerase. The mammalian enzyme possesses a pH maximum at 6.0, has a K_m for the Δ^3-isomer of 4×10^{-6} M, is activated by Mn^{++}, and catalyzes a reversible isomerization, the equilibrium for which lies toward the Δ^2-isomer (135). Consequently, after formation of the Δ^3-compound from MVA 5-pyrophosphate, the next step in the biosynthetic sequence must be the isomerization, as shown in Scheme 4.10. The mechanism of isomerization is not yet clear.

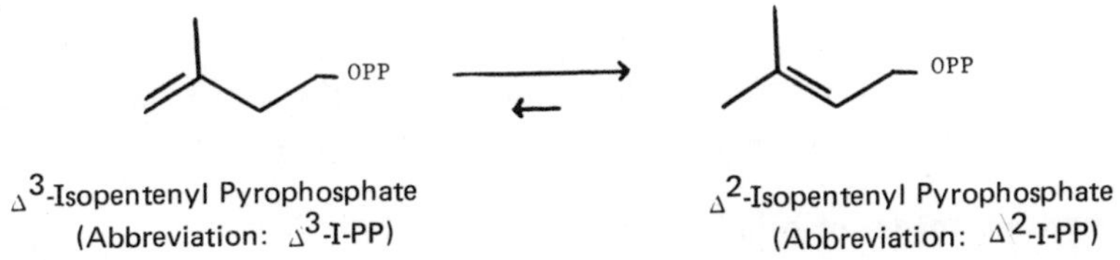

Δ^3-Isopentenyl Pyrophosphate Δ^2-Isopentenyl Pyrophosphate
(Abbreviation: Δ^3-I-PP)   (Abbreviation: Δ^2-I-PP)

Scheme 4.10. The C_5 unit pair and their interconversion.

The intermediate formation of an enzyme-bound form (joined through a sulfur link) has been suggested (133), as has a more direct double-bond migration (addition and elimination of protons) (113). The mechanism is discussed further in Section D.3.

D. STEREOCHEMISTRY

1. Absolute Configuration of C_6 Compounds

Natural ($+$)-mevalonic acid [which yields a ($-$)-benzhydrylamide] has been shown to have the R configuration (136). By inference the configurations of the active enantiomers of HMG-CoA and of mevaldate must be analogous, as shown in Scheme 4.11, where all the structures are meant to imply that the methyl group points toward and the tertiary hydroxyl group away from an observer whose view of the molecule shows the COOH group to the left,

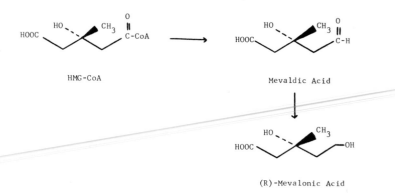

Scheme 4.11. Absolute configuration of isopentenoid precursors.

C-2, C-3, and C-4 in a plane (the plane of the paper) that is perpendicular to the direction of view, and the central carbon atom (C-3) up relative to the two CH$_2$ groups on either side.

Lactobacillus acidophilus biosynthesizes only (+)-mevalonate and will utilize only this enantiomer, the antipode remaining essentially unchanged (*109*). Similarly, when the radioactive racemate is fed to rats, about half of the label is excreted in the urine within 6 hr. The urinary product is (−)-mevalonic acid (*137*). The enzymic reduction of HMG-CoA and the phosphorylation of MVA are both demonstrably stereospecific (*121, 138*).

2. Stereochemistry of Elimination to Form C$_5$ Units

The formation of Δ^2-isopentenyl pyrophosphate occurs by a *trans*-elimination, as shown by Cornforth et al. (*139*) from studies of mevalonate that had been labeled stereospecifically with deuterium at the carbon atom (C-2) bearing the carboxyl group.

3. Stereochemistry of the Isomerization of the C$_5$ Units

Stereospecificity also arises in the isomerization of Δ^3- to Δ^2-isopentenyl pyrophosphate. This is apparent from the labeling pattern in squalene biosynthesized from [2-^{14}C]mevalonate (Scheme 4.6). Degradation (*50, 52, 77*) of squalene from both plants and animals has proved the position of the labeled carbon atoms in the central four isopentenoid units, but the location in the terminal units was first deduced from indirect evidence (*77*). Direct degradation yields methyl-labeled acetone in which the two methyl groups are equivalent. Consequently, one cannot discriminate between labeling in the *cis*- versus *trans*-positions of the original squalene. However, ergot alkaloids, e.g., agroclavine, biosynthesized from [2-^{14}C]mevalonate have the moiety and labeling pattern (*140, 141*) shown in Scheme 4.12. It will be apparent that localization

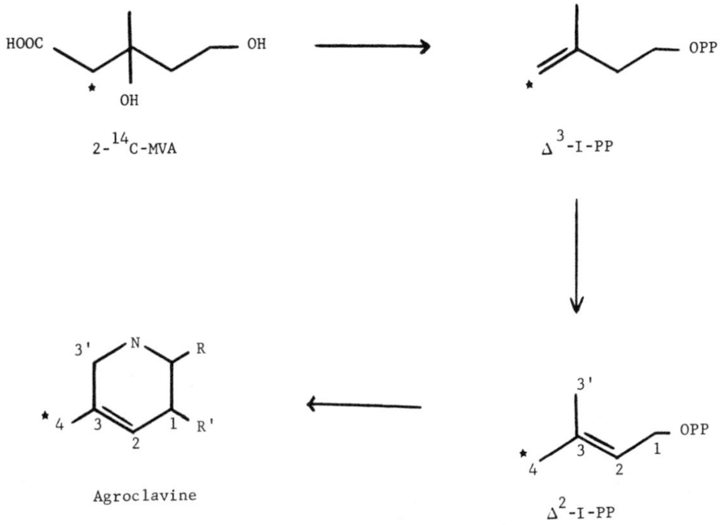

Scheme 4.12. Determination of labeling pattern in isopentenyl pyrophosphates.

of the label in the methyl group of the fungal alkaloid means (*77*) that the label in the intermediate Δ^2-isopentenyl pyrophosphate must be in the methyl group (C-4), which is *trans*-oriented to C-1. More recently, the proton magnetic resonance spectra of appropriately deuterium-labeled squalene confirm that C-2 of MVA becomes the *trans* carbon atom at the terminus (*142, 143*). This information, together with the data for the central four units, gives the complete labeling pattern for squalene (Scheme 4.6) and analogously for other linearly polymerized isopentenoids. However, labeling of only C-4 means in turn that during the isomerization there will have to be conformational control (*77*). As seen from Scheme 4.12, the Δ^3-isopentenyl pyrophosphate conformer possessing the labeled carbon atom in the position *trans*-oriented to C-1 will yield the observed results, but, as shown in Scheme 4.13, a conformer with the labeled carbon atom in the *cis*-orientation will not. In the latter case, C-3' rather than C-4 will be labeled. In agroclavine, for instance, under these circumstances the methyl group would not be labeled. Instead, the CH$_2$ group joined to the nitrogen atom would be labeled. As far as can be seen, the conformational nature of the isomerization will determine the labeling pattern regardless of the mechanism of isomerization. The argument presented here assumes a proton addition-elimination, but an addition-elimination of a sulfhydryl group, etc., would require analogous consideration. Further evidence for conformational control has come from

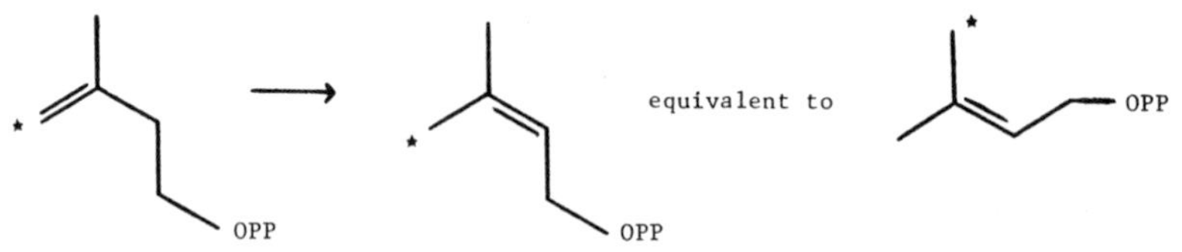

Scheme 4.13. Labeling pattern from *cis*-conformer of Δ^3-isopentenyl pyrophosphate.

studies of isopentenyl pyrophosphate homologs, and a model for the active site has been suggested (*144*). Other data (e.g., *145*), reviewed in detail by Bentley (*146*), also indicate the same stereospecificity. It should be noted, however, that while no randomization of the label occurs in lanosterol (*142*) or β-amyrin (*143*), it has been reported in several cases of terpenes and alkaloids. The literature has been reviewed by Bentley (*146*), but no consistent or certain explanation of the lack of stereospecificity in some cases is yet available.

Studies (*132, 134*) with water and mevalonate that have been labeled with isotopic hydrogen have revealed that a proton originating from water is incorporated onto C-4 of the isopentenyl pyrophosphates in the isomerization of the Δ^3- to the Δ^2-isomer and at C-2 in the reverse reaction. During short incubations, label appears only at C-4, but after long ones it appears at both positions, as would be expected for establishment of a dynamic equilibrium. 4(*R*)-Mevalonate possessing deuterium or tritium at C-4 leads to retention and the (4*S*)-diastereoisomer to loss of the label in both plants and animals (*147–151*), when the isopentenoid produced has or is formed via an intermediate, e.g., squalene, which has *trans*-oriented double bonds. This means the proton removed from C-2 of the C₅ unit must have the *pro-R* configuration; i.e., when the Δ^3-molecule has the fully extended conformation with all of the carbon atoms lying in the plane of the paper with C-1 at the right as shown in Scheme 4.14, the proton eliminated at C-2 is on the side of the paper away from the observer.

The *pro-R* hydrogen at C-2 of Δ^3-isopentenyl pryrophosphate is, unfortunately, equivalent to the *pro-S* hydrogen at C-4 of mevalonate as a result of the way groups are chosen in the Cahn-Ingold-Prelog sequence rule (*152*, *a*, *b*). A *pro-R* hydrogen is the one which, if replaced by tritium or deuterium on a CH₂ group, would render the carbon asymmetric with the *R* configuration. The configurational designation is further determined by a convention of weighting the remaining two groups. Although the Cahn-Ingold-Prelog sequence rule is independent of conformation and one's view of the molecule and thus has many important uses, it would be convenient for the biochemistry of isopentenoids to have a stereochemical designation which is consistent for a given side of the molecule regardless of the reactions it undergoes. For most cases this is possible by adopting the steroidal α,β-convention (substituents to the rear are α-oriented, etc.) under the assumption that an acyclic molecule is considered to be in the fully extended conformation with C-1,

C-2, C-3, and C-4 of the C_5 unit in the plane of the paper, the original or incipient *gem*-dimethyl group at the left, and C-2 of the C_5 unit down relative to the carbons on either side. The appropriate conformation and view are given in Scheme 4.14. Such a convention would mean, considering the

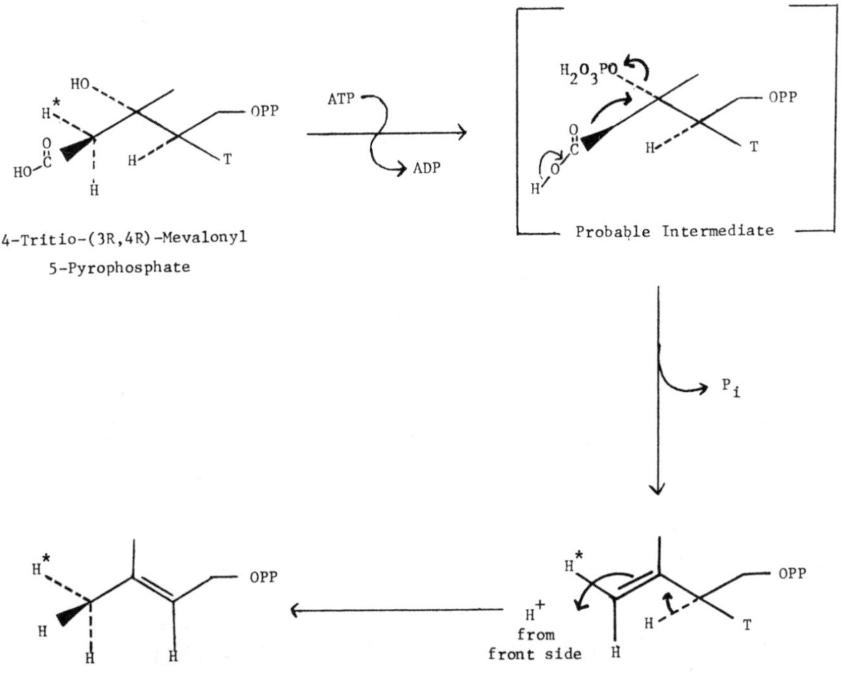

4-Tritio-(3R,4R)-Mevalonyl
5-Pyrophosphate

Probable Intermediate

Scheme 4.14. Stereochemistry of formation of isopentenyl pyrophosphates.

evidence in the foregoing paragraph, that the biosynthetically active (R)-mevalonic acid possesses a 3β-methyl group and the 4β-hydrogen is retained during further metabolism. We could also say that 4β-tritiomevalonate yields 2β-tritio-Δ^3-isopentenyl pyrophosphate without coping with reversal of configurational nomenclature. Since the carboxyl and hydroxyl groups eliminated from mevalonyl pyrophosphate are on opposite sides of the molecule and are eliminated apparently in a concerted process (*153*), it follows that in the conformer reacting the carboxyl group is on the front face (β face).

The remaining problem of the orientation of the proton added to C-4 had been considered earlier by Popjak and Cornforth (*154*) and has recently been resolved by Cornforth and his associates (*155-157*). The protons being removed from and added to C-2 and C-4, respectively, are different and on opposite sides of the isopentenyl pyrophosphate when C-1 through C-4 lie in the same plane.

LITERATURE CITED

1. H. J. Channon, Biochem. J. 20:400 (1926).
2. I. M. Heilbron, E. D. Kamm, and W. M. Owens, J. Chem. Soc. 1630 (1926).
3. M. Tsujimoto, J. Ind. Eng. Chem. 8:889 (1916).
4. M. Tsujimoto, Chem. Zentralblatt I:638, 1048 (1918).
5. M. Tsujimoto and K. Kimura, Chem. Zentralblatt II:1042 (1927).
6. A. Ch. Chapman, J. Chem. Soc. 111:56 (1917).
7. I. M. Heilbron, W. M. Owens, and I. A. Simpson, J. Chem. Soc. 873 (1929).
8. P. Karrer, A. Helfenstein, H. Wehrli, and A. Wettstein, Helv. Chim. Acta 13:1084 (1930).
9. P. Karrer and A. Helfenstein, Helv. Chim. Acta 14:78 (1931).
10. R. Robinson, J. Soc. Chem. Ind. 53:1062 (1934).
11. K. Bloch, in R. S. Harris, G. F. Marrian, and K. V. Thimann (eds.), Vitamins and Hormones. Vol. XV. Academic Press, New York, 1957. p. 120.
12. R. Sonderhoff and H. Thomas, Liebig's Ann. 530:195 (1937).
13. D. Rittenberg and R. Schoenheimer, J. Biol. Chem. 121:235 (1937).
14. K. Bloch and D. Rittenberg, J. Biol. Chem. 143:297 (1942).
15. K. Bloch and D. Rittenberg, J. Biol. Chem. 145:625 (1942).
16. J. Bonner and B. Arrequin, Arch. Biochem. Biophys. 21:109 (1949).
17. B. Arrequin and J. Bonner, Arch. Biochem. Biophys. 26:178 (1950).
18. B. Arrequin, J. Bonner, and B. J. Wood, Arch. Biochem. Biophys. 31:234 (1951).
19. J. Bonner, J. Chem. Ed. 26:628 (1949).
20. J. Wuersch, R. L. Huang, and K. Bloch, J. Biol. Chem. 195:439 (1952).
21. E. C. Grob, G. G. Poretti, A. von Muralt, and W. H. Schroepfer, Experientia 7:218 (1951).
22. R. G. Langdon and K. Bloch, J. Biol. Chem. 200:129 (1953).
23. R. G. Langdon and K. Bloch, J. Biol. Chem. 200:135 (1953).
24. G. Popjak, Ann. Rev. Biochem. 27:533 (1958).
25. J. W. Cornforth, Brit. Med. Bull. 14:221 (1958).
26. J. W. Cornforth, G. D. Hunter, and G. Popjak, Biochem. J. 54:597 (1953).
27. J. W. Cornforth, I. Gore, and G. Popjak, Biochem. J. 65:94 (1957).
28. J. W. Cornforth, Revs. Pure and Appl. Chem. (Australia) 4:275 (1955).
29. I. Zabin and K. Bloch, J. Biol. Chem. 185:131 (1950).
30. R. O. Brady and S. Gurin, J. Biol. Chem. 189:371 (1951).
31. H. Rudney, in G. E. W. Wolstenholme, and M. O'Connor (eds.), Biosynthesis of Terpenes and Sterols. Little, Brown, Boston, 1959. p. 75.
32. J. L. Rabinowitz and S. Gurin, J. Biol. Chem. 208:307 (1954).
33. H. J. Klosterman and F. Smith, J. Am. Chem. Soc. 76:1229, (1954).
34. R. Adams and B. L. Van Duuren, J. Am. Chem. Soc. 75:2377 (1953).
35. B. K. Bachhawat, W. G. Robinson, and M. J. Coon, J. Biol. Chem. 219:539 (1956).
36. H. Rudney, J. Am. Chem. Soc. 76:2595 (1954).
37. H. Rudney, J. Am. Chem. Soc. 77:1698 (1955).
38. A. F. Novak and S. M. Hague, J. Biol. Chem. 174:647 (1948).
39. K. Folkers, C. H. Shunk, B. O. Linn, F. M. Robinson, P. E. Wittreich, J. W. Huff, J. L. Gilfillian, and H. R. Skeggs, in G. E. W. Wolstenholme and M. O'Connor (eds.), Biosynthesis of Terpenes and Sterols. Little, Brown, Boston, 1959. p. 20.

40. W. H. Ott, A. M. Dickinson, A. van Inderstine, A. W. Page, and K. Folkers, J. Nutr. 64:525 (1958).

41. H. R. Skeggs, L. D. Wright, E. L. Cresson, G. D. E. MacRae, C. H. Hoffman, D. E. Wolf, and K. Folkers, J. Bact. 72:519 (1956).

42. D. E. Wolf, C. H. Hoffman, P. E. Aldrich, H. R. Skeggs, L. D. Wright, and K. Folkers, J. Am. Chem. Soc. 78:4499 (1956).

43. L. D. Wright, E. L. Cresson, H. R. Skeggs, G. D. E. MacRae, C. H. Hoffman, D. E. Wolf, and K. Folkers, J. Am. Chem. Soc. 78:5273 (1956).

44. D. E. Wolf, C. H. Hoffman, P. E. Aldrich, H. R. Skeggs, L. D. Wright, and K. Folkers, J. Am. Chem. Soc. 79:1486 (1957).

45. C. H. Hoffman, A. F. Wagner, A. N. Wilson, E. Walton, C. H. Shunk, D. E. Wolf, F. W. Holly, and K. Folkers, J. Am. Chem. Soc. 79:2316 (1957).

46. C. H. Shunk, B. O. Linn, J. W. Huff, J. L. Gilfillian, H. R. Skeggs, and K. Folkers, J. Am. Chem. Soc. 79:3294 (1957).

47. G. Tamura, J. Gen. Microbiol. 2:431 (1956).

48. P. A. Tavormina, M. H. Gibbs, and J. W. Huff, J. Am. Chem. Soc. 78:4498 (1956).

49. P. A. Tavormina and M. H. Gibbs, J. Am. Chem. Soc. 78:6210 (1956).

50. J. W. Cornforth, R. M. Cornforth, G. Popjak, and I. Y. Gore, Biochem. J. 69:146 (1958).

51. G. Popjak in G. E. W. Wolstenholme and M. O'Connor (eds.), Biosynthesis of Terpenes and Sterols. Little, Brown, Boston, 1959. p. 148.

52. F. Dituri, S. Gurin, and J. L. Rabinowitz, J. Am. Chem. Soc. 79:2650 (1957).

53. F. Lynen, H. Eggerer, U. Henning, and I. Kessel, Angew. Chem. 70:738 (1958).

54. E. Capstack, Jr., D. J. Baisted, W. W. Newschwander, G. A. Blondin, N. L. Rosin, and W. R. Nes, Biochemistry 1:1178 (1962).

55. H. J. Nicholas, J. Biol. Chem. 237:1485 (1962).

56. D. A. Beeler, D. G. Anderson, and J. W. Porter, Arch. Biochem. Biophys. 102:26 (1963).

57. H. J. Nicholas, Nature 189:143 (1961).

58. D. J. Baisted, E. Capstack, Jr., and W. R. Nes, Biochemistry 1:537 (1962).

59. H. J. Nicholas, J. Biol. Chem. 237:1476 (1962).

60. H. J. Nicholas, J. Biol. Chem. 237:1481 (1962).

61. D. F. Johnson, E. Heftmann, and G. V. C. Houghland, Arch. Biochem. Biophys. 104:102 (1964).

62. R. D. Bennett, E. Heftmann, W. H. Preston, Jr., and J. R. Haun, Arch. Biochem. Biophys. 103:74 (1963).

63. E. J. Horbert and G. W. Kirby, Tetrahedron Lett. 1505 (1963).

64. J. A. Waters and D. F. Johnson, Arch. Biochem. Biophys. 112:387 (1965).

65. A. J. Birch, R. J. English, R. A. Massy-Westropp, and H. Smith, Proc. Chem. Soc. 233 (1957).

66. A. J. Birch, R. J. English, R. A. Massy-Westropp, and H. Smith, J. Chem. Soc. 369 (1958).

67. J. Fishman, E. R. H. Jones, G. Lowe, and M. C. Whiting, Proc. Chem. Soc. 127 (1959).

68. R. G. Stanley, Nature 182:738 (1958).

69. D. Arigoni, Experientia 14:153 (1958).

70. R. B. Park and J. Bonner, J. Biol. Chem. 233:340 (1958).

71. G. D. Braithwaite and T. W. Goodwin, Biochem. J. 66:31P (1957).

72. G. D. Braithwaite and T. W. Goodwin, Biochem. J. 67:13P (1957).
73. E. C. Grob, Chimia (Zurich) 11:338 (1957).
74. D. E. M. Lawson, D. R. Threfall, J. Glover, and R. A. Morton, Biochem. J. 79:201 (1961).
75. U. Gloor, O. Schindler, and O. Wiss, Helv. Chim. Acta 43:2089 (1960).
76. V. C. Joshi, J. Jayaraman, and T. Ramasarma, Biochem. Biophys. Res. Commun. 18:108 (1965).
77. E. Capstack, Jr., N. Rosin, G. A. Blondin, and W. R. Nes, J. Biol. Chem. 240:3258 (1965).
78. O. Isler, R. Ruegg, J. Wursch, K. F. Gey, and A. Pletscher, Helv. Chim. Acta 40:2369 (1957).
79. W. J. Steel and S. J. Gurin, J. Biol. Chem. 235:2778 (1960).
80. E. Heftmann, R. D. Bennett, and J. Bonner, Arch. Biochem. Biophys. 92:13 (1961).
81. M. J. Bryson and M. L. Sweat, Arch. Biochem. Biophys. 96:1 (1962).
82. E. Caspi, R. I. Dorfman, B. T. Khan, G. Rosenfeld, and W. Schmid, J. Biol. Chem. 237:2085 (1962).
83. R. B. Billiar, A. Oriol-Bosch, and K. B. Eik-Nes, Biochemistry 4:457 (1965).
84. K. H. Seifart and W. Hansel, Endocrinology 82:232 (1968).
85. A. Salonkangas, H. C. Rilling, and L. T. Samuels, Biochemistry 4:1606 (1965).
86. T. W. Goodwin, in T. W. Goodwin (ed.), Chemistry and Biochemistry of Plant Pigments. Academic Press, New York, 1965. pp. 167-169.
87. D. J. Baisted and W. R. Nes, J. Biol. Chem. 238:1947 (1963).
88. G. M. Jacobsohn and R. C. Corley, Fed. Proc. 16:200 (1957).
89. H. Rudney and T. G. Farkas, Fed. Proc. 14:757 (1955).
90. D. K. Bloomfield and K. Bloch, J. Biol. Chem. 235:337 (1960).
91. N. L. R. Bucher, J. Am. Chem. Soc. 75:498 (1953).
92. N. L. R. Bucher and K. McGarrahan, J. Biol. Chem. 222:1 (1956).
93. J. L. Rabinowitz and S. Gurin, Biochim. Biophys. Acta 10:345 (1953).
94. P. R. Stewart and H. Rudney, J. Biol. Chem. 241:1212 (1966).
95. H. Rudney, J. Biol. Chem. 227:363 (1957).
96. H. Rudney, P. R. Stewart, P. W. Majerus, and P. R. Vagelos, J. Biol. Chem. 241:1226 (1966).
97. G. M. Fimognari and V. W. Rodwell, Abstracts of the Sixth International Congress of Biochemistry, 1964, IUB Vol. 32, p. 573.
98. J. D. Brodie, G. Wasson, and J. W. Porter, J. Biol. Chem. 238:1294 (1963).
99. J. D. Brodie, G. Wasson, and J. W. Porter, J. Biol. Chem. 239:1346 (1964).
100. M. J. P. Higgins and R. G. O. Kekwick, Biochem. J. 134:295 (1973).
101. H. Y. Neujahr and L. Bjork, Acta Chem. Scand. 24:2361 (1970).
102. A. N. Klimov, O. K. Dokusova, L. A. Petrova, and E. D. Polyakova, Biochemistry (Engl. Transl.) 36:379 (1971).
103. J. J. Ferguson and H. Rudney, J. Biol. Chem. 234:1072 (1959).
104. H. Rudney and J. J. Ferguson, J. Biol. Chem. 241:1076 (1959).
105. P. R. Stewart and H. Rudney, J. Biol. Chem. 234:1222 (1966).
106. H. M. Miziorko, K. D. Clinkenbeard, W. D. Reed, and M. D. Lane, J. Biol. Chem. 250:5768 (1975).
107. Deleted in proof.
108. H. J. Knauss, J. W. Porter, and G. Wasson, J. Biol. Chem. 234:2839 (1959).
109. F. Lynen, H. Eggerer, U. Henning, J. Knappe, I. Kessel, and E. Ringel-

man, *in* G. E. W. Wolstenholme and M. O'Connor (eds.), Biosynthesis of Terpenes and Sterols. Little, Brown, Boston, 1959. p. 116.

110. I. F. Durr and H. Rudney, J. Biol. Chem. 235:2572 (1960).
111. J. Knappe, E. Ringelmann, and F. Lynen, Biochem. Z. 332:195 (1959).
112. M. E. Kirtley and H. Rudney, Biochemistry 6:230 (1967).
113. G. Popjak and J. W. Cornforth, Adv. Enzymol. 22:281 (1960).
114. J. Retey, E. Von Stetton, U. Coy, and F. Lynen, Eur. J. Biochem. 15:72 (1970).
115. R. C. Hughes, W. T. Jenkins, and E. H. Fischer, Proc. Natl. Acad. Sci. U.S.A. 48:1615 (1962).
116. D. E. Metzler, M. Ikawa, and E. E. Snell, J. Am. Chem. Soc. 76:648 (1954).
117. F. Lynen, B. W. Agranoff, H. Eggerer, U. Henning, and E. M. Moslein, Angew. Chem. 71:657 (1959).
118. G. Popjak, L. Gosselin, I. Y. Gore, and R. G. Gould, Biochem. J. 69:238 (1958).
119. B. H. Amdur, H. Rilling, and K. Bloch, J. Am. Chem. Soc. 79:2647 (1957).
120. T. T. Tchen, J. Am. Chem. Soc. 79:6344 (1957).
121. T. T. Tchen, J. Biol. Chem. 233:1100 (1958).
122. S. Chaykin, J. Law, A. H. Phillips, T. T. Tchen, and K. Bloch, Proc. Natl. Acad. Sci. U.S.A. 44:998 (1958).
123. K. Bloch, S. Chaykin, A. H. Phillips, and A. de Waard, J. Biol. Chem. 234:2595 (1959).
124. A. de Waard, A. H. Phillips, and K. Bloch, J. Am. Chem. Soc. 81:2913 (1959).
125. M. Lindberg, C. Yuan, A. de Waard, and K. Bloch, Biochemistry 1:182 (1962).
126. C. Yuan and K. Bloch, J. Biol. Chem. 234:2605 (1959).
127. T. N. R. Varma and C. O. Chichester, Arch. Biochem. Biophys. 96:265 (1962).
128. H. Yokoyama, T. O. M. Nakayama, and C. O. Chichester, J. Biol. Chem. 237:681 (1962).
129. H. Rilling, T. T. Tchen, and K. Bloch, Proc. Natl. Acad. Sci. U.S.A. 44: 167 (1958).
130. H. R. Levy and G. Popjak, Biochem. J. 75:417 (1960).
131. J. Bataille and W. K. Loomis, Biochim. Biophys. Acta 51:545 (1961).
132. U. Henning, E. M. Moslein, and F. Lynen, Arch. Biochem. Biophys. 83: 259 (1959).
133. B. W. Agranoff, H. Eggerer, U. Henning, and F. Lynen, J. Biol. Chem. 235:326 (1960).
134. D. H. Shah, W. W. Cleland, and J. W. Porter, J. Biol. Chem. 240:1946 (1965).
135. P. W. Holloway and G. Popjak, Biochem. J. 106:835 (1968).
136. M. Eberle and D. Arigoni, Helv. Chim. Acta 43:1508 (1960).
137. R. H. Cornforth, K. Fletcher, H. Hellig, and G. Popjak, Nature 185:923 (1960).
138. J. J. Ferguson, Jr., I. F. Durr, and H. Rudney, Proc. Natl. Acad. Sci. U.S.A. 45:499 (1959).
139. J. W. Cornforth, R. H. Cornforth, G. Popjak, and L. Yengoyan, J. Biol. Chem. 241:3970 (1966).
140. S. Bhattacharji, A. J. Birch, A. Brack, A. Hoffman, H. Kobel, D. C. C. Smith, H. Smith, and J. Winter, J. Chem. Soc. 421 (1962).

141. R. M. Baxter, S. I. Kandel, and A. Okany, Tetrahedron Lett. 596 (1961).
142. K. J. Stone, W. Roeske, R. B. Clayton, and E. E. van Tamelen, J. Chem. Soc. D 530 (1969).
143. T. Suga and T. Shishibori, Phytochemistry 14:2411 (1975).
144. T. Koyama, K. Ogura, and S. Seto, J. Biol. Chem. 248:8043 (1973).
145. D. Arigoni, in G. E. W. Wolstenholme and M. O'Connor (eds.), Biosynthesis of Terpenes and Sterols. Little, Brown, Boston, 1959.
146. R. Bentley, Molecular Asymmetry in Biology. Vol. II. Academic Press, New York, 1970. p. 267.
147. B. L. Archer, D. Barnard, E. G. Cockbain, J. W. Cornforth, R. H. Cornforth, and G. Popjak, Proc. Roy. Soc. London, Ser. B 163:519 (1966).
148. J. W. Cornforth, R. H. Cornforth, C. Donninger, and G. Popjak, Proc. Roy. Soc. London, Ser. B 163:492 (1966).
149. K. J. Stone and F. W. Hemming, Biochem. J. 104:43 (1967).
150. H. H. Rees, E. I. Mercer, and T. W. Goodwin, Biochem. J. 99:726 (1966).
151. J. W. Cornforth, R. H. Cornforth, C. Donninger, G. Popjak, Y. Shimizu, S. Ichii, E. Forchielli, and E. Caspi, J. Amer. Chem. Soc. 87:8224 (1965).
152a. R. S. Cahn, J. Chem. Ed. 41:116 (1964).
152b. R. S. Cahn, C. K. Ingold, and V. Prelog, Angew. Chem. Int. Ed. Engl. 5:385 (1966).
153. J. W. Cornforth, R. H. Cornforth, G. Popjak, and L. Yengoyan, J. Biol. Chem. 241:3970 (1966).
154. G. Popjak and J. W. Cornforth, Biochem. J. 101:553 (1966).
155. K. Clifford, J. W. Cornforth, R. Mallaby, and G. T. Phillips, J. Chem. Soc. D 1599 (1971).
156. J. W. Cornforth, Chem. Rev. 2:1 (1973).
157. J. W. Cornforth, K. Clifford, R. Mallaby, and G. T. Phillips, Proc. Roy. Soc. London, Ser. B 182:277 (1972).

Chapter 5

Polymerization of the C₅ Unit

A. General Considerations 171
  1. *Structure and Nomenclature of the Polymers* 171
  2. *Relationship to Other Polymers* 174
  3. *Naturally Occurring Polymers* 174
B. Biosynthesis 182
  1. *Energetics* 182
  2. *Enzymology* 184
  3. *Mechanisms* 184
  4. *Regulation of Chain Length* 187
  5. *Stereochemistry* 188
C. Biochemical Role of Polymers 191
  1. *Intermediates for Biosynthesis of Steroids and Carotenoids* 191
  2. *Intermediates for Quinone Cofactors and Other Isopentenylated Molecules* .. 191
  3. *Intermediates in Chlorophyll Biosynthesis* 192
  4. *Carbohydrate Carriers* 193
  5. *Juvenile Hormone* 194
  6. *Pheromones* 196
Literature Cited 201

A. GENERAL CONSIDERATIONS

1. Structure and Nomenclature of the Polymers

Isopentenoid polymers are considerably varied in structure, and many of them have now been isolated and characterized. Except in a few rare cases, they are the resultant of "head-to-tail" polymerization, which produces the structure shown in Scheme 5.1. For simplicity we shall adopt the symbol I (capital "i") to designate the C_5 unit (the I unit) regardless of its chemical functionality or stereochemistry. This allows us to write the dimer as I_2, the trimer as I_3, etc. In most cases beyond the dimer stage, when a double bond is present in the I unit, it occurs in the positions shown in Scheme 5.1, i.e., extending from the isopropyl group toward the "head" of the

$$
\begin{array}{ccc}
\overset{\displaystyle CH_3}{\underset{\displaystyle |}{}} & & \overset{\displaystyle CH_3}{\underset{\displaystyle |}{}} \\
CH_3-C = CH-CH_2 & \vdots & CH_2-C = CH-CH_2 - - - - - \\
\text{tail} \qquad\qquad \text{head} & \vdots & \text{tail} \qquad\qquad \text{head} \\
\text{I Unit} & \vdots & \text{I Unit}
\end{array}
$$

Normal Arrangement

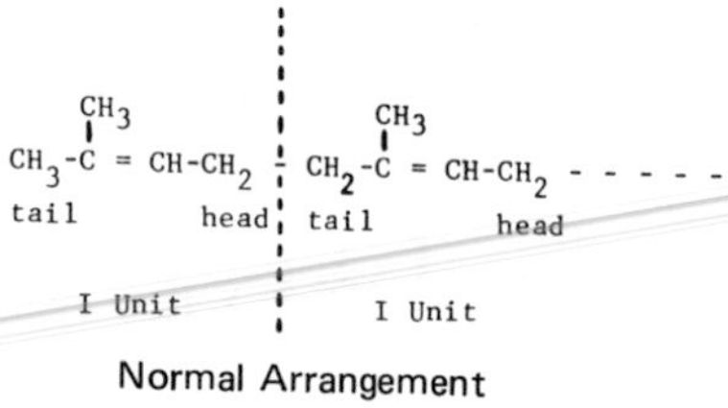

Scheme 5.1. General structure of isopentenoid polymers.

unit. This will be designated the "normal arrangement." Two other arrangements of importance are the one in which the double bond of the unit in the *gem*-dimethyl or tail end of the polymer proceeds from one of the terminal carbon atoms, and the one in which the double bond in the unit at the head end of the polymer is between the terminal two carbon atoms. These two other arrangements will be designated, respectively, "allo$_t$-" and "allo$_h$-arrangements." In the older literature, the normal and allo$_t$-structures were referred to as β and α forms, respectively. This convention will not be used, since it contrasts with configurational notations with Greek letters.

The structures shown in Schemes 5.1 and 5.2 do not indicate any stereo-

$$
\begin{array}{ccc}
\overset{\displaystyle CH_3}{\underset{\displaystyle |}{}} & & \overset{\displaystyle CH_3}{\underset{\displaystyle |}{}} \\
CH_2 = C-CH_2-CH_2 & \vdots & CH_2-C = CH-CH_2 - - - - - \\
\end{array}
$$

allo$_t$ - Arrangement

$$
\begin{array}{ccc}
\overset{\displaystyle CH_3}{\underset{\displaystyle |}{}} & & \overset{\displaystyle CH_3}{\underset{\displaystyle |}{}} \\
CH_3-C = CH-CH_2 - - - - - - CH_2-\underset{\displaystyle OR}{\overset{\displaystyle |}{C}}-CH = CH_2 \\
\end{array}
$$

allo$_h$ - Arrangement

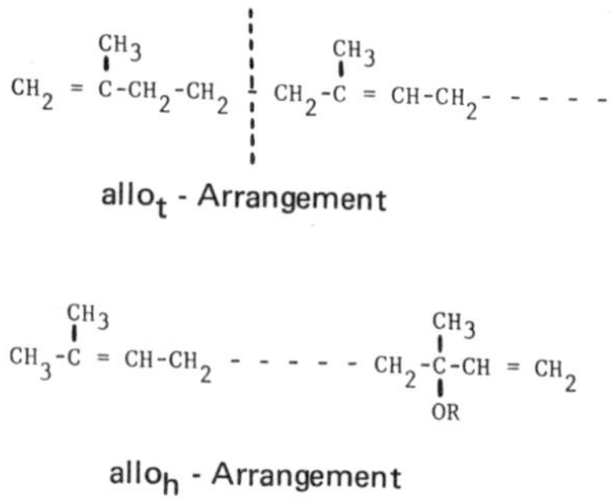

Scheme 5.2. Alternative structures of isopentenoid polymers.

chemistry. However, it will be seen by inspection of Scheme 5.3 that the normal arrangement allows formal *cis*- and *trans*- isomerism at the double

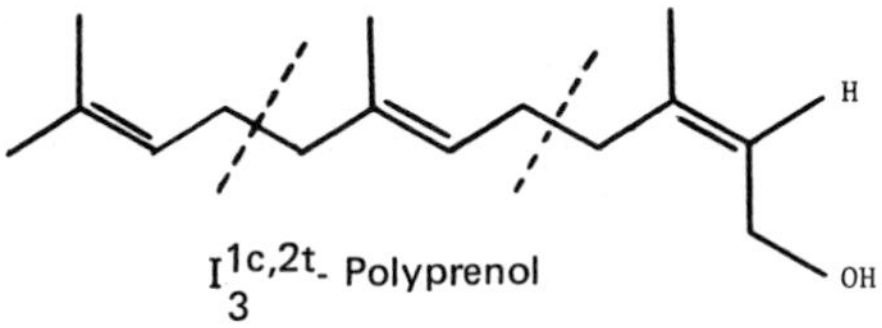

$I_3^{1c,2t}$- Polyprenol

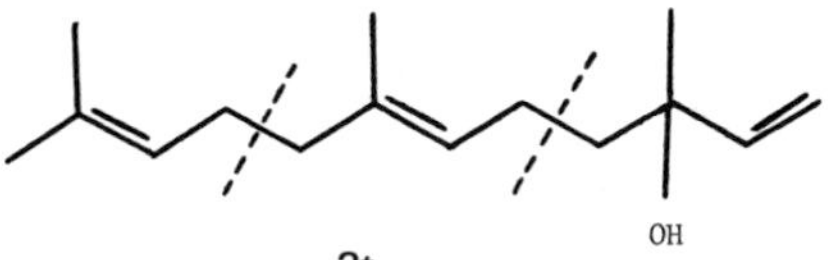

$allo_h$-I_3^{2t}- Polyprenol

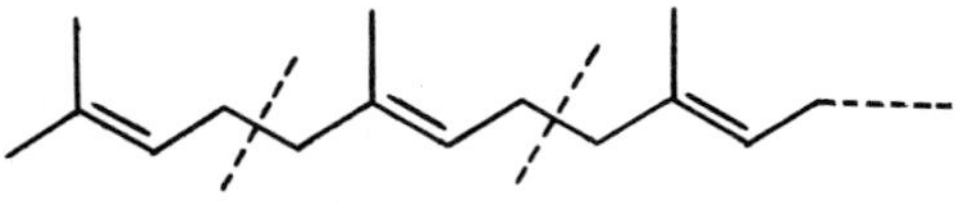

All-*trans*-I_n- or I_n^{at}- Polyprenol

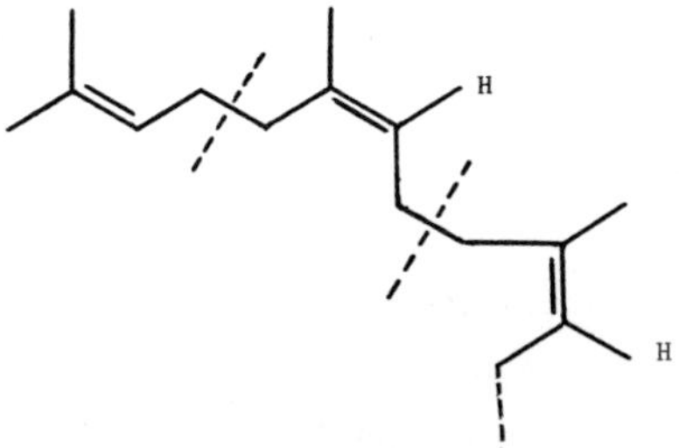

All-*cis*-I_n- or I_n^{ac}- Polyprenol

Scheme 5.3. Stereochemical variations.

bonds in all of the I units except for the one at the tail end. This stereo-chemical variability is known naturally. If we adopt the existing terminology "polyprenol" for the isopentenoid alcohols, then the terms allo$_t$- and allo$_h$-polyprenol can be used for the alcohols of the other arrangements. The stereochemistry and chain length can be designated by superscripts and subscripts, as shown in Scheme 5.3. Thus, the I_3^{at}-polyprenol is the normal trimer bearing *trans*-oriented (t) double bonds (*trans* with respect to carbon atoms in the chain) in all (a) of the units. The trimer in which the double bond in the first unit (counting from the alcoholic or head-end) is *cis* (c) and the one in the second is *trans* would be designated the $I_3^{1c,2t}$-polyprenol, etc.

Similarly, the allo series can be designated by the appropriate prefix (Scheme 5.3). The absence of double bonds can be shown by the letter "s" for "saturated" as a superscript. The completely reduced trimer would be the I_3^{as}-polyprenol, while the one bearing only a *trans*-double bond in the second unit would be the $I_3^{1s,2t,3s}$-polyprenol, etc.

A second nomenclature involves numbering the carbon atoms from the head end of the polymer. Thus, the $I_3^{1s,2t,3s}$-polyprenol is also the $\Delta^{trans-6}$-polyprenol, and the methyl group in the second unit contains C-7' and is located on C-7. Finally, nomenclature can be based systematically on the parent, unbranched hydrocarbon (Scheme 5.4).

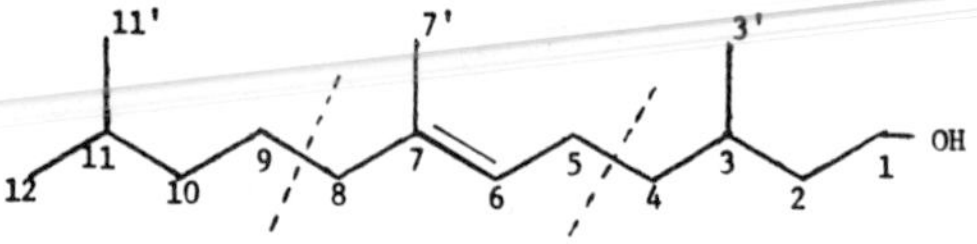

$I_3^{1s,2t,3s}$-Polyprenol

$\Delta^{trans-6}$ -Polyprenol

3,7,11-Trimethyl-*trans*-Δ^6-dodecenol

3,7,11-Trimethyldodec-6(*trans*)-en-1-ol

Scheme 5.4. Examples of nomenclature.

2. Relationship to Other Polymers

The isopentenoid polymers have much in common with other polymers in that (1) they are composed of a repeating unit of a general structure (the isopentane skeleton comparable to a carbohydrate, amino acid, or nucleotide unit); (2) the structure of the unit can be varied in detail (by double bonds, etc. in the isopentenoid case), giving rise to sequencing; (3) the chain length can vary from a few to a great many; and (4) conformational aspects of the molecule are real and of importance biochemically. They are unlike the other natural polymers in that (1) a C—C bond links the units together; and (2) they are relatively nonpolar, belonging to the lipid class. The covalent linking of the isopentenoid units imposes a "one-way metabolism." Once formed, the polymers do not revert to the monomeric state, as do polysaccharides, etc.

3. Naturally Occurring Polymers

The known polymers are listed in Tables 5.1 and 5.2. Some have trivial names. Others do not, and in some cases, such as "rubber," the name does not imply a distinct chemical entity but rather a polymer of a given range of

Table 5.1. Natural oligo- and polymeric prenols retaining all isopentenoid double bonds^a.

Structural designation	Trival name	Remarks
I_1	Δ^2-Isopentenol (Dimethylallyl alcohol)	Occurs as the pyrophosphate ester in all MVA-metabolizing cells. Also found as a cysteine adduct, felinine, in feline urine. Lacking the OH group, the I_1 unit is bound by a C—N link to adenine in a plant kinetin, and by a C—C link to a benzoquinone in ubiquinone-1. By other links it forms a part of certain alkaloids.
allo$_h$-I_1 I_2^t	Δ^3-Isopentenol (Isopentenol) Geraniol	Occurs as the pyrophosphate ester in all MVA-metabolizing cells. Occurs as the pyrophosphate ester in all cells producing steroids, carotenoids, $I_n^{(n-1)t}$-polyprenols, trans-rubber, and certain terpenes from MVA. Also found as the free alcohol or various esters (acetate, etc.) in citronella oil, rose oil, lemon grass oil, orange and jasmine blossom oil, camphor oil, geranium plants, Douglas fir, green tea, etc. Lacking an HO group and bound by a C—C link, forms a part of ubiquinone-2, etc.

continued

175

Table 5.1. Continued.

Structural designation	Trivial name	Remarks
I_2^c	Nerol	First isolated from orange blossom oil (neroli) but also found in the fruit as well as in Alpen violets and as a companion to geraniol in various oils, e.g., rose oil. As pyrophosphate ester may occur as biosynthetic intermediate in cells producing *cis*-isopentenoids, e.g., *cis*-rubber and cyclic compounds.
$allo_h$-I_2	Linalool	Both enantiomers occur naturally, the (+) form in orange oil, Brazilian rose wood oil, coriander oil, lavender oil, etc., and the (−) form in linaloa oil, Ceylon cinnamon oil, orange leaf oil, lavender oil, etc. The epoxide (2nd I unit) is reported free or esterified in lavender oil, grapefruit juice, etc.
$allo_t$-I_2	—	While not unquestionably natural, reported as a minor companion of geraniol and nerol.
I_3^{at}	Farnesol	As pyrophosphate ester occurs in all cells producing steroids, carotenoids, $I_n^{(n-1)t}$-polyprenols, *trans*-rubber, and certain terpenes from MVA. Also found in many flowers, Australian sandalwood oil, *Hibiscus abelmoschus* seeds, etc. Lacking an HO group and bound by a C—C link, forms part of ubiquinone-3, etc.
$allo_h$-I_3^{2t}	Nerolidol	First isolated from Peruvian balsam, later from orange blossom oil (neroli), *Myrospernum erythroxylon* wood, orange oil, etc.
$allo_{t,h}$-I_3^{2t}	"α-form" of Nerolidol	Reported as a minor companion of nerolidol isolated from *Myocarpus frondosus*.

continued

Table 5.1. Continued.

Structural designation	Trivial name	Remarks
I_4^{at}	Geranylgeraniol	As the pyrophosphate ester occurs in all cells producing carotenoids from MVA and presumably in cells producing various diterpenes, trans-rubber, other polyprenols with trans-double bonds in I units Nos. $(n-1)$, $(n-2)$, and $(n-3)$, and terpenoid metabolites of them. Lacking the HO group and bound by a C—C link, is a part of ubiquinone-4, etc.
I_5	—	Known only in the form of the side chain of ubiquinone-5.
I_{6-9}	Betulaprenols	Found in the wood of Betula verrucosa. Lacking the HO-group and bound by a C—C link, also found in ubiquinone-6-9 etc. In addition, the I_9 compound is present in the leaves of sugar beets and decorative rubber plants and traces in the leaves of the horse chestnut tree. See also the I_9^{at} compound (solanesol).
I_9^{at}	Solanesol	Found in tobacco leaves. Lacking an HO group and bound by a C—C link, also a part of ubiquinone-9, etc. Presumably the polyprenol as the pyrophosphate is an intermediate to Q9, trans-rubber, etc., and occurs in appropriate cells.
I_{10}	Castaprenol-10	Found in leaves of sugar beet and decorative rubber plants and traces in leaves of horse chestnut trees. Based on co-occurrence with castaprenol-12, probably has a mixture of cis- and trans-double bonds.
I_{11}	Castaprenol-11	See remarks for castaprenol-10.

continued

Table 5.1. Continued.

Structural designation	Trivial name	Remarks
I_{11}	Bactoprenol Antigen carrier lipid Carbohydrate carrier lipid	Isolated from *Salmonella* bacteria as an ester (linked through a pyrophosphate group to carbohydrate). Is tentatively believed to have the all-*trans*-structure. A similar I_{11}-polyprenol occurs in *Micrococcus lysodeikticus*, where it occurs as a somewhat different ester (linked through a pyrophosphate group to a disaccharide and oligopeptide).
I_{12}	Castaprenol-12	Principal (82%) polyprenol of horse chestnut leaves. Also found in leaves of the sugar beet and decorative rubber plants. I unit No. 1 has a *trans*-double bond and I units 2-11 contain six *cis*- and four *trans*- double bonds. Castaprenol-like alcohols detected in many mono- and dicotyledonous angiosperms.
I_{13} I_{13-14}	Castaprenol-13 Castaprenol-13-14	See remarks for castaprenol-10. Partial identification in *Chlorella pyrenoidosa*, but may represent higher homologs with saturated double bonds.
I_{10^3}	Rubber	Occurs in thousands of plants among the *Euphorbiaceae, Moraceae, Apocynaceae, Compositae, Asclepiadaceae*, etc. Both *cis*- and *trans*-forms are known. The commercial variety is *cis*, obtained principally from *Hevea brasiliensis*. The structure of the first I unit is not known and may be dehydrated. The number of I units in the chain ranges from 700 to 5,000 with molecular weights as high as 3×10^5.

[a]For leading recent references see text, and for older literature see W. Karrer, Konstitution und Vorkommen der Organischer Pflanzenstoffe, Birkhäuser Verlag, Basel, 1958.

Table 5.2. Natural oligo- and polymeric prenols bearing reduced double bonds[a]

Structural designation	Trivial name	Remarks
I_2^{1s}	Citronellol	Occurs as both enantiomers: The (+) form (yacarol) in geranium, rose, and citronella oils, etc. The (−) form (rhodinol) in pelargonium and rose oils, the wood of *Xanthorrhoea preissii*, etc. Also reported in alligators.
$I_4^{1t,2-4s}$	Phytol	Occurs as the ester moiety of the chlorophylls in both higher and lower plants.
I_{11}	Bactoprenol Dihydrobactoprenol	Isolated from *Lactobacillus casei*. Contains 10 double bonds. The one reduced is probably not in either of the terminal I units.
I_{16-22}	Dolichols	Isolated from pig liver, human kidney, and baker's yeast. Contains a saturated double bond in the first I unit. The remaining double bonds are predominantly *cis*-oriented.
I_{18-24}	Hexahydropolyprenols	Isolated from *Aspergillus fumigatus*. Only two of the double bonds are *trans*-, the rest being *cis*-oriented. The first, last, and penultimate I units are saturated.

[a] For leading recent references see text, and for older literature see W. Karrer, Konstitution und Vorkommen der Organischer Pflanzenstoffe, Birkhäuser Verlag, Basil, 1958.

179

I units. Polyprenols are found more or less ubiquitously, having been isolated from bacteria, algae (both prokaryotic and eukaryotic), gymnosperms,
angiosperms, birds, and mammals. They may well be required constituents
of all living cells. Their roles (Section 5.C) are varied and, in many known
cases, demonstrably essential to life.

The polyprenols occur naturally as the free alcohols, and also as esters,
e.g., the pyrophosphates, amines (RNH replacing OH), or simple oxidation
products (polyprenals and polyprenoic acids). The nature of the chemical
functionality depends on the biochemical role played (Section 5.C). The
polymeric chains also occur bound through a covalent C—C bond to another
moiety, especially a quinone (Scheme 5.5). In the latter case, the unsaturated I_n chains constitute a portion of the structure of the ubiquinones and
plastoquinones. The $I_n^{n,(n-1),(n-2)s}$ chains are found in the vitamins K and

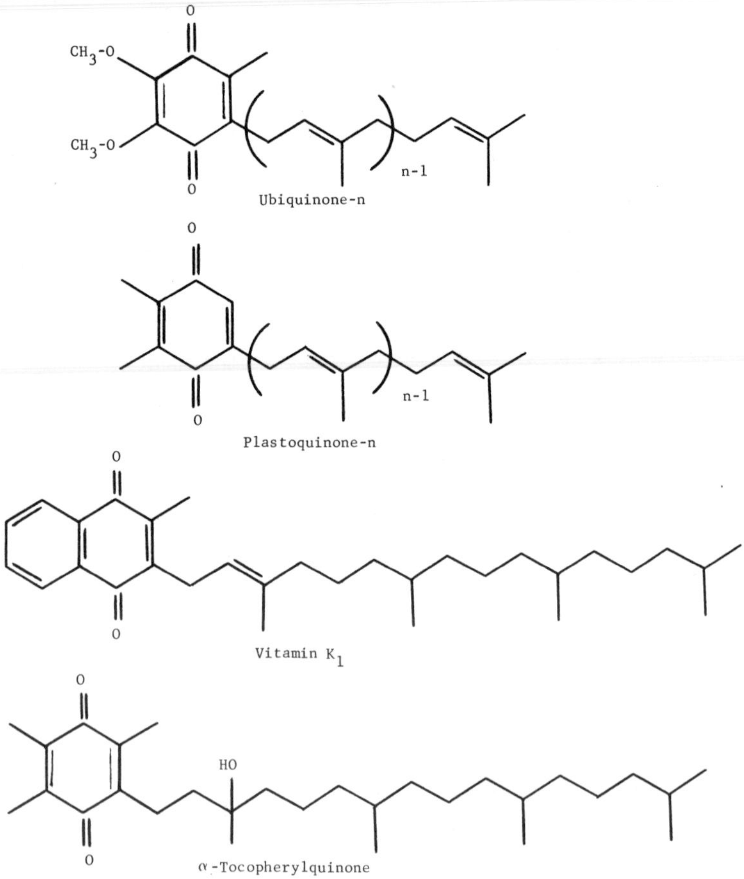

Scheme 5.5. I chains bound through C—C links.

the $I_n{}^{as}$ chains in the tocopherols. Ubiquinones with I_n side chains have been found with all values of n from 1 to 10 (1–3). Each of the I units retains its double bond. In both the ubiquinones and plastoquinones, the double bonds are probably *trans*-oriented. Thus, the $I_9{}^{at}$-polyprenol, which is called solanesol, lends its carbon chain to plastoquinone-10 (Q_{10}) from which its systematic name, 2,3-dimethyl-5-solanesylbenzoquinone, is derived.

Polyprenols with but a few isopentenoid residues (oligoprenols) have been known since the latter part of the last century. Jacobsen (4) isolated the *trans*-dimer, geraniol, from Turkish geranium oil as early as 1871. By 1888 the natural occurrence of its aldehyde, citral-a, was recognized, and it was prepared synthetically from geraniol 2 years later (5). During the 1890s the $allo_h$-isomer of geraniol, linalool (6), and the derivative of geraniol reduced in the first unit, citronellol (7), as well as the latter's aldehyde, citronellal (8), were all isolated. The following decade witnessed the discovery of the *cis*-isomer of geraniol, nerol (9), the trimer, farnesol (10), and the partially reduced tetramer, phytol (11). During the following years, the rather wide distribution of these and related compounds became evident, and stereochemical and other structural aspects were investigated. Then in 1956 the first polyprenol beyond the I_4 stage of condensation was discovered by Rowland, Latimer, and Giles (12) in tobacco leaves. It was named solanesol and proved to have the $I_9{}^{at}$ structure (13–15). At about the same time the structures of several new isopentenoid quinones were coming to light, and, even more importantly, in the period 1957–1959 such quinones were shown to be involved in electron transport (16–20). This elicited a concerted search for polyprenols, and several laboratories were successful in finding new ones. Lindgren and Hemming and his associates isolated I_n alcohols with n values from 6 to 13 from a variety of plants. Thus, the wood of the silver birch (*Betula verrucosa*) contains the betulaprenols (I_{6-9}) (21, 22), and sugar beets, the decorative rubber plant, and horse chestnut contain the castaprenols (I_{9-13}) (23). Castaprenol-like substances have also been found in a wide variety of other Phanerogams as well as in Cryptogams (24). While no fully saturated examples are known, except in fossil deposits (25–28), partly reduced compounds do occur. The tetramer bearing only one double bond, phytol, is a part of the chlorophyll molecule in higher plants (29), brown and blue-green algae (30), and certain bacteria (31, 32). It has also become clear that bacterial microorganisms have both fully unsaturated as well as partly saturated polyprenols of considerably larger size than I_4. The first of these to be recognized was bactoprenol, which is an I_{11} alcohol in which the first I unit is saturated. It was discovered by Thorne and Kodicek (33) in a strain of *Lactobacillus* (*L. casei*). Shortly afterward the fully unsaturated I_{11} polyprenol was isolated from *Salmonella* (34) and from *Micrococcus lysodeikticus* (35) in a study designed to identify a lipid component recognized as a "carbohydrate carrier" in the biosynthesis of polysaccharides of the bacterial cell wall. This "carrier lipid" has also been called "bactoprenol," and the suggestion was made that Kodicek's bactoprenol be called "dihydrobactoprenol" (35). Two other series of reduced polyprenols have been characterized by Hemming and others. They are the dolichols (36–39), originally isolated from pig liver, and the $\alpha\psi\omega$-hexahydropolyprenols (40) found in plants. In the former case, the double bond in the first I unit is saturated, and, except for possible stereochemical differences, the dolichols and the dihydrobactoprenols form a homologous series. The $\alpha\psi\omega$-hexahydropolyprenols are more fully reduced, having not only the first [the "α-unit" (40)] but the last [the "ω-unit" (40)] as well as the penultimate [the "ψ-unit" (40)] I units reduced. They are found in the mycelium of Aspergillus fumigatus.

The existence of cis- and trans-isomers is found at all levels of polymerization from the I_2 pair, geraniol and nerol, to the very large polymers, cis-rubber and trans-rubber (gutta-percha or balata). In the case of the dolichols and other I_{14-24}-polyprenols, cis- and trans-double bonds are also found mixed in the same molecule, leading to a sequence problem complicated by the presence of saturated I units. None of the sequences is as yet fully known. The dolichols are a homologous series in which the first I unit is saturated, and the hexahydropolyprenols are such a series in which the first, last, and penultimate I units are saturated. In both series most of the remaining double bonds are cis-oriented.

B. BIOSYNTHESIS

1. Energetics

In principle, the formation of polymers is an up-hill process energetically. This is the resultant of the Second Law of Thermodynamics, which requires that a system will tend toward greater randomness (increased entropy). The forming of monomeric units into a polymer restricts their independence, results in less entropy, and consequently requires an energy input. The isopentenoid polymers not only follow these general rules, but the manner in which the energy is injected is entirely analogous to the way it is done in other biological polymerizations, viz., through a phosphate bond introduced from ATP.

Since the monomeric unit is the pair of isopentenols, the apparently simplest process would be to phosphorylate them as needed. Actually, in the investigated cases nature proved to have chosen to phosphorylate them just prior to their formation, i.e., at the mevalonate stage (Section 4.C.1). During polymerization, a pyrophosphate ion is eliminated. The greater stability of pyrophosphate as an independent, hydrated ion (loss of energy) is the immediate source of the energy for C—C bond formation during polymerization. The ultimate source traces back through the anhydride existence of the phosphoryl moiety of ATP, and thence, of course, to the origins of ATP.

Little or no information on the energetics is available at a quantitative thermodynamic level. However, the concepts are illustrated in the energy diagram in Scheme 5.6 and by the stoichiometry in Scheme 5.7. The latter is reasonably well established.

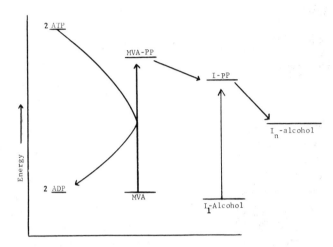

Scheme 5.6. Schematic representation of energy relationships.

Individual Steps

Equation 1 n MVA $\xrightarrow[\text{2n ADP}]{\text{2n ATP}}$ n MVA-PP $\xrightarrow[\substack{nADP + nP_i \\ + nCO_2}]{n\ \text{ATP}}$ n I-PP

Equation 2 n I-PP $\xrightarrow[n-1\ PP_i]{}$ I_n-PP

Overall Reaction

Equation 3 n MVA $\xrightarrow[3n\ ADP\ +\ n\ P_i\ +\ n\ CO_2\ +\ n-1\ PP_i]{3n\ ATP}$ I_n-PP

Scheme 5.7. Formation of isopentenoid polymer.

2. Enzymology

The polymerizing enzymes (synthetases or prenyltransferases) are soluble and have been partially purified in several animal (*41, 42*), plant (*43–46*), and microbial (*47, 48*) cases. Farnesyl pyrophosphate synthetase (EC 2.5.1.1), for instance, isolated from pig liver, can be obtained free of isopentenyl pyrophosphate isomerase and will convert 100 nmol of geranyl pyrophosphate and isopentenyl pyrophosphate into farnesyl pyrophosphate per minute per milligram of protein (*42*). Geranylgeranyl pyrophosphate synthetase has been purified from *Micrococcus lysodeikticus* (*47*), and the same organism has yielded another synthetase which will accept the I_{1-4}-pyrophosphates as substrates for the formation of a family of I_{7-10}-pyrophosphates (*48*).

3. Mechanisms

The polymerization proceeds by a mechanism first appreciated in detail by Lynen and his associates (*49*). It is a type of reaction, relatively rare in biochemistry, that Cornforth has classed as "olefin alkylation" (*50*). The presence of a C—C double bond adjacent (allylic) to the C—O ester bond of the pyrophosphate ester of Δ^2-isopentenyl pyrophosphate lowers the energy of activation for cleavage of the C—O bond and allows formation of the pyrophosphate ion. During the process, the now electron-deficient carbon atom is neutralized and stabilized by the π electrons of Δ^3-isopentenyl pyrophosphate, which in turn is neutralized and stabilized by loss of a proton. The resultant dimer, geranyl or neryl pyrophosphate, depending on the stereochemistry of elimination of a proton, still possesses the allylic ester functionality of the Δ^2-monomer, and, consequently, still possesses the polymerization characteristic of the Δ^2-monomer. Repetition of the reaction with the Δ^3-monomer yields the trimer. The trimer also has the requisite allylic ester characteristics, and continued repetition yields the tetramer, etc. Such polymerization is illustrated in Scheme 5.8 for the formation of *trans*-compounds through the I_3 stage.

An alternate process (mechanism 2) is also illustrated in Scheme 5.8. It involves isomerization of Δ^2-isopentenyl pyrophosphate to the tertiary ester (allo$_h$-Δ^2-isopentenyl pyrophosphate), which one can also envision coupling with Δ^3-isopentenyl pyrophosphate. The second mechanism requires isomerizations not only of the phosphorylated Δ^2-monomer but also of the dimer and at each succeeding stage of monomer addition. These allo$_h$-isomers, e.g., linalool at the I_2 stage and nerolidol at the I_3 stage, actually occur in nature. It is not yet entirely clear whether they represent the operation of the alternative mechanism. Current opinion is that they probably do not.

The existence in nature of the allo$_t$-isomers raises still another unsettled question. It will be recalled (Section A.1) that the allo$_t$-compounds possess a terminal methylene group. Δ^3-Isopentenyl pyrophosphate is the simplest

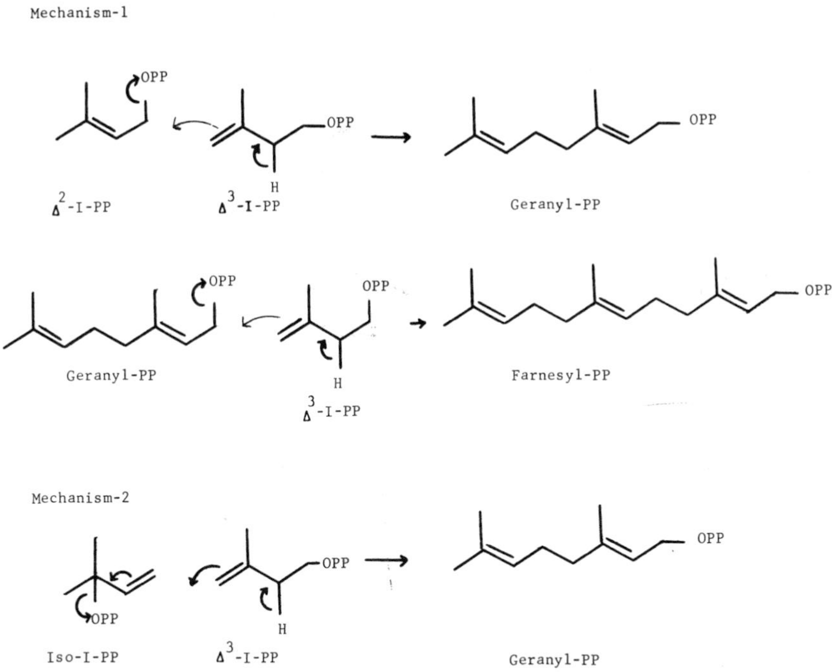

Mechanism-1

Scheme 5.8. Possible mechanisms of polymerization.

case, but they exist at many levels. For instance, the I_3-alcohol, nerolidol, is known in its $allo_t$ form. The question raised by these isomers is whether or not the I unit added is at the head or tail of the chain. In Scheme 5.8, the addition is shown to the head end by utilization of the $allo_t$-monomer. However, if an isomerase acted on the dimer (instead of the monomer) to give the $allo_t$-dimer, the $allo_t$-dimer could react with Δ^2-isopentenyl pyrophosphate (instead of with Δ^3-isopentenyl pyrophosphate) to give the trimer, etc. (mechanism 3, Scheme 5.9). Indeed, the dimeric (trimeric, etc.) $allo_t$-isomer could well react with the $allo_h$-monomer giving still a fourth mechanism (Scheme 5.9). Whether or not the $allo_t$-isomers (other than at the monomeric stage) have any bearing on the mechanism of polymerization, their existence suggests the presence of an isomerase for the normal to $allo_t$ structures, unless the polymerization is initiated at the tail end by Δ^3-isopentenyl pyrophosphate. While the latter is certainly mechanistically possible and may represent a fifth mechanism, it would require the less preferable homoallylic stabilization of the transition state of coupling.

Three main kinds of evidence exist to discriminate between the alternative pathways. Lynen and his colleagues (51, 52) purified the isomerase for the interconversion of the Δ^3- and Δ^2-isopentenyl pyrophosphates and showed that it was inhibited by iodoacetamide. They also demonstrated

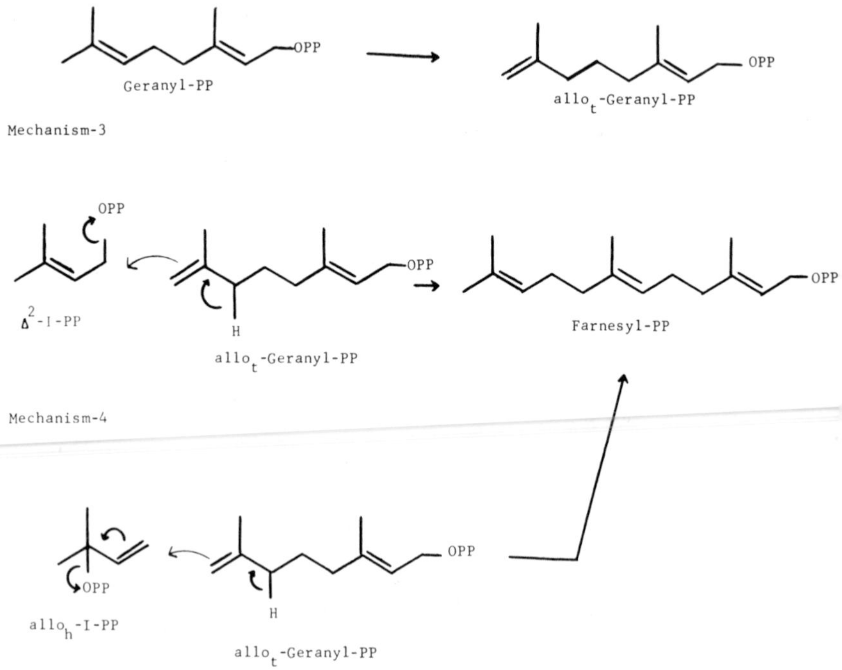

Scheme 5.9. Alternative mechanisms of polymerization.

that in a complete enzymatic system from yeast for the conversion of me-valonate to farnesyl pyrophosphate, the use of iodoacetamide leads to accumulation of Δ^3-isopentenyl pyrophosphate. Thus, both the Δ^3- and the Δ^2-isomers are necessary. Secondly, Popjak and his associates (41, 42) have purified the polymerizing enzyme, prenylsynthetase, from liver. In the presence of radioactive Δ^3-isopentenyl pyrophosphate, no reaction occurs, but labeled farnesyl pyrophosphate is formed when unlabeled geranyl pyrophosphate is also added. Consequently, chain elongation must occur by addition of the Δ^3-monomer to the head end of the molecule, and mechanism 1 is presumably the correct one (Scheme 5.8). Finally, the mechanisms involving the allo$_t$-isomers and chain elongation by the addition of an I unit to the tail end of the molecule are suggestively eliminated by the fact that the derivative of geranyl pyrophosphate in which the two terminal methyl groups are replaced by hydrogen adds an I$_l$ unit from the head end despite the availability of a terminal methylene group (44). More importantly, elongation from the tail end is essentially eliminated as a possibility by the finding (42) that the I$_2$-pyrophosphate lacking a double bond in the second I unit (6,7-dihydrogeranyl pyrophosphate) is readily alkylated at the head end by Δ^3-isopentenyl pyrophosphate (42) to give 10,11-dihydrofarnesyl pyrophosphate (Scheme 5.10). In this case the saturated I unit not only

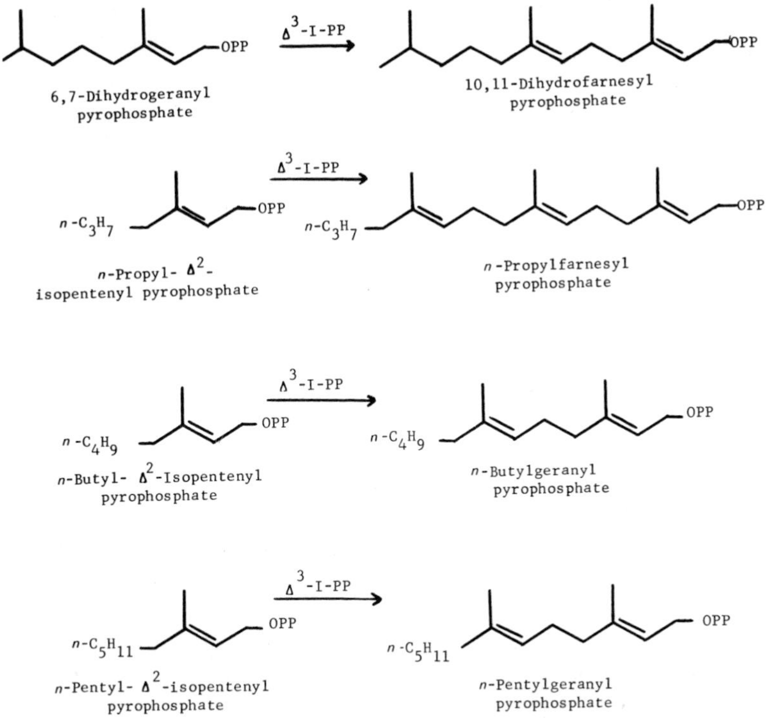

6,7-Dihydrogeranyl
pyrophosphate

Δ^3-I-PP

10,11-Dihydrofarnesyl
pyrophosphate

n-C$_3$H$_7$

Δ^3-I-PP

n-Propyl- Δ^2-
isopentenyl pyrophosphate

n-C$_3$H$_7$

n-Propylfarnesyl
pyrophosphate

n-C$_4$H$_9$

Δ^3-I-PP

n-Butyl- Δ^2-Isopentenyl
pyrophosphate

n-C$_4$H$_9$

n-Butylgeranyl
pyrophosphate

n-C$_5$H$_{11}$

Δ^3-I-PP

n-Pentyl- Δ^2-isopentenyl
pyrophosphate

n-C$_5$H$_{11}$

n-Pentylgeranyl
pyrophosphate

Scheme 5.10. Structural features determining extent of chain elongation.

serves as a marker of the tail end of the dimer, but it also allows one to conclude that no π-electrons are necessary at this end for elongation to occur. Consequently, isomerization to the allo$_t$ form has no significance. It is interesting to note in this regard that uneven labeling of, say, farnesyl pyrophosphate is sometimes found when a labeled precursor is used as substrate. While in some cases this can be interpreted in terms of alternative mechanisms, the more probable explanation is the existence of an endogenous pool of an intermediate. Thus, in the presence of a geranyl pyrophosphate pool, [2-^{14}C]MVA would yield highly labeled Δ^3-monomer to add to it, producing greater specific activity in the first of the three units of the trimer.

4. Regulation of Chain Length

Purification of the synthetase has allowed a study of substrate and product characteristics from which it can be concluded that chain length in both plant (*43,44a*) and mammalian cases (*42*) is controlled by the size of the product. The alternative would be the number of double bonds. Discrimination was made by the use of artificial substrates (Scheme 5.10). Thus, when the partially reduced $I_2^{2s,1t}$-pyrophosphate (6,7-dihydrogeranyl pyrophosphate) was the substrate for the liver synthetase normally yielding the I_3^{at}-compound, farnesyl pyrophosphate, the analogously reduced $I_3^{3s,1t,2t}$-pyrophosphate (10,11-dihydrofarnesyl pyrophosphate) was produced by the addition of one I unit (*42*). Had the synthetase recognized the number of double bonds, the monenic $I_2^{2s,1t}$-substrate should not have reacted or should have added two I units. Similarly, when the structure of Δ^2-isopentenyl pyrophosphate was extended from the tail end by a *n*-Δ^3-propenyl group (CH_2=CH—CH_2—), two I units were still added, yielding the tetraenic *n*-propenylfarnesyl pyrophosphate (*44a*). The enzyme clearly took little notice of the additional double bond. On the other hand, when *n*-butyl or *n*-pentyl homologs of Δ^2-isopentenyl pyrophosphate were incubated with Δ^3-isopentenyl pyrophosphate and the pumpkin synthetase, the corresponding I_2-polyprenols, *n*-butyl and *n*-pentylgeranyl pyrophosphates, were formed as the major and only products, respectively, but use of the *n*-propyl-Δ^2-isopentenyl pyrophosphate led to the *n*-propyl-I_3-compound as the sole product (*43*). Obviously, the pumpkin synthetase recognized the C_3-I_1 unit as a simple I_1 unit as had the liver enzyme, but recognized the C_4-I_1 and the C_5-I_1 units as I_2 units. In extension of this work (*44b*) it was found that, while C_7- and C_8-I units were recognized as I_2 units, C_9- and C_{11}-I units were recognized as I_3 units and did not react with Δ^3-isopentenyl pyrophosphate in the presence of farnesyl synthetase.

5. Stereochemistry

Since mevalonic acid is demonstrably the precursor of both the *cis*- and the *trans*-oriented double bonds, e.g., respectively, in *cis*-rubber and farnesol, and since the mechanism of chain elongation appears to be through the successive additions of Δ^3-isopentenyl pyrophosphate (Sections B.3 and B.4), the stereochemistry of the final double bonds must depend only on the conformation of the Δ^3-isopentenyl pyrophosphate adsorbed on the synthetase. If C-1 is oriented *cis* to C-4, a *cis*-double bond will result, and conversely a *trans*-conformation (also called *anti*-conformation) will lead to a *trans*-double bond. This is illustrated in Scheme 5.11 for the I_2 cases.

On the assumption that the synthetase actively abstracts the proton from C-2 of the adding Δ^3-monomer, rigid control of the conformation would require the abstraction to be from only one of the two sides of the molecule. At C-2 there is an H atom on each of these sides, one having the *pro-R* configuration and one having the *pro-S* configuration derived, respectively, from the *pro-S* and *pro-R* H atoms on C-4 of MVA (Chapter 4, Section D.3, Scheme 4.14). The synthesis and incubation of stereospecifically labeled MVA and other precursors have been accomplished by Cornforth and Popjak. Cornforth has reviewed this elegant achievement (*50*). The work has demonstrated that the *pro-R* H atom at C-2 of the Δ^3-monomer is removed and the *pro-S* H atom is retained in the formation of the *trans*-

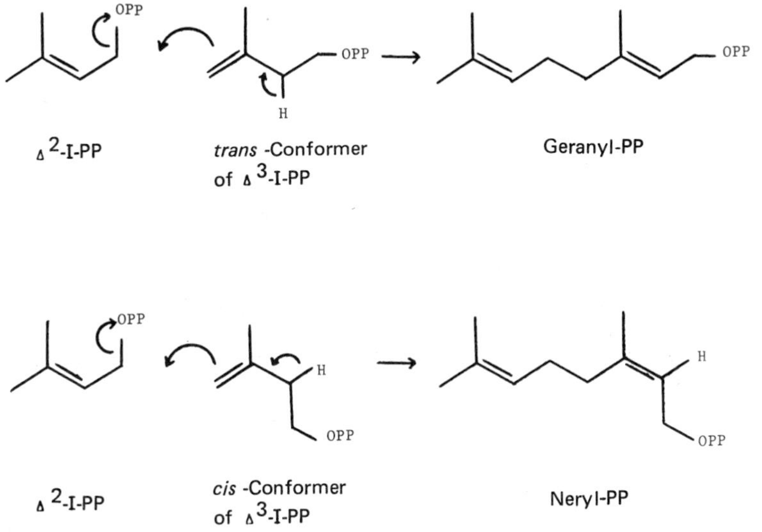

Δ^2-I-PP   trans -Conformer   Geranyl-PP
             of Δ^3-I-PP

Δ^2-I-PP   cis -Conformer   Neryl-PP
             of Δ^3-I-PP

Scheme 5.11. Conformational regulation of configuration.

double bond. The stereospecificity is identical to that in the isomerization of the Δ^3- to the Δ^2-monomer, which means, as is experimentally found, that the *pro-R* H atom at C-4 of MVA is retained through both the isomerization and polymerization in the *trans*-series in both animals (*50, 53–55*) and plants (*56,57*). One would guess that the reverse would be true in the *cis*-series, i.e., that the *pro-R* H atom at C-4 of MVA would be lost, on the assumption that the active site of the synthetase maintained the proton-abstracting group at the same point relative to the polymer as a whole with rotation about the C-2,C-3 bond having occurred as a result of a new arrangement of the appropriate binding points for the Δ^3-monomer (e.g., to the pyrophosphate group). While the experimental data are in accord with this in the biosynthesis of *cis*-rubber, 4-H$_R$ rather than 4-H$_S$ of MVA being eliminated (*58*), the reverse is true for nerol and *cis*-Δ^2-farnesol (*59*).

The *pro-R* H atom at C-4 of MVA is the one pointing toward the observer in the staggered conformation shown in Scheme 4.14. During chain elongation, as shown in Scheme 5.12, it is this nearest H atom (*pro-S* of Δ^3-I-PP) which is retained, and the proton-abstracting group on the enzyme must then be on the other or rear side of the plane of the five carbon atoms of the I unit being added to give a *trans*-double bond.

Cornforth (*50*) has postulated that the alkylation occurs in a two-step process ("the X-group mechanism") in which C-4 of the Δ^3-monomer is attacked by C-1 of the Δ^2-I$_n$-pyrophosphate from below the plane of the paper when the structure is written as shown in Scheme 5.12. Some group

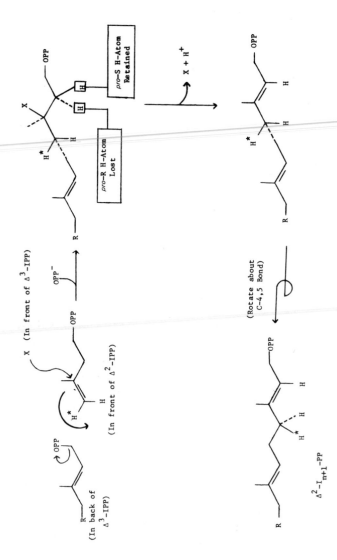

Scheme 5.12. Stereochemistry of chain elongation to give a *trans*-double bond illustrated with Cornforth's "X-group mechanism."

(X) simultaneously attacks C-3 of the Δ^3-monomer from the top to give the X-intermediate which undergoes a *trans*-elimination of HX yielding the final I_{n+1}-pyrophosphate with a *trans*-double bond. For various reasons Cornforth favors the two-step mechanism over an alternative he has discussed (50) which involves an addition of the Δ^2-I_n-pyrophosphate to the Δ^3-monomer producing a nonclassical, bridged carbonium ion.

C. BIOCHEMICAL ROLE OF POLYMERS

1. Intermediates for Biosynthesis of Steroids and Carotenoids

The all-*trans*-trimer, farnesyl pyrophosphate, is the obligatory source of the isopentenoid carbon atoms for the biosynthesis of steroids. The isopentenoid carbon atoms are all the carbon atoms except for substituents (C-28 and C-29) at C-24 in phytosterols. However, a portion of the side chain of certain steroids (the C_{23}-cardenolides and C_{24}-bufadienolides) are derived by oxidative cleavage of the C_{27}-steroidal side chain between C-20 and C-22 and resynthesis of C-22 and C-23, and of C-22, C-23, and of C-24, respectively, from other, as yet unknown, units (60–66). Farnesyl pyrophosphate is also an intermediate for the carotenoid hydrocarbons and their oxygenated derivatives. In the steroid case, polymerization ceases at the farnesyl stage and two I_3-pyrophosphates are condensed through reactions involving the first I unit of each molecule. In the carotenoid case, polymerization continues to the I_4^{at} stage to give geranylgeranyl pyrophosphate, two molecules of which condense at C-1 of each one to give the C_{40}-backbone of the carotenoid family. These condensations are discussed in detail in Chapter 6.

2. Intermediates for Quinone Cofactors and Other Isopentenylated Molecules

There are several molecular types in nature, some apparently ubiquitous, such as the ubiquinones, in which a polyprenyl side chain exists. The structures of some of these (quinone cofactors) are shown in Scheme 5.5. A number of others exist, e.g., in aromatic compounds (67, 68) and kinetins. The final molecules are derived by the isopentenylation of some intermediate. The side chains are experimentally derivable from mevalonic acid, as already discussed, and presumably the preformed I_n chain becomes attached to a nucleophilic site on an intermediate. An example of a reasonable mechanism is the *ortho*- (Scheme 5.13), or its allylic extension, the *para*-directed condensation of phenol with a polyprenyl pyrophosphate to give a polyprenylated ketone which on enolization would yield the more stable, benzenoid polyprenylated phenol. 2-Octaprenylphenol (Scheme 5.13, polyprenylphenol where $n = 8$) is actually isolable from an *E. coli* mutant, as is the corresponding carboxylic acid, 3-octaprenyl-4-hydroxy-

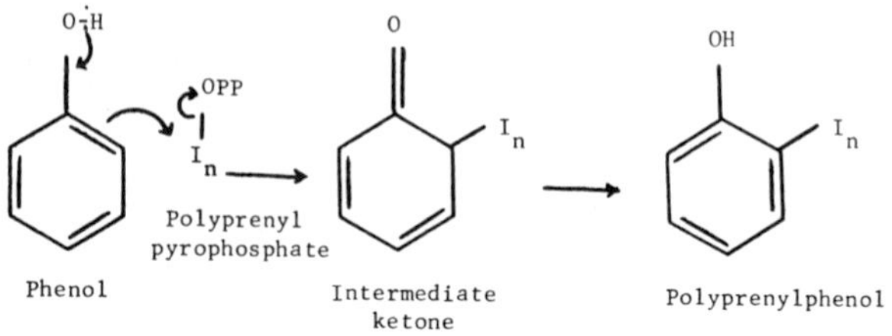

Scheme 5.13. Example of isopentenylation.

benzoic acid (*69*). If, as is thought to be the case, the benzoyl moiety is present as the CoA derivative, the same mechanism as shown in Scheme 5.13 would operate with 4-hydroxybenzoyl-CoA as the substrate to give, after hydrolysis, the observed 3-octaprenyl-4-hydroxybenzoic acid which, by decarboxylation, would yield the observed 2-octaprenylphenol. Superimposition of other sorts of metabolism on this sort of pathway, i.e., addition of other reactions before or after the ones mentioned, leads to the ubiquinones, plastoquinones, etc., the biosynthesis of which has been the subject of much investigation. 4-Hydroxybenzoic acid, derived by the shikimic acid pathway in plants and microorganisms and from tyrosine in rats, appears to be commonly involved in ubiquinone biosynthesis, and a detailed pathway has been suggested (*70*) and examined (*71–73*).

3. Intermediates in Chlorophyll Biosynthesis

The chlorophylls of all photosynthetic systems bear an ester side chain in which the alcohol residue is an oligoprenol. In higher plants (*29*), *Chlorophyta* (*74–76*), as well as brown and the procaryotic blue green algae (*30*), the oligoprenol is phytol; in certain bacteria (*Chlorobium*) phytol is replaced by farnesol (*77, 78*). Phytol seems to be derived by reduction after the I_4^{at} stage of condensation is reached, since experimentally MVA (*79*) and geranygeraniol (*80*) are incorporated into chlorophyll as phytol. The mechanism and sequence of events are not yet clear. A simple possibility would be hydrolysis of geranylgeranyl pyrophosphate, three reductions, and reaction with the CoA ester of the porphyrin carboxylic acid. Although the reaction sequence with respect to the isopentenoid molecule is not known, it has been found that the introduction of the I_4 moiety occurs during the very last stages of chlorophyll biosynthesis, never being earlier than the protochlorophillide stage (*81*). The suggestion has therefore been made (*30*) that evolution of the phytol pathway occurred parallel with or later than that of the porphyrin pathway but that both pathways evolved earlier than did the kind of subcellular membranes characteristic of eukaryots.

4. Carbohydrate Carriers

The cell envelope of bacteria is composed of a mixed polymer of amino acids and sugars that is known as a peptidoglycan. Associated with this peptidoglycan on the cell surface is another polysaccharide which is responsible for the substance responsible for antigenic action produced by infection with gram-positive organisms. The biosynthesis of both kinds of polymer requires the participation of polyprenols. The discovery and elucidation of their role were stimulated by the medical importance of antigenicity and by the originally puzzling and fortuitous observation that bacteria utilize mevalonic acid as a vital substrate despite the absence of an obvious end product (Chapter 4.A.3). Thorne and Kodicek (82), investigating the latter phenomenon, showed that MVA did not lead in quantity to sterols, carotenoids, ubiquinones, vitamin K, or tocopherols in four different species of *Lactobacillus*. Having eliminated such compounds, they studied the remaining lipids, and an I_{11}-polyprenol was isolated and named bactoprenol (33). At essentially the same time, several other laboratories were investigating the antigen problem and the nature of cell wall formation. This led to the isolation from *Micrococcus lysodeikticus* (35) and from *Salmonella anatum* (34) of an I_{11}-polyprenol containing all 11 isopentenoid double bonds, which are tentatively believed to have the *trans*-configuration. If further work establishes the configuration, the compound becomes a solanesol extended by two unsaturated I units, and represents a dehydroderivative of Kodicek's bactoprenol. The suggestion has therefore been made (35) that the nomenclature be bactoprenol for this compound and dihydrobactoprenol for Kodicek's. Owing to its relationship to antigenicity, the I_{11} compound has also been called the "antigen carrier lipid" or ACL. However, since antigenicity is a phenomenon derived after the fact of biosynthesis and ignores the peptidoglycan, a better term would be something like "carbohydrate carrier lipid."

The polyprenol plays its role by being involved in the assembly and transfer of the repeating unit of the polysaccharide. Thus, in *Salmonella* the antigenic polysaccharide has a polytriose structure (mannosy-rhamnosyl-galactosyl)$_n$, and the polyprenol is found attached through its pyrophosphate group to exactly this triose giving the structure, I_{11}-P-P-Gal-Rh-Man (34). Evidence (83, 84) has been obtained for the polymerization of the undecyl-prenylpyrophosphoroxytriose to give I_{11}-P-P-(Gal-Rh-Man)$_n$ with elimination of $(n-1)$ phosphate ions and $(n-1)$ molecules of I_{11}-phosphate. The I_{11}-P-P-polysaccharide in a final reaction with a "core" and elimination of P_i and I_{11}-P yields the completed polysaccharide. The original I_{11}-P-P-triose is formed from uridine diphosphoroxygalactose and the I_{11}-monophosphate. Rhamnose and mannose are added sequentially from the corresponding thymidine and guanosine derivatives, respectively. The full sequence as presently understood (34) is shown in Scheme 5.14.

$$\text{UDP-Gal} + I_{11}^{at}\text{-P} \longrightarrow I_{11}^{at}\text{-P-P-Gal} + \text{UMP}$$

$$I_{11}^{at}\text{-P-P-Gal} + \text{TDP-Rh} \longrightarrow I_{11}^{at}\text{-P-P-Gal-Rh} + \text{TDP}$$

$$I_{11}^{at}\text{-P-P-Gal-Rh} + \text{GDP-Man} \longrightarrow I_{11}^{at}\text{-P-P-Gal-Rh-Man} + \text{GDP}$$

$$n\ I_{11}^{at}\text{-P-P-Gal-Rh-Man} \longrightarrow I_{11}^{at}\text{-P-P-(Gal-Rh-Man)}_n + (n-1)P_i + (n-1)I_{11}^{at}\text{-P}$$

$$I_{11}^{at}\text{-P-P-(Gal-Rh-Man)}_n + \text{"Core"} \longrightarrow \text{"Core"-(Gal-Rh-Man)}_n + P_i + I_{11}^{at}\text{-P}$$

Scheme 5.14. Role of undecylpolyprenol in biosynthesis of *Salmonella* cell surface polysaccharide.

Work on the biosynthesis of the peptidoglycan of *M. lysodeikticus* has shown the operation of an analogous process which is different primarily as a reflection of a different structure of the polymer. The polyprenol is found joined as a pentapeptidodisaccharide pyrophosphate, I_{11}-P-P-GlcNAc-MurNAc-L-Ala-D-Glu-L-Lys-D-Ala-D-Ala (*35*). Its biosynthesis requires a particulate enzyme, Mg^{++}, and appropriate uridine diphosphate derivatives, UDP-MurNAc-pentapeptide and UDP-GlcNAc (*35*). The I_{11}-P-P-disaccharide-pentapeptide then adds glycine to the free carboxyl group of the glutamic acid residue through the action of an ATP-dependent, particulate enzyme. Finally, the resulting I_{11}-P-P-disaccharide-branched hexapeptide is used for insertion of the repeating units of the forming peptidoglycan by sequential transfer of the disaccharide-branched hexapeptide moiety to an acceptor. In other organisms investigated, the I_{11}-P-P-disaccharide-pentapeptide intermediate is the same but is metabolized in a slightly different fashion.

Bacitracin is a specific inhibitor of the conversion of lipid pyrophosphate to lipid phosphate, and in its presence the pyrophosphate accumulates and peptidoglycan synthesis is consequently inhibited (*85*) (cf. Scheme 5.14).

5. Juvenile Hormone

Insects go through several morphologic stages of development the exact nature of which depends on the type of insect. At each stage orderly development is necessary, and in several cases the regulatory processes have been associated with hormones. Of special interest to our discussion of polyprenols is the observation that the brain-like tissue (corpus allatum) of insects secretes an I_3 compound functioning to prevent metamorphosis from the larval to the pupal stage. Since it maintains the insect in an immature state, it is called "juvenile hormone." In 1956 Williams (*86*) found that the abdomen of the male silkmoth, *Platysamia cecropia*, was particularly rich in such activity, and subsequently Röller and his colleagues (*86–90*) showed the *cecropia* hormone to be the methyl ester of *trans-trans-cis*-10-epoxy-7-ethyl-3,11-dimethyl-2,6-tridecadienoic acid (Scheme 5.15). This is tantamount to farnesoic acid with extra methyl groups added to

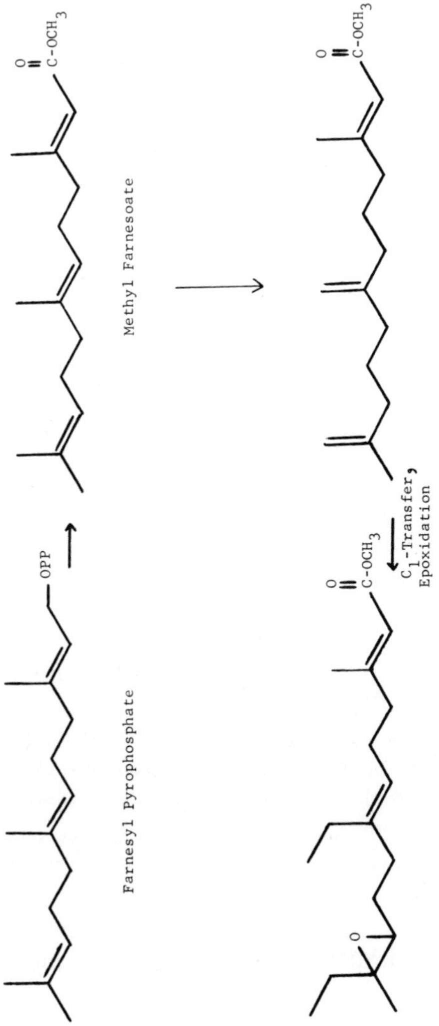

Scheme 5.15. Juvenile hormone and its hypothetical origin.

the protruding methyl groups of I units 2 and 3 and with the third double bond epoxidized. Farnesol itself and various derivatives are biologically active (91-94).

It is not known how the extra methyl groups are derived. Two possibilities come to mind. One is their origin in the carboxyl group of mevalonic acid, and the other is their addition by C_1 transfer from S-adenosylmethionine via the $allo_t$-type of methylene derivative. The latter route (Scheme 5.15) seems more probable, since the observed carbon skeleton could be arrived at without alteration of the general isopentenoid pathway by the relatively simple addition of two types of reaction (isomerization and alkylation) which are, in fact, already known in isopentenoid biochemistry. It is interesting to note that the I unit lacking an extra methyl group is the one with a conjugated double bond less prone to the isomerization required for alkylation.

As is also true for the molting hormone (which is steroidal), there is an ecological involvement in the biology of juvenile hormone, since plants possess related and active molecules. This was observed through serendipity. Williams and Sláma (95) transported *Pyrrhocoris apterus* from Prague to Boston and found surprisingly that no metamorphosis occurred. The trip itself was shown not to be the factor but rather a particular paper towel placed in the rearing jars at the start of the trip. Upon further examination *The New York Times, The Wall Street Journal,* and *Science* were all active, but *The Times* and *Nature* from England were not! The American paper originated in balsam fir, *Abies balsamea,* and Bowers and his colleagues (96) showed the active ingredient to be an I_3 compound, (+)-juvabione (the methyl ester of todomatuic acid) (Scheme 5.16). From Czechoslovak fir, Černý et al. (97) subsequently isolated the same substance and its slightly less active dehydroderivative.

The plant "hormone" is believed to play a physiological role as a defense against predation of insects through the induction of a pathological growth pattern in the invading organism (98). At a biochemical level the true insect juvenile hormone has been shown to induce biosynthesis of the "yolk protein" (known as vitellogenin) in the monarch butterfly (99).

6. Pheromones

Interorganismic communication has been found to be mediated by a variety of relatively small molecules called "pheromones" by Karlson and Lüscher. Karlson (100, 101) has reviewed the early work. More recent literature has been reviewed by Regnier (102). Oligoprenols and their simple metabolites are frequently found among these hormones. The so-called "recruiting pheromones" of insects are nearly all I_2 compounds. About half of the "alarm pheromones" are either I_2 compounds or their seeming metabolites, as is true for a few of the "aggregating pheromones." In fact, about half of all the pheromones in the three categories mentioned are isopentenoid.

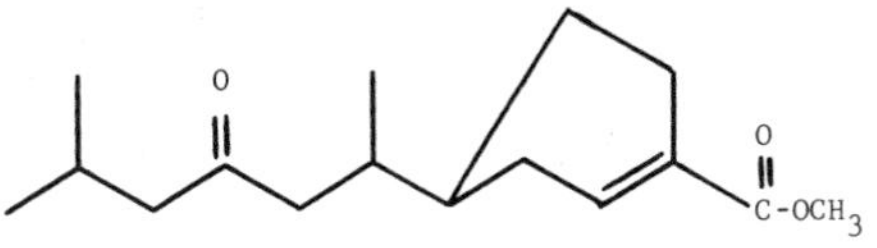

Juvabione

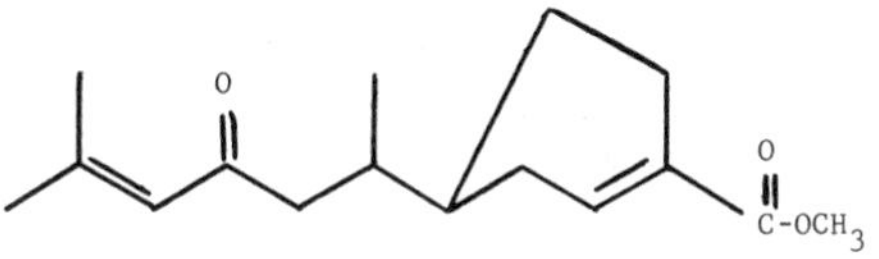

Dehydrojuvabione

Scheme 5.16. Plant products with juvenile hormone activity. Structures are drawn in a way to emphasize relationship to insect hormone.

The ones not oligoprenols per se (or simple metabolites derived by oxidation or oxidative cleavage) are cyclized derivatives, e.g., limonene or α-pinene. This is in some contrast to the "sex pheromones," since none of the molecules endowed only with sex-attractant activity are isopentenoid. Cyclic derivatives of geraniol, (+)-cis-2-isopropenyl-1-methylcyclobutane-ethanol and cis-3,3-dimethy-Δ$^{1,\beta}$-cyclohexaneethanol, and of geranial, cis-3,3-dimethyl-Δ$^{1,\alpha}$-cyclohexaneacetaldehyde and its trans-isomer, are the female attractants produced by the male boll weevil (Anthonomus grandis Boheman), but in the spring and fall they exhibit aggregating activity by attracting both sexes (103).

The "recruiting pheromones" of the honey bee (Apis mellifera) are geraniol, its aldehyde and acid, geranial and geranoic acid, respectively, and nerol and its acid, nerolic acid. In the honey bee the state of oxidation and stereochemistry appear to be less important to activity than is the gross I$_2$ structure. This structural type also has alarm activity in several insect families, but a carbonyl group is more common than a hydroxyl group. Thus, geranial, its 2,3-dihydroderivative, citronellal, and 2,6-dimethylhept-5-en-1-al (and the corresponding alcohol), clearly derived by oxidative cleavage at the double bond of the first I unit of an I$_2$ compound, e.g., geraniol, are alarm pheromones in Formiciae. Removal of still another C atom to give 2-methylhept-2-en-6-one yields the alarm pheromone of the Dolichoderinae. Among the "aggregating hormones" of the bark beetle (Ips confusus), one finds I$_2$ compounds in which the oxygen function at C-1 has been removed by dehydration and a new hydroxyl group introduced on

C-5 yielding the structure $(CH_3)_2CH-CH_2-CH(OH)-CH_2-C(=CH_2)-CH=CH_2$ (2-methyl-6-methyleneoct-7-en-4-ol). The dihydroderivative in which reduction has occurred in the second I unit (*gem*-dimethyl end) is a similar pheromone.

It is interesting to note that, while not a simple polyprenol or oxidative derivative, the bicyclic I_2 compound, nepetalactone, is the active ingredient (feline attractant) of the catnip plant *Nepta cataria*, which attracts the domestic cat (*104, 105*). The compound is oxidatively metabolized by the animal and excreted in the urine (*106*). A simple derivative (the adduct of cysteine) of Δ^{2-} or Δ^3-isopentenol (felinine) derived from MVA (*107*) might also be classed as a pheromone, since it gives feline urine a part of its characteristic odor, and since some large members of the feline family are thought to delineate their territory by urination at strategic points of its periphery. Examples of insect pheromones and feline attractants are given in Scheme 5.17, and naturally occurring oligoprenyl hydrocarbons, aldehydes, and acids are listed in Tables 5.3 and 5.4.

Recruiting Pheromones	I_2-alcohols, I_2-aldehydes, and I_2-acids, e.g., geraniol, its stereoisomer, and oxidation products.
Alarm Pheromones	I_2-aldehydes, e.g., geranial, related ketones, and cyclic I_2-hydrocarbons, e.g., limonene and α-pinene.
Aggregating Pheromones	Unusual I_2-alcohols, e.g., and cyclic I_2-alcohols, e.g., verbenol.
Catnip attractant for cats	Nepetalactone
Feline urine principle	Felinine

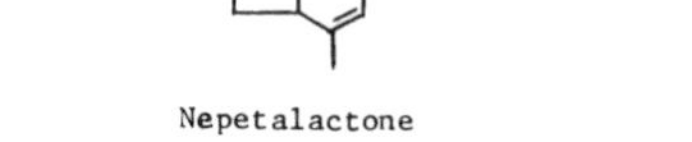

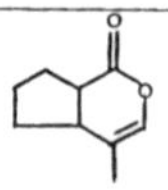

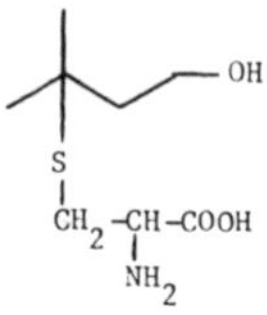

Scheme 5.17. Examples of insect pheromones and feline attractants.

Table 5.3. Natural acyclic oligoprenyl hydrocarbons.

Structure	Name	Remarks
I$_1$	Isoprene	Not yet known to occur naturally.
I$_2$	Ocimene	Occurs in leaves of *Ocimum gratissimum*, fruits of *Evodia rutaecarpa*, and oils from *Heracleum mantegazzianum*, *Salvia sclarea*, etc.
I$_2$	Myrcene	Occurs in leaves of *Pimenta acris*, hop oils from *Humulus lupulus*.
I$_2$	Cosmene	Occurs in *Cosmos bipinnatus*, *Coreopsis verticillata*, other *Compositae*, and roots and leaves of *Amellus strigosus*.
I$_3$	Farnesene	Occurs in hop oil, and either farnesene or its ocimene-like double bond isomer (or both) occur in *Matricaria indora*, buds of *Populus balsamifera*, Ylang-ylang oil, etc.

Table 5.4. Natural oligoprenals and prenoic acids

Structural Designation	Name	Remarks
I_1-acid	Dimethylacrylic acid β-Methylcrotonic acid	Bacterial, liver, etc., metabolite. First isolated from rhizomes of *Senecio kaempferi*. Also found in fruit of *Omphalea diandra*. Probably not always a true isopentenoid, since derivable in ways other than from isopentenol.
I_2^t-aldehyde	Geranial (Citral-a)	Occurs in lemon grass oil and many other plants.
I_2^c-aldehyde	Neral (Citral-b)	Occurs in lemon grass oil and many other plants.
I_2^t-acid I_2^{1s}-acid	Geranioic acid Citronellic acid	Obtained by liver and in vivo incubation of I_2^t-pyrophosphate. Occurs in both enantiomeric forms. The (+) form was isolated first from oil of *Barosoma pulchellum*. Also present in lemon grass and geranium oils and fruits of *Xanthoxylum piperitum*. The (−) form was isolated first from the wood of *Callitris glanca*. Later found in *Chamaecyparis obtusa* and *Thujopsis dolabrata*.
I_3-acid $I_4^{n-(n-2)s}$-acid	Farnesoic acid Phytanic acid	Obtained both from MVA and I_3^{at}-pyrophosphate by liver and in vivo incubations. Pathologic human metabolite of phytol. Deposited as abnormal fat in Refsum's disease.

LITERATURE CITED

1. G. Daves, Jr., R. F. Muraca, J. S. Wittick, P. Friis, and K. Folkers, Biochemistry 6:2861 (1967).
2. P. Friis, G. D. Daves, Jr., and K. Folkers, Biochem. Biophys. Res. Commun. 24:252 (1966).
3. R. L. Lester and F. L. Crane, J. Biol. Chem. 234:2169 (1959).
4. O. Jacobsen, Liebigs Ann. Chem. 157:232 (1871).
5. F. W. Semmler, Ber. Deutsch. Chem. Gesellschaft 23:3556 (1890).
6. F. W. Semmler, Ber. Deutsch. Chem. Gesellschaft 24:201 (1891).
7. A. Hesse, J. pr. Chem [2] 53:238 (1896).
8. F. W. Semmler, Ber. Deutsch. Chem. Gesellschaft 24:208 (1891).
9. O. Zeitschel, Ber. Deutsch. Chem. Gesellschaft 39:1780 (1906).
10. M. Kerschbaum, Ber. Deutsch. Chem. Gesellschaft 46:1732 (1913).
11. R. Willstätter and F. Hocheder, Liebigs Ann. Chem. 354:205 (1907).
12. R. L. Rowland, P. H. Latimer, and J. A. Giles, J. Am. Chem. Soc. 78: 4680 (1956).
13. R. H. Bates, R. H. Carnighan, R. O. Rakutis, and J. H. Schauble, Chem. Ind. (London) 1020 (1962).
14. R. E. Erickson, C. H. Shunk, N. R. Trenner, B. H. Arison, and K. Folkers, J. Am. Chem. Soc. 81:4999 (1959).
15. M. Kofler, A. Langemann, R. Ruegg, U. Gloor, U. Schweiter, J. Wuersch, O. Wiss, and O. Isler, Helv. Chim. Acta 42:2252 (1959).
16. A. F. Brodie, M. M. Weber, and C. T. Grey, Biochim. Biophys. Acta 25: 448 (1957).
17. F. L. Crane, Y. Hatefi, R. L. Lester, and C. Widmer, Biochim. Biophys. Acta 25:220 (1959).
18. R. L. Lester and F. L. Crane, J. Biol. Chem. 234:2169 (1959).
19. F. L. Crane, Plant Physiol. 34:546 (1959).
20. N. L. Bishop, Proc. Natl. Acad. Sci. U.S.A. 45:1696 (1959).
21. B. O. Lindgren, Acta Chem. Scand. 18:836 (1964).
22. B. O. Lindgren, Acta Chem. Scand. 19:1317 (1965).
23. A. R. Wellburn and F. W. Hemming, in T. W. Goodwin (ed.), Biochemistry of the Chloroplast. Vol. I. Academic Press, New York, 1966. p. 173.
24. A. R. Wellburn and F. W. Hemming, Phytochemistry 5:969 (1966).
25. M. Calvin, Proc. Roy. Soc. (London), Ser. A 288:441 (1965).
26. P. E. Cloud, Jr., J. W. Gruner, and H. Hagen, Science 143:1713 (1965).
27. A. Albrecht and G. Ourisson, Angew. Chem. (Intl. Ed. Engl.) 10:209 (1971).
28. E. D. McCarthy and M. Calvin, Tetrahedron 23:2609 (1967).
29. R. Willstätter, F. Hocheder, and E. Hug, Liebigs Ann. Chem. 371:1 (1909).
30. N. J. de Souza and W. R. Nes, Phytochemistry 8:819 (1969).
31. A. S. Holt, D. W. Hughes, H. J. Kende, and J. W. Purdie, Plant Cell Physiol. 4:49 (1963).
32. I. Iwata and Y. Sakurai, Agr. Biol. Chem. (Tokyo) 27:253 (1963).
33. K. J. I. Thorne and E. Kodicek, Biochem. J. 99:123 (1966).
34. A. Wright, M. Dankert, P. Fennessey, and P. W. Robbins, Proc. Natl. Acad. Sci. U.S.A. 57:1798 (1967).
35. Y. Higashi, J. L. Strominger, and C. C. Sweeley, Proc. Natl. Acad. Sci. U.S.A. 57:1878 (1967).
36. J. Burgos, P. H. W. Butterworth, F. W. Hemming, and R. A. Morton, Biochem. J. 91:22P (1964).
37. J. Burgos, F. W. Hemming, J. F. Pennock, and R. A. Morton, Biochem. J. 88:470 (1963).

38. K. J. Stone, P. H. W. Butterworth, and F. W. Hemming, Biochem. J. 102: 443 (1967).
39. P. J. Dunphy, J. D. Kerr, J. F. Pennock, K. J. Whittle, Chem. Ind. (London) 1549 (1966).
40. K. J. Stone, P. H. W. Butterworth, and F. W. Hemming, Biochem. J. 102: 443 (1967).
41. P. W. Holloway and G. Popjak, Biochem. J. 104:57 (1967).
42. G. Popjak, P. W. Holloway, and J. M. Baron, Biochem. J. 111:325 (1969).
43. K. Ogura, T. Nishino, T. Koyama, and S. Seto, J. Am. Chem. Soc. 92: 6036 (1970).
44. (a) T. Nishino, K. Ogura, and S. Seto, J. Am. Chem. Soc. 93:794 (1971); (b) 94:6849 (1972).
45. J. E. Graebe, Science 157:73 (1967).
46. P. Benveniste, G. Ourisson, and L. Hirth, Phytochemistry 9:1073 (1970).
47. A. A. Kandutsch, H. Paulus, E. Levin, and K. Bloch, J. Biol. Chem. 239: 2507 (1969).
48. C. M. Allen, W. Alworth, A. Macrae, and K. Bloch, J. Biol. Chem. 242: 1895 (1967).
49. F. Lynen, H. Eggerer, U. Henning, and I. Kessel, Angew. Chem. 70:738 (1958).
50. J. W. Cornforth, Angew. Chem. (Intl. Ed. Engl.) 7:903 (1968).
51. F. Lynen, B. W. Agranoff, H. Eggerer, U. Henning, and E. M. Moslein, Angew. Chem. 71:657 (1959).
52. B. W. Agranoff, H. Eggerer, U. Henning, and F. Lynen, J. Biol. Chem. 235:326 (1960).
53. J. W. Cornforth, R. H. Cornforth, C. Donninger, and G. Popják, Proc. Roy. Soc. (London), Ser. B. 163:492 (1966).
54. J. W. Cornforth, R. H. Cornforth, G. Popják, and L. S. Yengoyan, J. Biol. Chem. 241:3970 (1966).
55. G. Popják and J. W. Cornforth, Biochem. J. 101:553 (1966).
56. K. J. Stone and F. W. Hemming, Biochem. J. 104:43 (1967).
57. H. H. Rees, E. I. Mercer, and T. W. Goodwin, Biochem. J. 99:726 (1966).
58. B. L. Archer, D. Barnard, E. G. Cockbain, J. W. Cornforth, R. H. Cornforth, and G. Popjak, Proc. Roy. Soc. (London), Ser. B 163:519 (1966).
59. E. Jedlicki, G. Jacob, F. Faini, and E. Cori, Arch. Biochem. Biophys. 152: 590 (1972).
60. T. Reichstein, Naturwiss. 54:53 (1967).
61. R. Tschesche, Angew. Chem. 73:727 (1961).
62. E. Leete, H. Gregory, and E. G. Gros, J. Am. Chem. Soc. 87:3475 (1965).
63. E. Leete and E. G. Gros, J. Am. Chem. Soc. 87:3479 (1965).
64. J. A. F. Wickramasinghe, E. P. Burrows, R. K. Sharma, and E. Caspi, Phytochemistry 8:1433 (1969).
65. A. M. Porto and E. G. Gros, Experientia 26:11 (1970).
66. R. Tschesche and B. Brassat, Z. Naturforsch. 20b:707 (1965).
67. A. J. Birch, J. Schonfield, and H. Smith, Chem. Ind. (London) 1321 (1958).
68. A. J. Birch, Fortschr. d. Chem. Org. Naturstoffe, Springer Verlag, Vienna 14:186 (1957).
69. G. B. Cox, I. G. Young, L. M. McCann, and F. Gibson, J. Bact. 99:450 (1969).
70. P. Friis, G. D. Daves, and K. Folkers, J. Am. Chem. Soc. 88:4754 (1966).
71. R. S. Raman, H. Rudney, and N. K. Buzzelli, Arch. Biochem. Biophys. 130:164 (1969).

72. G. R. Whistance, F. E. Field, and D. R. Threlfall, Eur. J. Biochem. 18: 46 (1971).
73. H. G. Nowicki, G. H. Dialameh, B. L. Trumpower, and R. E. Olson, Fed. Proc. 28:884 (1969).
74. R. Willstätter, F. Hocheder, and E. Hug, Liebigs Ann. Chem. 371:1 (1909).
75. I. Iwata, H. Nakata, M. Mizushima, and Y. Sakurai, Agr. Biol. Chem. (Tokyo) 25:319 (1961).
76. I. Iwata and Y. Sakurai, Agr. Biol. Chem. (Tokyo) 27:253 (1963).
77. H. Rapoport and H. P. Hamlow, Biochem. Res. Commun. 6:134 (1961).
78. A. S. Holt, D. W. Hughes, H. J. Kende, and J. W. Purdie, Plant Cell Physiol. 4:49 (1963).
79. H. J. Perkins and W. H. Vogel, Proc. Can. Soc. Plant Physiol. 8:55 (1967).
80. C. Costes, Abstracts of the 6th International Biochemical Congress, New York, 1964, p. 569.
81. L. Bogorad and R. F. Troxler, in P. Bernfeld (ed.), Biogenesis of Natural Compounds. 2nd Ed. Pergamon, Oxford, 1967. pp. 261-272.
82. K. J. I. Thorne and E. Kodicek, Biochim. Biophys. Acta 59:280 (1962).
83. M. J. Osborn and I. M. Weiner, Fed. Proc. 26:70 (1967).
84. P. W. Robbins, A. Wright, and M. Dankert, J. Gen. Physiol. 49:331 (1966).
85. G. Siewert and J. L. Strominger, Proc. Natl. Acad. Sci. U.S.A. 57:767 (1967).
86. C. M. Williams, Nature 178:212 (1956).
87. H. Röller and J. S. Bjerke, Life Sci. 4:1617 (1965).
88. H. Röller, J. S. Bjerke, and W. H. McShan, J. Insect Physiol. 11:1185 (1965).
89. H. Röller, K. H. Dahm, C. C. Sweeley and B. M. Trost, Angew. Chem. 79: 190 (1967).
90. K. H. Dahm, H. Roller, and B. M. Trost, Life Sci. 7:129 (1968).
91. C. Hintze-Podufal, Z. Naturforsch. 26b:154 (1971).
92. M. Schwarz, P. E. Sonnet, and N. Wakabayashi, Science 167:191 (1970).
93. W. S. Bowers, Science 161:895 (1968).
94. W. S. Bowers, Science 164:323 (1969).
95. C. M. Williams and K. Sláma, Biol. Bull. 130:247 (1966).
96. W. S. Bowers, H. M. Fales, M. J. Thompson, and E. C. Uebel, Science 154:1020 (1966).
97. V. Černý, L. Dolejas, L. Labler, F. Sorm, and K. Sláma, Coll. Czech. Chem. Commun. 32:3926 (1967).
98. D. B. Carlisle, P. E. Ellis, Z. Brettschneiderova, and V. J. A. Novak, J. Endocrinol. 35:211 (1966).
99. M. L. Pan and G. R. Wyatt, Science 174:503 (1971).
100. P. Karlson, 4th International Congress of Biochemistry, XII:37 (1959).
101. P. Karlson, Ergeb. Biol. 22:212 (1960).
102. F. E. Regnier, Biol. Reproduction 4:308 (1971).
103. J. H. Tumlinson, D. D. Hardee, R. C. Gueldner, A. C. Thompson, and P. A. Hedin, Science 166:1010 (1969).
104. S. M. McElvain, R. D. Bright, and P. R. Johnson, J. Am. Chem. Soc. 63: 1558 (1941).
105. N. B. Todd, J. Hered. 53:54 (1962).
106. G. R. Waller, G. H. Price, and E. D. Mitchell, Science 164:1281 (1969).
107. P. V. Avizonis and J. C. Wriston, Biochim. Biophys. Acta 34:279 (1959).

Chapter
6

Head-to-Head Coupling of Isopentenoid Polymers

A. General Considerations 205
B. Biosynthesis of Squalene 208
   1. *Farnesyl Pyrophosphate as Precursor* 208
   2. *Presqualene Pyrophosphate as an Intermediate* 208
   3. *Mechanism of Condensation and Reduction* 211
   4. *Enzymology* 217
C. Biosynthesis of Phytoene 219
   1. *General Comments* 219
   2. *Biosynthesis* 220
   3. *Enzymology* 222
   4. *Stereochemistry and Mechanism* 222
Literature Cited 225

A. GENERAL CONSIDERATIONS

I$_n$ polymers resulting from head-to-tail polymerization of I-pyrophosphate units possess a reactive primary ester group at the head end. Instead of a continuation of the polymerization by attack of this head end on the terminal double bond of Δ^3-isopentenyl pyrophosphate, it is possible for the head end to attack a nonterminal double bond of another molecule. In principle, this could be either another isopentenoid or essentially any other substance with appropriate nucleophilic centers. Such a process is known as "isopentenylation" and some very important molecules, e.g., quinone cofactors, with expected structures are known in nature (Scheme 6.1; see also Scheme 5.5).

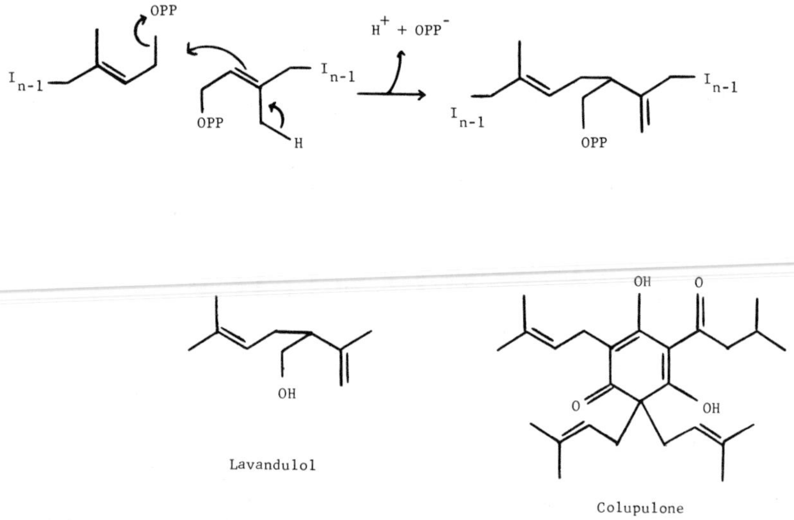

Lavandulol

Colupulone

Scheme 6.1. Examples of isopentenylation.

The structure of lavandulol (*1, 2*) illustrates the attack of Δ^2-isopentenyl pyrophosphate, followed by hydrolysis. Colupulone (*3*) illustrates isopentenylation of a non-isopentenoid. It must be noted, however, that isopentenylation of a double bond situated internally in an isopentenoid polymer must of necessity lead to a molecule with one or more C atoms as a side chain, as in the case of the CH_2—OH group of lavandulol, which represents C-1 of the I_1-pyrophosphate. If attack were on, say, the double bond in the third unit of an I_3-pyrophosphate, then the side chain would have 11 carbon atoms (the first two I units and the first C atom of the third). Consequently, it is surprising at first sight to find exceedingly important molecules in nature that are derived from coupling of two isopentenoid polymers in a head-to-head arrangement such that no side chain is extruded.

From a simple mechanistic standpoint the usual allylic cleavage of the C—O bond with elimination of pyrophosphate anion, which occurs both in head-to-tail polymerization and in isopentenylation, would be regarded as the most characteristic reaction of an ester of a strong acid (pyrophosphoric acid) and an α,β-unsaturated primary alcohol. This process would yield two electrophilic carbon atoms at C-1 of two I_n-pyrophosphate polymers (Scheme

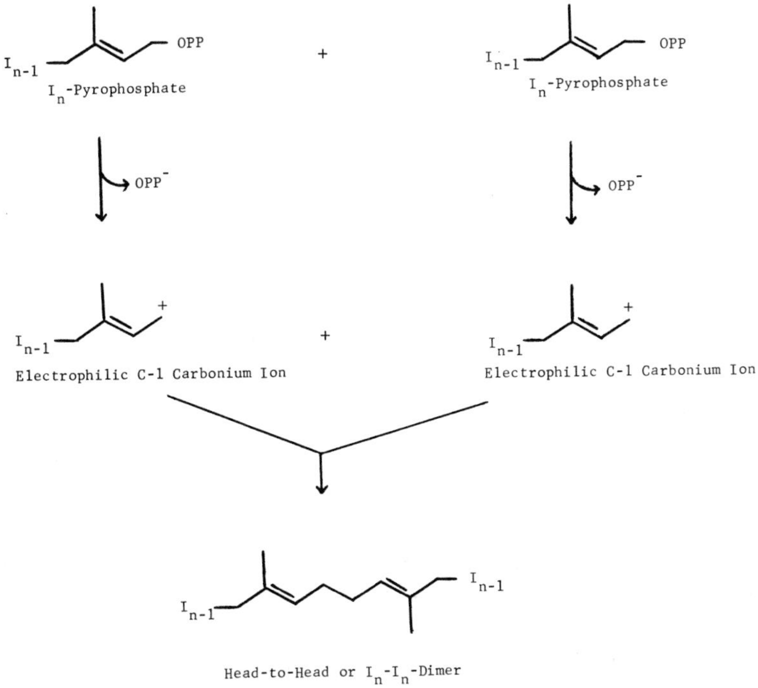

Scheme 6.2. Impossible process of coupling of I_n-pyrophosphate polymers.

6.2), which could not possibly couple, because of charge repulsion. The only way coupling could occur would be by elimination of pyrophosphate anion and a proton, i.e., by a process of the dehydration type. This is shown without regard to mechanism in Scheme 6.3. Either a coupled product still bearing one of the pyrophosphoroxy groups (an I_n-I_n-pyrophosphate) or one bearing a double bond in its place would result (an unsaturated I_n-I_n-dimer). If reduction were superimposed on the elimination reactions, a dimer lacking any pyrophosphoroxy groups could be formed in which the I_n-polymers have been brought together through a single bond joining the two C-1 atoms (a reduced I_n-I_n-dimer). However, a detailed mechanism for such processes has little precedent. Despite this, both the reduced and unsaturated I_n-I_n-dimers exist in nature and in fact comprise the route of metabolism leading in the former case to steroids and many other cyclic compounds and in the latter to carotenoids. Owing to this great significance, much work has been done to elucidate the problem, and some success has been achieved, as described in what follows.

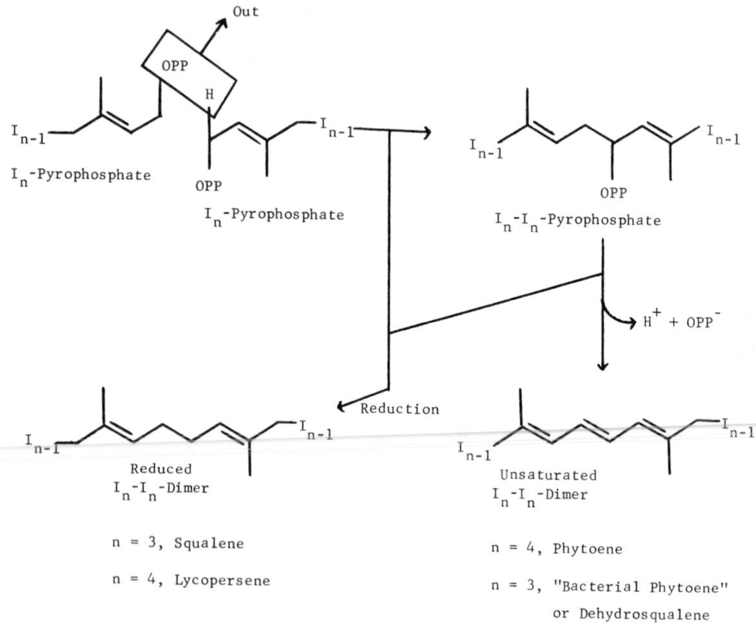

Scheme 6.3. Concept of coupling by elimination of pyrophosphoric acid.

B. BIOSYNTHESIS OF SQUALENE

1. Farnesyl Pyrophosphate as Precursor

Because the formation of farnesyl pyrophosphate (the $I_3{}^{at}$-isopentenoid pyrophosphate, Chapter 5, Sections A and B and Scheme 5.8) was achieved in a cell-free system quite early, and because it requires no oxidation-reduction cofactors, it was among the first of the intermediates to be discovered and examined. Lynen and his associates (4) found that in the absence of reduced pyridine nucleotide yeast enzyme preparations led to the $I_3{}^{at}$-pyrophosphate, but, when NADPH was present, the hydrocarbon, squalene, appeared instead. This hydrocarbon was already known to have a structure corresponding to a reduced $I_3{}^{at}$-$I_3{}^{at}$-dimer (Chapter 4, Section A.1, Scheme 4.1, and Scheme 6.3), and it had already been shown to be on the steroid pathway (Chapter 4, Section A.1). It was now obvious from the kinetic data that it must arise by some set of condensative events from two farnesyl pyrophosphate molecules. A recent demonstration of this is the incubation of [³H]farnesyl pyrophosphate with [¹⁴C]farnesyl pyrophosphate, which yielded doubly labeled squalene (5).

2. Presqualene Pyrophosphate as an Intermediate

Rilling (6–8) subsequently showed that the elimination of NADPH from the yeast enzyme system also led to a C_{30} pyrophosphate that yielded squalene upon reincubation with NADPH. This intermediate was named "presqualene" (7), but recent usage is to describe the free alcohol as presqualene alcohol and the pyrophosphate ester as presqualene pyrophosphate (PSPP).

Considerable controversy has surrounded PSPP. A cyclopropyl structure was proposed (6) and discarded (9), as was a gycolyl structure (10). Reinvestigation by Rilling and his associates (7, 8) led to the proposal of a second cyclopropyl structure (Scheme 6.4). Synthesis of this pyrophosphate

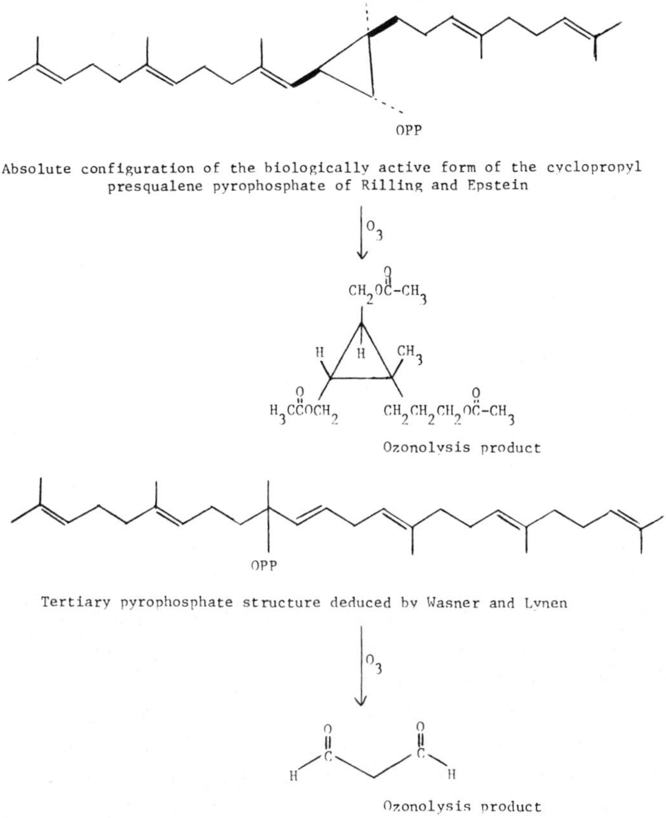

OPP

Absolute configuration of the biologically active form of the cyclopropyl presqualene pyrophosphate of Rilling and Epstein

Ozonolysis product

OPP

Tertiary pyrophosphate structure deduced by Wasner and Lynen

Ozonolysis product

Scheme 6.4. Proposed structure and degradation products of presqualene PP.

and the alcohol has been reported by three laboratories (11–14); in addition, the absolute configuration of the biologically active conformer depicted in Scheme 6.4 was established recently (15, 16). Chemical and physical characterization of Rilling's PSPP has been carried out primarily with the synthetic alcohol, the alcohol derived from $LiAlH_4$ reduction of the pyrophosphate, or the alcohol produced by enzymatic depyrophosphorylation of the natural product. Great effort has been expended to demonstrate that these processes do not produce a rearranged product, a phenomenon that is not unknown when $LiAlH_4$ is the reductant (8, 15). Results from mass spectrometry show a molecular weight of 426 for the alcohol and fragments at M^+ -18 and M^+-31 indicative of the loss of water and CH_2OH, respectively (8, 12–15). These data are evidence for, but not absolute proof of, the presence of a primary alcohol group. Absorptions at 1,010 cm^{-1} in the far infrared and 1.65–1.80 μm in the near infrared are attributed to the resonance of cyclopropane ring deformation and the first overtones of cyclopropane CH stretching, respectively (15). NMR of the alcohol results in a sharp singlet at τ 8.84–8.98 indicative of the cyclopropyl methyl group as well as a group of unresolved resonances in the region τ 8.4–9.12 indicative of the cyclopropyl hydrogen and a CH_2 group adjacent to the cyclopropane ring (8, 12–15). The presence of double bonds similar to those in squalene was indicated by NMR and mass spectrometry (7, 8, 15). Popjak and co-workers deduced that PSPP probably has five double bonds from an increase of 10 mass units of the catalytically hydrogenated alcohol (15). Ozonolysis of the alcohol derived biosynthetically from a mixture of $[4,8,12-^{14}C_3]FPP$ and $[1-^3H_2]$- or $[1-D_2]FPP$ yielded isopropyl alcohol, pentane-1,4-diol acetate, and a C_{15} cyclopropane fragment after reduction and acetylation of the ozonolysis products. Only the C_{15} portion contained deuterium or tritium (15).

Synthetic and/or natural PSPP incubated in the presence of NADPH produces squalene in an average of 65% yield in yeast systems (8, 12–14) or 10% yield in pea systems (17). When PSPP is prepared from yeast enzymes incubated with $[1-^3H_2]$- or $[1-D_2]FPP$, PSPP retains three of the four atoms of isotopic hydrogen (8, 15). Similarly, squalene biosynthesized from labeled PSPP and/or NADPH retains the expected labeling pattern of isotopic hydrogen (18–20).

Wasner and Lynen also isolated a C_{30}-pyrophosphate from incubations of $[^{14}C]FPP$ with yeast cell-free systems starved for NADPH (21). Hydrolysis of the pyrophosphate produced an alcohol with molecular weight 426. NMR and the mass spectrum indicated the presence of double bonds with most arranged as in squalene. Absorptions in the τ 9.0 region of NMR were not noted. Acid hydrolysis cleaved the pyrophosphate group and water from PSPP. Ozonolysis of PSPP biosynthesized in yeast from $[1-^{14}C]FPP$ yielded radioactive malondialdehyde. Consequently, Wasner and Lynen proposed from their data the structure shown in Scheme 6.4, containing a tertiary pyrophosphate group, and which did not indicate the presence of a cyclopropane ring. Incubation of this PSPP with yeast in the presence of NADPH resulted in the biosynthesis of squalene in 90% yield.

It has been suggested (22–24) that PSPP may not be a free intermediate or that it may be formed as a result of a reversible side reaction in the absence of NADPH (i.e., the lack of available reductant promotes formation of the side product, PSPP). Rilling and his associates have reported the isolation of PSPP from intact rat liver and yeast microsomes in the presence of NADPH (25). However, identification of their product is based solely on retention of a radioactive product by a Dowex 1-X8 formate column. Rigorous chemical and physical identification of the compound was not reported.

The questions of the actual structure of PSPP and its intermediacy have still not been fully resolved. There is a wealth of evidence presented above that points to the cyclopropyl structure. On the other hand, the tertiary pyrophosphate compound has not been examined in similar detail. Various mechanisms can be derived for the formation of both structures from FPP (and their reduction to squalene). Conflicting kinetic evidence indicates on one hand that PSPP dissociates from the enzyme and reattaches to another site for reduction, and, on the other hand, that PSPP may not be a "free" intermediate or that it may be an artifact of NADPH deprivation. Answers to these problems will come from more thorough investigation and the preparation of more highly purified squalene synthetase preparations.

3. Mechanism of Condensation and Reduction

The elegant studies of Cornforth and Popjak with stereospecifically labeled MVA have established the fate of the protons at C-1 of FPP during condensation for the formation of squalene. Squalene biosynthesized from $[5,5-^2H_2]$ MVA or $[2-^{14}C,1,1-^2H_2]$FPP retains all but one of the possible deuterium atoms in the central portion of the squalene molecule (26, 27). Further experimentation provided evidence that: 1) the source of the hydrogen transferred to the central portion of squalene was NADPH, 2) the transfer of hydrogen from NADPH was a stereospecific process occurring from one side of the pyridine ring (the B side), 3) the configuration of the hydrogen eliminated from C-1 of FPP was pro-S, and 4) the configuration of the hydrogen atom in the central portion of squalene added from NADPH was pro-R (19, 20, 26, 27). Scheme 6.5 depicts the orientation of the hydrogen atoms at the center of squalene.

The direct head-to-head union of two molecules of FPP is rather difficult to conceive mechanistically. Popjak and Cornforth (19, 28) suggested that there might be a prior rearrangement of one molecule of FPP to the isomer, nerolidyl pyrophosphate (NPP), which would then condense with an unrearranged molecule of FPP. The advantage of such an intermediate is that it has a reactive π electronic system on C-1 that can donate bonding electrons to the electrophilic C-1 of FPP when the latter loses a pyrophosphate anion. Several mechanisms can readily be imagined that can lead to a presqualene pyrophosphate structure of the sort proposed by Wasner and Lynen (21). All of these mechanisms depend on pyrophosphate anion from FPP functioning as an electron sink with C-1 to C-1 σ bond formation arising from the σ bond between C-1 and C-2 of NPP. What is not easy to predict is the detail of how the proton is lost. It seems unlikely for it to be removed concomitantly with C-C bond formation, since electron flow on C-1 would

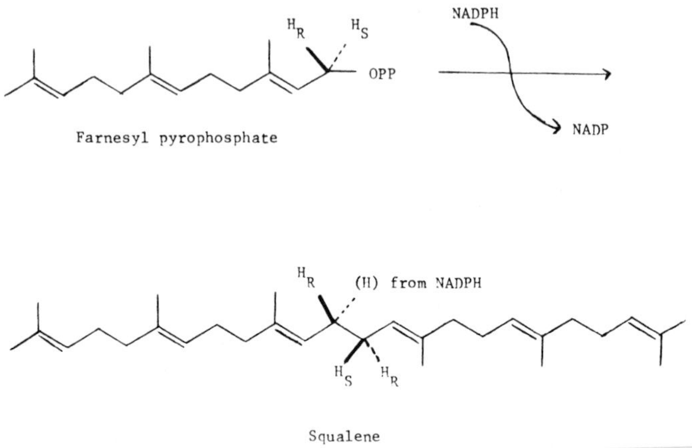

Scheme 6.5. Stereochemistry of squalene biosynthesis from farnesyl pyrophosphate.

become confused. More likely, there might be a charged transition state or neutral intermediate of the sorts shown in Scheme 6.6. Of these, a neutral intermediate formed by bond formation with the enzyme is particularly attractive.

While the biosynthesis of NPP has been reported (29) in rat liver, which also forms squalene, nonenzymatic divalent cation (Mn^{++} particularly) catalysis of its formation from FPP has also been reported (30). Whether such catalysis is really the source of the experimental formation (29) of the isomer remains to be determined with certainty, but a far more serious indictment of its intermediate role is the finding that, in a squalene synthesizing system: (1) farnesyl and nerolidyl pyrophosphates are not interconvertible, (2) radioactivity from [1-^{3}H$_2$]nerolidyl pyrophosphate is not converted to squalene, and (3) the presence of unlabeled nerolidyl pyrophosphate does not alter the relative loss of hydrogen atoms from farnesyl pyrophosphate during the latter's conversion to squalene (5). Nevertheless, there remain the very attractive, almost compelling, mechanistic reasons for invoking the tertiary structure, and a report actually exists of its depressing incorporation of FPP into squalene (31). Perhaps what is actually happening is the formation of an enzyme-bound form of NPP. One can easily imagine several ways in which this could occur, e.g., by a nucleophilic group from the enzyme feeding into C-3 of FPP as the pyrophosphate anion leaves or prior formation of an ester between the FPP and the enzyme with intramolecular rearrangement and formation of an active enzyme-bound NPP that does not readily equilibrate with free NPP (Scheme 6.7).

The identification of a PSPP having a cyclopropyl structure that is formed from FPP has led to the suggestion of several mechanisms for the direct head-to-head union of two molecules of FPP with the assistance of nucleo-

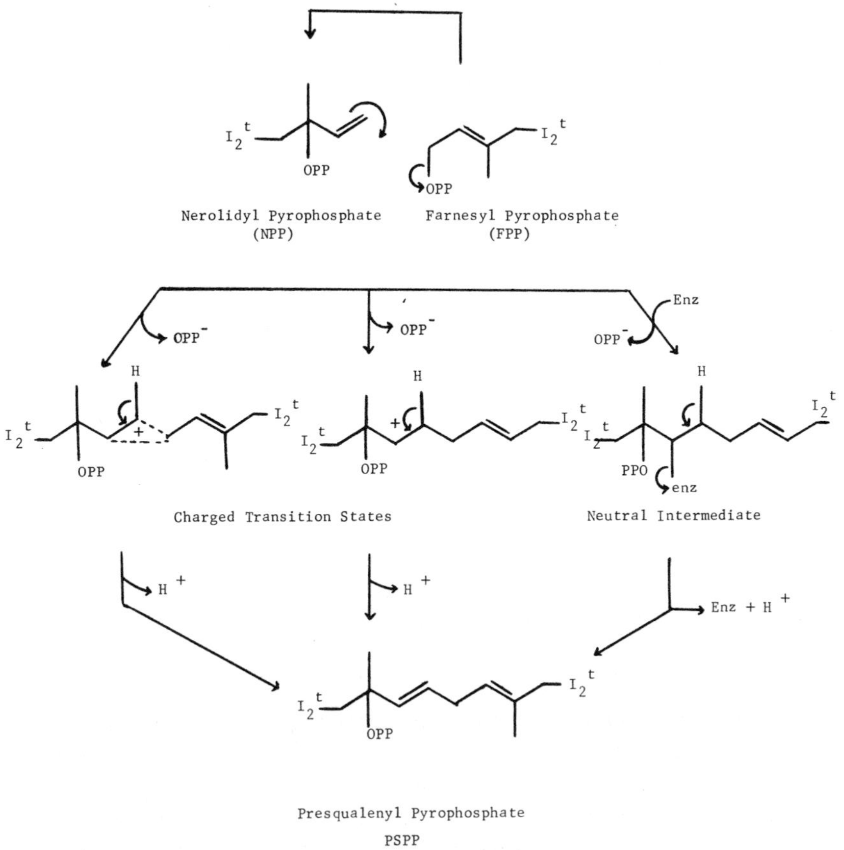

Scheme 6.6. Reasonable mechanisms for formation of Lynen's presqualene pyrophosphate.

philic groups (from the enzyme) in one or more steps (*8, 15, 32-34*). These mechanisms are in many ways similar to the mechanism of the well-studied prenyl transfer reaction of DMAPP and IPP (discussed in Chapter 5, Section B) for head-to-tail condensation in the formation of polyisoprenoids. Porter and his associates (*33*) have proposed a mechanism that agrees with their results from kinetic studies of purified yeast and liver (*35*) squalene synthetases. Their data indicated that the binding of the first molecule of FPP to the enzyme is irreversibly connected to the binding of NADPH and to the binding of the second FPP molecule. Consequently, it can be envisioned that an S_N2 displacement of the PP$_i$ by a nucleophilic group on the enzyme yields an enzyme-bound form of FPP. With the assistance of another nucleophilic moiety on the enzyme, the electron-rich π system of the second FPP molecule displaces the enzyme from C-1 of the farnesyl-enzyme. Isomerization of the double bond, in a manner similar to the isomerization of IPP to

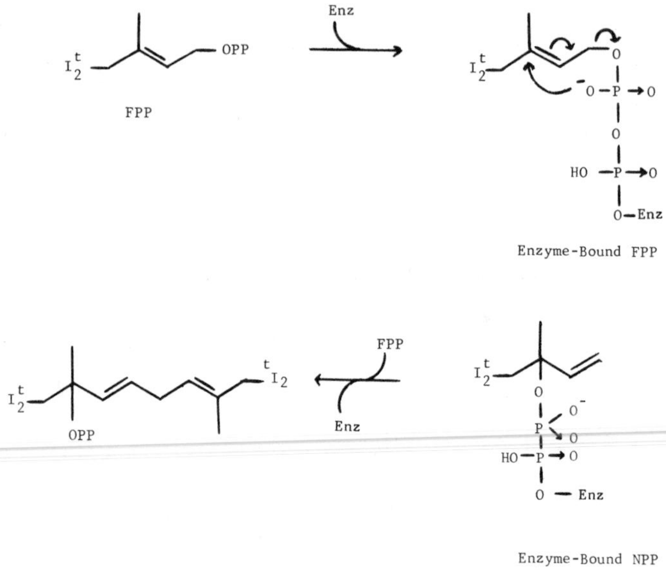

Scheme 6.7. Conceivable involvement of enzyme-bound form of nerolidyl pyrophosphate in head-to-head coupling.

DMAPP, forms a homoallylic system. This is followed by intramolecular S$_N$2 displacement of the enzyme by the new π electron system resulting in closure of the cyclopropane ring, as shown in Scheme 6.8. Cyclopropane ring closure from a homoallylic system has precedent (34) and, in fact, can be demonstrated biogenetically in the terpene family. Cyclogeranyl mesylate, when heated at 50° for 45 min in aqueous acetone over CaCO$_3$, produces a major product with a cyclopropyl group (34). A mechanism similar to the one for formation of the cyclopropane ring in PSPP can be rationalized (Scheme 6.9) for the formation of this compound.

Reasonable mechanisms for the reduction of the two PSPP structures by NADPH in agreement with the known stereochemistry of the hydrogen atoms at the central carbons of squalene are possible to predict. Reduction of the tertiary pyrophosphate structure for PSPP could occur in one step with the attack of hydride ion (from NADPH) on the C atom at the end of the allylic pyrophosphate ester system with elimination of pyrophosphate anion and migration of the double bond (Scheme 6.10). A mechanism proposed by Popjak and co-workers (15) for the reduction of cyclopropyl PSPP is in agreement with kinetic evidence for squalene synthetase (33) in which NADPH is bound first by the enzyme followed by PSPP. The order or release of products has been found to be: 1) PP$_i$, 2) squalene, and 3) NADP. Ring expansion of cyclopropyl PSPP to the tautomeric cyclobutyl compound coupled with migration of the pyrophosphate anion and followed by attack

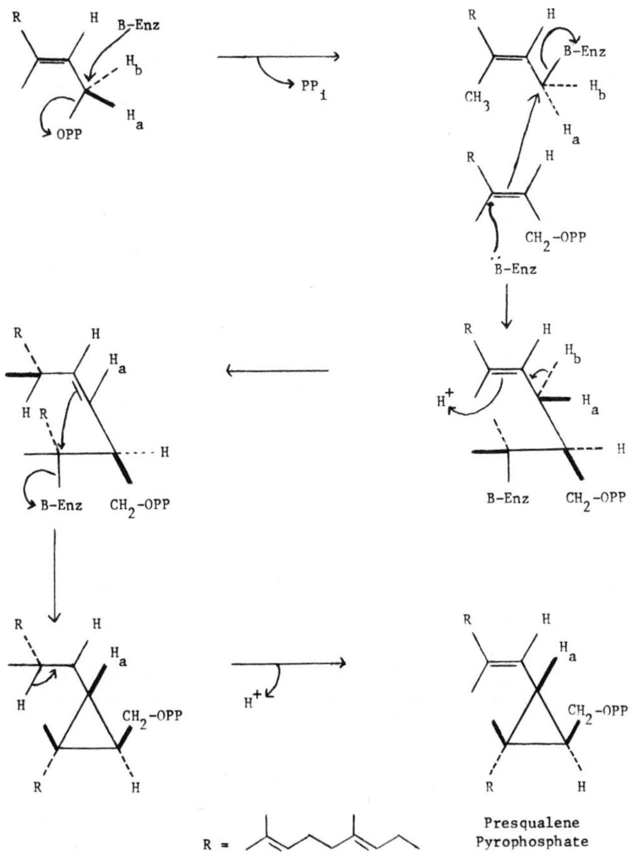

Scheme 6.8. Mechanism for the formation of Rilling's presqualene PP proposed by Porter and co-workers.

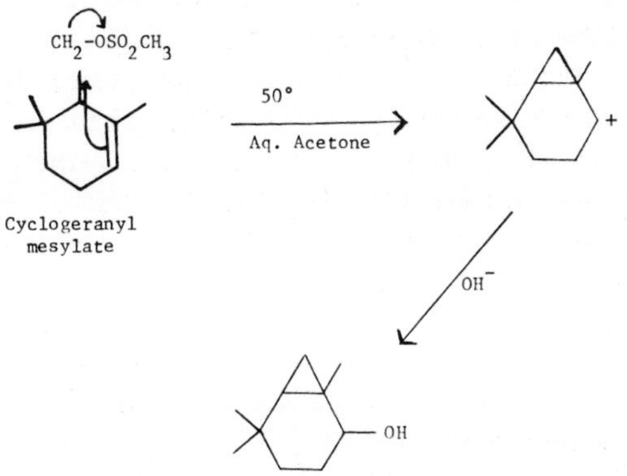

Scheme 6.9. Biogenetic closure of a cyclopropane ring from a homoallylic system.

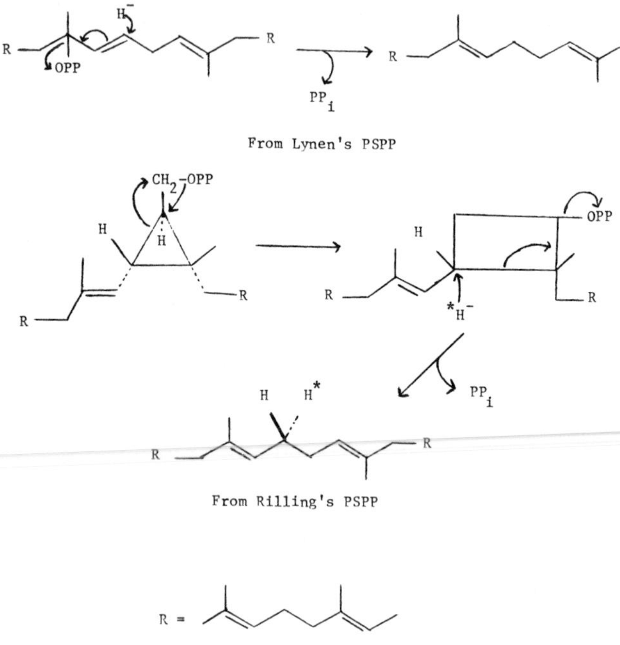

Scheme 6.10. Possible mechanisms for the formation of squalene from PSPP (hydride ion from NADPH). (Mechanism for Rilling's PSPP proposed by Popjak and co-workers.)

of hydride ion (from NADPH) could produce ring cleavage with concomitant generation of the double bond and elimination of pyrophosphate (Scheme 6.10). Several other mechanisms propose ring contraction of the cyclobutyl intermediate to a rearranged cyclopropyl compound before reduction to squalene (*12, 32, 34, 36*). Biogenetic studies of compounds similar to PSPP indicate that the enzyme must provide selective assistance in order to suppress other types of rearrangements because the proposed cyclopropyl rearrangement via the cyclobutyl intermediate is not normally stereoselective (*37*).

The various mechanistic considerations for the condensation and reduction do not in any way depend on the length of the isopentenoid chain that should be controlled by the polymerase, e.g., farnesyl pyrophosphate synthetase or geranyl-geranyl pyrophosphate synthetase, and by the recognition centers for chain length on the dimerizing and reducing enzymes. Thus, there could be isopentenylogs of squalene with longer or shorter chains. One is known synthetically, lycopersene (Scheme 6.3), with four I^{at} units on each half of the molecule. However, despite earlier reports of its existence (*38, 39*) it does not appear to arise naturally (*40–45*).

Scheme 6.11 summarizes the entire biosynthetic route to squalene and traces the fate of some pertinent atoms.

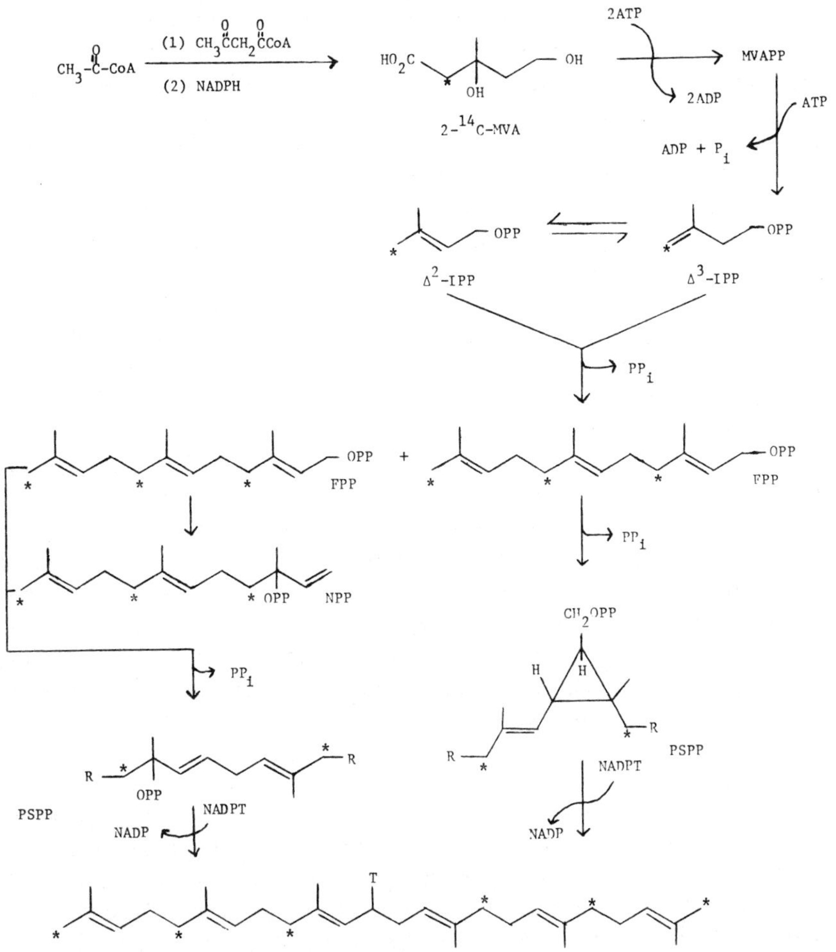

Scheme 6.11. Biosynthesis of squalene from [2-^{14}C]acetate, unlabeled acetoacetate, ATP, and [4-^{3}H$_1$]NADPH.

4. Enzymology

Squalene synthetase, which catalyzes the formation of squalene from two molecules of farnesyl pyrophosphate in the presence of NADPH, occurs in a wide variety of organisms, including yeast (46, 47), liver (29, 48, 49), pea (50), tobacco (51), and carrot root and tomato (52). This particular enzyme is associated with membrane particles in yeast (6) and tobacco (53) and microsomes in liver (29, 48). Enzymes of this type are especially difficult to solubilize from membrane fragments. Two research groups have recently reported the successful solubilization of yeast (22, 54) and liver (35) squalene synthetases by sonication, treatment with detergent, or high-density sucrose solution followed by purification with retention of biological activity. The purified yeast enzyme apparently exists in a polymeric form that can be dissociated to the protomeric form in the presence of low concentrations of glycerol (54). The overall condensation of two units of FPP to squalene is catalyzed by the polymer, whereas the protomer produces only presqualene pyrophosphate from FPP. Reassociation of the protomer results in a loss of activity of the reassociated form in comparison with the activity of the orig- inal undissociated preparation. Divalent cation [Mn^{++} being better than Mg^{++} at low concentration, but the reverse being so at high concentration (31, 33)] and a pH of 7.3 to 7.5 (29, 31, 33) are required. Similar divalent cation phenomena have been observed in at least one other enzyme that utilizes phosphorylated intermediates, mevalonate kinase (55). Squalene for- mation is inhibited by a concentration of FPP or NPP greater than 1×10^{-4} M for the liver enzyme (31) and a similar concentration for the yeast enzyme (33). Also, detergents such as deoxycholate markedly inhibit squalene syn- thetase (22). Inhibition of the enzyme by N-ethylmaleimide, p-hydroxy- mercuribenzoate, or monoiodoacetamide (29, 31, 33, 56, 57), in addition to the requirement for 2-mercaptoethanol (22) for enzyme stabilization, indicates that a sulfhydryl group is probably necessary for enzyme activity.

Porter and co-workers have been able to determine the order of binding of substrates and release of products in the first partial reaction terminating in presqualene PP from kinetic studies with their purified hog liver (35) and yeast (33) squalene synthetase preparations. The results indicate a "ping-pong" mechanism in which the binding of the first molecule of FPP to the enzyme is irreversibly connected to the binding of NADPH and of the second FPP molecule. Kinetic analysis of the second partial reaction in yeast systems, i.e., the conversion of PSPP to squalene in the presence of NADPH, led to the conclusion that this reaction is sequentially ordered (33). From their data Porter and his associates have proposed the mechanism in Scheme 6.12 for the order of binding of substrates and release of products. Isolation of enzyme-bound intermediates, for example, an enzyme-bound farnesol derivative, would provide more direct evidence for this mechanism. This evidence may already be available, since enzyme-bound C_{15} intermedi- ates have been reported that are acid labile (31). The mechanism in Scheme 6.12 and the kinetic results obtained by Porter et al. are in agreement with the isolation of PSPP as a free intermediate in squalene biosynthesis. Schechter and Bloch (22), on the other hand, have observed that, while PSPP no doubt exists as a stabilized intermediate, it does not satisfy the kinetic criteria for a free, dissociable intermediate, since squalene formation proceeds two or three times more quickly from FPP than from PSPP, depending on the cofactor.

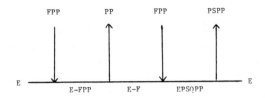

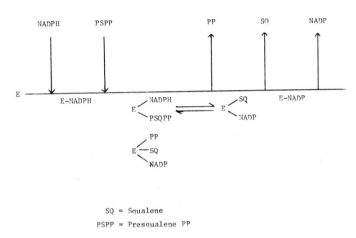

SQ = Squalene

PSPP = Presqualene PP

Scheme 6.12. Mechanism for the binding of substrates and the release of products proposed by Porter and co-workers for yeast squalene synthetase.

BIOSYNTHESIS OF PHYTOENE

1. General Comments

Head-to-head coupling without reduction would lead to a dehydrosqualene if two I_3-pyrophosphates condensed. The resultant compound, "bacterial phytoene," has been reported present in *Staphylococcus aureus* (*58*). Much more important, however, and more extensively studied is phytoene itself, which is formed in the chloroplast of higher photosynthetic plants. It was first isolated by Porter and Zscheile in 1946 from tomatoes (*59*) and a decade later Rabourn and Quackenbush established its structure (*60*). Phytoene has four I^{at} units joined head-to-head through a central double bond.

2. Biosynthesis

The identity of the first C_{40} product of the condensation of two I_4 units has been the subject of some controversy. Lynen and co-workers (*38*) observed the enzymatic biosynthesis of lycopersene from the I_4 precursor, geranyl-geranyl pyrophosphate (GGPP), in a cell-free system from *Neurospora crassa*. Subsequent studies with the same strain of *N.crassa* were unable to confirm the formation of lycopersene (*41*), although evidence has been obtained for the natural occurrence of lycopersene in red and white carrots (*61*). In addition, phytoene accumulates during anaerobic incubation in the absence of oxidation-reduction cofactors (*62*). Phytoene and not lycopersene also accumulates in a variety of systems in which its further metabolism is inhibited

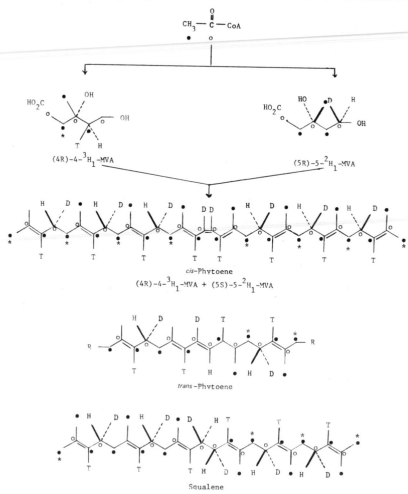

Scheme 6.13. Stereospecific fate of H atoms from MVA during phytoene and squalene biosynthesis.

by a suitable chemical or genetic block (*63, 64*), and no unequivocal isolation of lycopersene has been made (*40, 64, 65*). Moreover, three groups (*45, 66, 67*) have found that [^{14}C]GGPP is converted only to phytoene in various systems. In contrast, a recent study by Porter and his associates (*68*) reports the isolation (and careful characterization) of [^{14}C]lycopersene biosynthesized from [^{14}C]GGPP in tomato enzyme systems. They also found that [^{14}C]lycopersene gave rise to phytoene and lycopene in 22–40% conversion. Gregonis and Rilling (*69*) have suggested that lycopersene may have been produced by squalene synthetase, since it is known that this enzyme will synthesize lycopersene from GGPP (*70*). This phenomenon is not unexpected, since squalene is identical with lycopersene with the exception of the length of the isoprenoid chain. Therefore, it is probable that 2 units of GGPP could be condensed to lycopersene in a process which is mechanistically similar to squalene formation from FPP. The full explanation for the conversion of lycopersene to phytoene must await purification of phytoene synthetase which is free of squalene synthetase activity.

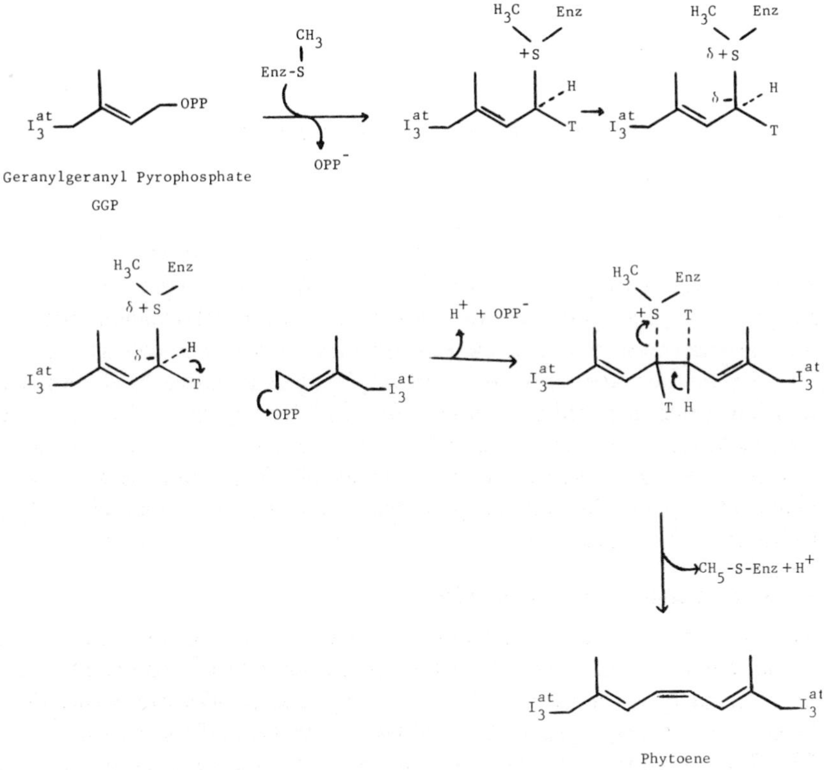

Scheme 6.14. Possible ylide-type mechanism for phytoene biosynthesis.

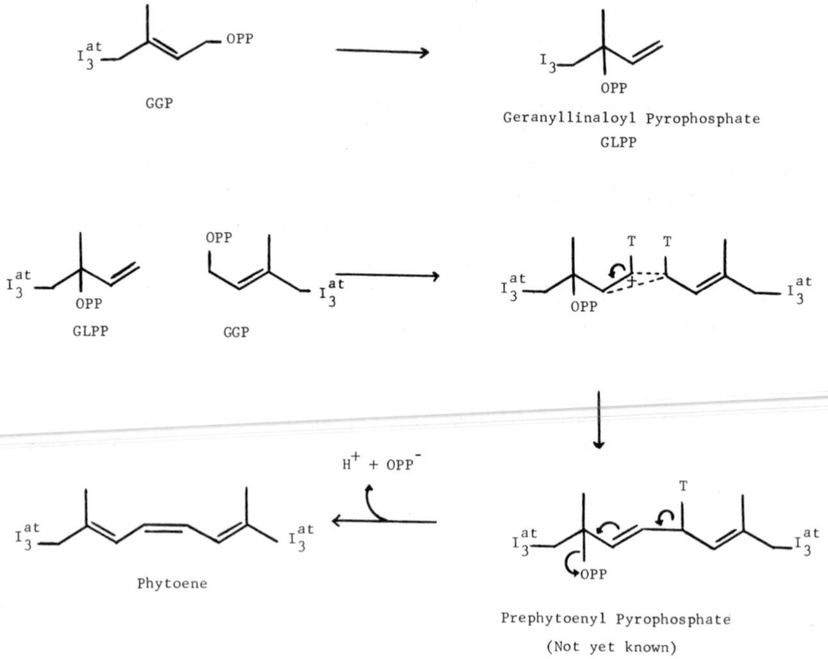

GGP

Geranyllinaloyl Pyrophosphate
GLPP

GLPP   GGP

$$H^+ + OPP^-$$

Phytoene

Prephytoenyl Pyrophosphate
(Not yet known)

Scheme 6.15. Possible mechanism for phytoene biosynthesis based on analogy to squalene biosynthesis.

3. Enzymology

Phytoene synthetase is an enzyme obtainable from chloroplasts which have been ruptured with glass beads (71) or sonication (72). Thin slices of ripe fruit will also yield phytoene from MVA (73). When chloroplastic preparations are used, the particles are best isolated by a non-aqueous technique (74). The synthetase can also be obtained (71) by suspending the chloroplasts in buffer which is added to acetone. The resulting powder is then extracted with buffer and the extract centrifuged at 105,000 × g. The supernatant contains the enzyme which has been further purified by ammonium sulfate precipitation (71). The data suggest that the synthetase is a soluble enzyme within the chloroplast.

4. Stereochemistry and Mechanism

Natural phytoene from higher plants is believed to have the cis-configuration at the central double bond (75, 76), while phytoene from some bacteria may have the trans-configuration (77). From experiments with stereospecifically labeled precursors, e.g., (5R)-[5-³H₁]MVA, in Goodwin's laboratory (45, 72, 73) it has been concluded that both pro-S H atoms are eliminated from C-1 of each of the geranylgeranyl pyrophosphate molecules utilized for coupling. It is interesting to note, and at the least serves as a useful mnemonic, that all the *pro-R* H atoms at both C-4 and C-5 of the eight MVA molecules metabolized are retained in *cis*-phytoene, and in the extended conformation of MVA these H atoms are on the same side of the molecule (toward the viewer with carboxyl on the left, Scheme 6.13). Gregonis and Rilling (*69*) have recently shown that when (1S)-[1-^{3}H]GGPP is the substrate for enzyme

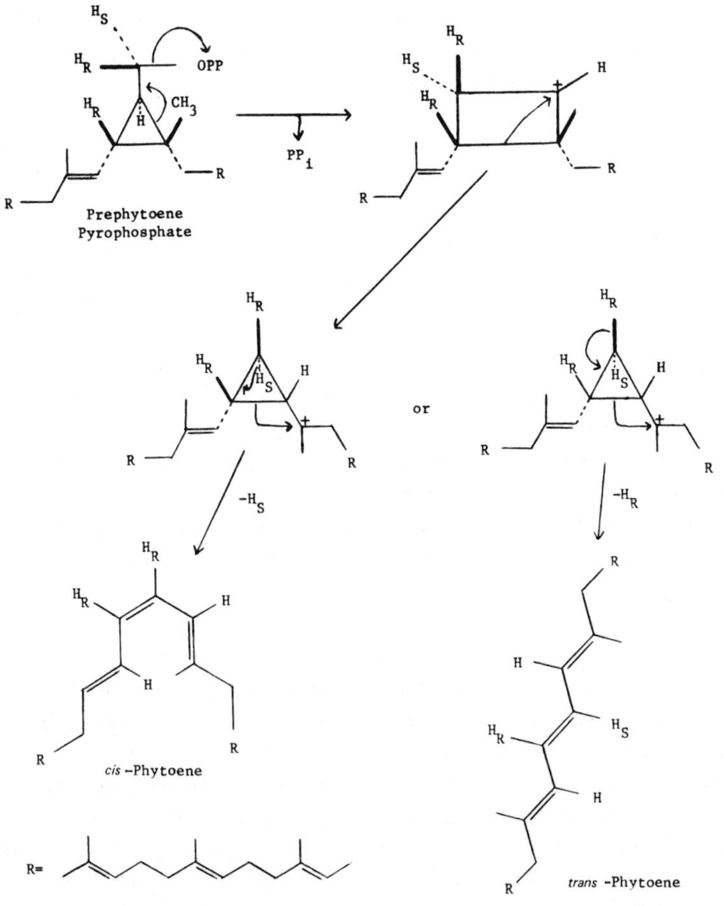

Scheme 6.16. Mechanism for the formation of *cis*- and *trans*-phytoenes from cyclopropyl prephytoene pyrophosphate proposed by Gregonia and Rilling.

from *Mycobacterium sp.*, only one of the two tritium atoms is retained in the biosynthesized *trans*-phytoene. Therefore, 1 *pro-R* and 1 *pro-S* hydrogen from GGPP are retained during the formation of *trans*-phytoene.

As shown by Popjak, Cornforth, and Goodwin and their associates, the fate of the C-4 and C-5 hydrogen atoms from MVA in *cis*-phytoene is the same for squalene biosynthesis in both animals and plants (*45, 78, 79*). However, presqualene pyrophosphate retains only three H atoms in the two central carbon atoms (*15, 21*), which means that one of the H atoms from

C-5 of one of the MVA molecules must actually have been lost. Which one is evident from the labeling pattern of squalene (*19, 20, 78*), which shows retention of five *pro-R* H atoms and a loss of one *pro-S* H atom from C-5 of MVA, a retention of all *pro-R* H atoms from C-4, and the introduction of one H atom onto one of the two central C atoms from the B side of NADPH (Scheme 6.13). Consequently, in the coupling of two-I₃ units to form PSPP, one *pro-S* H atom from C-5 of MVA must be lost, and all *pro-R* H atoms from both C-4 and C-5 must have been retained up to and including the coupling and reduction.

A mechanism has been suggested (*45*) for the head-to-head coupling of two molecules of GGPP that depends on enzyme-bound sulfonium formation. The positive charge of this complex then induces C-1 to bear a partial negative charge (ylide), thus allowing electron flow to the pyrophosphate group of the second molecule, C—C bond formation, and overall elimination of the elements of two moles of pyrophosphoric acid (Scheme 6.14). No direct evidence is available for such a mechanism, and the intermediacy of the isomer, geranyllinaloyl PP, cannot be excluded as a possibility. However, free geranyllinaloyl PP could not be detected in cell-free systems of *Phycomyces blakesleeanus* incubated with [¹⁴C]GPP (*80*). An enzyme-bound intermediate was isolated from the reaction mixture which could be converted to phytoene upon reincubation in the same system.

One can write a series of perfectly reasonable steps (Scheme 6.15) which are analogous to squalene biosynthesis but which substitute allylic elimination of H⁺ and OPP⁻ for addition of H⁻ and removal of OPP⁻. Such a series of reactions would predict the existence of a prephytoene pyrophosphate with an isopentenylogous structure to presqualene pyrophosphate with a tertiary pyrophosphate group. The existence of a prephytoene PP (PPPP) structure analogous to cyclopropyl PSPP can also be predicted. In fact, Rilling and his associates (*81*) have isolated a C₄₀ pyrophosphate from incubation of [³H]GGPP with a cell-free system from a photoinduced *Mycobacterium sp.* Ozonolysis and acetylation of the C₄₀ pyrophosphate produced an isopropyl fragment which is identical to the cyclopropyl fragment from ozonolysis of PSPP (*15, 32*). In addition, the C₄₀ pyrophosphate (named "prephytoene pyrophosphate") can be converted to carotenoids in 34–45% yield. Synthetic PPPP, which differs from cyclopropyl PSPP only in the number of isoprenoid groups, has been prepared by two groups (*81, 82*) and converted in 34–45% yield to carotenoids by *Mycobacterium sp.* (*81*). A cyclopropyl PPPP has also been identified in tomato enzyme systems and as the product of yeast squalene synthetases incubated with GGPP (*68, 70*). Gregonis and Rilling (*69*) have proposed the mechanism shown in Scheme 6.16 for the elimination of hydrogen atoms from PPP in the formation of *cis*- and *trans*-phytoenes.

LITERATURE CITED

1. H. Schinz and J. P. Bourquin, Helv. Chim. Acta 25:1591 (1942).
2. H. Schinz and G. Schaeppi, Helv. Chim. Acta 30:1483 (1947).
3. G. A. Howard, J. R. A. Pollock, and A. R. Tatchell, J. Chem. Soc. 174 (1955).
4. F. Lynen, H. Eggerer, U. Hemming, and I. Kessel, Angew. Chem. 70:738 (1958).
5. S. S. Sofer and H. C. Rilling, J. Lipid Res. 10:183 (1969).
6. H. C. Rilling, J. Biol. Chem. 241:3233 (1966).
7. H. C. Rilling and W. W. Epstein, J. Am. Chem. Soc. 91:1041 (1969).
8. W. W. Epstein and H. C. Rilling, J. Biol. Chem. 245:4597 (1970).
9. E. J. Corey and P. O. de Montellano, Tetrahedron Lett. 5113 (1968).
10. G. Popjak, J. Edmond, K. Clifford, and V. Williams, J. Biol. Chem. 244: 1897 (1969).
11. R. V. M. Campbell, L. Crombie, and G. Pattenden, Chem. Commun. 218 (1971).
12. L. J. Altman, R. C. Kowerski, and H. C. Rilling, J. Am. Chem. Soc. 93: 1782 (1971).
13. R. M. Coates and W. H. Robinson, J. Am. Chem. Soc. 93:1785 (1971).
14. R. V. M. Campbell, L. Crombie, and G. Pattenden, J. Chem. Soc. D 218 (1971).
15. J. Edmond, G. Popjak, S. Wong, and V. P. Williams, J. Biol. Chem. 246: 6254 (1971).
16. G. Popjak, J. Edmond, and S. Wong, J. Am. Chem. Soc. 95:2713 (1973).
17. G. H. Beastall, H. H. Rees, and T. W. Goodwin, FEBS Lett. 28:243 (1972).
18. C. Donninger and G. Popjak, Proc. Roy. Soc. (London), Ser. B 163:465 (1966).
19. J. W. Cornforth, R. H. Cornforth, C. Donninger, and G. Popjak, Proc. Roy. Soc. (London), Ser. B 163:492 (1966).
20. J. W. Cornforth, R. H. Cornforth, C. Donninger, G. Popjak, G. Ryback, and G. J. Schroepfer, Jr., Proc. Roy. Soc. (London), Ser. B 163:436 (1966).
21. H. Wasner and F. Lynen, FEBS Lett. 12:54 (1970).
22. I. Schechter and K. Bloch, J. Biol. Chem. 246:7690 (1971).
23. J. W. Cornforth, Chem. Soc. Rev. 2:1 (1973).
24. R. C. Ebersole, W. O. Godtfredsen, S. Vangedal, and E. Caspi, J. Am. Chem. Soc. 95:8133 (1973).
25. F. Muscio, J. P. Carlson, L. Kuehl, and H. C. Rilling, J. Biol. Chem. 249: 3746 (1974).
26. G. Popjak, D. S. Goodman, J. W. Cornforth, R. H. Cornforth, and R. Ryhage, J. Biol. Chem. 236:1934 (1961).
27. G. Popjak, J. W. Cornforth, R. H. Cornforth, R. Ryhage, and D. S. Goodman, J. Biol. Chem. 237:56 (1962).
28. G. Popjak and J. W. Cornforth, Advan. Enzymol. 22:281 (1960).
29. D. W. S. Goodman and G. Popjak, J. Lipid Res. 1:286 (1960).
30. C. G. Nasciemento, R. P. Lezica, and O. Cori, Biochem. Biophys. Res. Commun. 45:119 (1971).
31. G. Krishna, H. W. Whitlock, Jr., D. H. Feldbruegge, and J. W. Porter, Arch. Biochem. Biophys. 114:200 (1966).
32. H. C. Rilling, C. D. Poulter, W. W. Epstein, and B. Larsen, J. Am. Chem. Soc. 93:1783 (1971).

33. E. Beytia, A. A. Qureshi, and J. W. Porter, J. Biol. Chem. 248:1856 (1973).
34. E. E. van Tamelen and M. A. Schwartz, J. Am. Chem. Soc. 93:1780 (1971).
35. R. E. Dugan and J. W. Porter, Arch. Biochem. Biophys. 152:28 (1972).
36. R. M. Coates and W. H. Robinson, J. Am. Chem. Soc. 94:5920 (1972).
37. C. D. Poulter, O. J. Mascio, and R. J. Goodfellow, Biochemistry 13:1530 (1974).
38. E. C. Grob, K. Kirschner, and F. Lynen, Chimia 15:308 (1961).
39. E. C. Grob and A. Boschetti, Chimia 16, 15 (1962).
40. E. I. Mercer, B. H. Davies, and T. W. Goodwin, Biochem. J. 87, 317 (1963).
41. B. H. Davies, D. Jones, and T. W. Goodwin, Biochem. J. 87, 326 (1963).
42. S. S. Scharf and K. L. Simpson, Biochem. J. 106, 311 (1968).
43. D. G. Anderson and J. W. Porter, Arch. Biochem. Biophys. 97:509 (1962).
44. J. W. Porter and D. G. Anderson, Ann. Rev. Plant Physiol. 18:197 (1967).
45. T. W. Goodwin, Biochem. J. 123:293 (1971).
46. F. Lynen, H. Eggerer, U. Henning, and I. Kessel, Angew. Chem. 70:738 (1958).
47. B. H. Amdur, H. C. Rilling, and K. Bloch, J. Am. Chem. Soc. 79:2647 (1957).
48. G. Popjak, L. Gosselin, I. Youhotsky-Gore, and R. G. Gould, Biochem. J. 69, 238 (1958).
49. D. G. Anderson, M. S. Rice, and J. W. Porter, Biochem. Biophys. Res. Commun. 3:591 (1960).
50. J. W. Graebe, Phytochemistry 8:2003 (1968).
51. P. Benveniste, G. Ourisson, and L. Hirth, Phytochemistry 9:1073 (1970).
52. D. A. Beeler, D. G. Anderson, and J. W. Porter, Arch. Biochem. Biophys. 102:26 (1963).
53. M. Ferne, P. Benveniste, and M. E. Stoeckel, C. R. Hebd. Séances Acad. Sci. Paris 272:2385 (1971).
54. A. A. Qureshi, E. Beytia, and J. W. Porter, J. Biol. Chem. 248:1848 (1973).
55. E. Beytia, J. K. Dorsey, J. Marr, W. W. Cleland, and J. W. Porter, J. Biol. Chem. 245:5450 (1970).
56. H. Hellig and G. Popjak, J. Lipid Res. 2:235 (1961).
57. H. C. Rilling, J. Lipid Res. 11:480 (1970).
58. G. Suzue, K. Tsukada, and S. Tanaka, Biochim. Biophys. Acta 144:186 (1967).
59. J. W. Porter and F. P. Zscheile, Arch. Biochem. Biophys. 10:547 (1946).
60. W. J. Rabourn and F. W. Quackenbush, Arch. Biochem. Biophys. 61:111 (1956).
61. E. Nusbaum-Cassuto and J. Villoutreix, C. R. Hebd. Acad. Séances, Paris 260:1013 (1965).
62. H. C. Rilling, Biochim. Biophys. Acta 65:156 (1962).
63. C. O. Chichester and T. O. M. Nakayama, in P. Benfield (ed.), Biogenesis of Natural Products. Pergamon, Oxford, 1963.
64. T. W. Goodwin, Chemistry and Biochemistry of Plant Pigments. Academic Press, New York, 1965. p. 151.
65. J. F. Pennock, F. W. Hemming, and R. A. Morton, Biochem. J. 82:11P (1962).
66. D. V. Shah, D. H. Feldbruegge, A. R. Houser, and J. W. Porter, Arch. Biochem. Biophys. 127:124 (1968).
67. T. C. Lee and O. Chichester, Phytochemistry 8:603 (1969).
68. F. J. Barnes, A. A. Qureshi, E. J. Semmler, and J. W. Porter, J. Biol. Chem. 248:2768 (1973).
69. D. E. Gregonis and H. C. Rilling, Biochemistry 13:1538 (1974).

70. A. A. Qureshi, F. J. Barnes, E. J. Semmler, and J. W. Porter, J. Biol. Chem. 248:2755 (1973).
71. F. B. Jungalwala and J. W. Porter, Arch. Biochem. Biophys. 119:209 (1967).
72. M. J. Buygy, G. Britton, and T. W. Goodwin, Biochem. J. 114:641 (1969).
73. R. J. H. Williams, G. Britton, J. M. Charlton, and T. W. Goodwin, Biochem. J. 104:767 (1967).
74. J. M. Charlton, K. J. Treharne, and T. W. Goodwin, Biochem. J. 105:205 (1967).
75. J. B. Davis, L. M. Jackman, P. T. Siddons, and B. C. L. Weedon, Proc. Chem. Soc. (London) 261 (1961).
76. F. B. Jungalwala and J. W. Porter, Arch. Biochem. Biophys. 110:241 (1965).
77. O. B. Weeks, in T. W. Goodwin (ed.), Aspects of Terpene Biochemistry. Academic Press, New York, 1971. p. 291.
78. G. Popjak and J. W. Cornforth, Biochem. J. 101:553 (1966).
79. T. W. Goodwin and R. J. H. Williams, Proc. Roy. Soc. (London), Ser. B 163:515 (1966).
80. T. Lee, T. H. Lee, and C. O. Chichester, Phytochemistry 11:681 (1972).
81. L. J. Altman, L. Ash, R. C. Kowerski, W. W. Epstein, B. R. Larsen, H. C. Rilling, F. Muscio, and D. E. Gregonis, J. Am. Chem. Soc. 94:3257 (1972).
82. R. V. M. Campbell, L. Crombie, D. A. R. Findley, R. W. King, G. Pattenden, and D. A. Whiting, J. Chem. Soc., Perkin 1:897 (1975).

Chapter
7

Cyclization
of
Squalene

A. **General and Historical Comments** 230
   1. *Robinson Hypothesis* 230
   2. *Historical Role of Lanosterol* 231
   3. *Folding Pattern* 231
   4. *Hydroxylation and the Role of Squalene Oxide* 232
B. **Mechanism of Cyclization** 234
   1. *Fundamental Rules* 234
   2. *Protosteroid Cation* 236
   3. *Evidence for Protosteroid Cation* 238
   4. *Steroid Formation from Protosteroid Cation* 239
   5. *Evidence for Protosteroid Cation in Steroid Formation* 242
   6. *Protoeuphoid Cation* 243
   7. *Hopenyl Cation* 246
   8. *Lupenyl Cation* 248
   9. *Direct Cyclization of Squalene* 250
  10. *Mono- and Bicycle Formation* 251
  11. *Stereochemistry at C-20* 253
C. **Absolute Configurational Control by Cyclases** 256
   1. *Ubiquity of Absolute Configuration* 256
   2. *Asymmetric Induction* 258
   3. *Asymmetric Conformation of Squalene* 258
   4. *Asymmetric Conformation of Squalene Oxide* 260
D. **Enzymology** 262
   1. *Squalene Oxidase* 262
   2. *Cyclases* 262
   3. *Carrier Protein* 264
E. **Summary** 264
Literature Cited 267

A. GENERAL AND HISTORICAL COMMENTS

1. Robinson Hypothesis

As early as 1934, Robinson (*1*) suggested that the squalene molecule could assume a folding pattern which placed its carbon atoms in positions more or less equivalent to those of the carbon atoms of cholesterol (Scheme 7.1).

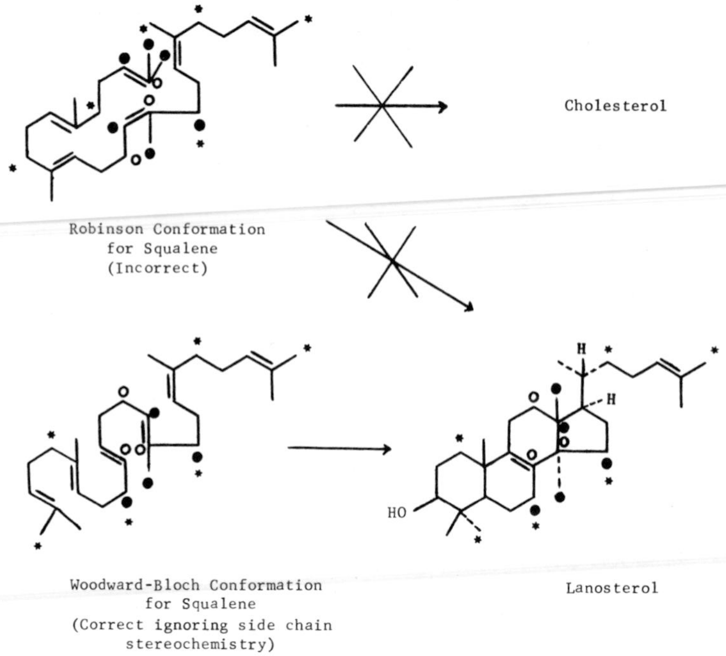

Robinson Conformation
for Squalene
(Incorrect)

Cholesterol

Woodward-Bloch Conformation
for Squalene
(Correct ignoring side chain
stereochemistry)

Lanosterol

Scheme 7.1. Comparison of the Robinson and Woodward-Bloch views of the cyclization of squalene. ●, CH₃ of Acetate; ○, CO of Acetate; ✳, C-2 of MVA.

Moreover, in this pattern one or more double bonds appear at positions where ring closure could take place to form the tetracyclic system of steroids. This was the first detailed attempt to rationalize the origins of steroids from squalene. It was most remarkable for its time, because our understanding of conformations and of reaction mechanisms was only nascent in 1934, and the science of enzymology was at best fetal. For these and other reasons, not the least of which was the absence of isotopic methodology, there was no way to examine the idea experimentally until two decades later when Woodward and Bloch (*2*) proved Robinson to be right in essence although wrong in detail (Section A.3).

2. Historical Role of Lanosterol

Lanosterol proved to be the clue to the folding of squalene. A crude preparation, named "isocholesterol," was isolated along with cholesterol from wool fat in 1872 (3). In 1930 Windaus and Tschesche (4) further purified it, naming the major component lanosterol (wool sterol, Latin *lana*, wool) which is now known (5) to co-occur with the $\Delta^{7,9(11),24}$-derivative (agnosterol) and the 24,25-dihydro derivatives of both lanosterol and agnosterol. Lanosterol was found to be identical with "cryptosterol" from yeast (6). After much effort in a number of laboratories [reviewed by Fieser and Fieser (7)], the structure was finally proved by 1952. While it will be seen from Scheme 7.1 that lanosterol retains all 30 of the squalene carbon atoms, they are not all in their original positions. However, the mechanistic and biochemical genius of Woodward and Bloch (2) immediately saw that squalene, by appropriate folding, electrophilic attack, and ring closures with Wagner-Meerwein rearrangements, could lead to exactly this structure (Scheme 7.1). The actual intermediacy of lanosterol was established shortly afterwards by Bloch and his associates by achieving its biosynthesis both from acetate (8, 9) and squalene (10, 11) and its conversion to cholesterol (12).

3. Folding Pattern

Since lanosterol proved to be the (mammalian) product of cyclization (2, 8–10), Robinson's folding pattern (1) for squalene was unlikely. For instance, it does not place a *gem*-dimethyl group at C-4. Direct evidence for the Woodward-Bloch conformation (2) was brought forward by labeling experiments (2). The experiments depended on methyl- or carboxyl-labeled acetate (the substrate) leading to a definite labeling pattern in biosynthesized squalene. The required pattern is shown in Schemes 6.13 and 7.1, from which it will be seen that the Robinson and Woodward-Bloch alternatives yield different origins (at C-7, C-8, C-12, and C-13 of the steroid) of the squalene carbon atoms in the cyclized product. For instance, C-13 of lanosterol derived from the Woodward-Bloch conformation would come from the methyl group of acetate but from the carboxyl group in the Robinson scheme. A steroid was therefore obtained from biosynthesis with labeled acetate as precursor, and C-13 was degradatively isolated. It proved to be derived from the methyl group of acetate. It will also be seen (Schemes 6.13 and 7.1) that [2-^{14}C]MVA would lead to different labeling patterns in the steroid. For example, label in ring A would appear at C-3 by the Robinson postulate and C-1 by the Woodward-Bloch proposal. Results from the laboratories of Cornforth and Popjak (13, 14), Bloch (15), and others (16–18) from very extensive degradation of sterols biosynthesized from acetate or MVA, fully verified the Woodward-Bloch pattern of folding.

4. Hydroxylation and the Role of Squalene Oxide

Essentially all steroids possess an oxygen atom at C-3, which implies some sort of association between its introduction and the art of forming steroids. The Woodward-Bloch ideas (2) together with the more mechanistic considerations of the Swiss school (19) (Section B) require electrophilic attack on the squalene precursor at C-3 (steroid numbering) for cyclization to occur. The nucleophilic character of the double bonds renders them susceptible to such an attack by an electrophile, resulting in electron delocalizations which promote cyclization. Electrophiles can be added in one of three ways. 1) Electrophilic addition of a proton is perhaps the simplest, a process that accounts for the existence of several 3-desoxy triterpenes, e.g., tetrahymanol and fern-9-ene. However, this process does not reasonably account for the ubiquity of oxygen at C-3 of steroids and most triterpenes. Subsequent introduction of oxygen should depend exclusively on positional orientation and the enzyme active site, factors that would be expected to reflect evolutionary divergence in biosynthetic pathways. Despite these arguments, the idea of an initial proton attack on squalene in sterol biosynthesis was held by some investigators (20) until quite recently. 2) Electrophilic addition of an electron-deficient oxygen group and cyclization might occur simultaneously. Such a process is extremely attractive, but it would require an enormously complicated enzyme to direct both the attack of the oxygenated species as well as the stereochemistry of the cyclization. 3) Electrophilic attack of a proton might follow a previous, separate oxygenation step. Addition of the proton to the oxygen atom would initiate cyclization. The latter view is the correct one for the majority of cases examined (the 3-oxygenated steroids and triterpenes). Prior oxygenation at some other position, e.g., C-11, as opposed to oxygenation at C-3, would not lead to an electronic condition that could yield steroids and, while perhaps occurring, this would not be useful.

A very extensive literature (21) was developing in the 1950s that indicated that molecular oxygen could undergo a reduction with reduced pyridine nucleotide (usually NADPH), leading to an electrophilic species capable of introducing oxygen atoms into unsaturated (and even saturated) molecules. Although the precise nature of the electrophilic grouping is as yet unknown, it is convenient to regard it as a species acting as if it were HO^+ without implying the existence per se of a free, positively charged hydroxyl ion. It may be bonded, for instance, to ferrous iron on the enzyme. A large variety of substrates (22) have been found to undergo such oxygenations (the enzyme system being an oxygenase), and there is an association between evolution and the development of the enzymatic system (23). The process requires that the final oxygen atom be derived from molecular oxygen.

Using incubations in an atmosphere of $^{18}O_2$, Bloch (24) showed that the steroidal hydroxyl group (at C-3) was labeled. This excluded the utilization of water, established the existence of the HO^+ mechanism at some stage, and was consistent with, but did not prove, the induction of cyclization

by HO⁺ rather than H⁺ (alternative 2). Depending on the substrate's structure and enzymatic choices for deprotonation, the HO⁺ mechanism (hydroxylation mechanism) could theoretically lead to a saturated alcohol, a saturated
oxide, an unsaturated alcohol, or a ketone (Scheme 7.2). The first two pos-

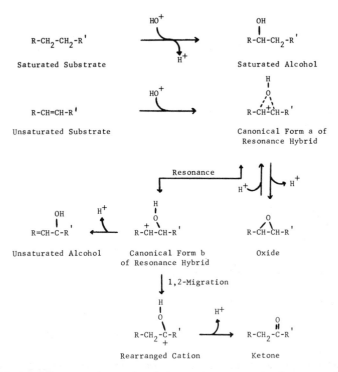

Scheme 7.2. Possible products from hydroxylative attack on saturated and unsaturated products
and deprotonation.

sibilities have been extremely well documented. Incubation of steroidal
substrates bearing a $\Delta^{9(11)}$-double bond with the fungus *Curvularia lunata*
leads to $9\beta,11\beta$-oxidosteroids (*25*), while incubation of steroids bearing a
saturated bond between C-9 and C-11 with the same organisms leads to
11β-hydroxy derivatives (*26*). The oxides are of some theoretical interest,
because upon protonation they could lead back to the same positively charged
species which one would write for HO⁺ attack on a double bond (canonical
Form b, Scheme 7.2). The importance of this is that the hydroxylative and
cyclizative steps could theoretically be separated (alternative 3) without violating the initiation of cyclization by an electrophile.

Experiments by Corey, Clayton, van Tamelen, and their associates
demonstrated successfully that the oxidation and cyclization of squalene
are separate steps. Their experiments also firmly established the role of

squalene-2,3-oxide as the intermediate in the conversion of squalene to lanosterol. Several years following the synthesis of squalene-2,3-oxide (*28*), several laboratories obtained conversion of this epoxide to lanosterol. The principal findings from these experiments included: 1) the conversion of squalene-2,3-oxide to lanosterol and other metabolites by liver homogenates, 2) the trapping of squalene-2,3-oxide in the presence of carrier squalene, 3) the accumulation of squalene-2,3-oxide during lanosterol biosynthesis in the presence of 2,3-iminosqualene (cyclization inhibitor), and 4) the origin of the 3β-OH of lanosterol from the oxygen of squalene-2,3-oxide (*29–33*). The S isomer of squalene-2,3-oxide is the exclusive precursor of lanosterol in pig liver, lanosterol and ergosterol in yeast, and β-amyrin, lupeol, and cycloartenol in pea seedlings (*34*).

Van Tamelen (*27, 28*) found that in certain solvents (polar environments) squalene assumes a "bunched" conformation, with the terminal double bonds exposed. It was possible to achieve preferential attack at one or both of the terminal double bonds nonenzymatically under these conditions. Squalene epoxidase apparently does not distinguish between the terminal double bonds even though, in a biosynthetic sense, squalene is an asymmetric molecule. The C_{15} halves are not identical biosynthetically since one contains a hydrogen atom donated by NADPH (see Chapter 6, Section B). Fusidic acid biosynthesized by *Fusidium coccineum* from $(3RS,5S)$-[2-^{14}C,5-^{3}H]MVA contains tritium distributed equally between the 11β and 12α positions, carbons which have their origins in the central portion of squalene (*35*). These results are in agreement with an earlier publication (*36*) which indicated that the distribution of tritium at C-11 and C-12 of lanosterol biosynthesized from [^{14}C]FPP and NAPT in pig liver could only have resulted from random cyclization of squalene.

Squalene epoxidase appears to be sensitive to the overall configuration of the squalene molecule (*37*). Substrate analogs with modified squalene chains (i.e., shortened by two isoprenoid units partially cyclized at one end), some with modifications remote from the site of epoxidation, markedly reduced epoxidase activity. The enzyme does not appear to be unduly sensitive to the number of double bonds. Alternation of the *gem*-dimethyl groups only reduced epoxidase activity slightly. These results indicate specific binding of the substrate to the enzyme, lack of sensitivity to steric factors at the site of oxidation, and an insensitivity to the nucleophilic character of the double bond at the oxidation site.

B. MECHANISM OF CYCLIZATION

1. Fundamental Rules

Eschenmoser, Ruzicka, Jeger, and Arigoni (*19*), in a classic paper published in 1955, were able to arrive a priori at the structures of a large variety of known polycyclic triterpenoids in full stereochemical detail by assuming squalene to be the precursor. Their ideas were closely similar to those used by Woodward and Bloch (2) in arriving at the formation of lanosterol, and two major conclusions, which now have been extensively verified and extended experimentally, arose immediately. They are: 1) that squalene has several ways in which it can be cyclized, and that in consequence it acts as the precursor of many different kinds of cyclic isopentenoids, and 2) that the process of cyclization can be understood and predicted owing to the operation of certain fundamental rules surrounding electrophilic attack. A rapid flowering of biochemical and chemical sophistication in the intervening two decades has further refined the original concepts. Our current view of the rules is as follows:

1. Squalene can be cyclized directly by proton attack, or it can first be oxygenated, yielding squalene mono- or diepoxide, which then can be cyclized by proton attack. Mechanistically, the alternatives are much the same, but the nature, position, and origin of any oxygen appearing in the product become quite different.
2. The position of proton attack, governed by an appropriate group on the enzyme, is one of several factors determining the structure of the product. In the great majority of cases it is at the end of the molecule, and it must occur at a nucleophilic center, either a double bond or an oxygen atom.
3. The extent of cyclization, i.e., the number of rings formed, and certain other structural details, notably stereochemical ones, in the product are governed by the conformation of squalene or its oxide, which is bound to the cyclase. This conformation is almost certainly controlled by the nature and position of binding groups on the protein at the active site and bears no simple relationship to the ordinarily preferred conformation(s) in true solution. The possible positions of atoms in the structure that is bound to the cyclase are, however, limited by the rigid *trans*-configuration of the double bonds; i.e., binding energies for formation of the substrate-enzyme complex are not sufficient to twist a double bond to any major degree and major variations in the positioning of atoms must have their origin only in rotations about single bonds.
4. In addition to the rules discussed above which influence the outcome of squalene cyclization, the final structure of the cyclized product is determined by the site of removal of the positive charge remaining from the original protonation step. The nature of the nucleophile at the enzyme active site which donates these electrons also influences the structure of the product. Two nucleophiles appear to exist, one a proton acceptor, and the other a source of a species acting as if it were hydroxyl ion (OH^-). The latter has its origins in water, experimentally. In this case, it is probable that the enzyme active site involves a proton acceptor with the exception that the proton is extracted from water rather than the cyclized product.

5. Migrations of various atoms (H or C), together with an octet of electrons, i.e., a group acting as if it were R⁻, may occur from one position to the next adjacent one. These migrations are governed, however, by strict limitations. They must be initiated by and form an integral part of an electron flow from the position of proton attack to the position of proton removal or OH⁻ addition. In fact, the capacity for such migrations determines whether a given position of a nucleophile at the active site of the enzyme will or will not be successful in determining product stereochemistry. Migrations of H and CH₃ take place with one atom attacking another on the side opposite from that of any atom leaving the one attacked, i.e., a *trans*-process must occur. Furthermore, no atom itself can move from one side of the system to the other. It is not known whether the migrations are assisted by the enzyme, but it may well be so.

2. Protosteroid Cation

If the structure of a steroid product is examined in the light of the preceding discussion, it becomes apparent that the substrate must assume a conformation when bound to the cyclase (Scheme 7.3) which approximates the structure of   *trans-syn-trans-anti-trans-anti*-1,2-cyclopentanoperhydrophenanthrene

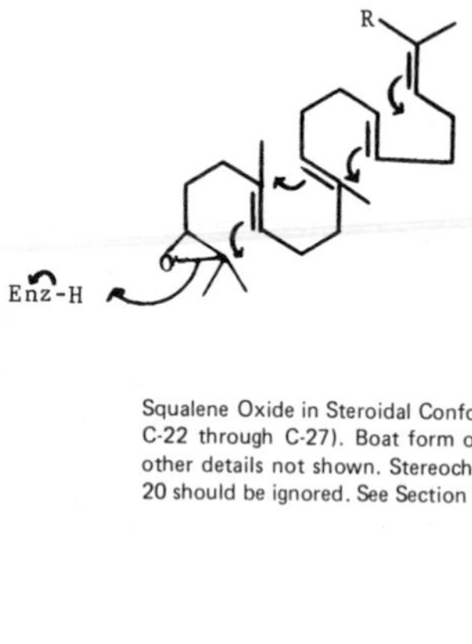

Squalene Oxide in Steroidal Conformation (R = C-22 through C-27). Boat form of Ring B and other details not shown. Stereochemistry of C-20 should be ignored. See Section B-11.

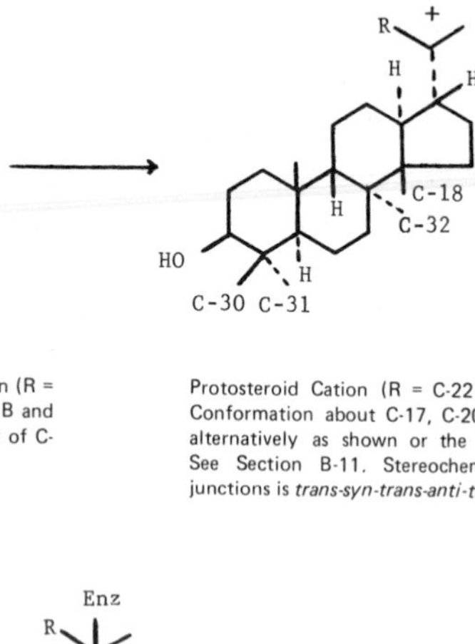

Protosteroid Cation (R = C-22 through C-27). Conformation about C-17, C-20-bond may be alternatively as shown or the 180° rotamer. See Section B-11. Stereochemistry at ring junctions is *trans-syn-trans-anti-trans-anti*.

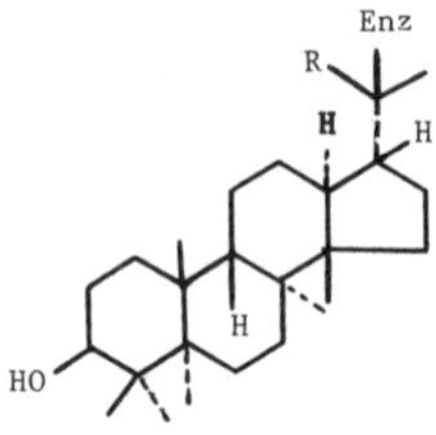

Structure of Conceivable Protosteroid-Enzyme Complex. Stereochemistry of C-20 is ignored. See Section B-11.

Scheme 7.3. Formation of protosteroid cation.

with a side chain. *Trans* and *cis* refer to the opposite and the same configuration, respectively, of atoms that form the junction between two rings, i.e., the configuration at C-5 and C-10 that forms the A/B junction. *Anti* and *syn* refer to the opposite or the same configuration, respectively, of two atoms on the same ring that participate in two separate ring junctions, i.e., the relationship of the configuration at C-10 and C-9 that is called the A/C junction. Protonation on the oxygen atom would then lead by electronic redistribution to a cation (carbonium ion) bearing a positive charge at C-20 and possessing the familiar tetracyclic ring system of steroids, but with some skeletal and stereochemical differences. This cation is known as the protosteroid cation—"protosteroid" because it arises prior to or without the skeletal rearrangements necessary for true steroid formation. In particular, C-18 and C-32 are not in their "correct" places, and most of the ring junctions (A/C, B/C, B/D, C/D, and C-13/C-17) have inverted configurations. Corey (*39*) has proposed the term "protosterol" for compounds with a tetracyclic skeleton corresponding directly to this cation in which no migration has occurred. We shall call compounds protosteroids if they are derived directly from this cation without migration of any carbon atoms.

What uncertainties there are about the existence of this cation reside in some details. It may represent a real energy minimum with higher energy states between it and both substrate and product. In a precise chemical sense, it then represents a charged intermediate with a distinct lifetime. Such stabilization could come from a variety of sources, e.g., dipole interaction with charges on the enzyme. Stabilization of the general structure could also arise through conversion to a neutral intermediate by bond formation at C-20 from a nucleophile (electron source) at the active site of the enzyme. This would yield a condition very properly described as a protosteroid-enzyme complex (Scheme 7.3), but such a term could also be reasonably ascribed to the condition of dipole stabilization. As described in detail in Section B.11, there are cogent theoretical reasons for believing that a bond of some sort is indeed formed at C-20 between the substrate and enzyme, and that there is a real period of existence. On the other hand, the cations that have no lifetime at all and only represent some nonminimum portion of the energy diagram, especially those that represent a maximum of energy, would properly be described as transition states. We do not know what the reality of this situation is in most cases, but it is clearly convenient, as an accounting process at the least, to regard cations per se as being involved. In the event that they do not represent true energy minima, they still will remain useful as tools for intellectually following the course of cyclization in much the same way as canonical forms of a resonance hybrid are useful intellectually. The subtle problem of time in a cation's existence is related to the problem of whether at an exacting level squalene oxide can really assume a conformation with atomic nuclei so disposed as to allow complete reaction to occur instantaneously, the so-called "nonstop" or "synchronous" hypothesis (*19*). Actually, since all the carbonium ions that one can write, starting with protonation of the oxide's oxygen atom and proceeding stepwise to lanosterol, possess extensive capacity for hyperconjugative stabilization, each such step may well be a true step, with each carbonium ion representing an energy minimum and a pause in time. Somewhat similar questions arise in regard to what, if any, assistance the enzyme provides to a migrating group. These are very esoteric and difficult questions to examine. For the time being it is convenient to regard a nonstop process from the bound acyclic conformer to the protosteroid cation (complexed with the enzyme at C-20) as occurring with a pause for the cation followed by a nonstop rearrangement to give the final product. The nonenzymatic cyclization has been examined in some depth by van Tamelen and others (39a and Ref. cited therein) who conclude that rings A, B, and C are formed either in an entirely concerted manner or with the involvement of "frozen" mono- and bicyclic carbonium ions.

3. Evidence for Protosteroid Cation

The evidence for the existence of the protosteroid cation in some form is substantial and is of two major kinds: 1) the structures of products and 2) labeling patterns.

1. If the cyclase possessed a deprotonating agent oriented adjacent to C-13, C-17, C-21, or C-22, an olefin would result, bearing the skeleton and stereochemistry of the protosteroid cation. Such compounds exist. Two examples (Schemes 7.4 and 7.5) are the alisols, which are a series of $\Delta^{13(17)}$-protosteroids (40–42), presumably derived from $\Delta^{13(17)}$-protosterol, and fusidic acid (43, 44), which is a $\Delta^{17(20)}$-31-norprotosteroid presumably derived from $\Delta^{17(20)}$-protosterol. Both of the final products possess the predicted skeleton and stereochemistry, although other metabolism (such as hydroxylation) has occurred subsequent to cyclization. Other important structural evidence lies in the conversion of 10,15-dinorsqualene (squalene lacking the two central methyl groups) by rat liver to the corresponding $\Delta^{20(22)}$-dinorprotosterol (45, 46). The absence of the two methyl groups [but not of one (47)] for reasons not entirely clear (48) prevents the normal rearrangement of the protosteroid cation. Also, if a double bond is introduced in conjugation with the two terminal double bonds of squalene oxide (Δ^{22}, steroid numbering), the dehydrosubstrate yields a protosteroid with an HO group in the side chain (49). Again, it is not quite clear why HO^- addition to the cation should be favored over the normal deprotonation, but for our present purposes the formation of these compounds is fortunate, since it provides strong evidence for the intermediacy of the protosteroid cation in the well-investigated mammalian system for true steroid biosynthesis.

2. Fusidic acid is especially important because it has been examined biosynthetically. Mulheirn and Caspi (48) examined the labeling pattern of fusidic acid produced from (4R) -[2-^{14}C, 4-^{3}H]MVA. The product contained six ^{14}C and four ^{3}H atoms. By degradation the tritium was located at positions

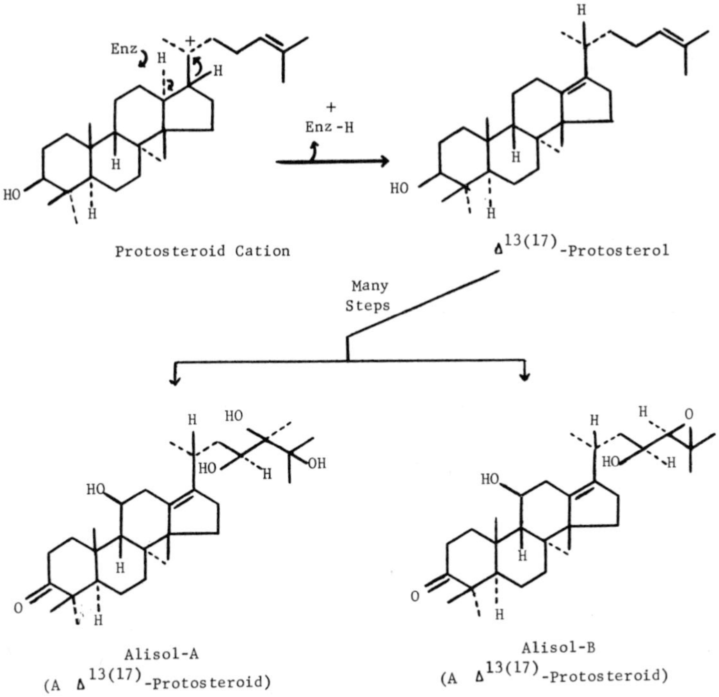

Scheme 7.4. Formation of $\Delta^{13(17)}$-protosteroids.

5α, 9β, 13α, and 24 as required for the formation of the protosteroid cation without rearrangement according to the rules of cyclization followed by the processes: hydroxylation, oxidation, decarboxylation, acetylation, and reduction of an intermediate 3-ketone to the 3α-hydroxy derivative. Furthermore, the structures of lanosterol and its metabolite, cholesterol, and the labeling patterns obtained from them are interpreted reasonably by assumption of the existence of the protosteroid cation (Sections B.4 and B.5).

4. Steroid Formation from Protosteroid Cation

If the cyclase deprotonates the protosteroid cation at C-9, which bears a β-H atom, a series of *trans*-1,2-migrations can occur that yield electronic neutralization of the charge at C-20 (Scheme 7.6). The product is lanosterol. If, on the other hand, the cyclase donates electrons from the α face of the protosteroid cation to C-9, this would induce the 9β-H to migrate to the 8β position, inducing in turn the same series of migrations as found for lanosterol but production in this case of a steroid-enzyme complex (Scheme 7.7). Such a complex exists between glucose and the enzyme responsible for formation of maltose from UDPG (50). In the latter case the C atom is believed to be inverted in the complex and again inverted in the subsequent formation

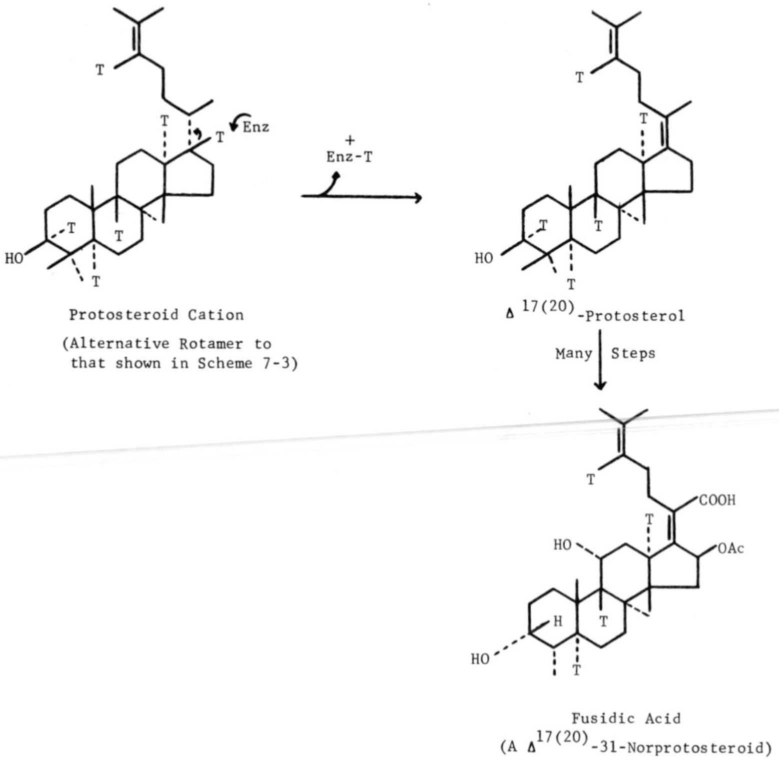

Protosteroid Cation

(Alternative Rotamer to
that shown in Scheme 7-3)

$\Delta^{17(20)}$-Protosterol

Many | Steps

Fusidic Acid
(A $\Delta^{17(20)}$-31-Norprotosteroid)

Scheme 7.5. Formation of fusidic acid showing fate of 4-*pro*-R H atom (T) from MVA.

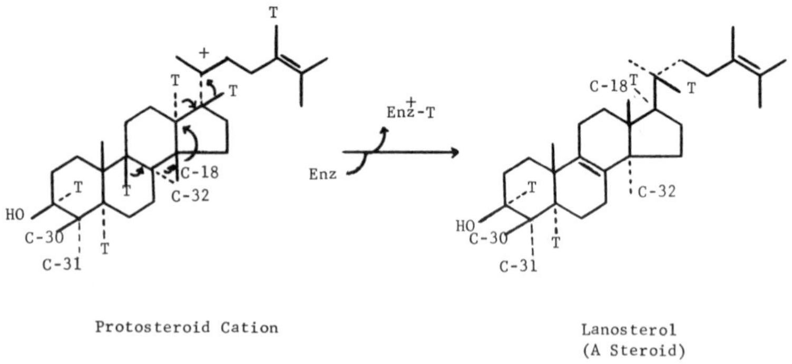

Protosteroid Cation

Lanosterol
(A Steroid)

Scheme 7.6. Steroid formation from the protosteroid cation showing labeling derived from the 4-*pro*-R H atom (T) of MVA.

of product leading to a total of double inversion. If the steroid-enzyme complex underwent deprotonation at C-19, C-19 could attack C-9 with analogous inversion, and cycloartenol retaining the original configuration at C-9 would

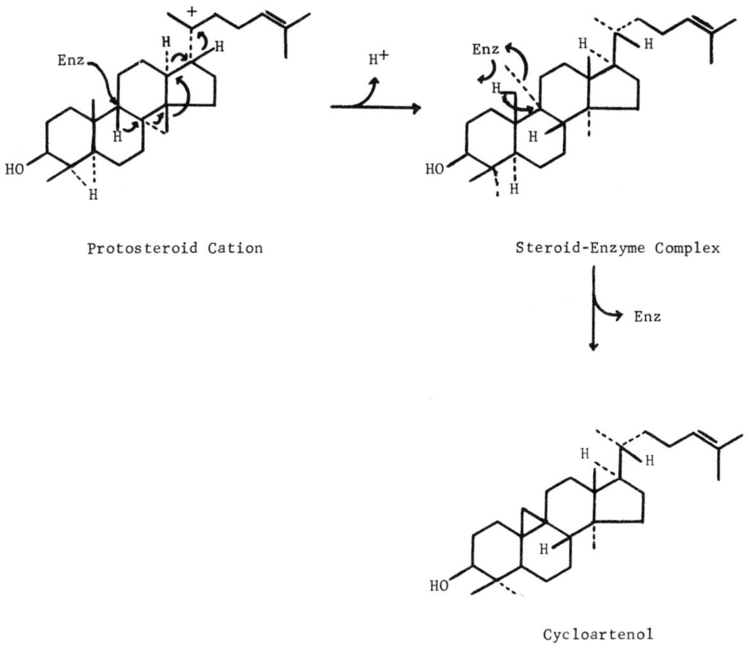

Protosteroid Cation   Steroid-Enzyme Complex

Cycloartenol

(A steroid)

Scheme 7.7. Formation of cycloartenol via hypothetical steroid-enzyme complex.

result as a consequence of double inversion at C-9. Both lanosterol (*30, 51, 52*) and cycloartenol (*53, 54*) are experimental products of the cyclization of squalene oxide, but the existence of the suggested enzyme complex has yet to be examined experimentally.

The protosteroid cation must be involved in some form in the synthesis of cycloartenol or lanosterol, because the stereochemistry and labeling patterns of the products cannot otherwise be accounted for. Consequently, we shall describe any compound which is derived biosynthetically through the protosteroid cation by electron addition in whatever form (HO$^-$ addition, proton abstraction, etc.) to C-7, C-8, C-9, C-11, or C-19 as a steroid. This definition implies precise stereochemical and skeletal arrangements and requires that both lanosterol and cycloartenol be steroids. It is worthy of note that both are intermediates to the common Δ^5-sterols of nature. It also suggests, for instance, that the Δ^7- and $\Delta^{9(11)}$-isomers of lanosterol might exist. They do exist (and we shall call them steroids), although it is not yet certain whether they are true products of cyclization or metabolites of lanosterol. The $\Delta^{9(11)}$-isomer is known as parkeol (*55*).

Deprotonation of the protosteroid cation at C-6 and C-15 is conceivable. In the latter case the stereochemistry may not be quite favorable because of the puckered shape of ring D, but the possibility of the removal of a 6β-H atom cannot be eliminated. Deprotonation at C-15 would yield a Δ^{14}-"steroid" retaining the methyl group at C-8. This structure might be called an ante-steroid, since only C-18 would have migrated. On the other hand, deproto-nation should be quite favorable from the axially oriented 6β-H, and indeed precisely the expected structure has been found in nature in a series of com-pounds. They differ in skeleton from the true steroids in that C-19 is attached to C-9, as is required for electron flow from C-6 to C-20. In view of this additional migration we shall call them poststeroids. Several (the cucur-bitacins) have been isolated from the Cucurbitaceae (55) (Scheme 7.8).

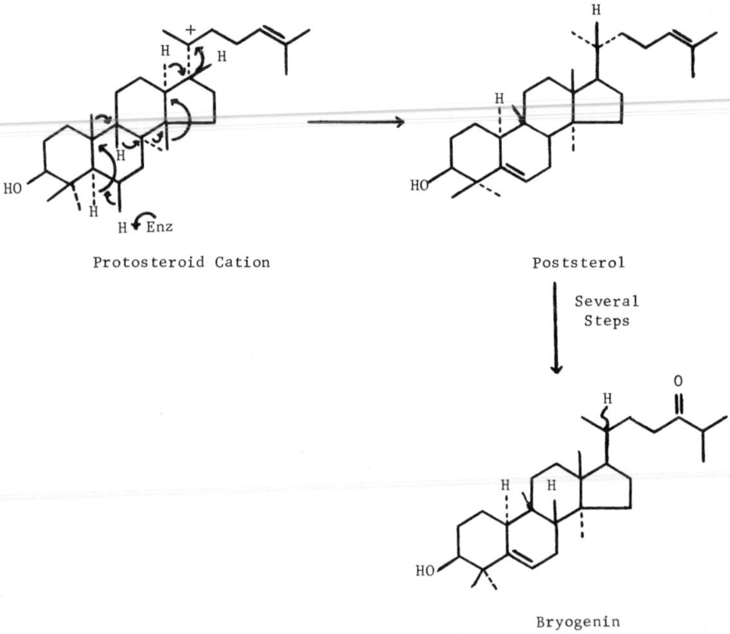

Scheme 7.8. Poststeroid formation from protosteroid cation.

5. Evidence for Protosteroid Cation in Steroid Formation

If the detailed uncertainties discussed in Sections B.1 to B.4 are accepted as not violating the concept of the existence of a protosteroid cation, then deprotonation of the cation with concomitant 1,2-migrations during steroid formation can be imagined. Such a process has some precise implications in the labeling patterns of the steroids that have been verified. In particular, the six 4-*pro-R*-H-atoms of six MVA molecules should appear in squalene, as shown in Scheme 6.13. Upon formation of the protosteroid cation, they should appear at positions 3α, 5α, 9β, 13α, 17β, and 24, as is shown in Scheme 7.6. Finally, conversion to lanosterol should yield the labeling pattern (3α, 5α, 17α, 20, and 24, the 9β-H having been eliminated) shown in Scheme 7.6. Cornforth et al. (56) showed that lanosterol derived from (4R)-[4-^{3}H]MVA in rat liver homogenates retains the expected five of six tritium atoms. By degradation the one that should have been seen at C-13 in the protosteroid cation and migrated to C-17 was indeed located at C-17 (56), the one originally at C-17 was found as predicted at C-20 (56, 57), and one remained as it should have at C-24 (56, 57). Cholesterol retained only the latter three (56), which is consistent with our view of its formation from lanosterol (Section B). In addition, C-18 and C-32 should have migrated to their final positions, which requires, among other things, that C-13 and C-18 of steroids should both have their origin in the methyl group of acetate. This and related requirements of the origin of the C atoms have been documented (2, 13–18). In the formation of cycloartenol, all the labeling data should be the same as for lanosterol except that the H atom (derived from a 4-pro-R H atom of MVA), which is lost from C-9 in the latter case, should be retained and should appear at the 8β position. Goodwin and co-workers (58) incubated (4R) -[2-^{14}C, 4-^{3}H$_1$]MVA with chopped leaves of Solanum tuberosum. Cycloartenol isolated from these incubations retained a ^{3}H/^{14}C atomic ratio of 6:6, showing that no tritium had been lost during cyclization. Isomerization of this cycloartenol produced lanosterol with a ratio of 5:6 and parkeol with a 6:6 ratio, confirming that the hydrogen atom from C-9 of the protosteroid cation had indeed migrated to C-8 during cycloartenol formation. For more extensive considerations of the protosteroid cation, the folding pattern of squalene and its oxide, and related questions, and for a key to the literature, the discussions of Cornforth (56, 59), Caspi (48, 57, 60), Bentley (61), Barton (62), and van Tamelen and Clayton (63, 64) should be consulted. Similar problems arise with respect to the cations described in the following sections.

6. Protoeuphoid Cation

Euphol, first isolated by Newbold and Spring (65) in 1944 and found in a number of species of the genus Euphorbia (55), has the same tetracyclic structure as lanosterol except that C-13, C-14, and C-17 have inverted configurations. This condition is possible if squalene oxide folds into a conformation approximating the structure of the all-trans-anti-stereoisomer of 1,2-cyclopentanoperhydrophenanthrene bearing the appropriate side chain on the five-membered ring. This will yield a C-20 cation (the protoeuphoid cation, Scheme 7.9) that is epimeric to the protosteroid cation at C-8, C-9, C-13, C-14, and C-17. As with the protosteroid cation, deprotonation at C-13, C-17, C-21, or C-22 would lead without rearrangement to an olefin, and HO$^-$ addition at C-20 would lead to a diol. Such structures are known (Scheme 7.10). The Δ^{20}-olefin (Δ^{20}-protoeuphol, also known as dammara-dienol) and the 20-epimeric hydroxy derivatives (protoeuphadiols, also known as the dammarenediols) were discovered by Mills and Werner (66) in the

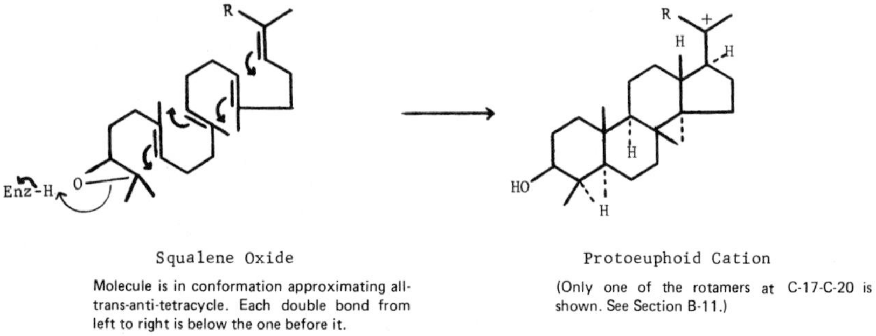
R
Enz-H
O
R
H
H
H
HO
H
Squalene Oxide
Molecule is in conformation approximating all-trans-anti-tetracycle. Each double bond from left to right is below the one before it.
Protoeuphoid Cation
(Only one of the rotamers at C-17-C-20 is shown. See Section B-11.)

Scheme 7.9. Formation of the protoeuphoid cation.

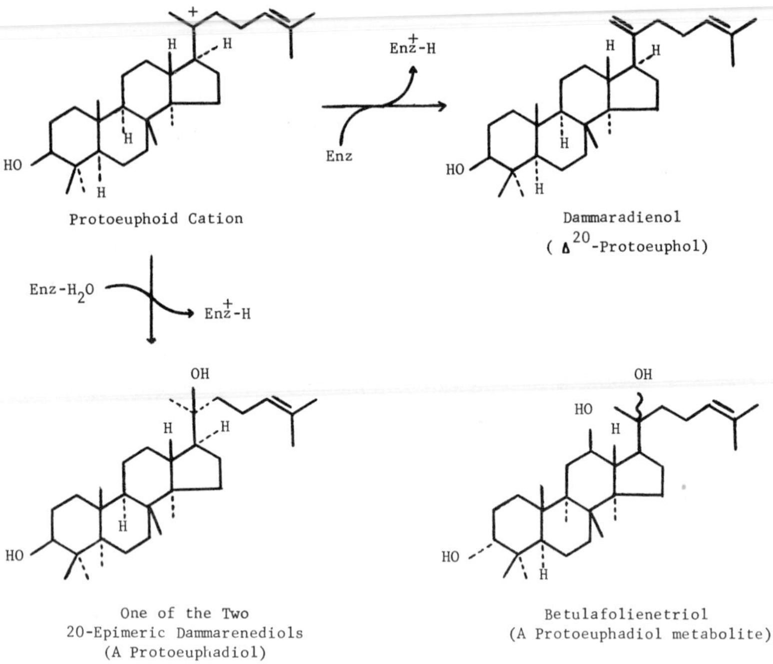
HO
Protoeuphoid Cation
Enz-H
Enz
HO
Dammaradienol
(Δ20-Protoeuphol)
Enz-H2O
Enz-H
OH
HO
One of the Two
20-Epimeric Dammarenediols
(A Protoeuphadiol)
OH
HO
HO
Betulafolienetriol
(A Protoeuphadiol metabolite)

Scheme 7.10. Protoeuphoid formation from protoeuphoid cation.

Dipterocarpaceae, notably in the so-called "Dammar resins." Similarly, apparent metabolites of the initial protoeuphadiols are known (*55*), such as betulafolientriol (*67, 68*) in birch leaves (*Betula alba*), which appears to be derived by 11β-hydroxylation and oxidation-reduction at C-3. On the other hand, deprotonation at C-9, as in lanosterol formation, would lead to rear-

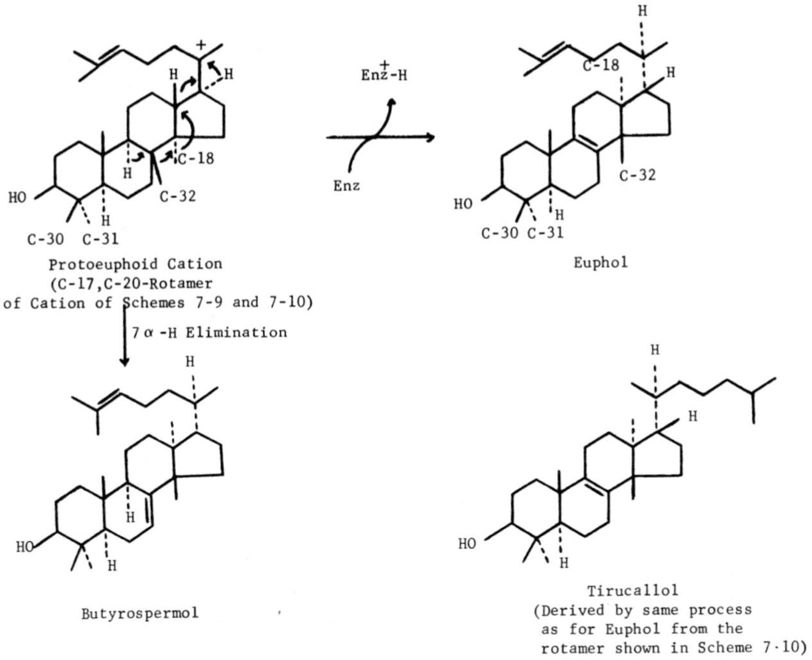

Protoeuphoid Cation
(C-17,C-20-Rotamer
of Cation of Schemes 7-9 and 7-10)

Euphol

7α-H Elimination

Butyrospermol

Tirucallol
(Derived by same process
as for Euphol from the
rotamer shown in Scheme 7·10)

Scheme 7.11. Euphoid formation from protoeuphoid cation.

rangement, and euphol itself or its 20-epimer would result (Scheme 7.11). The epimer, tirucallol, is also found in *Euphorbia* species (55), and the Δ⁷-isomer, butyrospermol, occurs in the genera *Butyrospermum, Artocarpus,* and *Maclura* (55). These and related tetracyclic compounds derived through the protoeuphoid cation with migration of C-18 and C-32 will be called euphoids in analogy to the term steroid. Butyrospermol was the first discovered (69). It will be recalled (Section B.4) that antesteroids are conceivable through migration only of C-18 induced by deprotonation at C-14 (HO⁻ addition at C-13). Exactly such compounds are known in the euphoid series (Scheme 7.12), which by analogy we will call anteuphoids. While Δ¹⁴-anteuphol or its 20-epimer, antetirucallol, itself has not yet been discovered, apparent metabolites (the limonin group of compounds) have been found in heartwoods of *Guarea, Khaya,* and other genera (55). Cedrelone, for instance, in *Cedrela toona* would represent Δ¹⁴-anteuphol in which hydroxylation (HO⁺ mechanism) and other oxidations have led to the epoxidation of the Δ¹⁴-bond as well as to introduction of oxygen at positions 7 and 8, and to cleavage and cyclization of a portion of the side chain. Posteuphoids could conceivably exist also.

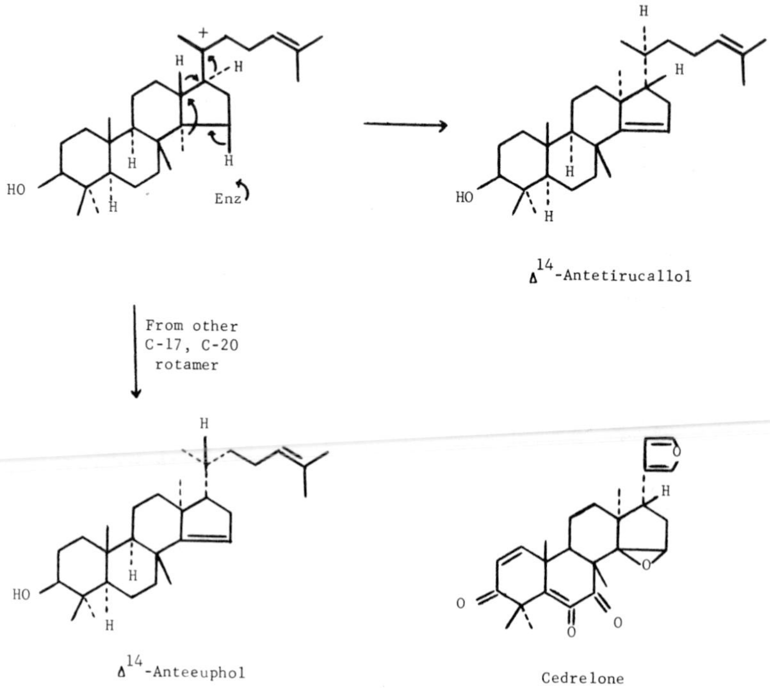

Δ^{14}-Antetirucallol

From other
C-17, C-20
rotamer

Δ^{14}-Anteeuphol

Cedrelone

Scheme 7.12. Anteuphoid formation from protoeuphoid cation.

7. Hopenyl Cation

Further folding of squalene oxide than is achieved for formation of the proto-steroid and protoeuphoid cations is possible, and it occurs, as is seen in the structures of many pentacyclic products. The simplest intermediate cation would possess the all-*trans*-*anti*-arrangement, as is found in the protoeuphoid cation. Indeed, the two would be the same except for the presence of a five-membered ring E. We shall call this pentacyclic analog the hopenyl cation (or the desoxyhopenyl cation, if it is from squalene directly) in deference to the names of known compounds derived from it (Scheme 7.13). In the 3-desoxy series the product of proton elimination from one of the terminal methyl groups is known as hopene-b and arises in bacteria (70), and other hopenoids, e.g., hopene-I, the $\Delta^{17(24)}$-analog of hopene-b (71), have been found in ferns and lichens (72). As with the other cations, deprotonation or HO$^-$ addition at some remote site is possible with rearrangement. An example again in the desoxyca-tion series is HO$^-$ addition to C-24, which includes enlargement of ring E and formation of tetrahymanol in *Tetrahymena pyriformis* (Scheme 7.14). Alter-natively, Caspi et al. (73, 74) have proposed a mechanism for the direct cyclization of tetrahymanol with squalene folded into six six-membered rings in the *trans*-*anti* configuration. The origin of the carbon atoms is the same

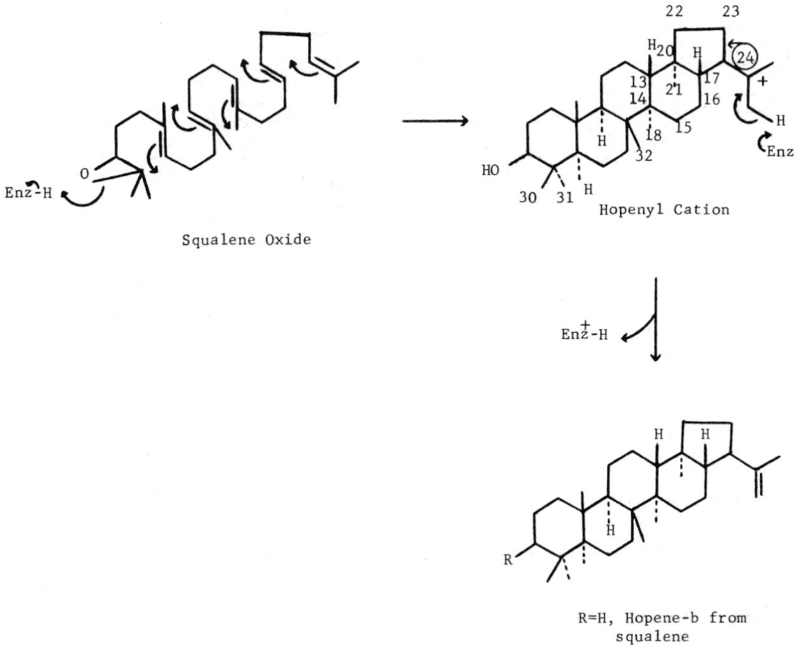

Scheme 7.13. Formation of the hopenyl cation.

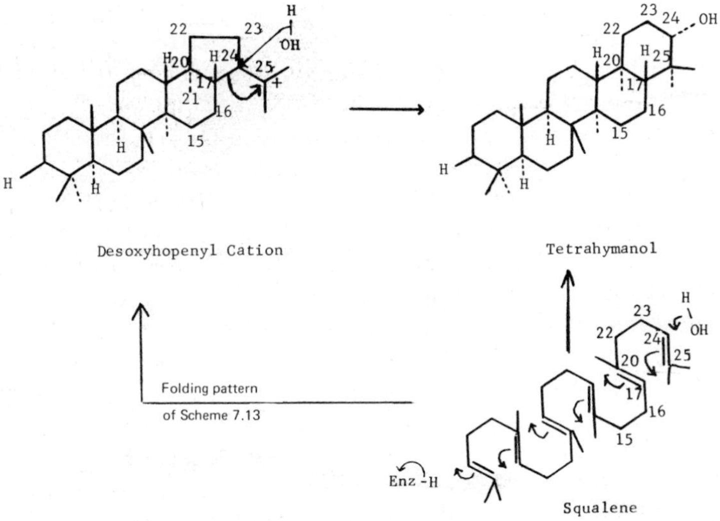

Scheme 7.14. Conversion of squalene to tetrahymanol (steroid numbering).

in either case. *T. pyriformis* also contains diplopterol, which results from addition of OH⁻ to the desoxyhopenyl cation at C-25 without rearrangement.

8. Lupenyl Cation

Another sort of pentacyclic product can be formed by rearrangement of a cation other than the hopenyl cation. While the new cation probably arises directly from cyclization, it can be visualized as arising from the protoeuphoid cation by migration of C-16 instead of the 17α-H atom to C-20 with concomitant attack of the Δ^{24}-electrons onto the electron-deficient site produced at C-17 (Scheme 7.15). This would yield the lupenyl cation, which should

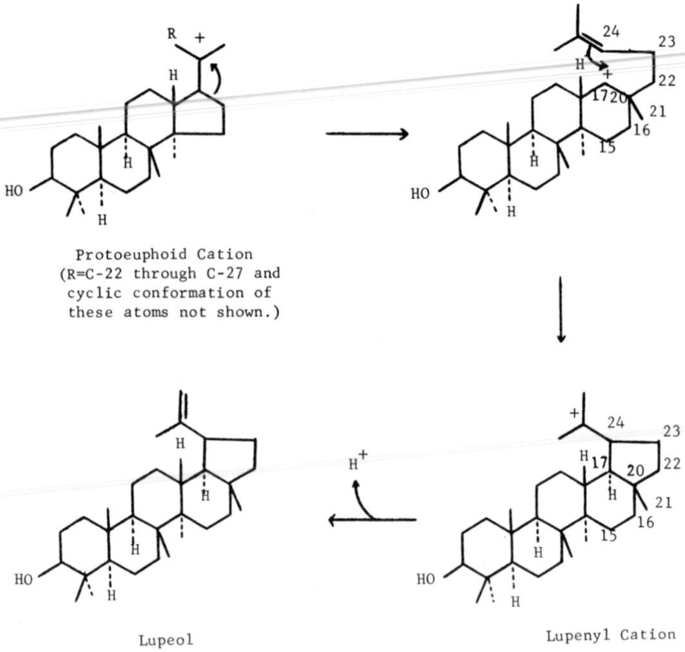

Protoeuphoid Cation
(R=C-22 through C-27 and cyclic conformation of these atoms not shown.)

Lupeol   Lupenyl Cation

Scheme 7.15. Formation of lupeol through the lupenyl cation.

be stabilized by maximal hyperconjugation from the six H atoms on C-26 and C-27 acting in part as a driving force for its formation. A large number of known structures (75) are derived (19) from the lupenyl cation. The most obvious would be elimination of a proton from C-26 or C-27. This product, known as lupeol, was first found in 1889 in *Lupinus albus* and is widely distributed, occurring in at least 13 plant families (75). All compounds bearing this structure will be called lupoids if no C migrations have occurred.

As with other cations, remote deprotonation could induce rearrangement, which, in fact, occurs widely (75). For instance, deprotonation of the

12α-H atom induces a series of 1,2 migrations, with concomitant enlargement of ring E to the more stable six-membered system (Scheme 7.16). This product is the widely occurring β-amyrin. Other compounds possessing the β-amyrin skeleton will be designated β-amyroids.

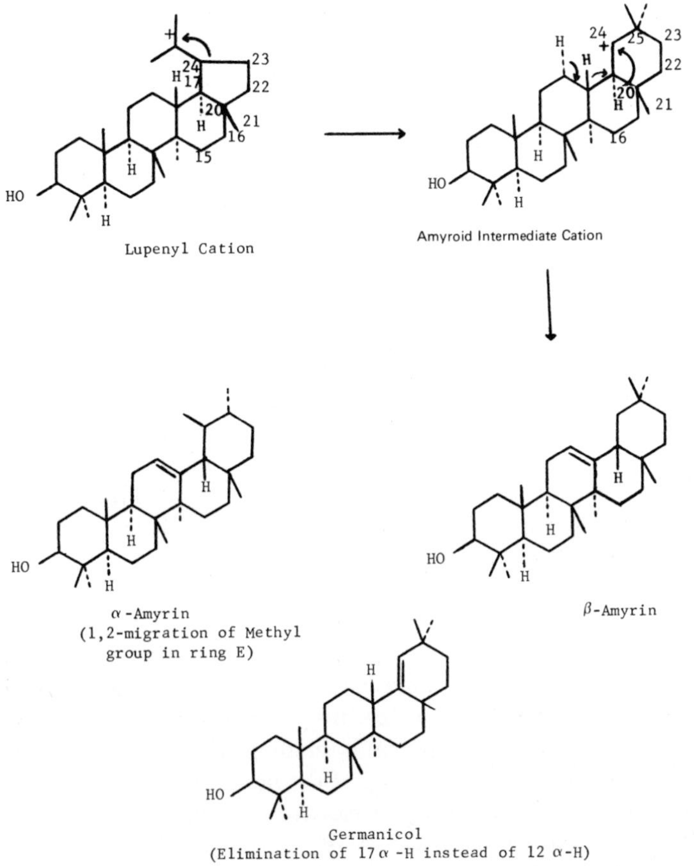

Lupenyl Cation

Amyroid Intermediate Cation

α-Amyrin
(1,2-migration of Methyl
group in ring E)

β-Amyrin

Germanicol
(Elimination of 17α-H instead of 12 α-H)

Scheme 7.16. Amyroid formation from lupenyl cation.

It is a most subtle but important point that on thermodynamic grounds the lupenyl cation would be expected to have the stable all-*trans*-*anti*-arrangement (from the stereochemistry of lupeol). This in turn would require that the *trans*-migration yielding β-amyrin invert C-17 but not C-20. Thus, the *trans*-D/E ring junction should become *cis*-fused, and indeed such is the stereochemistry of β-amyrin, adding much weight to the general mechanisms (2, 19). β-Amyrin is also interesting in that it was historically the first pentacyclic compound to be obtained experimentally from squalene. In 1965 this was achieved by Nes and his associates (76) through aerobic incubation of biosynthetically labeled squalene with a cell-free enzyme preparation from peas. Following the availability of squalene oxide, the cyclase was enriched from the same source by Corey et al. (77), who were able to demonstrate the oxide's intermediacy also for the first time in the pentacyclic series through an anaerobic incubation that converted it to β-amyrin.

The mechanistic origin of α-amyrin is much less clear. It has the same structure as β-amyrin except that one of the gem-dimethyl groups on ring E has migrated to C-24. While this is clearly allowable, there is a mystery about how migration or no migration is controlled. One might imagine an intrinsic proclivity for migration at some quantitative level such that α- and β-amyrin mixtures are always obtained, but such does not appear to be the case. Some plants contain both, but some are reported to contain only one or the other (78), which suggests enzymatic control of the 1,2-migration. A push-pull process involving S-adenosylmethionine does not appear to be involved (78).

A number of other pentacyclic triterpenes (75) are derivable from the lupenyl cation (19). Thus, deprotonation at C-15 would induce migration of the methyl group from C-14 to C-13 to yield the compound taraxerol found in dandelions and other plants (75). Perhaps the most dramatic illustration of the impact of the site of deprotonation is the removal of the original proton added to squalene oxide. This should lead (Scheme 7.17) to a ketone lacking a methyl group between rings A and B (as in poststeroids) and a 1,2-dimethyl instead of a gem-dimethyl arrangement on ring A. Exactly this compound is known. It is friedelin, found in cork, etc. (75). This structure incidentally adds some weight to the possibility of the existence of intermediate cations, since the concept of elapsed time between addition and abstraction of the same proton is attractive. However, proponents of the nonstop hypothesis could argue that all that happens is binding of a given conformation of squalene oxide followed by touching of the proton to the oxygen atom, with instantaneous redistribution of the electrons yielding an H-bonded ketone that desorbs as the ketone itself. A related ketone, alnusenone, found in the bark of black alder (75), retains the 4,4-dimethyl group and bears a Δ^5-bond and must be derived by elimination of the 6β-H atom. It is one level higher in oxidation than friedelin (which does not have a C=C grouping). This and the mechanistic considerations indicate the carbonyl group arises by separate oxidation rather than as an integral part of cyclization.

9. Direct Cyclization of Squalene

Squalene could theoretically cyclize directly by proton attack without passing through the oxide (79). A desoxycation would result, which would be similar in general principle to the hydroxycations (protosteroid, etc.). A number of products with expected structures are known (71, 80). Examples include zeorin (81), ambrein (82), diplopterol (83), dustanin (84), serratene (85),

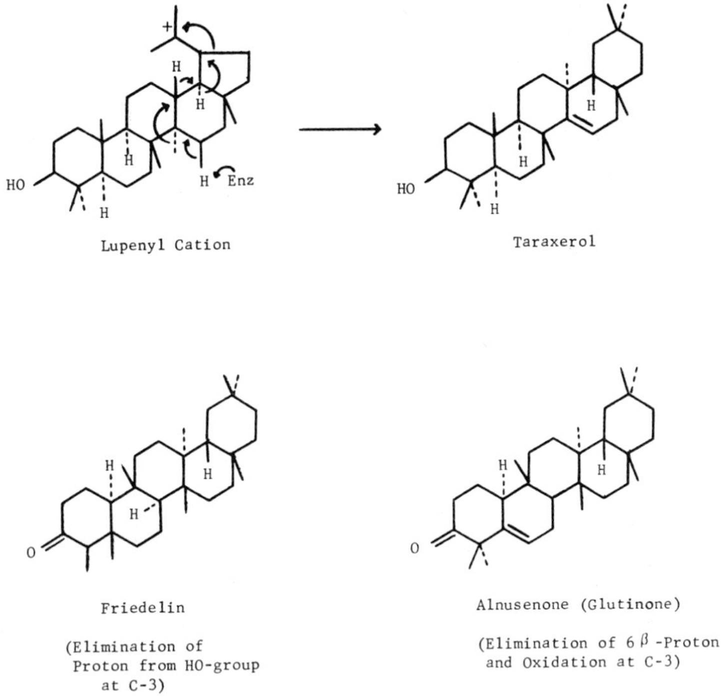

Lupenyl Cation   Taraxerol

Friedelin   Alnusenone (Glutinone)

(Elimination of   (Elimination of 6 β -Proton
Proton from HO-group   and Oxidation at C-3)
at C-3)

Scheme 7.17. Formation of rearranged β-amyroids (post-β-amyroids).

hopene-b (*70*), fernene (*86*), and tetrahymanol (*73, 87*). Tetrahymanol in
the protozoan *Tetrahymena pyriformis* and fernene in the fern *Polypodium
vulgare* have been studied biosynthetically by Caspi, Conner, Mallory, and
Barton and their associates. Squalene oxide leads to neither product but
squalene acts as the precursor in both cases (*73, 86*). The labeling pattern
(*88*) of tetrahymanol derived from (4*R*)-[^{3}H, 2-^{14}C]MVA is consistent with
the route shown in Schemes 7.14 and 7.17. The fact that tetrahymanol is
accompanied by diplopterol (*74*) (Scheme 7.18) is further evidence for a
route through the desoxyhopenyl cation. Incorporation of deuterium from
^{2}H$_2$O (*60, 89*) and ^{18}O from H$_2$^{18}O (*60, 90*) into tetrahymanol agrees with
proton-initiated cyclization terminated by nucleophilic attack by a species
acting as if it were HO$^-$.

10. Mono- and Bicycle Formation

Since the extent of folding of squalene or its oxide, governed by the cyclase,
determines the number of rings formed, it is theoretically possible for less
than the previously discussed four or five rings to arise. While formation of
the smaller polycycles appears to be quite rare, there are two well-documented
examples. In one of these, ambrein, the structure (*75*) indicates direct cycliza-

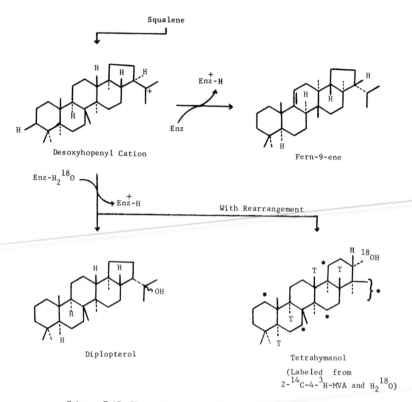

Scheme 7.18. Examples of nonoxidative cyclization of squalene.

tion of squalene with monocyclic formation at one end and bicycle formation at the other. No biosynthetic work has been done, leaving such questions as the number of steps (and cyclases) open. The compound is found in the ambergris of sperm whales. Ambergris is an intestinal secretion that sometimes appears on the surface of the ocean, especially in the southern hemisphere. The intestinal origin and the apparent biosynthesis directly from squalene (Scheme 7.19) rather than an oxide strongly indicate that it is biosynthesized by intestinal microorganisms. Bicyclic metabolism of an oxide is also known in the biosynthesis of α-onocerin in some species of *Ononis* and in *Lycopodium clavatum* (*75*). α-Onocerin is cyclized at both ends of the molecule, as in ambrein, but, unlike ambrein, both ends contain a bicycle and squalene-2,3,22,23-diepoxide acts experimentally as the precursor in *Ononis spinosa* (*91*) (Scheme 7.19). The molecule is optically active, does not possess a plane of symmetry, and the two ends are identical and possess exactly the same absolute configurations.

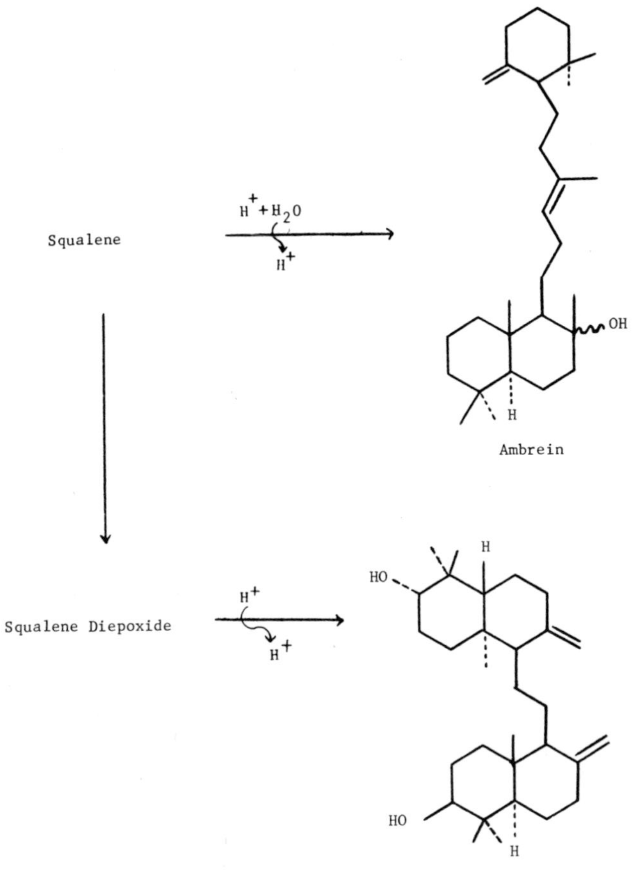

Squalene

$\overset{+}{H} + H_2O$

$\overset{+}{H}$

Ambrein

Squalene Diepoxide

H^+

H^+

α -Onocerin

Scheme 7.19. Mono- and bicyclic metabolism of squalene and its diepoxide. (The solid and interrupted lines are in the spatial not steroid convention. Thus, in α-onocerin the absolute configurations of the two bicyclic systems are identical).

11. Stereochemistry at C-20

Extensive evidence exists for the R configuration at C-20 (α-H atom) of cholesterol (92), and it has recently been possible to show (92a) that this configuration requires the side chain to lie to the right (C-22 trans-oriented to C-13) (Scheme 7.20 and Scheme 2.15). Of the rotational isomers about the 17(20)-bond, the eclipsed forms can automatically be discounted. There then remain three skew isomers as possible candidates, viz., those with C-22 to the right, to the left, and in front. The latter two will place C-21 and C-22, respectively, in a 1,3-diaxial relationship with C-18, while the first will place the 20-H atom in this position. Since the smallest group (H) opposing C-18

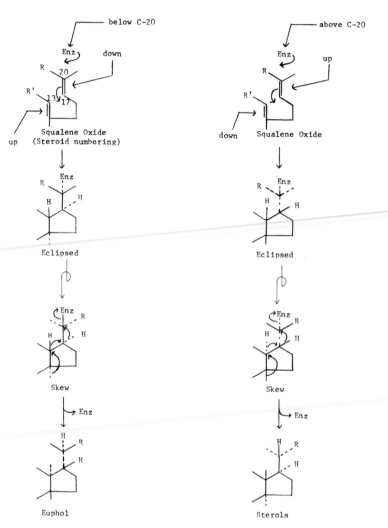

Scheme 7.20. Cyclization of squalene oxide to euphol and sterols.

will be energetically favored, the right-handed isomer clearly will represent the preferred conformation. Three lines of evidence corroborate the conformational analysis. X-ray diffraction indicates a lengthwise dimension of 20 Å for cholesterol, which can only be satisfied by the right-handed conformer. Monolayer studies of the 1930s that led to the correct formulation of the nuclear structure require the molecule to be flat. The conformer with C-22 in front would place too much of the side chain on the β face to be consistent with the results. Finally, recent (92a, 92b) studies of the proton magnetic resonance spectra (PMR) of sterols lead to a preference for the right-handed conformer. When C-22 is fixed rigidly to the right, as in (E)-17(20)-dehydrocholesterol, the PMR signal (1.68 ppm) from C-21 (on the left) is downfield (larger number) compared to the opposite condition (C-22 on the left and C-21 on the right, as in (Z)-17(20)-dehydrocholesterol with C-21 giving a signal at 1.55 ppm).

In the absence of a double bond at C-20, sterols with a 20α-H atom should exist as the right-handed skew conformer, while the left-handed rotamer should be the preferred skew conformer if a 20β-H atom is present (Scheme 2.15). When the PMR signals from cholesterol and its epimer, 20-isocholesterol, were measured (92a), the former had the downfield signal (0.91 and 0.81 ppm, respectively, both being shifted upfield because of the absence of the $\Delta^{17(20)}$-bond). Consequently, cholesterol must have the right-handed and 20-isocholesterol the left-handed conformation in agreement with the a priori considerations of the relative stabilities of the rotamers. Since the configuration dictates the conformation and the conformation dictates the PMR signal, PMR spectroscopy becomes a way of determining the configuration at C-20. The spectra of sterols have been examined (92a) from an array of lower and higher organisms, e.g., cholesterol of animals, 24α- and 24β-methylcholesterol of Tracheophytes, 24β-methylcholesterol derived from ergosterol of yeast, 24α-ethylcholesterol and its Δ^{22}-derivative of Tracheophytes, and 24β-ethylcholesterol and its Δ^{22}-derivative of algae. In all cases, the signal from C-21 agrees with the presence of a 20α-H atom.

Knowing the configuration at C-20 has allowed Nes et al. (92a) to make a theoretical analysis of the events just before and after the formation of the protosteroid cation during the cyclization of squalene oxide. Since the $\Delta^{17(20)}$-bond (steroid numbering) of the substrate lies above the $\Delta^{13(14)}$-bond (Scheme 7.20) when the two condense the $\Delta^{17(20)}$-bond will have been attacked from below (the α-face of the nucleus). An antiparallel reaction will then require that something else attack from the front. The 17β-H (of the protosteroid cation produced) lies in front, but its attack on C-20 would yield the wrong configuration. This means the enzyme must attack. The resulting protosteroid-enzyme complex will then have an eclipsed conformation. To relieve the repulsive interactions, rotation of 180° should occur about the 17(20) bond to give the right-handed, skew conformer. This also places the 17β-H atom antiparallel to the enzyme at C-20, permitting a trans-migration of the H atom to occur from C-17 to C-20 with elimination of the enzyme and induction of the remaining steps in steroid formation. The product (lanosterol, etc.) will have the observed stereochemistry at C-20 (right-handed conformer with the 20-H atom in front). It should be remembered from Chapter 2 that when we take the right-handed conformer as a standard for nomenclature, groups on the front side of the chain are given the α-designation and those in back are considered to be β-oriented, which is the reverse of the convention in the nucleus. Thus, the 17β-H atom becomes the 20α-H atom, i.e., the designation is reversed even though no stereochemical change has occurred.

The foregoing explanation also accounts for the configuration at C-20 of euphol. In the protoeuphoid cation ring D, the side chain and the stereochemistry of the enzyme C-20 bond will be the mirror image of that in the protosteroid cation. The enantiomeric condition (17β-H, 20β-H, right-handed conformer) therefore will arise in the product. This is indeed the accepted stereochemistry of euphol, but the problem has not been examined yet by PMR spectroscopy.

It is very attractive to assume that the observed stereochemistry at C-20 of euphol and steroids is a necessary result of minimization of energies (preferred conformations) during the cyclization of squalene oxide. If the enzyme is bound to C-20, such an analysis would predict that the epimeric condition could not exist. However, 20-isoeuphol (tirucallol) is believed to occur (55), as are haliclonasterol and 20-isofucosterol (sargasterol) (93, 94). Verification of the occurrence of the latter has been attempted without success (see Chapter 10), and re-examination of the others would be worthwhile. The occurrence of what are believed to be epimeric 20-hydroxyprotoeuphoids (dammarenediols, Scheme 7.10) also would be interesting to re-examine. If the protoeuphoid epimers really do exist, they can be tolerated theoretically on the assumption that they arise through a true, racemized carbonium ion that is not bonded at C-20 to the enzyme. Under such circumstances attack on C-20 could occur from either side. The euphol-tirucallol pair is not so easily explained. The protoeuphoid cation should have to exist long enough to undergo rotation, since the 17α-H atom is fixed in space. A more plausible explanation is that tirucallol arises by a concerted cyclization, bypassing the protoeuphoid-enzyme complex, and that the intermediacy of the complex leads to the epimer (euphol). The epimeric 20-hydroxy compounds could also be explained in this way.

C. ABSOLUTE CONFIGURATIONAL CONTROL BY CYCLASES

1. Ubiquity of Absolute Configuration

All cyclases giving rise to tetra- or pentacyclic products, regardless of the organism containing them, bind squalene or squalene oxides in such a way that the same enantiomeric series at the A/B ring junction is always produced. Without exception the A/B ring junction arises in a *trans* arrangement for which two enantiomeric possibilities exist. While mechanistic reasons inherent in double-bond chemistry dictate the *trans*-junction, it is the enzyme that must dictate the enantiomeric choice by asymmetric induction. With C-3 to the left and down, the C-10 methyl group can be either away from the observer or toward him. In all products of cyclization of squalene or of either of its oxides, the latter condition exists, as is shown in Schemes 7.6, 7.7, 7.10, etc. All of the cations have exactly the same absolute configurations at C-5 and C-10 (compare the protosteroid, protoeuphoid, and other cations). However, the rearranged products of these cations may not have the same configuration at these centers. Friedelin (Scheme 7.21) and alnusenone

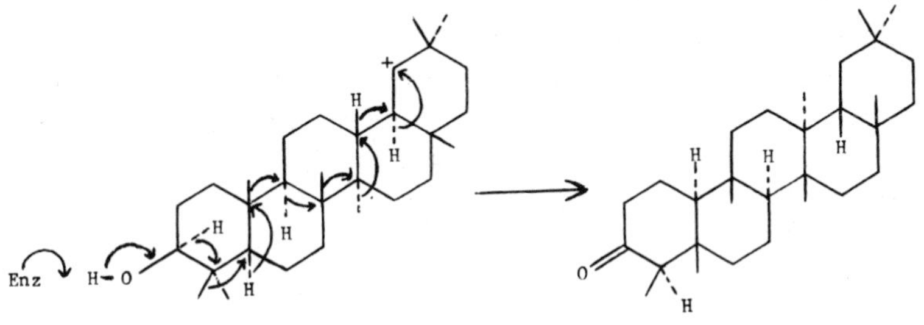

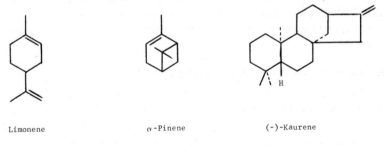

Amyroid Intermediate
Cation

(cf. Scheme 16)

Friedelin

Scheme 7.21. Mechanism of formation of friedelin.

(Scheme 7.17) most notably do not. The configurations at C-5 and C-10 of friedelin and alnusenone are derived from the same enantiomeric condition at the A/B ring junction for squalene oxide that produces lanosterol (compare the lupenyl and protosteroid cations). During the course of cyclization, as a result of *trans*-1,2-migrations, the configuration at C-5 and C-10 in friedelin and alnusenone has been inverted.

The configurational control that is exerted in the cyclization of squalene and its oxides is quite remarkable and not necessarily expected. As discussed in greater detail elsewhere (*95*), such complete discrimination is not made in cyclizations at other levels of isopentenoid polymerization (Scheme 7.22).

Limonene

α-Pinene

(-)-Kaurene

Scheme 7.22. Examples of compounds known in nature in enantiomeric forms.

In particular, cyclization at the I₂ level leads frequently both to racemates in some organisms or to one or the other enantiomer in other organisms.

Limonene, for instance, occurs as the racemate as well as the (+) or the (−) form, and α-pinene occurs either as the (+) or the (−) form. Greater selectivity exists as the molecular size increases, but even at the I_4 level enantiomers are known [(+)- and (−)-kaurene, etc.].

2. Asymmetric Induction

Asymmetry, the condition that allows the existence of nonsuperimposable mirror images of molecules, arises from the lack of any of the following three properties in a molecule: a plane of symmetry, a center of symmetry, or an alternating axis of symmetry. A carbon atom with four different substituents is also asymmetric, and there may be several such centers in a given molecule; e.g., MVA substituted at C-2, -4, and -5 with tritium has four asymmetric centers, including C-3 (Scheme 7.23). Squalene itself is a symmetric

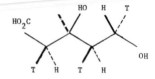

2R, 3R, 4R, 5S–Mevalonic Acid

Scheme 7.23. Asymmetric centers of mevalonic acid.

molecule, but the introduction of an (S)-epoxide group renders squalene asymmetric.

Because of the asymmetry in the α-amino acid residues of proteins, only a given conformation of the substrate will fit or match with the appropriate asymmetrically oriented binding groups at the active site of the enzyme. Thus, the enzyme can select, hold, and induce reaction in one out of many conformations. This process by which an asymmetric substance interacts with a formally nonasymmetric substance producing formal asymmetry in the product of the latter is known as asymmetric induction. It has been achieved in and extensively studied in nonliving systems, but life is its principal milieu.

3. Asymmetric Conformation of Squalene

In the squalene case, the absolute configurations and mechanism of origin of the products make clear what sort of asymmetric conformation must be bound by the cyclase. It is a spiral, with one of the terminal isopropylidene groups pointed toward the observer, and alternating clockwise and counterclockwise loops arranged to the right and away from the observer. This can be seen from Scheme 7.24, which shows the atoms that become rings A and B. Using steroid numbering, we see that the attack of C-4 from above onto C-5 forces the 5-H atom down (α), while the attack of C-10 onto C-9 below

R continues to loop or spiral in alternating directions away from the observer:

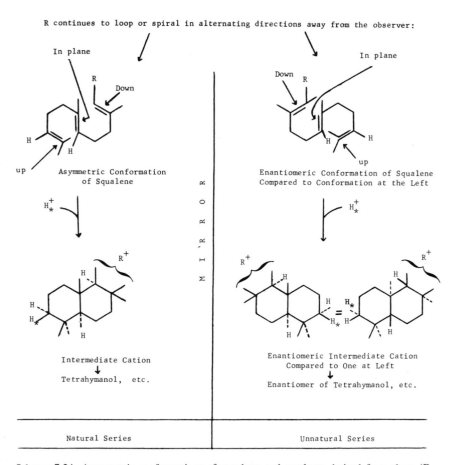

Scheme 7.24. Asymmetric conformations of squalene and products derived from them (R, remainder of squalene molecule).

it forces the 10-methyl (C-19) up (β). No other possibility exists for this conformer, and conversely the configurations obtained at C-5 and C-10 could not have arisen in some other way. These are the natural configurations, and therefore the conformer described is the one bound naturally. The mirror-image spiral would lead to the enantiomeric configuration. The use of models will also reveal that the *cis*-oriented methyl group at C-4 is above and cannot pass C-5, while the *trans*-oriented one is free to do so. Consequently, the *trans*-one, which is derived from C-2 of mevalonate, must become α-oriented, with the *cis*-one remaining on the front or β face. It also follows from the natural conformation that the H atom at C-9 must be α-oriented and a *trans-anti*-arrangement must be produced, as is found, for instance, in tetrahymanol. In order to produce the full pentacyclic structure, the conformation shown is simply extended in the alternating clockwise-counterclockwise way already described with each incipient ring from left to right below the one before it. All-*trans-anti*-stereochemistry must be produced as found, for the same reasons described for rings A and B. The desoxyprotoeuphoid and desoxyhopenyl cations are formed in this way. A more precise analysis of the acyclic conformation shows that it approximates an all-chair structure, and the resulting cations would actually have the all-chair conformations. The formation of the desoxylupenyl cation requires only slight conformational modification at the right-hand end of the molecule.

The origin of the protosteroid cation and hence of steroids is a bit more complex. While the same conformation of squalene oxide must exist relative to ring A, i.e., C-4 up and the molecule spiraling down and to the right, which accounts for the *trans*-A/B junction as in other modes of cyclization and the same absolute configuration at C-3, C-5, and C-10, the incipient ring B must assume a boat type of conformation by rotations about the 5,6-, 6,7-, and 7,8-bonds (steroid numbering) (Scheme 7.25). These rotations place the opposite side of the 8,9-double bond toward the 5,10-double bond that is found with the incipient chair-chair arrangement. *Trans*-cyclization of the chair-boat type of system will then produce a 9β-H instead of a 9α-H. If the atoms forming rings C and D are arranged in the usual overlapping chair-chair type of arrangement below and to the right of the boat form of ring B, the protosteroid cation results with *trans-syn-trans-anti-trans-anti*-stereochemistry.

The *trans-syn*-system is energetically less favorable than the *trans-anti*-system because of diaxial and other steric interactions brought about by the boat form required of ring B. Steric strain is relieved in the ensuing re-arrangement of the protosteroid cation to lanosterol, which has the all-chair stereochemistry except for a slight perturbation inherent in the Δ^8-bond. The complication of the system passing through an energetically unfavorable state is finally compensated for by arrival at a final state that is not only energetically favored but also, unlike the case with the euphoids, has all but two (4α- and 14α-methyl groups) carbon substituents on a single side (the β face) of the four rings. The α-oriented substituents are then removed by further metabolism and the all-chair structure is retained in the process. The product (cholesterol, etc.) is unique in now possessing all of the axial substituents on one side of a flat molecule. Nature's development of the more complicated cyclase is probably an evolutionary feedback or selection related to the superior role that such a structure can play biologically. Since sterols are components of the layered structure of membranes, it may well be this that has functioned to select a cyclase producing as thin and flat a molecule as possible.

4. Asymmetric Conformation of Squalene Oxide

The situation with squalene oxide is entirely analogous. A spiral conformer of the same sort must exist with the oxido end of the molecule toward the

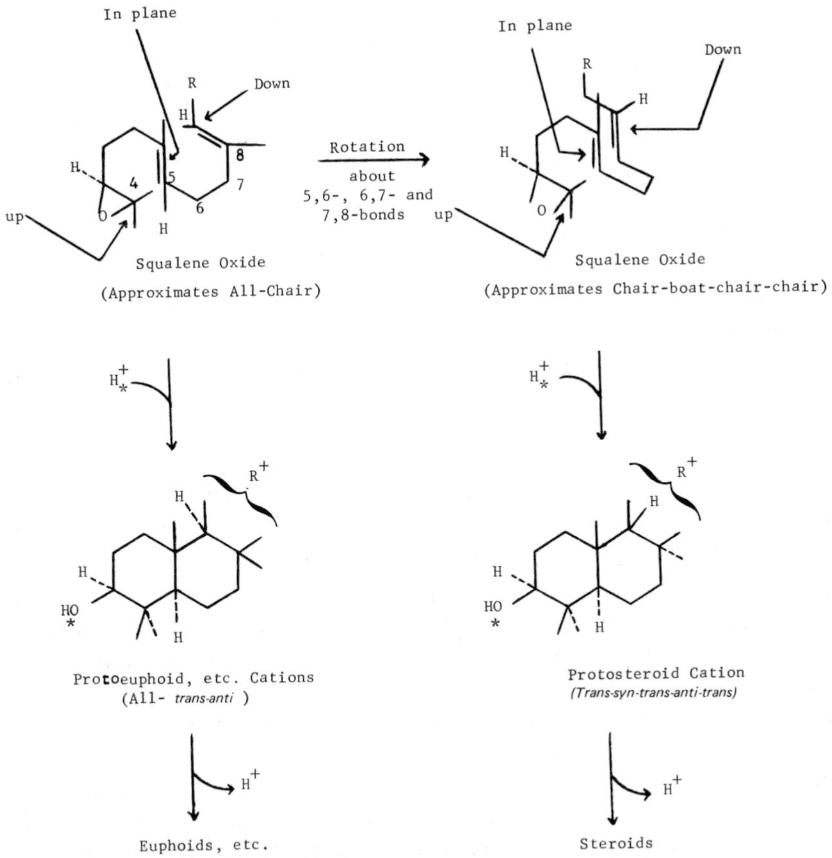

In plane

R   Down

H

R

8

4   5

7

6

H

up

O

H

Rotation

about

5,6-, 6,7- and

7,8-bonds

In plane

R   Down

H

H

up

O

Squalene Oxide

(Approximates All-Chair)

Squalene Oxide

(Approximates Chair-boat-chair-chair)

H⁺
*

H⁺
*

H   R⁺

H

H

HO
*

H

H   R⁺

H

H

HO
*

H

Protoeuphoid, etc. Cations

(All- *trans-anti*)

Protosteroid Cation

(Trans-syn-trans-anti-trans)

H⁺

H⁺

Euphoids, etc.

Steroids

Scheme 7.25. Natural asymmetric conformations of squalene oxide (R, remainder of molecule, and it loops or spirals in alternating directions away from observer in squalene oxide).

observer and the rest of the chain spiraling down and to the right. In addition, however, there is presumably asymmetric introduction of the oxido group. This cannot be deduced from the cyclized products, since only the oxide (*S* configuration) with the oxygen atom toward the observer in the natural conformation could lead mechanistically to *trans*-cyclization, production of the natural A/B configuration, and 3β-oriented hydroxyl group. Thus, the *R*-oxide if present would not react, but the generality of asymmetric induction and, more importantly, the economy of living systems lead one to expect that only the *S*-oxide is produced. Indeed, Barton et al. (*34*) have shown experimentally that only (*S*)-squalene-2,3-oxide and not the *R* isomer is the precursor of lanosterol and ergosterol in yeast, lanosterol in pig liver, and cycloartenol, β-amyrin, and lupeol in germinating peas.

D. ENZYMOLOGY

1. Squalene Oxidase

The enzyme system(s) for the introduction of the oxido linkage to give 2,3-oxidosqualene (29-31) or 2,3,22,23-dioxidosqualene (91) have not been studied in any detail. However, it is known that the enzyme that forms squalene-2,3-oxide is microsomal (96). Ono and Bloch (97) have isolated a microsomal system from rat liver that catalyzes squalene epoxidation. The enzyme system requires molecular oxygen, NADPH, and FAD, as well as a supernatent protein and phospholipids. There is no evidence for the participation of cytochromes P-450 or b$_5$. Enzyme activity occurs in two fractions and the activity of the combined fractions is five times the sum of the activity of each fraction alone. The second fraction appears to be identical with flavoprotein NADPH-cytochrome c reductase. The inhibitors, CO and KCN, are ineffective.

The apparently low concentration of the oxide and frequently much higher concentration of squalene suggest that the epoxidation is physiologically a rate-limiting step in sterol formation. Squalene is epoxidized from either end of the molecule (35, 98, 99) to give the monoepoxide, contraindicating the possibility that newly formed squalene is attacked by a neighboring particulate oxidase without first dissociating and becoming free of squalene synthetase (35, 99). The squalene found in tissues probably then acts as a precursor pool. Based on the occurrence of cyclized products bearing oxygen at C-3, the oxidase is found in plants, animals, and generally in higher forms of life with the probable exceptions of insects and terrestrial annelids (100, 101). It is also present in algae and other lower forms with the possible exception of some bacteria. However, Methylococcus capsulatus apparently possesses the oxidase, since squalene and sterols can be isolated from cells grown on methane (102). Procaryotic blue-green algae also must possess the oxidase, since several species grown on synthetic media contain sterols (102, 103).

2. Cyclases

Cyclases either for squalene or its oxides are apparently ubiquitous, with the exception of those in mycoplasma (38), insects (100) (and perhaps other Arthropoda), and terrestrial annelids (101), from which the Arthropoda are conceivably derived in an evolutionary sense. In the latter two cases, the lack probably represents a deletion, since both eukaryotic (53) and prokaryotic (103, 104) algae possess a cyclase, as do fungi (52, 105-107) and protozoa (73, 74), all of which presumably are more primitive than terrestrial annelids and insects. Bacteria, frequently believed to lack a cyclase, have one at least in some cases. Squalene has been isolated from Methylococcus capsulatus (102), its oxidative cyclization product, sterols, from the same source (102), and its direct cyclization product, hopene-b, from a thermophilic bacterium in the volcanic area of Naples (*70*).

Three types of substrate have been identified: squalene itself (*74, 86*), 2,3-oxidosqualene (*51, 105-108*), and 2,3,22,23-dioxidosqualene (*91*). Squalene-2,3-oxide is known to possess the *S* configuration at the carbon atoms joined to oxygen (*34*) and the diepoxide is thought to also have the *S* configuration (*38*). This conclusion is based in part on the configuration at C-3 of the cyclized products. The cyclases are named (*38*) according to the form "substrate-product cyclase"; we have, for instance, squalene-tetrahymanol cyclase, 2,3-(*S*)-oxidosqualene-lanosterol cyclase, or 2,3-(*S*),22,23-(*S*)-dioxidosqualene-α-onocerin cyclase. Some 17 cyclases, reviewed by Dean (*38*), are under current examination. In all cases cyclization occurs anaerobically and proceeds without observable cofactors. However, purification of none of the enzymes has yet been achieved in a really satisfactory manner enzymologically. Frequently (but not always) they are associated with the endoplasmic reticulum. The yeast enzyme is found in the soluble fraction of cell homogenates, but the enzymes from *Ochromonas malhamensis* (*107*) and the liver enzyme (*106*) are associated with the microsomes. Disruption of the membranous material without alterations in the enzyme is extremely difficult. It has forced investigators to deal with entities that are believed to represent a variety of particle sizes, perhaps retaining part of the membrane, and to obtain results of a puzzling and inconsistent nature. For instance, while the liver cyclase leading to lanosterol and the cycloartenol cyclase from *O. malhamensis* will tolerate concentrations of many detergents, the cyclase for α-onocerin formation and the yeast enzyme for lanosterol formation are sensitive to detergent. The liver and algal enzymes require continuous exposure to desoxycholate, but this does not appear to be true of all cyclases.

The 2,3-(*S*)-oxidosqualene-lanosterol cyclase of liver has been obtained from microsomes and purified by ammonium sulfate precipitations (*51*). It possesses a specific activity of 1.5-2.0 nmol of substrate converted per minute per milligram of protein. It is unaffected by EDTA, ascorbate, fluoride, iodoacetate, glutathione, cyanide, nicotinamide, thiocyanate, azide, or $CaCl_2$ at concentrations of 10^{-3} M. It is completely inactivated by organic solvents, to a 20% extent by 10^{-3} M *N*-ethylmaleimide, markedly by the imino analog and slightly by the sulfur analog of the substrate. Even though the properties of the algal cyclase have not been investigated as thoroughly, it is known (*107*) that the enzyme has a specific activity of 17 μmol per hour per milligram of protein, is stimulated by dithiothreitol and inhibited by *p*-hydroxymercuribenzoate, and is inhibited by 2,3-iminosqualene but not as extensively as the liver cyclase. To the extent that they have been examined (*77*), the properties of the cyclase from peas for β-amyrin formation are much the same. In the several cases that have been carefully investigated, notably for cyclases leading to lanosterol, cycloartenol, and β-amyrin, which represent three rather different and biologically important modes of cyclization of the same substrate, only a single product is produced with a given enzyme. Since cycloartenol can be isomerized to lanosterol (by acid catalysis), proving the latter to be the more stable, the production of cycloartenol in the absence of its more stable isomer proves unequivocally that the cyclases are different. The pH optima for liver, brain, algal, and *O. spinosa* cyclases are similar (7.3 ± 0.1), despite very different products produced (lanosterol, cycloartenol, and α-onocerin). The Michaelis constants for the liver, brain, and algal cyclases are, however, substantially different (10^{-4}, 10^{-6}, and 10^{-4}, respectively) for the same substrate squalene oxide leading to the products lanosterol and cycloartenol. The cyclase leading to cycloartenol has been obtained in a cell-free system from a gymnosperm (*108a*).

Current classification of the cyclases is based on substrate structure and product stability (*38*). Class I and class II enzymes utilize oxido- or dioxido-squalene, while class III enzymes utilize squalene itself. Classes I and II differ in that the former produces products that do not give skeletal rearrangements ("backbone rearrangements") by acid catalysis while products formed through the latter do. Class I enzymes yield lanosterol, cycloartenol, β-amyrin, α-onocerin, etc. Class II enzymes yield friedelin, campanulin, etc. Class III enzymes yield tetrahymanol, perhaps the fernenes, etc. The classification attempts to imply mechanism in that class II enzymes presumably utilize an incipient all-chair conformation of substrate, while class I enzymes utilize substrate folded in a form approximating cyclized conformations possessing a boat form of one of the rings.

3. Carrier Protein

The mammalian utilization of squalene and sterols for further metabolism has been found by Dempsey and Scallen and their co-workers (*109, 110*) to require a soluble protein generally called a squalene and sterol carrier protein (SCP). SCP has also been isolated from *T. pyriformis* (*111*). Its properties are similar to the liver protein. More recently, Rilling (*112*) has reported that presqualene pyrophosphate (but not farnesyl pyrophosphate) is also bound by SCP. The liver protein has a molecular weight of 16,000 aggregating to 150,000, forms non-covalent bonds with the substrate, and binding constants for many substrates have been measured (*109*). The protein is not thought to have intrinsic enzymatic activity of its own, but to act in concert with the enzymes by solubilizing water-insoluble materials. Additional functions in sequencing brought about by the quantitative nature of the binding constants may also be involved.

E. SUMMARY

The cyclization of squalene (giving rise to 3-desoxy products) or of its oxide(s) (giving rise to 3β-hydroxy products) is governed by two major factors: 1) the conformation bound to the cyclase, and 2) the nature and position of deprotonation or HO^- addition to a cation that is produced by protonation of the bound conformer. Four principal cations appear to exist. Two are tetracyclic ones (the protosteroid and protoeuphoid cations) and two are pentacyclic (the hopenyl and lupenyl cations). All four possess five or six H atoms adjacent to the positive charge, which could offer hyperconjugative stabilization. While the details of cation stabilization by the enzyme and of the cations' lifetimes remain to be elucidated, these four cations allow all known facts about structure, steric orientation, and labeling pattern of all tetra- and pentacyclic products to be understood.

The steroids are formed through the protosteroid cation (in which ring B is in the boat form) by elimination of a proton from C-7, C-9, C-11, or C-19, yielding, respectively, $\Delta^{7,24}$-lanostadienol, lanosterol, parkeol, or cycloartenol. Lanosterol and cycloartenol have both been shown to be on the pathway to the common Δ^5-sterols. Only one configuration is found in steroids at C-20 (20-H pointed toward the observer with C-22 on the right, which is the preferred conformation).

All tetra- and pentacyclic products are of the same enantiomeric series in all organisms in that the two carbon atoms (C-5 and C-10) at the juncture of rings A and B of all four primary cations have the same absolute configuration (C-19 toward the observer and 5-H atom away when viewed with ring A to the left). Stereochemical differences reside exclusively in diastereoisomeric differences in the cations at other centers and the extent of migrations of H or C atoms. The enantiomer of none of the products of cyclization has been found in nature.

The cyclization of squalene or its oxide occurs at all levels of biological evolution from prokaryotic blue-green algae and bacteria through eukaryotic fungi and algae to higher plants and animals, but a few organismic types, e.g., the Arthropoda, appear to have lost the capacity for it. The formation of lanosterol occurs in nonphotosynthetic organisms (fungi, animals), while cycloartenol is produced in photosynthetic organisms (algae, gymnosperms, angiosperms, etc.). The pentacyclic products have not been found in man, but they arise in some protozoa, some bacteria, and very commonly in plants.

The cyclases do not have observable cofactors and are frequently microsomal. Cyclization in all cases is an anaerobic process. However, the formation of squalene oxide, which has the S configuration, is aerobic, with molecular oxygen being reduced in an NADPH-dependent reaction. The oxygen appears in the oxide and ultimately in the steroids and other compounds formed from the oxide.

In addition to the steroids and pentacyclic compounds various other products of cyclization occur. The various possibilities are summarized in Scheme 7.26.

A carrier protein (SCP) has been isolated from animals and evidence exists for it in plants. It seems to bind presqualenyl pyrophosphate and its

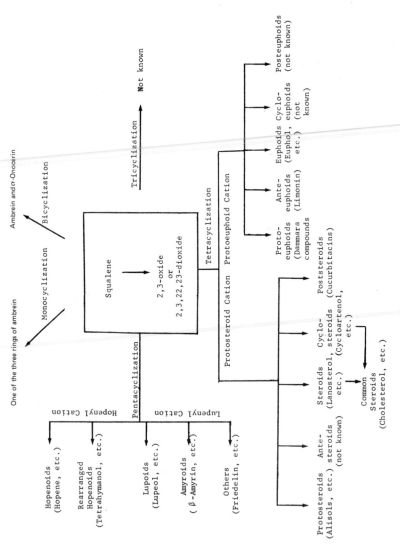

Scheme 7.26. Summary of cyclization.

subsequent metabolites (squalene, lanosterol, etc.). SCP is a soluble, non-catalytic protein, the apparent function of which is to solubilize the substrate and deliver it to the enzyme.

LITERATURE CITED

1. R. Robinson, Chem. Ind. 53:1062 (1934).
2. R. B. Woodward and K. Bloch, J. Am. Chem. Soc. 75:2023 (1953).
3. E. Schulze, Ber. Deutsch. Chem. Gesellshaft 5:1075 (1872).
4. A. Windaus and R. Tschesche, Hoppe Zeller's Z. Physiol. Chem. 190:51 (1930).
5. L. Ruzicka, E. Rey, and A. C. Muhr, Helv. Chim. Acta 27:472 (1944).
6. L. Ruzicka, R. Denss, and O. Jeger, Helv. Chim. Acta 29:204 (1946).
7. L. F. Fieser and M. Fieser, Steroids. Reinhold, New York, 1959. pp. 364–379.
8. R. B. Clayton and K. Bloch, J. Biol. Chem. 218:305 (1956).
9. R. B. Clayton and K. Bloch, J. Biol. Chem. 218:319 (1956).
10. T. T. Tchen and K. Bloch, J. Biol. Chem. 226:921 (1957).
11. T. T. Tchen and K. Bloch, J. Biol. Chem. 226:931 (1957).
12. T. T. Tchen and K. Bloch, J. Am. Chem. Soc. 77:6085 (1955).
13. J. W. Cornforth, R. H. Cornforth, A. Pelter, M. G. Horning, and G. Popjak, Proc. Chem. Soc. (London) 112 (1958).
14. J. W. Cornforth, I. Y. Gore, and G. Popjak, Biochem. J. 65:94 (1957).
15. R. K. Maudgal, T. T. Tchen, and K. Bloch, J. Am. Chem. Soc. 80:2589 (1958).
16. W. G. Dauben and T. W. Hutton, J. Am. Chem. Soc. 78:2647 (1956).
17. W. G. Dauben, T. W. Hutton, and G. A. Boswell, J. Am. Chem. Soc. 81:403 (1959).
18. O. Isler, R. Ruegg, J. Wursch, K. F. Gey, and A. Pletscher, Helv. Chim. Acta 40:2369 (1957).
19. A. Eschenmoser, L. Ruzicka, O. Jeger, and D. Arigoni, Helv. Chim. Acta 38:1890 (1955).
20. D. H. R. Barton and G. P. Moss, Chem. Commun. 261 (1966).
21. O. Hayaishi (ed.), Oxygenases. Academic Press, New York, 1962.
22. M. Hayano, in O. Hayaishi (ed.), Oxygenases. Academic Press, New York, 1962. p. 182.
23. K. Bloch, Fed. Proc. 21:1058 (1962).
24. T. T. Tchen and K. Bloch, J. Am. Chem. Soc. 78:1516 (1956).
25. B. M. Bloom and G. M. Shull, J. Am. Chem. Soc. 77:5767 (1955).
26. G. M. Shull and D. A. Kita, J. Am. Chem. Soc. 77:763 (1955).
27. E. E. van Tamelen, Accounts of Chem. Res. 1:111 (1968).
28. E. E. van Tamelen and T. J. Curphey, Tetrahedron Lett. 121 (1962).
29. E. E. van Tamelen, J. D. Willett, R. B. Clayton, and K. E. Lord, J. Am. Chem. Soc. 88:4752 (1966).
30. J. D. Willett, K. B. Sharpless, K. E. Lord, E. E. van Tamelen, and R. B. Clayton, J. Biol. Chem. 242:4182 (1967).
31. E. J. Corey and W. E. Russey, J. Am. Chem. Soc. 88:4750 (1966).
32. E. E. van Tamelen, J. D. Willett, and R. B. Clayton, J. Am. Chem. Soc. 89:3371 (1971).
33. E. J. Corey, W. E. Russey, and P. R. Ortiz de Montellano, J. Am. Chem. Soc. 88:4750 (1966).
34. D. H. R. Barton, T. R. Jarman, K. G. Watson, D. A. Widdowson, R. B. Boar, and K. Damps, J. Chem. Soc., Chem. Commun. 861 (1974).

35. R. C. Ebersole, W. O. Godtfredsen, S. Vangedal, and E. Caspi, J. Am. Chem. Soc. 95:8133 (1973).
36. A. H. Etemadi, G. Popjak, and J. W. Cornforth, Biochem. J. 111:445 (1969).
37. E. E. van Tamelen and J. R. Heys, J. Am. Chem. Soc. 97:1252 (1975).
38. P. D. G. Dean, Steroidologia 2:143 (1971).
39. E. J. Corey, P. R. Ortiz de Montellano, and H. Yamamoto, J. Am. Chem. Soc. 90:6254 (1968).
39a. E. E. van Tamelen, R. G. Lees, and A. Grieder, J. Am. Chem. Soc. 96, 2255 (1974).
40. T. Murata and M. Miyamoto, Chem. Pharm. Bull. (Tokyo) 18:1354 (1970).
41. T. Murata, M. Shinohara, and M. Miyamoto, Chem. Pharm. Bull. (Tokyo) 18:1369 (1970).
42. K. Kamiya, T. Murata, and M. Nishikawa, Chem. Pharm. Bull. (Tokyo) 18:1362 (1970).
43. W. O. Godtfredsen, W. von Daehne, S. Vangedal, A. Marquet, D. Arigoni, and A. Melera, Tetrahedron 21:3505 (1965).
44. A. Cooper and D. C. Hodgkin, Tetrahedron 24:909 (1968).
45. E. J. Corey, P. R. Ortiz de Montellano, and H. Yamamoto, J. Am. Chem. Soc. 90:6254 (1968).
46. E. J. Corey and H. Yamamoto, Tetrahedron 27:2385 (1970).
47. E. E. van Tamelen, R. P. Hanzlik, K. B. Sharpless, R. B. Clayton, W. J. Richter, and A. L. Burlingame, J. Am. Chem. Soc. 90:3284 (1968).
48. L. J. Mulheirn and E. Caspi, J. Biol. Chem. 246:2494 (1971).
49. E. J. Corey, K. Lin, and H. Yamamoto, J. Am. Chem. Soc. 91:2132 (1969).
50. A. White, P. Handler, and E. L. Smith, Principles of Biochemistry. 4th Ed. McGraw-Hill, New York, 1968. p. 267.
51. S. Yamamoto, K. Lin, and K. Bloch, Proc. Natl. Acad. Sci. U.S.A. 63:110 (1969).
52. E. I. Mercer and M. W. Johnson, Phytochemistry 8:2329 (1969).
53. H. H. Rees, L. J. Goad, and T. W. Goodwin, Biochim. Biophys. Acta 176: 892 (1969).
54. H. H. Rees, L. J. Goad, and T. W. Goodwin, Tetrahedron Lett. 723 (1968).
55. G. Ourisson, P. Crabbe, and O. R. Rodig, Tetracyclic Triterpenes. Holden-Day, San Francisco, 1964. pp. 134-176.
56. J. W. Cornforth, R. H. Cornforth, C. Donninger, G. Popjak, Y. Shimizu, S. Ichii, E. Forchielli, and E. Caspi, J. Am. Chem. Soc. 87:3224 (1965).
57. L. J. Mulheirn and E. Caspi, J. Biol. Chem. 246:3948 (1971).
58. H. H. Rees, L. J. Goad, and T. W. Goodwin, Biochem. J. 107:417 (1968).
59. J. W. Cornforth, Angew. Chem. 7:903 (1968).
60. J. M. Zander, J. B. Grieg, and E. Caspi, J. Biol. Chem. 245:1247 (1970).
61. R. Bentley, Molecular Asymmetry. Vol. II. Academic Press, New York, 1970. p. 267.
62. D. H. R. Barton, G. Mellows, D. A. Widdowson, and J. J. Wright, J. Chem. Soc. 1142 (1971).
63. E. E. van Tamelen, J. B. Willett, and R. B. Clayton, J. Am. Chem. Soc. 89:3371 (1967).
64. E. E. van Tamelen, R. B. Hanzlik, R. B. Clayton, and A. L. Burlingame, J. Am. Chem. Soc. 92:2137 (1970).
65. G. T. Newbold and F. S. Spring, J. Chem. Soc. 249 (1944).
66. J. S. Mills and A. E. A. Werner, J. Chem. Soc. 3132 (1955).

67. F. G. Fischer and N. Seiler, Liebig's Ann. Chem. 644:146 (1961).
68. F. G. Fischer and N. Seiler , Liebig's Ann. Chem. 644:162 (1961).
69. I. M. Heilbron, G. I. Moffet, and F. S. Spring, J. Chem. Soc. 1583 (1934).
70. M. de Rosa, A. Gambacorta, and L. Minale, Chem. Commun. 619 (1971).
71. H. Fazakerley, T. G. Halsall, and E. R. H. Jones, J. Chem. Soc. 1877 (1959).
72. G. Berti and F. Bottari, Progr. Phytochem. 1:589 (1968).
73. E. Caspi, J. M. Zander, J. B. Greig, F. B. Mallory, R. L. Conner, and J. R. Landrey, J. Am. Chem. Soc. 90:3563 (1968).
74. J. M. Zander, J. B. Greig, and E. Caspi, J. Biol. Chem. 245:1247 (1970).
75. P. de Mayo, in K. W. Bentley (ed.), The Chemistry of Natural Products. Vol. III. The Higher Terpenoids, Interscience, New York, 1959.
76. E. Capstack, Jr., N. Rosin, G. A. Blondin, and W. R. Nes, J. Biol. Chem. 240:3258 (1965).
77. E. J. Corey and P. R. Ortiz de Montellano, J. Am. Chem. Soc. 89:3362 (1967).
78. W. R. Nes and J. W. Cannon, Phytochemistry 7:1321 (1968).
79. T. T. Tchen and K. Bloch, J. Biol. Chem. 226:931 (1957).
80. T. G. Halsall and R. T. Aplin, Fortschr. Chem. Org. Naturstoffe 22:153 (1964).
81. D. H. R. Barton, P. de Mayo, and J. C. Orr, J. Chem. Soc. 2239 (1958).
82. P. Dietrich and E. Lederer, Helb. Chim. Acta 35:1548 (1952).
83. Y. Tsuda, A. Morimoto, T. Sano, Y. Inubushi, F. B. Mallory, and J. T. Gordon, Tetrahedron Lett. 1427 (1965).
84. Y. Tsuda and K. Isobe, Tetrahedron Lett. 3337 (1965).
85. G. Berti, F. Bottari, A. Marsili, I. Morelli, and A. Mandelbaum, Chem. Commun. 50 (1967).
86. D. H. R. Barton, A. F. Gosden, G. Mellows, and D. A. Widdowson, Chem. Commun. 184 (1969).
87. Y. Tsuda, A. Morimoto, T. Sano, Y. Inubushi, F. B. Mallory, and J. T. Gordon, Tetrahedron Lett. 19:1427 (1965).
88. F. B. Mallory, R. L. Conner, J. R. Landrey, J. M. Zander, J. B. Greig, and E. Caspi, J. Am. Chem. Soc. 90:3564 (1968).
89. E. Caspi, J. B. Greig, and J. M. Zander, Chem. Commun. 28 (1969).
90. J. M. Zander and E. Caspi, Chem. Commun. 209 (1969).
91. M. G. Rowan, P. D. G. Dean, and T. W. Goodwin, FEBS Lett. 12:229 (1971).
92. L. F. Fieser and M. Fieser, Steroids. Reinhold, New York, 1959. pp. 337–338.
92a. W. R. Nes, T. E. Varkey, and K. Krevitz, J. Am. Chem. Soc. 99:260 (1977).
92b. W. R. Nes, T. E. Varkey, D. R. Crump, and M. Gut, J. Org. Chem. 41:3429 (1976).
93. T. Tsuda and K. Sakai, Chem. Pharm. Bull. 8:554 (1960).
94. K. Tsuda, R. Hayatsu, Y. Kishida, and S. Akagi, J. Am. Chem. Soc. 80:921 (1958).
95. W. R. Nes, D. J. Baisted, E. Capstack, Jr., W. W. Newschwander, and P. T. Russell, in T. W. Goodwin (ed.), Biochemistry of Chloroplasts. Vol. II. Academic Press, New York, 1967. p. 274.
96. S. Yamamoto and K. Bloch, in T. W. Goodwin (ed.), Natural Substances Formed Biologically from Mevalonic Acid, Biochemical Society Symposium No. 29. Academic Press, New York, 1970. p. 35.

97. T. Ono and K. Bloch, J. Biol. Chem. 250:1571 (1975).
98. B. Samuelson and DeW. S. Goodman, J. Biol. Chem. 239:98 (1964).
99. A. H. Etemadi, G. Popjak, and J. W. Cornforth, Biochem. J. 111:445 (1969).
100. J. Clark and K. Bloch, J. Biol. Chem. 234:2589 (1959).
101. Deleted in proof.
102. C. W. Bird, J. M. Lynch, F. J. Pirt, W. W. Reid, C. J. W. Brooks, and B. S. Middleditch, Nature 230:473 (1971).
103. R. C. Reitz and J. G. Hamilton, Comp. Biochem. Physiol. 25:401 (1968).
104. N. J. de Souza and W. R. Nes, Science 162:363 (1968).
105. D. H. R. Barton, A. F. Gosden, G. Mellows, and D. A. Widdowson, Chem. Commun. 1067 (1968).
106. I. Schechter, F. W. Sweat, and K. Bloch, Biochim. Biophys. Acta 220:463 (1970).
107. G. H. Beastall, H. H. Rees, and T. W. Goodwin, FEBS Lett. 18:175 (1971).
108. P. D. G. Dean, P. R. Ortiz de Montellano, K. Bloch, and E. J. Corey, J. Biol. Chem. 242:3014 (1967).
108a. H. C. Malhotra and W. R. Nes, J. Biol. Chem. 247:6243 (1972).
109. M. C. Ritter and M. E. Dempsey, J. Biol. Chem. 246:1536 (1971).
110. T. J. Scallen, M. W. Schuster, and A. K. Dhar, J. Biol. Chem. 246:224 (1971).
111. T. Calimbas, Fed. Proc. 31:430 (1972).
112. H. C. Rilling, Biochem. Biophys. Res. Commun. 46:470 (1972).

Chapter
8

Cyclization
of
Other
Isopentenoids

A. General and Historical Comments 272
B. Cyclization at the I₂ Stage 273
   1. Mechanism 273
   2. Stereochemistry 279
   3. Metabolism of I₂ Compounds 282
C. Cyclization at the I₃ Stage 284
   1. Mechanism and Oxidative Metabolism 284
   2. Metabolism to Bi- and Tricyclic Products 287
   3. Cyclization With Methyl Migration 295
   4. Cyclization With Homoallylic Rearrangements 295
   5. Hydroxylative Cyclization 297
   6. Stereochemistry at the I₃ Stage 298
D. Cyclization and Metabolism at the I₄ Stage 301
   1. Formation of Monocycles 301
   2. Bi-, Tri-, and Tetracycle Formation 301
   3. Biosynthesis of Gibberellins 308
   4. Stereochemistry of the I₄ Stage 310
E. Cyclization of Neurosporene and Lycopene 313
   1. Origin of Acyclic Precursors 313
   2. Mechanism 315
   3. Stereochemistry 316
F. Enzymology 319
   1. I₂ Stage 319
   2. I₃ Stage 319
   3. I₄ Stage 319
   4. Carotenoid Stage 320
Literature Cited 320

A. GENERAL AND HISTORICAL COMMENTS

Considerations of the cyclization of isopentenoids other than squalene have a long and illustrious history dating back to the original ideas of Wallach a century ago (Chapter 1, Section C.2). However, very much less detailed biochemical progress has been made than with squalene. This is partially but not wholly the result of a smaller amount of experimental effort. Serious compartmentalization and other factors seem to have inhibited if not entirely prevented experimental attainment of biosynthetically active systems (1–4). In contrast to the cyclization of squalene and its oxide, cyclization of other isopentenoids tends to be rather restricted to particular types of cells or particular subcellular particles (plastids, etc.). Transport problems, the presence of pools of intermediates, volatility in the simpler cases, and a lack of specific knowledge of physiological parameters, e.g., information on the relationship of biosynthetic rate with morphologic, environmental, and developmental factors, and perhaps other factors, have led to great difficulty. On the other hand, from the work of Ruzicka (5–7) and others (8–10) an extremely good theoretical framework exists that is now greatly aided by what we know of the cyclization of squalene.

The extensive literature on the structures and occurrence of cyclized products (11–17) shows that cyclization at the I_2, I_3, and I_4 stages proceeds rather commonly in plants. Considerably less knowledge is available on the role of the compounds produced. At the lower levels of polymerization the idea of "waste products" has been suggested, but there is a growing feeling that this is not an adequate description of function. Among the reasons for believing this are the complicated and extensive control systems that operate in the biosynthesis and further metabolism of the products. A very clear role has been proven for the giberellins, which are cyclized I_4 compounds functioning as plant growth (18–20) and flowering (21) hormones. It may be that some cyclic isopentenoids function ecologically as a defense against invading insects and microorganisms. They are already known to function in a variety of hormonal ways in insects themselves (22–25). In some cases (euparotin, elephantin, vernolepin, etc.) antitumor activity has been reported (26, 27) as a mammalian pharmacologic property. The most fully studied physiological function is that of the carotenoids, which possess a condensed I_4-I_4 structure. They are active in the utilization of light during photosynthesis (28), in the phenomena of phototropism, phototaxis, and reproduction (29), and in the form of the carotenoid metabolite, vitamin A, in the visual process (30). While it is certainly true that cyclization of isopentenoids other than squalene and its oxides is rare in the animal kingdom, β-carotene is present, for unknown reasons, in the mammalian corpus luteum, and there is evidence (31) for its origin from acetate in this tissue. Moreover, mammalian liver is reported to possess geranylgeranyl pyrophosphate synthetase (32). Two possible functions for the I_4 product are as an intermediate to polyprenols for quinone cofactors and, in the present connection, for cyclized products such as the carotenoids.

B. CYCLIZATION AT THE I_2 STAGE

1. Mechanism

When the I_2 stage is reached, an isopentenoid has sufficient carbon atoms to form a six-membered ring. The proper stereochemistry is attainable either by neryl or linaloyl pyrophosphate, and C—O cleavage could yield an enzyme-bound "ion pair" (Scheme 8.1) in which condensation from

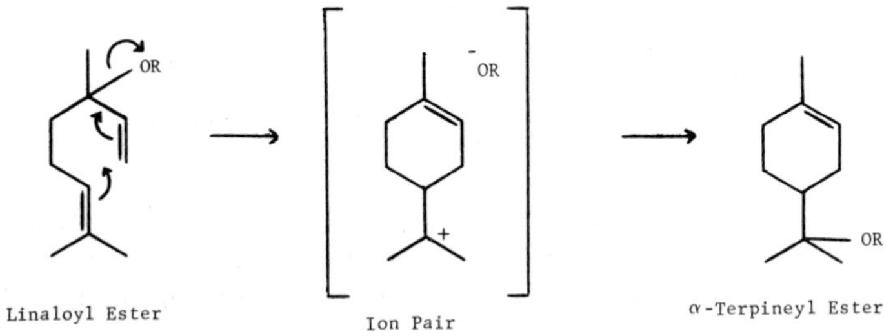

Linaloyl Ester	Ion Pair	α-Terpineyl Ester

Scheme 8.1. Winstein model for enzymatic cyclization. (In the nonbiological case, R is an aromatic ester; in biological systems it presumably would be the pyrophosphoroxy group.)

C-1 to C-6 has occurred. Nerol, presumably formed as the pyrophosphate, has actually been obtained from mevalonate in a cell-free system from *Pinus radiata* (*33*) which also converts mevalonate into the cyclic I_2-derivative, limonene (*34*). Nerol was isolated by oxygen-phosphorous cleavage with alkaline phosphatase and therefore probably represents a true metabolite and not an artifact. Although it remains to be proved whether the neryl or linaloyl system is the actual substrate for cyclization, Winstein (*35*) has made some important observations nonbiologically with the latter. He found that aromatic esters of linalool will undergo first-order cyclization in an aqueous medium to yield the corresponding ester of α-terpineol (Scheme 8.1) along with some α-terpineol itself. The conversion of the acyclic ester into the cyclic ester in the presence of water must have occurred intramolecularly without the ester anion completely departing from the immediate vicinity of the original molecule. If it had departed, water would have attacked the carbonium ion yielding the free alcohol. The work proves the intrinsic capacity for cyclization to occur through a mechanism in which the negative ester anion and the positive carbonium ion have remained together as an "ion pair." The extent to which this model can be applied to the enzymatic case has not yet been resolved. Unlike the model ester, neryl and linaloyl pyrophosphates bear an anionic end on the ester grouping that could conceivably undergo a concerted addition-elimination yielding the cyclized α-terpineyl pyrophosphate without ever passing through a real "ion pair" (Scheme 8.2). Furthermore, a concerted elimination of the

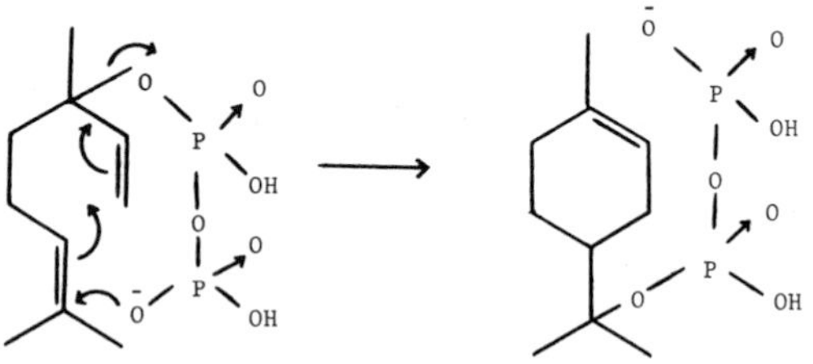

Linaloyl Pyrophosphate α-Terpineyl Pyrophosphate

Scheme 8.2. Conceivable mode of cyclization circumventing ion pair.

pyrophosphate anion and a proton could lead to a hydrocarbon, e.g., limonene, without passing through any true ionic condition. Still another possibility exists. At the moment of C—O cleavage, the enzyme may donate electrons to or otherwise stabilize the carbonium ion, e.g., by a dipole effect or by full covalent bond formation. Much work obviously remains to be done before these questions can be settled.

Thus, the uncertainties of the mechanism are much the same as in the case with squalene. However, there are some presumptive rules that must apply. In summary, they are (1) that the acyclic precursor is bound by the cyclase in a particular conformation; (2) cyclization is initiated either by protonation or by carbon-oxygen cleavage; and (3) the structure of the product is governed by the conformation together with the presence and nature of an electron-donating (HO⁻ from H_2O) or proton-abstracting group. At the very least, these rules allow one to rationalize the cyclic I_2 compounds that are known to exist (5-17). Important representatives, together with theoretical mechanisms, are shown in Schemes 8.3, 8.4, and 8.5. The α-terpineyl cation (Scheme 8.3) is assumed to play the sort of role that the protosteroid and other cations play in the squalene case, and as with these other cations we shall ignore, for the sake of simplicity, the uncertainties surrounding stabilization and origin. The principal difference between the formation of the α-terpineyl cation and those from squalene and its oxides is that in the latter cases cyclization is always proton-initiated, while in the present case it is frequently assumed to be initiated by C—O cleavage of the pyrophosphate. It must be noted that such an assumption may not represent reality. The cation might be produced in a two-step process, the first of which is C—O cleavage, with elimination of a proton,

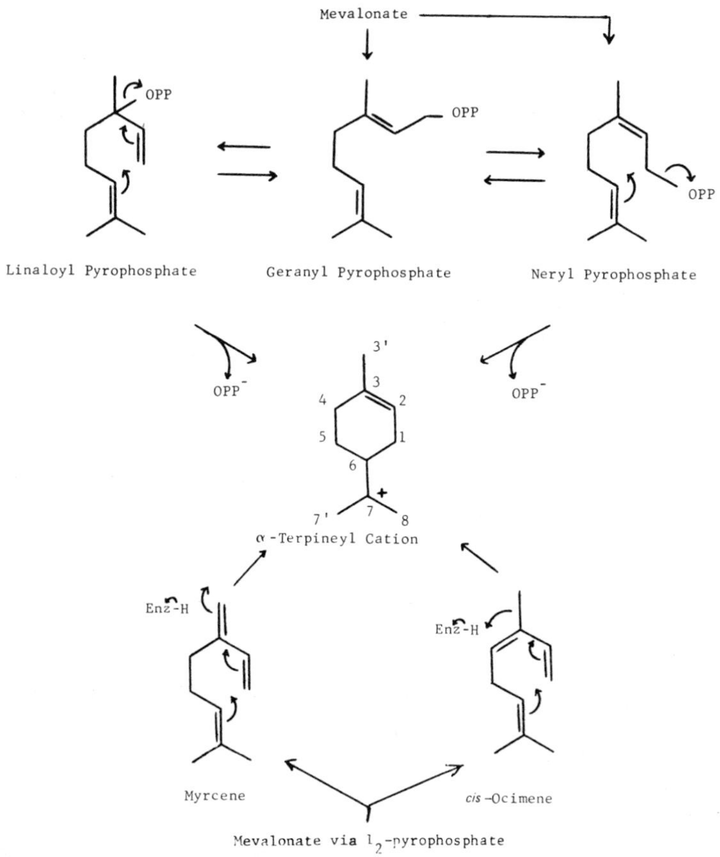

Mevalonate

OPP

OPP

OPP

Linaloyl Pyrophosphate   Geranyl Pyrophosphate   Neryl Pyrophosphate

3'

OPP⁻

3

4   2

5   1

6

OPP⁻

+

7'   7   8

α-Terpineyl Cation

Enz-H

Enz-H

Myrcene   *cis*-Ocimene

Mevalonate via 1₂-pyrophosphate

Scheme 8.3. Summary of possibilities for formation of α-terpineyl cation (numbering on cation is derived from that of acyclic precursor).

yielding a hydrocarbon that is subsequently reprotonated, as is shown in Scheme 8.3, bypassing the neryl-linaloyl argument. The expected hydrocarbons, myrcene and ocimene, are known in living systems and fairly widely distributed (*11*). The two-step process has the advantage of circumventing the problem of whether geranyl, neryl, or linaloyl pyrophosphate is the substrate for the cyclase. None may be, and the bifurcation in the pathway leading away from squalene, etc., may be in the C—O-cleaving enzyme producing the hydrocarbons rather than in the cyclase.

Sandermann and Schweers (*36*) have achieved the biosynthesis of α-pinene from [2-¹⁴C]mevalonic acid in *Pinus nigra austriaca* and have proven by degradation that no label was lost when the C—H group constituting part of the double bond was oxidatively removed. This proves that α-pinene has arisen by allylic closure of a three-membered ring from C-7 to

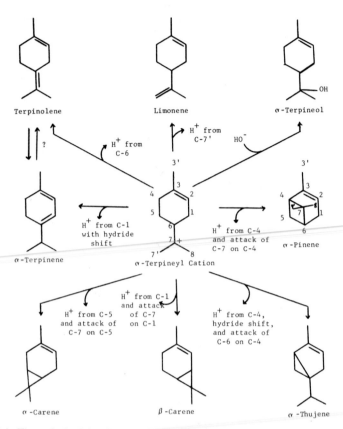

Scheme 8.4. Theoretical origin of some representative cyclic terpenes through the α-terpineyl cation (all products shown are naturally occurring).

C-4 as shown in Scheme 8.4 and not by attack of C-7 on C-2 with double-bond migration. Such an allylic process could also lead to the naturally occurring β-carene (Scheme 8.4), as was first proposed by Ruzicka (5); α-carene, which is also natural, could then arise either by double-bond migration or conceivably by direct electrophilic displacement at the non-allylic C-5. Electrophilic displacement at the allylic position also seems to account for the biosynthesis of thujene, since Sandermann and Schweers (37) were able to achieve the biosynthesis of the corresponding C-2 ketone (thujone) in *Thuja occidentalis* from [2-^{14}C]mevalonic acid and to present evidence that the closure of the three-membered ring is at C-6 and C-4 rather than at C-2 and C-4.

The cyclization could also conceivably take the course in which a charge is produced at C-2 by the bornyl cation, as shown in Scheme 8.5. Addition of HO$^-$ would lead to the naturally occurring borneol. The reac-

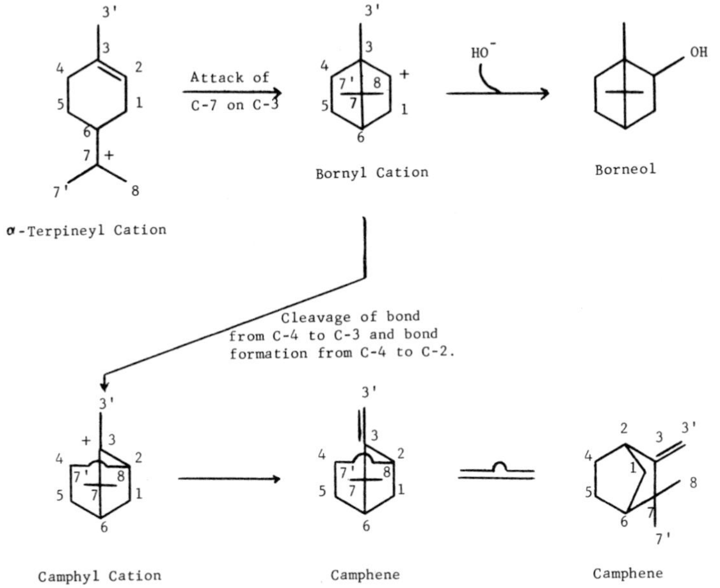

Scheme 8.5. Skeletal rearrangement of α-terpineyl cation (all products shown are naturally occurring).

tion might also take a course involving deprotonation, in which case there appears superficially to be a hydrocarbon, which could have a double bond between C-1 and C-2. Molecular models reveal, however, that this is a considerably strained structure, and it is not surprising that it has not been encountered naturally. On the other hand, the product of rearrangement, camphene, is known (Scheme 8.5).

In what has been discussed so far, all of the I₂ products of cyclization contain a six-membered ring, but just as formation of five-membered rings is encountered in the squalene case, so it is found at the simpler I₂ level. In fact, the products, called "cyclopentanoterpenoids" or "cyclopentanomonoterpenoids," are not uncommon. They are found in many insects (23) and plants (8, 10, 38, 39) and have a variety of detailed structures (38) derived from the 1,2-dimethyl-3-isopropylcyclopentyl skeleton. Many are bicyclic heterocycles (39) in which nitrogen or oxygen is included in a six-membered ring fused to the five-membered one. The carbon atoms of the six-membered ring are derived from the substituents on the cyclopropyl ring. Simple examples (Scheme 8.6) are the nonaromatic alkaloid skytanthine found in *Skytanthus actus* Meyen (40), the related aromatic alkaloid actinidine found in *Actinidia polygama* Miq. (41) with feline attractant activity, the O-heterocycles verbenalin found in *Verbena officinales* (42), and iridomyrmecin, found in *Iridomyrmex humulis* (43), which has antibiotic and in-

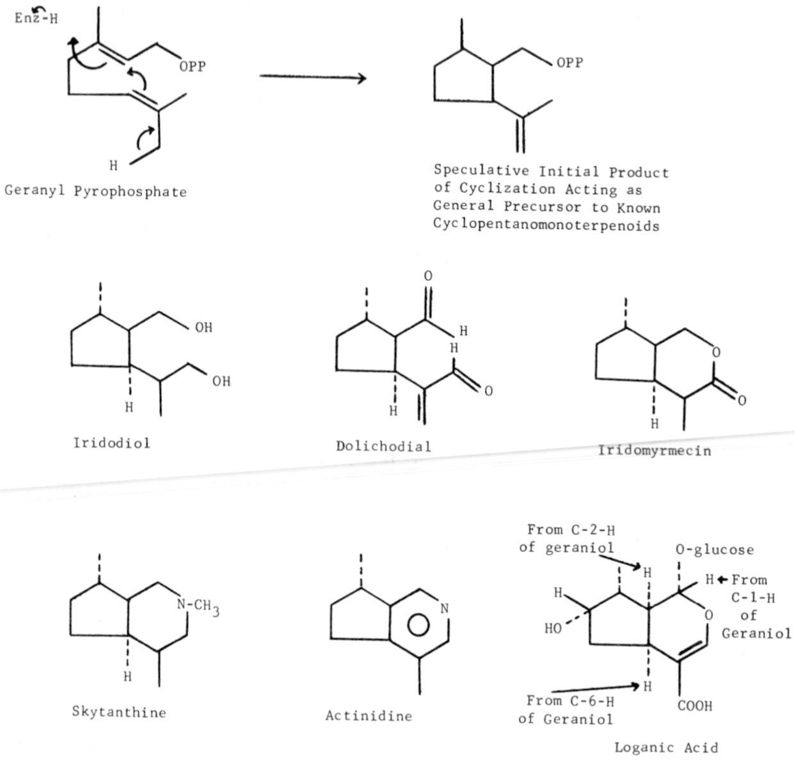

Geranyl Pyrophosphate

Speculative Initial Product
of Cyclization Acting as
General Precursor to Known
Cyclopentanomonoterpenoids

Iridodiol   Dolichodial   Iridomyrmecin

Skytanthine   Actinidine

From C-2-H
of geraniol   O-glucose

H ← From
C-1-H
of
Geraniol

From C-6-H
of Geraniol

Loganic Acid

Scheme 8.6. Some naturally occurring cyclopentano isopentenoids and their possible origin.

secticide activity and is believed to play a role in arthropod defense (23). More complicated metabolites are also well studied (Section C).

The precise origin of the cyclopentano compounds has not been established beyond the fact that they are indeed isopentenoid, since they are experimentally derivable from mevalonate (8) and geraniol (8). They are probably derived by proton-initiated cyclization (Scheme 8.6). Since C-1 of the acyclic precursor is frequently at the carbonyl stage of oxidation in the products, geranial or its reduction product citronellal have been invoked as a substrate for cyclization. Robinson (44) synthesized iridodial in 1959, taking advantage of carbonyl phenomena, and his work might serve as a model for the biosynthetic route. However, by analogy to the well-investigated squalene cases, proton-initiated cyclization of a simple geraniol derivative retaining two H-atoms at C-1 is probably the best speculative origin at the moment. Experiments by Battersby and his associates (8) with *Vinca rosea* plants have demonstrated that the single H atom at the glucosidic position in loganin (the methyl ester of loganic acid) is indeed derived from the H atom of C-1 of geraniol (Scheme 8.6). The H atoms at positions 2 and 6 are also retained. Loganin and its closely related precursors and metabolites are involved in the biosynthesis of many alkaloids, e.g., reserpine and quinine (Section C).

2. Stereochemistry

From a biochemical point of view, the most interesting stereochemical feature of the I_2 compounds is the fact that both enantiomeric forms of many of the representatives exist. This is in contrast to the high degree of stereospecificity that attends the biosynthesis and metabolism of amino acids, carbohydrates, steroids, etc., which usually are found in only one of the two possible optical configurations.

Among the I_2 compounds that occur as the (+) form in certain species and as the enantiomeric (−) form in others (11) are α-phellandrene, β-phellandrene, limonene, α-carene, sabinene, α-pinene, β-pinene, camphene, terpinenol-4, α-terpineol, fenchol, perilla alcohol, sobrerol, borneol, menthone, isomenthone, piperitone, carvone, fenchone, camphor, citronellal, perilla aldehyde, phellandral, and citronelloic acid. In addition, the following compounds occur in certain species as the racemic mixture: limonene, α-terpineol, fenchol, sobrerol, carvone, camphor, and citronelloic acid.

The absolute configuration of some of the I_2 compounds has been determined (45). Pertinent ones are shown in Schemes 8.6 and 8.7, which are derived in part from the work of Fredga, who correlated (−)-methylsuccinic acid with L-glyceraldehyde, and from the work of other investigators who carried out various interconversions among the I_2 compounds and correlated them with methylsuccinic acid. For example, (+)-pulegone has been converted both to (−)-menthone and to D-(+)-methylsuccinic acid, and (+)-limonene has been converted through (−)-carvone to (−)-menthone.

The absolute configurations and various signs of rotation of I_2 compounds considered together with the metabolic pathways which theoretically operate would require that a given tissue which biosynthesizes a given compound and then converts it to another one should yield the product with an appropriate sign of rotation compared to that of the precursor. Unfortunately, despite much work on isolation, the investigations have not always been done with defined species, the rotations have not always been determined, materials that were present in lower concentrations have rarely been examined, the age of the plant has usually not been recorded, different tissues of the same plant have not necessarily been investigated or were sometimes mixed, etc., and the present data are insufficient to allow a generalization that the predicted stereochemical relationships actually obtain. The difficulty in analyzing the available information is illustrated by the fact that (+)-α-pinene is reported to occur in the exudate (turpentine) from the trunk of many conifers, while the (−)-form has been isolated from the needles. Consequently, to obtain valid comparisons of absolute

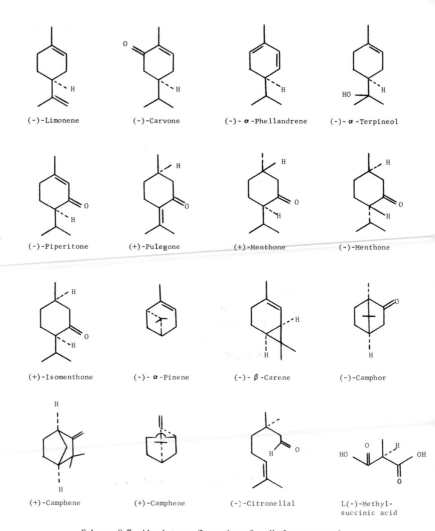

Scheme 8.7. Absolute configuration of cyclic I_2 compounds.

configurations in relation to a sequence of events, one should have, among other things, some knowledge of the site of biosynthesis.

The origin of opposite configurations in many of the cyclic I_2 compounds presumably has to do with the manner in which C-1 attacks the double bond at C-6. Thus, attack from the rear would lead to (+)-limonene and attack from the front would give (−)-limonene (Scheme 8.8), if a pseudo-chair conformation is involved. A boat form would invert the configuration as discussed in greater detail with the carotenoids (Section E.3). The control of the stereochemistry obviously resides in the asymmetry of

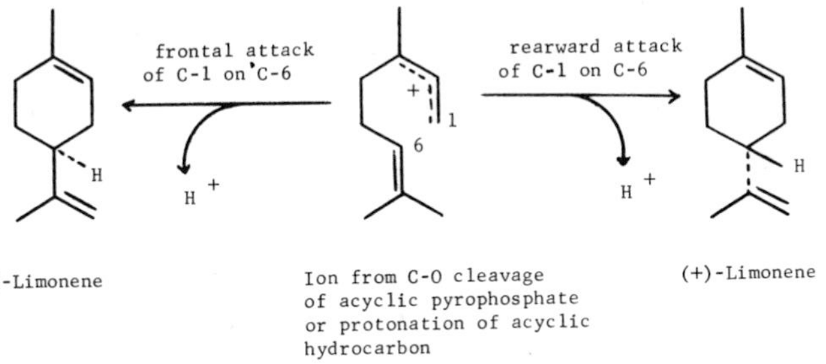

frontal attack
of C-1 on C-6

rearward attack
of C-1 on C-6

6
1

(-)-Limonene

Ion from C-O cleavage
of acyclic pyrophosphate
or protonation of acyclic
hydrocarbon

(+)-Limonene

Scheme 8.8. Stereochemistry of cyclization, assuming a conformation approximating the chair-form of the incipient ring (enantiomeric configurations would result from the boat-form).

the enzyme that catalyzes the cyclization. Such enzymatic control of the stereochemistry presumably also accounts for the formation of one or both of the epimeric *cis*- and *trans*-terpins (3-hydroxy-α-terpineol), both of which are natural. However, there is an alternative explanation, viz., that the *cis*-isomer results from linaloyl pyrophosphate through the intermediacy of the cyclic phosphate diester and that the *trans*-isomer is a consequence of a 1,2-diaxial addition of water to C-2 and C-3 of α-terpineol, which probably exists preferentially in the conformation with the isopropenyl group equatorially oriented. The two diastereoisomeric *cis*- and *trans*-forms of borneol are also natural. The isomer with the hydroxyl group *trans*-oriented to the bridge is borneol itself and the one with the hydroxyl group *cis*-oriented to the bridge is known as isoborneol (Scheme 8.9). Conforma-

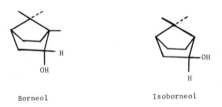

Borneol   Isoborneol

Scheme 8.9. Stereochemistry of borneol.

tional considerations reveal that in the *trans*-case (borneol) the hydroxyl group must be axially oriented to a boat form of the six-membered ring containing carbon atoms numbers 1–6, and borneol is then presumably the product formed initially by cyclization, because we would expect HO⁻ to be added in an axial *trans*-fashion when C-7 attacks C-3. This would suggest that isoborneol is a product either of equilibration or of stereo-specific reduction of camphor (Scheme 8.7). Similarly, menthol exists in two forms, menthol itself with the hydroxyl group *cis*-oriented to the isopropyl group and neomenthol in which the hydroxyl group is *trans*-oriented, and stereospecific reduction of the corresponding ketone may again be responsible for one or both of the epimers.

3. Metabolism of Cyclized I₂ Compounds

A very large number of substances are known that, based on their structures, must be derived by further metabolism of the initial cyclized I_2 compound(s). Simple examples are 1-methyl-4-isopropenylbenzene (*p*-cymene), 1-methyl-4-isopropylbenzene, 1-methyl-2-hydroxy-4-isopropylbenzene (carvacrol), and 1-methyl-2,3-oxido-3-oxo-4-isopropylidenecyclohexane (piperitenone oxide), which almost certainly are metabolites of limonene, terpinolene, or a related isomer. While these and many other of the simpler cases have not been the subject of biochemical study, the metabolism of piperitenone shown in Scheme 8.10 for the six-membered ring series has been demonstrated by Loomis and others (2). The existence of piperitenone strongly suggests that it arises from terpinolene by allylic hydroxylation fol-

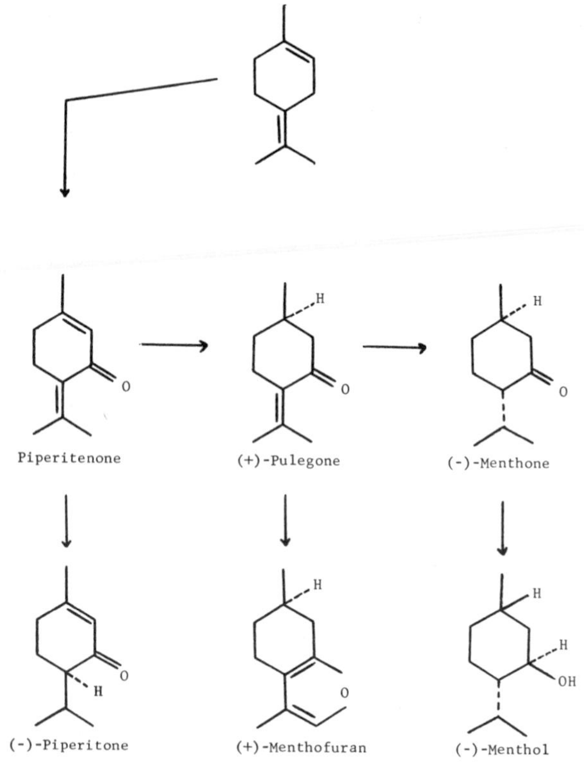

Scheme 8.10. Metabolism of piperitenone in peppermint plants.

lowed by pyridine nucleotide oxidation to the ketone. Its further metabolism to pulegone, menthone, and menthol presumably occurs by sequential reductions with NADH or NADPH. An allylic hydroxylation and oxidation also is the probable origin of carvone (from limonene, Scheme 8.11). This

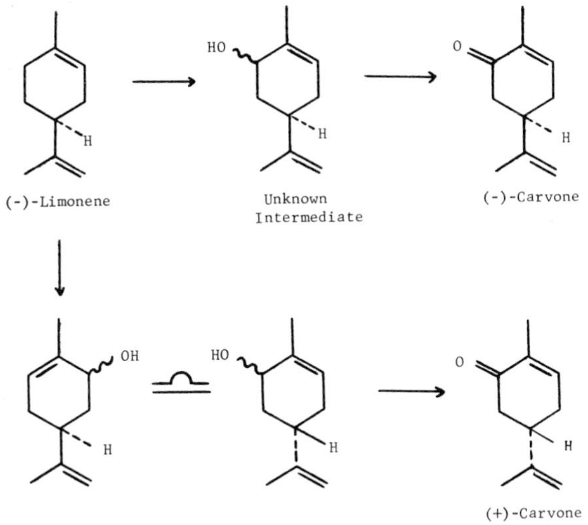

(-)-Limonene   Unknown   (-)-Carvone
                   Intermediate

(+)-Carvone

Scheme 8.11. Comparison of routes from limonene to carvone illustrating retention of configuration by allylic hydroxylation and inversion by attack on the double bond. (−)-Limonene and (−)-carvone occur in *Eucalyptus* species, while (+)-limonene and (+)-carvone are found in *Carum carvi*.

is supported by the fact that the absolute configurations of limonene and carvone are identical in the same plant. If hydroxylative attack had occurred on the double bond, the configurations would be inverted. Iridodiol (Scheme 8.6) may also be derived by allylic hydroxylation followed by reduction. Similarly, dolichodial is probably derived by pyridine nucleotide oxidation of the intermediate unsaturated diol, and allylic hydroxylations and pyridine nucleotide oxidations and reductions are presumably involved in the biosynthesis of loganin in a manner such as that shown in Scheme 8.12.

Considerable interest has surrounded the series bearing a five-membered ring, since many alkaloids with potent pharmacological characteristics possess a C_{10}-moiety, which is now known to be derived from the cyclopentano I_2 compounds. Battersby, who has recently reviewed (8) the work in his and other laboratories, has been especially active in this field. There can now be no doubt that loganin plays a key role as an intermediate by undergoing a cleavage between C-3 and C-4 and condensing with amino acid metabolites. This was first suggested by Thomas (46) and Wenkert (47) and has been fully documented (8). Thus, as shown in Scheme 8.13, loganin serves as the precursor of secologanin, sweroside, and gentiopicroside

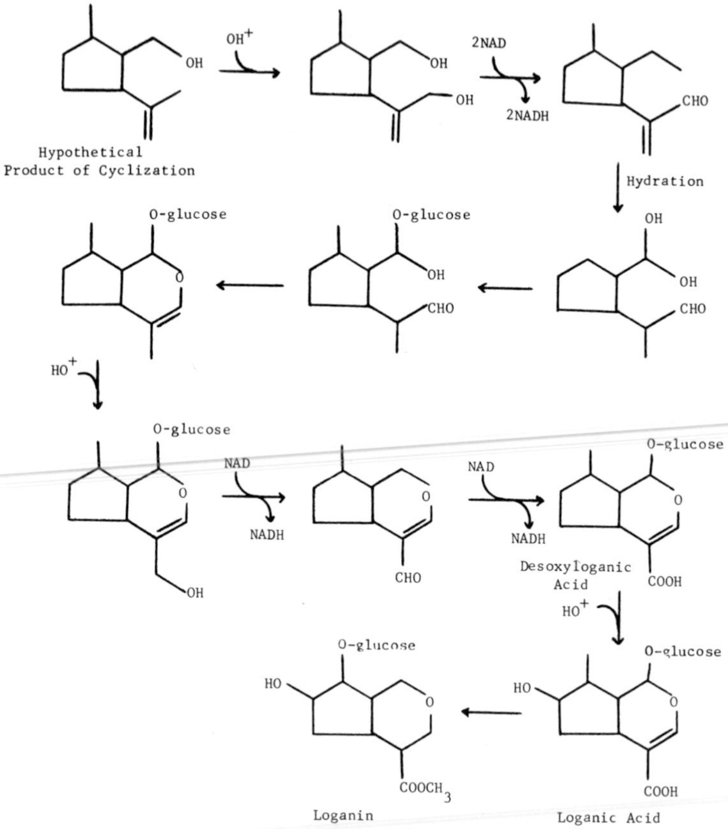

Scheme 8.12. Hypothetical origin of loganin.

as well as of alkaloids, among which are reserpine, quinine, serpentine, ajmalicine, perivine, and strychnine.

C. CYCLIZATION AT THE I₃ STAGE

1. Mechanism and Oxidative Metabolism

A group of cyclic I_3 compounds that have structures quite similar to the cyclic I_2 compounds are clearly present in nature (11, 12). At the I_3 stage the compounds are presumably derived from nerolidyl pyrophosphate or from the isomers of farnesyl pyrophosphate. We can imagine the existence of an intermediate cation (the bisabolenyl cation) having a structure analogous to the terpineyl cation. Elimination of a proton from C-6 would lead to an I_3 analog of terpinolene; a hydrocarbon with this skeleton and with the double bonds in precisely the positions expected is found in many plants

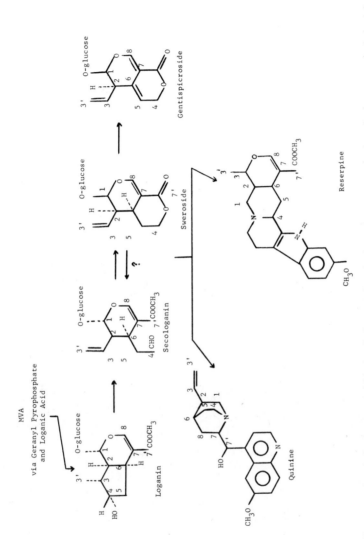

Scheme 8.13. Some experimentally documented biochemical conversions in the cyclopentano series (numbering system is derived from geraniol and represents theoretical possibilities).

and it is known as γ-bisabolene. Although the analog of limonene has not yet been clearly identified, the analog (bisabolol) of α-terpineol, the analog (γ-curcumene) of α-terpinene, the analog (β-curcumene) of γ-terpinene, and others are known to occur (Scheme 8.14).

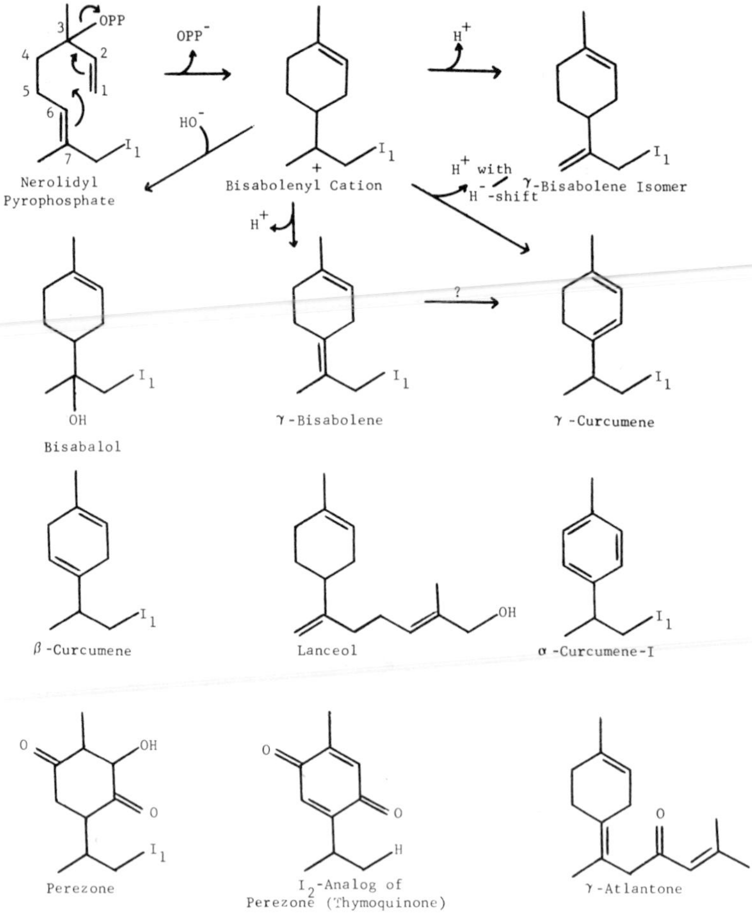

$$I_1 = (CH_3)_2C=CH-CH_2.$$

Scheme 8.14. Naturally occurring monocyclic I_3 compounds and their hypothetical origin.

It must be pointed out, however, that the origin of the monocyclic I_3 compounds cannot be assumed definitely to be directly from an acyclic I_3 precursor. It is theoretically possible that γ-bisabolene, for instance, is derived by isopentenylation of limonene, i.e., the sequence could be dimerization-cyclization-trimerization rather than trimerization-cyclization. This might account for the apparently wider occurrence of γ-bisabolene than of its isomer, since the conversion of limonene to γ-bisabolene could occur in a concerted process while the conversion of an acyclic precursor directly to γ-bisabolene would require a less probable nonconcerted process. It is also possible that, if an acyclic I_3-pyrophosphate is the precursor, then the primary product is bisabolol and γ-bisabolene is its metabolite. This too would account for the very wide occurrence of γ-bisabolene in comparison to its isomer. Unfortunately, no biochemical evidence is available on these important details, but there can be no doubt that the essence of the route shown in Scheme 8.14 is at least chemically reasonable, because Ruzicka and Capato (48) have been able to cyclize nerolidol to bisabolol by acid catalysis.

Just as further metabolism of the cyclic I_2 compounds is evident in various naturally occurring oxygenated derivatives, so there appears to be analogous metabolism at the I_3 stage. For instance, lanceol appears to have arisen by allylic hydroxylation of the I_3 analog of limonene. Several I_3-ketones are known, e.g., γ-atlantone which could have arisen by allylic hydroxylation, e.g., of bisabolene in the case at hand, followed by pyridine nucleotide dehydrogenation of the carbinol group. Allylic hydroxylation followed by dehydration (or direct dehydrogenation) of one of the dienes, however, probably accounts for the occurrence of α-curcumene-I, which is the I_3 analog of p-cymene, and a very considerable oxidation at the I_3 stage is obvious in perezone, which also has an analogy at the I_2 stage (thymoquinone).

A second type of monocyclic I_3 analog, the plant growth regulator abscisic acid, has a structure reminiscent of the ionone rings of the carotenoids. Labeled phytoene, however, is not a precursor (49). Analogous to carotenoid ionone ring formation (Section E.2), an enzyme-assisted cyclization of an I_3 precursor can be envisioned (Scheme 8.15). After formation of the ionone-type ring 1′,2′-epoxidation presumably occurs via a mixed function oxidase yielding an epoxide having the configuration shown in Scheme 8.15. This epimer, but not the opposite 1′,2′-epimer, is the precursor of abscisic acid in tomato shoots (50). An overall trans-elimination occurs during formation of the $\Delta^{4,5}$-bond (51). Hydroxylation and ketonization at C-4′ accompanied by epoxide cleavage and $\Delta^{2′,3′}$-bond introduction completes the biosynthesis of abscisic acid.

2. Metabolism to Bi- and Tricyclic Products

The bicyclic I_3 analogs of such I_2 compounds as borneol, the pinenes, and the carenes are unknown. This may result from steric hindrance of the extra I_1 group. On the other hand, there are known a number of bi- and tricyclic I_3 compounds that can have no analogies at the I_2 stage. At the

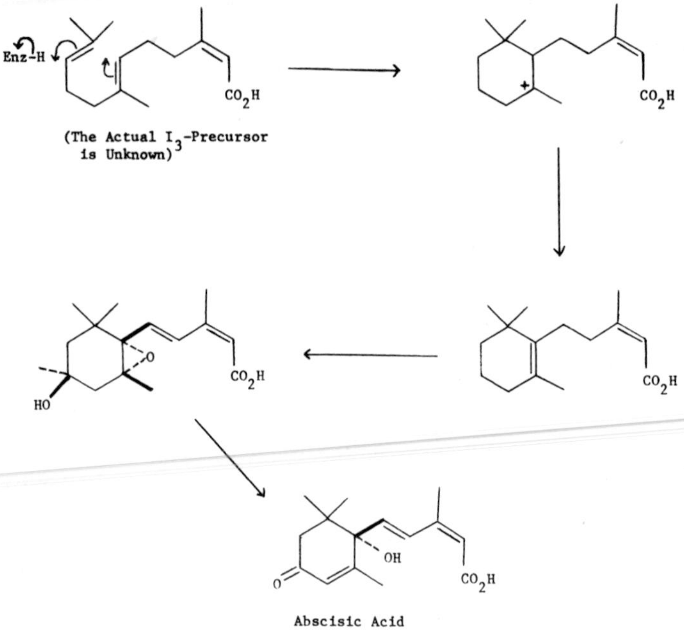

(The Actual I_3-Precursor is Unknown)

Abscisic Acid

Scheme 8.15. Possible mechanism for the cyclization of an I_3 precursor during abscisic acid biosynthesis.

I_3 stage, sufficient carbon atoms are available to form two six-membered rings fused together, as in naphthalene. Thus, the monocyclic β-curcumene can assume the conformation shown in Scheme 8.16. Protonation of the double bond in the terminal isopropylidene group could initiate a cyclization (process b) leading to the formal carbonium ion (cadinyl cation) which, upon elimination of a proton, would yield conjugated and unconjugated dienes. Neither of these dienes has yet been encountered, but closely related compounds are. If deprotonation or HO addition to the cadinyl cation occurred with an H shift, α-cadinene or β-cadinol would result. Both occur naturally (11). In fact, α-cadinene is the most widely distributed of the I_3 compounds. Unfortunately, biosynthetic data are lacking.

An alternative to protonation of the isopropylidene group of β-curcumene is protonation of one of the double bonds in the ring (process c in Scheme 8.16). The latter process could also lead to closure of a new ring in the same way as process a does, except that a double bond would appear exocyclic instead of endocyclic with respect to the new ring. There are several possible products that could arise from the ion (kiganyl cation). They include kiganene and kiganol. The natural occurrence (12) of the tricyclic cedrol and related hydrocarbons (the cedrenes) is consistent either with their being metabolites of bisabolene, as shown by process a in Scheme 8.16,

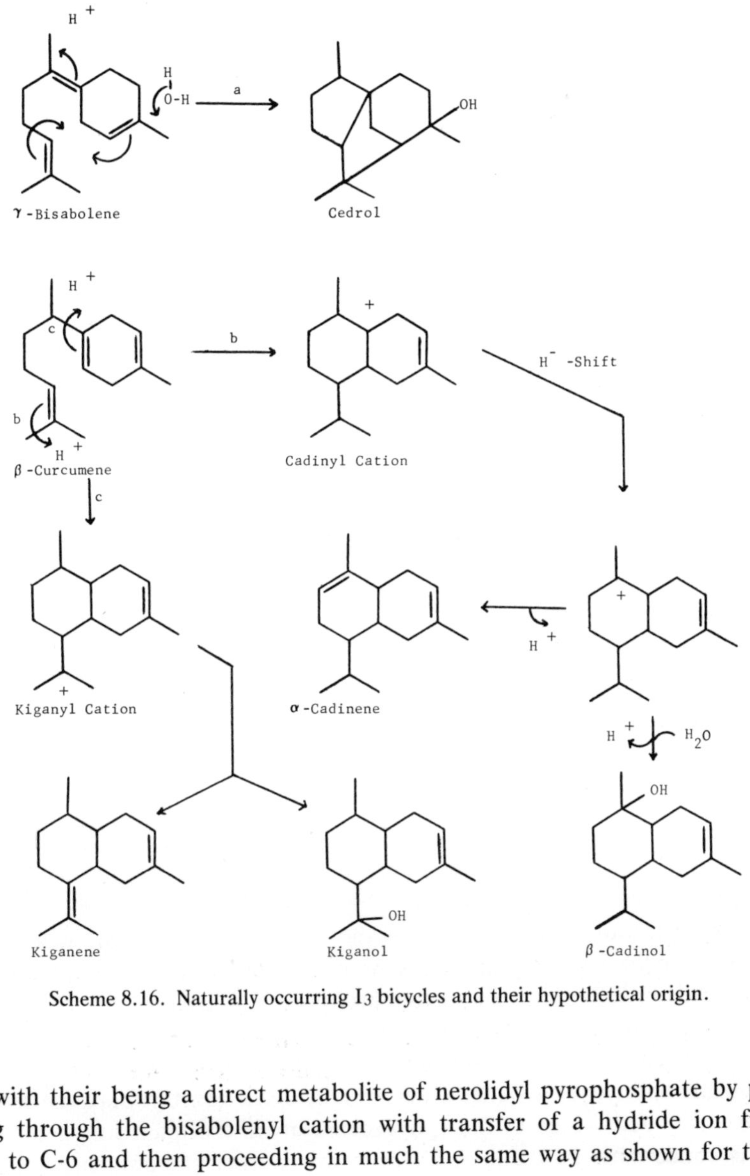

Scheme 8.16. Naturally occurring I₃ bicycles and their hypothetical origin.

or with their being a direct metabolite of nerolidyl pyrophosphate by passing through the bisabolenyl cation with transfer of a hydride ion from C-7 to C-6 and then proceeding in much the same way as shown for their origin in bisabolene.

In addition to cyclization of an acyclic I₃-pyrophosphate along the lines just discussed, several alternatives are possible. One of these is shown in Scheme 8.17, in which a formal ion is derived from either farnesyl pyrophosphate or from nerolidyl pyrophosphate by C—O cleavage. Attack of C-1 on C-11 would lead to closure of an 11-membered ring. Stabilization of the intermediate ion (humulenyl cation) by elimination of a proton would

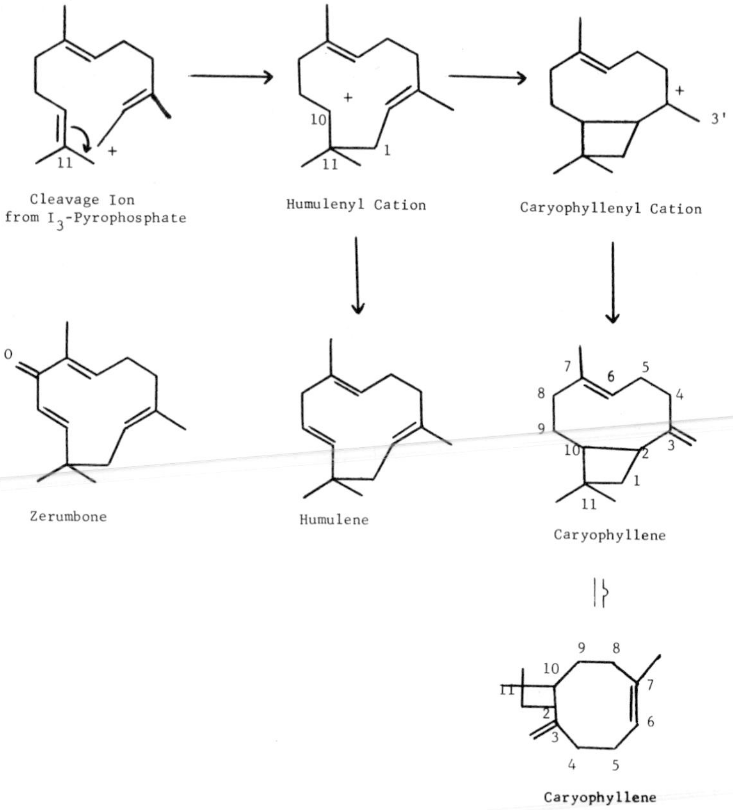

Scheme 8.17. Probable origin of macrocycles.

lead to a substance that has one of the structures compatible with other evidence for the naturally occurring humulene; alternatively elimination of a proton from C-3′, i.e., the methyl group on C-3, would lead to an additional ring closure between C-10 and C-2. The product has the structure that has been elegantly proved for the naturally occurring caryophyllene. Humulene and caryophyllene, which usually occur together, are the second most widely distributed of the I₃-hydrocarbons in the plant kingdom. One of the conceivable products of allylic hydroxylation of humulene followed by dehydrogenation of the carbinol group is a compound that probably represents the naturally occurring zerumbone.

Theoretically, another alternative for the cyclization of an acyclic I₃-pyrophosphate, e.g., nerolidyl pyrophosphate, is by attack at C-10 with elimination of a proton to give a hydrocarbon with a 10-membered ring (Scheme 8.18). This has not been encountered, but several of its apparent metabolites are known to be natural. If we imagine an additional ring

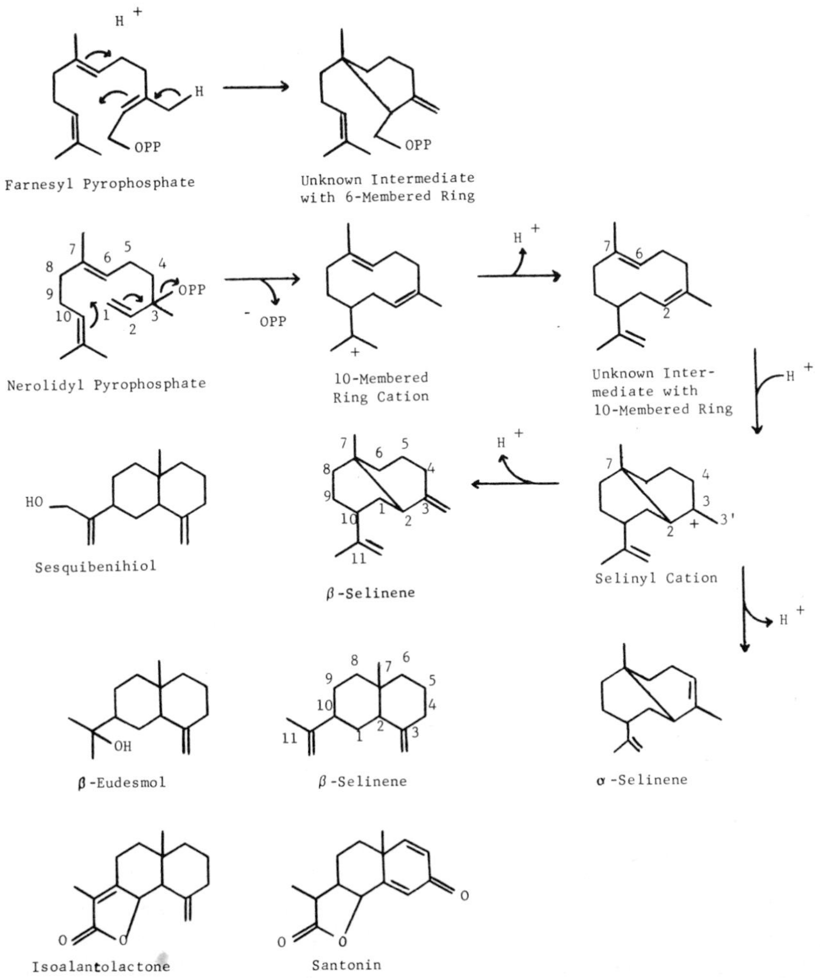

Farnesyl Pyrophosphate

Unknown Intermediate
with 6-Membered Ring

Nerolidyl Pyrophosphate

10-Membered
Ring Cation

Unknown Inter-
mediate with
10-Membered Ring

Sesquibenihiol

β-Selinene

Selinyl Cation

β-Eudesmol

β-Selinene

α-Selinene

Isoalantolactone

Santonin

Scheme 8.18. Reasonable origin of selinyl ring system.

closure between C-7 and C-2 by attack of a proton at C-7 to give a tertiary
carbonium ion (selinyl cation), elimination of a proton at C-4 or C-3′ leads,
respectively, to α-selinene and β-selinene, both of which are metabolites of
certain plants. The selinenes could conceivably also arise by a reverse sequence of events, i.e., through the unknown compound with a six-membered ring by attack of a proton at C-6 followed by closure of the second
six-membered ring by elimination of the pyrophosphate ion, but in this reverse sequence farnesyl pyrophosphate would probably have to be the precursor. It must be pointed out that a conceivable precursor also is α-farnesene
or β-farnesene (I_3-hydrocarbons analogous to ocimene and myrcene at the

I_2 stage), which could serve in a process analogous to that from nerolidyl pyrophosphate. Direct biosynthetic experimentation will have to be done before these questions can be settled, but initiation of the cyclization by elimination of the pyrophosphate ion followed by collapse of the 10-membered ring into the bicyclic system seems tentatively to be the more favored sequence from an energetic standpoint.

The selinenes are presumably subject to additional metabolism by hydroxylation, etc., in the same way as is apparent in other isopentenoids. Thus, we find naturally occurring the compound (β-eudesmol) corresponding to "hydration" of the Δ^{11}-bond either of β-selinene or of one of its precursors. Similarly, the analog (α-eudesmol) corresponding to α-selinene is known and the naturally occurring sesquibenihiol seems to have been derived by allylic hydroxylation. More highly oxidized derivatives of the selinenes are represented by isoalantolactone, santonin, and others. It is worthy of note that both oxygen functions in isoalantolactone are allylic, and all three of the oxygen functions in santonin could reasonably have been derived by an allylic process followed by loss of the bond in the five-membered ring through reduction in the α,β-position to the carbonyl group and introduction of one in the six-membered ring by dehydrogenation in the α,β-position (C-5,C-6) to the carbonyl group.

There remains a final way in which an acyclic I_3-pyrophosphate could cyclize, viz., by proceeding to the 10-membered ring cation as shown in Scheme 8.18 followed by elimination of a proton at C-10 to give the macrocycle shown in Scheme 8.19. This unknown macrocycle would have two alternatives for protonation with closure of a new ring. Protonation at C-3 (process a) could lead to ring closure and the intermediate formation of the tertiary carbonium ion (isoguajenyl cation). Alternatively, protonation at C-7 (process b) would lead through the tertiary carbonium ion (guajenyl cation) to the hydrocarbon that has the structure of δ-guajene-I. δ-Guajene-I and δ-guajene-II (which possesses a double bond at C-11,12 instead of C-10,11) are believed to be components of a mixture isolable from certain plants, and δ-guajene-II could reasonably be derived by process b proceeding from the presumed precursor of the selinyl cation. Similarly, α-chigadmarene, which is found naturally, may represent the occurrence of process a. Process a also appears to operate as the pathway leading to patchouliol, which is a known metabolite of certain plants and is in some respects an I_3 analog of the pinenes. The compounds shown in Scheme 8.19 can be depicted with alternative but equivalent drawings. This is illustrated with the two formulas shown for patchouli alcohol.

The compounds formed theoretically by the processes given should, like other isopentenoids, be subject to further metabolism. This seems to be the case. A number of highly oxygenated compounds exist, and they probably represent, among other things, allylic hydroxylation. Thus, if the Δ^6-bond of the precursor to the chigadmarenyl cation were to migrate

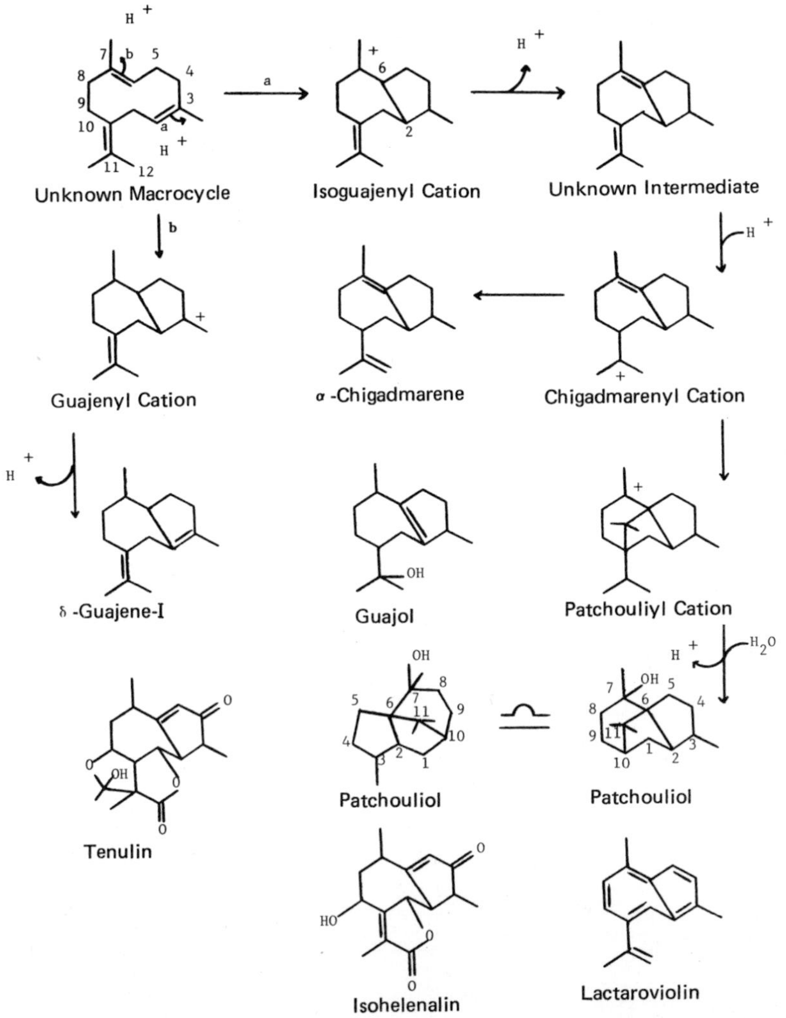

Unknown Macrocycle   Isoguajenyl Cation   Unknown Intermediate

Guajenyl Cation   α -Chigadmarene   Chigadmarenyl Cation

δ -Guajene-I   Guajol   Patchouliyl Cation

Tenulin   Patchouliol   Patchouliol

Isohelenalin   Lactaroviolin

Scheme 8.19. Bicyclic I₂ compounds and their possible origin.

to the 5-position and allylic hydroxylation at C-4, C-1, C-9, and C-12 were
to occur, the tetrahydroxylic derivative would be obtained. Dehydrogenation
of the primary alcoholic group of this derivative to the carboxyl stage,
lactonization, and dehydrogenation of the carbinol group at C-4 would
yield the naturally occurring isohelenalin. Reduction of the double bond
in the α,β position to the lactone-carbonyl group, acylation (by acetyl coenzyme A) in the enolic position (C-11), and hemi-ketal formation would
yield tenulin, which occurs in certain plants. Allylic hydroxylations and
dehydrations (perhaps via phosphorylation) would account for the naturally
occurring azulene, lactaroviolin, and 11,12-dihydro analog (guajazulene).

It is important to emphasize that some of the steps outlined in this section in which protonation is indicated conceivably may not actually occur as such. Instead, the carbonium ions can be derived by shifts of a hydride ion following the initial cleavage of the C—O bond of the pyrophosphate, i.e., the biosynthesis may take a concerted pathway rather than a stepwise one. This has been elegantly discussed by Hendrickson (9), who has carefully considered stereochemical implications, but the details of such problems are outside the scope of this book. Nevertheless, it is important that Hendrickson's analysis led him, as well as Ourisson (52), to predict that the humulenyl cation in Scheme 8.17 possessed the proper characteristics to undergo transfer of a hydride ion from C-1 to C-10 with further rearrangements as shown in Scheme 8.20 to give the naturally occurring longifolene. After the prediction of rearrangement was made, Sandermann and Bruns (53) achieved the biosynthesis of longifolene from carboxyl-labeled acetic acid and showed by degradation that the $=CH_2$

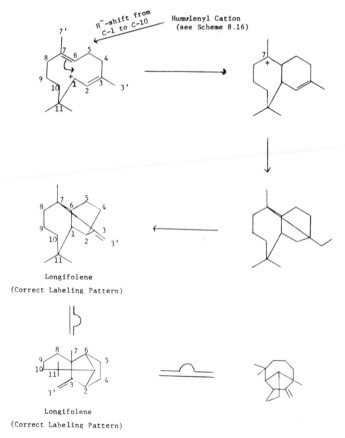

Longifolene
(Correct Labeling Pattern)

Longifolene
(Correct Labeling Pattern)

Scheme 8.20. Reasonable path to longifolene together with experimental labeling pattern.

group was not labeled. Carboxyl-labeled acetic acid would have yielded farnesyl pyrophosphate with C-1 labeled (but not C-3'), and consequently the $=CH_2$ group should be labeled.

3. Cyclization with Methyl Migration

As with squalene oxide, when a carbonium ion is formed and a methyl group is present on an adjacent carbon atom, there is the possibility for migration. It is highly probable that this happens in the biosynthesis of eremophilone. For instance, the formal carbonium ion (eremophilyl cation) is theoretically derivable from the selinyl cation by transfer of a hydride ion (or from a selinene itself with a Δ^2-bond by protonation). Migration of the methyl group from C-7 to C-2 would yield an intermediate, which by allylic hydroxylation and dehydrogenation of the carbinol group would give the observed structure (Scheme 8.21). Migrations of methyl groups appear

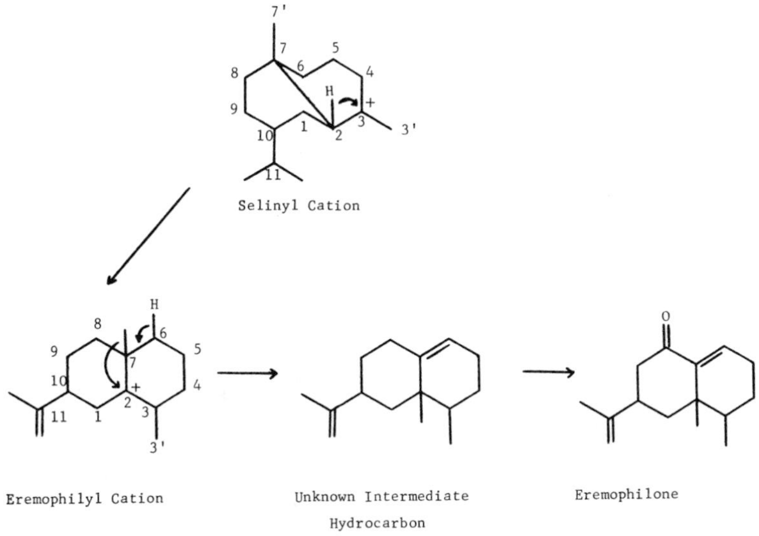

Selinyl Cation

Eremophilyl Cation

Unknown Intermediate
Hydrocarbon

Eremophilone

Scheme 8.21. Probable methyl migration in the biosynthesis of eremophilone.

to be rare at the I₂ and I₃ stages of isopentenoid metabolism, but they are quite common at the I₄ and higher stages, especially in the biosynthesis of steroids.

4. Cyclization with Homoallylic Rearrangements

We have already discussed the allylic rearrangement, e.g., of farnesyl pyrophosphate to nerolidyl pyrophosphate, in which the π-electrons of a double bond migrate to an adjacent position. If, however, the π-electrons migrate so as to form a new bond not with an adjacent carbon atom but with one once removed, a three-membered ring is produced and we speak of the reaction as a homoallylic rearrangement. It will be observed from Scheme 8.22 that the essential character of the two processes is the same, viz., the redistribution of the π-electrons.

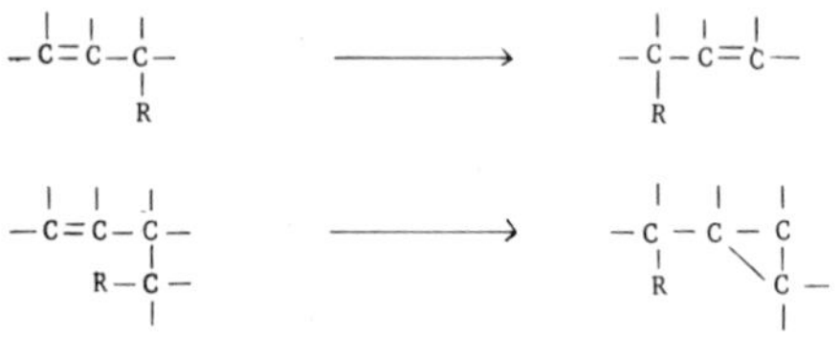

Scheme 8.22. Comparisons of allylic and homoallylic rearrangements.

As a first approximation, both types of rearrangement should be capable of proceeding by electrophilic attack on the original double bond as well as by other means, and acid-catalyzed migration of a double bond is a simple, demonstrable example in nonliving systems. In living systems, migration of double bonds has also been demonstrated, and either a proton is being delivered and one abstracted or, less probably, nucleophilic attack of some sort is aiding the intramolecular migration of a proton. While the acid-catalyzed homoallylic rearrangement has not been demonstrated, other kinds of homoallylic processes are well described, and it seems that under appropriate conditions the homoallylic rearrangements might occur by electrophic attack on the double bond with elimination of a proton. Indeed, there occur several compounds that are best understood biosynthetically by the assumption either of such a reaction or of an analogous one involving free radicals.

Maaliol is an I₃ compound with a structure closely related to the selinenes (Scheme 8.23). It differs importantly from them by the absence of one biosynthetically derived double bond and the presence of a three-membered ring. Two additional differences, the presence of an hydroxyl group, and the absence of a second double bond, are readily accounted for either by hydration or abstraction of an hydroxyl ion (or pyrophosphate ion) during cyclization. The first two differences could empirically be relegated to two unrelated processes, but it is more satisfying to assume that they, like the latter two, have a common origin. The common origin would be homoallylic rearrangement in which a positively charged C-10 (derived during cyclization of a pyrophosphate or afterwards by protonation) attacks C-1. The known stereochemistry of maaliol (54) is compatible with the process; the bicyclic system is *trans*-fused and the isopropyl group is attached to C-10 alpha and axially allowing elimination of the α-equatorial proton from C-1.

A completely similar situation is found with globulol, which is naturally occurring. Chemical investigations of the structure have led to the alterna-

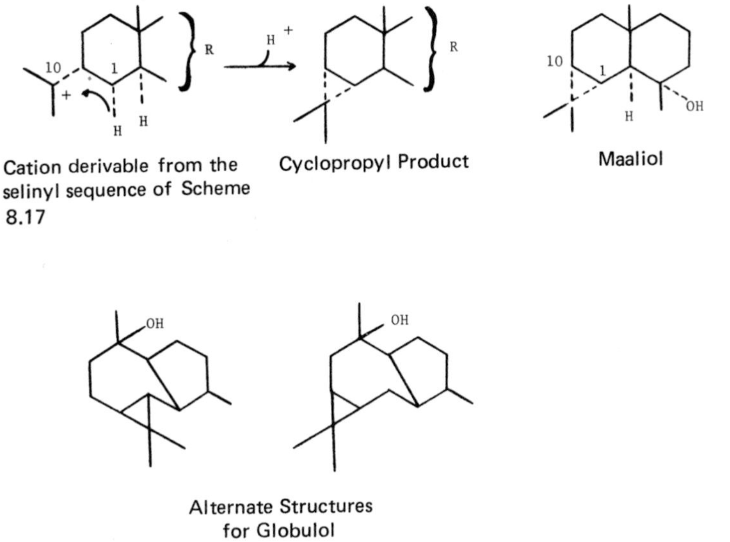

Cation derivable from the   Cyclopropyl Product   Maaliol
selinyl sequence of Scheme
8.17

Alternate Structures
for Globulol

Scheme 8.23. Probable example of homoallylic process in biosynthesis of maaliol.

tives shown in Scheme 8.23. The analog of globulol, lacking an hydroxyl group and with a double bond proceeding from C-7 to the methyl carbon atom (C-7′), is also known (aromadendrene). A variety of other I_3 compounds are known in which a biosynthetically derived double bond is replaced by a three-membered ring; they too may represent homoallylic reaction.

5. Hydroxylative Cyclization

In all the instances considered earlier, ring closure at the I_3 stage has appeared to occur by external attack of a proton (delivered presumably from the enzyme) on carbon or by internal attack of an electrophilic carbon atom; with the exception of the homoallylic reaction (Section C.4), the attack has been on an unsaturated carbon atom. Another way in which ring closure can be brought about is through initial attack of a species acting as if it were OH^+ (oxygenase reaction). The result would be, by analogy to squalene, the introduction of an oxido group that, upon protonation, would undergo cyclization.

A simple example would be the cyclization of farnesyl pyrophosphate; if the oxide assumes the conformation shown in Scheme 8.24 and the cyclase delivers H^+ to the oxygen atom, a concerted shift of electrons would give a bicyclic product. While this compound has not been encountered, its apparent metabolite, iresin, is naturally occurring. It almost certainly has arisen by hydroxylative cyclization, although it is not possible to ascertain

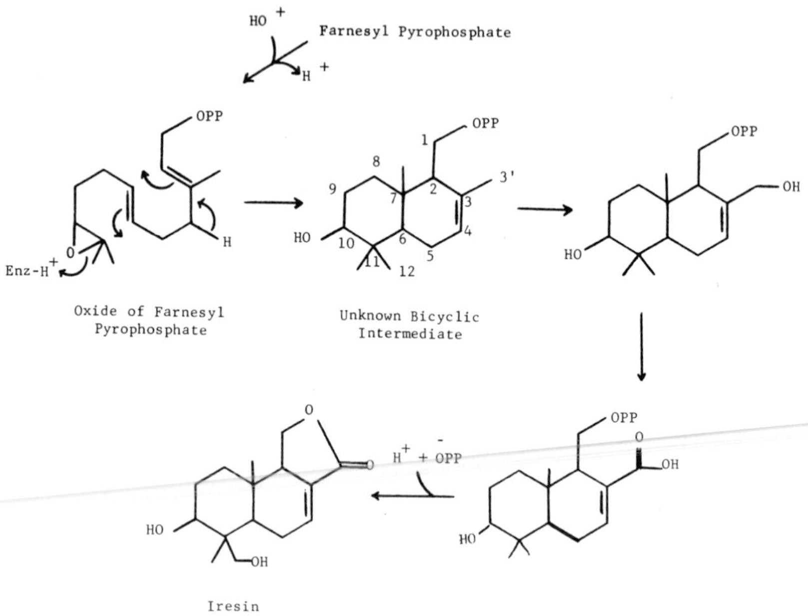

Scheme 8.24. Probable example of oxide intermediate.

with any degree of certainty at what stage the two oxygen functions on the methyl groups are introduced. The sequence of events depicted in Scheme 8.24 seems, however, to be a likely choice. In this sequence, we have invoked an allylic hydroxylation at C-3′ and oxidation of the allylic alcohol to the α,β-unsaturated acid, which is in keeping with the apparent reactions of compounds discussed previously. The introduction of the hydroxyl group onto the nonallylic C-12 is well described in the steroid series.

6. Stereochemistry at the I₃ Stage

Several stereochemical points are of significance biochemically. One of the most important of these is the influence of configuration and conformation on the outcome of a cyclization. This can be illustrated with the relatively simple example of γ-bisabolene. In the first place, one can probably conclude that a pseudo-chair conformation of farnesyl pyrophosphate is not the immediate precursor, because, with a *trans*-double bond in the 2,3-position, C-1 is too far removed from C-6 to allow bond formation unless the ion formed has a half-life considerably longer than would be expected. Usually, carbonium ions, if they are formed at all, do not exist sufficiently long for rotation about a bond to occur, as would be necessary to place C-1 close enough to C-6 for interaction. Farnesyl pyrophosphate could, however, cyclize in a pseudo-boat conformation. A fuller discussion of this is given in Section E.3. Nerolidyl pyrophosphate, on the other hand, can readily assume the proper pseudo-chair conformation (controlled by protein binding) in which C-1 is within bonding distance of C-6. Similarly, the 2,3-*cis*-isomer of farnesyl pyrophosphate could assume a proper conformation.

Experimentally, we do not yet know what the precursor of bisabolene is, but it is interesting to observe that, if nerolidyl pyrophosphate or the *trans-cis*-isomer of farnesyl pyrophosphate were the direct precursor, the γ-bisabolene formed would have a structure in which the acyclic I_1 unit is *cis*-oriented to the endocyclic double bond. Contrariwise, if the *cis-cis*-isomer of farnesyl pyrophosphate or the *cis*-isomer of nerolidyl pyrophosphate were the immediate precursor, the γ-bisabolene formed would have the structure in which the acyclic I_1 unit is *trans*-oriented to the endocyclic double bond. Unfortunately, unambiguous evidence is not available on the stereochemistry of natural bisabolene, and both configurations have been assumed by various authors. Ruzicka (48) has successfully obtained bisabolol by cyclization of nerolidol and has dehydrated it to a bisabolene with various properties identical with the natural substance, but the manner of comparison precludes definite stereochemical conclusions.

A second point of interest biochemically is that, although more work is needed to establish true generalities, there is reason to believe that somewhat more asymmetric induction operates between the enzymes responsible for catalysis of cyclization and further transformation than is so at the I_2 stage. For instance, α-cadinene, which, as mentioned previously, is the most widely distributed of the cyclic I_3 compounds in plants, is found preponderantly in the (−) form. Similarly, caryophyllene and β-selinene have been found exclusively in the (−) forms. Humulene and γ-bisabolene do not possess asymmetry and hence the question does not arise, but most of the other cyclic I_3 compounds that have been isolated have, when rotations were determined, been found to possess only one of the two possible enantiomeric forms. A striking exception is bisabolol, which has been isolated as the (−) form from *Matricaria chamomilla* and as the (+) form from *Populus balsamifera* (11).

The absolute configurations of several of the I_3 compounds have recently been elucidated, and the introduction of optical rotatory dispersion has been of particular value in many cases. (−)-Lanceol, which is the enantiomer so far found naturally, has the absolute configuration (55) shown in Scheme 8.25, which also shows caryophyllene and iresin in their absolute configurations (56).

Two things are of interest to note in the case of iresin, viz., (1) that the hydroxyl group at C-10 is equatorial, as in steroids, etc., but (2) the absolute configuration of rings A and B is enantiomeric to the steroids and other cyclization products of squalene and its oxides. On the other hand, this enantiomeric configuration is the same as that found in the few known I_4 compounds that possess the same type of bicyclic system and that have

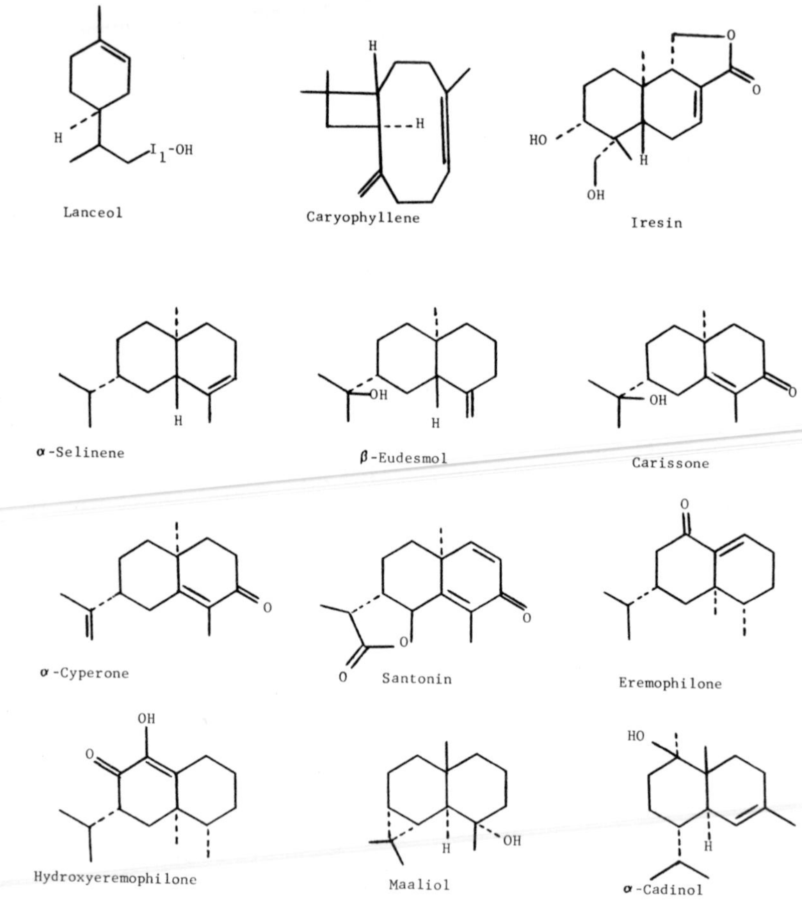

Lanceol

Caryophyllene

Iresin

α-Selinene

β-Eudesmol

Carissone

α-Cyperone

Santonin

Eremophilone

Hydroxyeremophilone

Maaliol

α-Cadinol

Scheme 8.25. Absolute configurations of some natural I₃ compounds.

an oxygen function at the analogous position. Thus, while the full significance of this is not clear, it seems that the stage of isopentenoid complexity can be correlated with the absolute configuration of the products derived by hydroxylative cyclization; one configuration, and one configuration only, is found in both plants and animals at the squalene stage, and this is the reverse of that found at the I₃ and I₄ stages.

The absolute configurations of several of the selinene group of compounds have been determined, and natural α-selinene (54, 55), β-eudesmol (57), carissone (58), α-cyperone (58), and santonin (59) all belong to the same enantiomeric series. Eremophilone and hydroxyeremophilone have also been shown (60) to have absolute configurations in agreement with a metabolic relationship to this series. On the other hand, maaliol (54) not only belongs to the enantiomeric series, but its C-11 is axially attached to

C-10, in contrast to an equatorial attachment in the other members of the selenine group.

The absolute configuration of α-cadinol is known (*61*); from this it can be seen that, like the other decalin-type compounds for which information is available, the two six-membered rings are *trans*-fused.

The absolute configurations of additional I_3 compounds, e.g., longifolene (*62*) and the guaianolide group (*63, 64*), are also known.

D. CYCLIZATION AND METABOLISM AT THE I_4 STAGE

1. Formation of Monocycles

Monocyclic diterpenes constitute only a small percentage of the diterpenes in plants. Several examples of the known types are shown in Scheme 8.26,

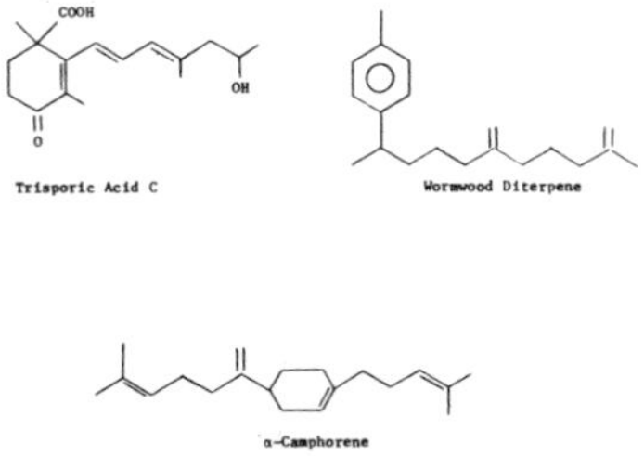

Scheme 8.26. Examples of monocyclic diterpenes containing small rings.

e.g., trisporic acid C (*65*), wormwood diterpene (*66*), and α-camphorene (*67*). Several macrocycles bearing a fourteen-membered ring are known also (*68–71*). They all possess the basic skeleton of cembrene isolated from certain pine species (*69*) and are closely related to the selinyl series (Scheme 8.18). The structure and probable origin of cembrene and its cyclopropyl analog, casbene, through the cembrenyl cation are shown in Scheme 8.27. The compounds have some general interest, because if we cleave C-12 from C-13 and add an I_2 unit to C-16, the proposed structure of casbene (*71*) becomes the cyclopropyl structure of Rilling (*72*) and Popjak (*73*) for presqualenyl pyrophosphate (Chapter 6, Section B.2). Biosynthetically, two I_3 units are replacing one I_4 unit. One can also mechanistically derive the structure of Wasner and Lynen (*74*) for presqualenyl pyrophosphate from the same type of process (Scheme 8.28). Casbene has been obtained from [2-^{14}C]mevalonate and ATP in a soluble system from *Ricinus communis* L. (*71*), and further studies may help elucidate not only its origin but also that of squalene.

2. Bi-, Tri-, and Tetracycle Formation

Cyclic I_4 compounds are quite common in nature (*11, 13, 75*) and their origin is discussed in what follows. If a tetraunsaturated acyclic I_4 alcohol

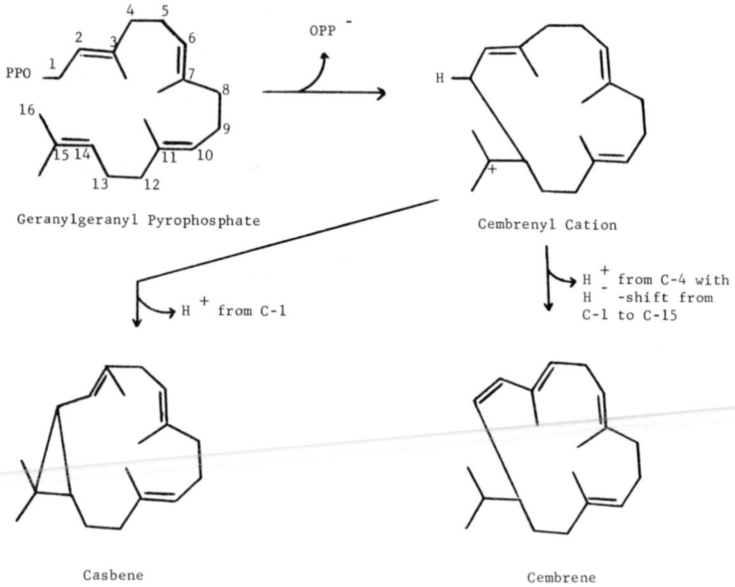

Scheme 8.27. Probable origin of 14-membered macrocycles (geranyllinaloyl pyrophosphate might replace geranylgeranyl pyrophosphate).

or ester, e.g., the I_4 analog of nerolidol (geranyllinalool), were to be bound to an enzyme in the conformation indicated in Scheme 8.29 and if the enzyme delivered a proton to C-14, we can imagine the formal production of a bicyclic carbonium ion (the manoyl cation). This ion, of course, has the implied uncertainties of the others we have discussed. There are several ways in which stabilization can occur. One of these is addition of OH⁻, in which case a diol would be produced. Alternatively, elimination of a proton from C-7' or from the hydroxyl group on C-3 would lead, respectively, to an internal ether or to a diunsaturated compound. All three of these substances are naturally occurring, their names being sclareol, manoyl oxide, and manool, and a pathway either as shown in Scheme 8.29 or one very close to it is clearly operating. There also does not seem to be an inherent reason why geranylgeraniol or its ester could not cyclize, leading to an analog of manool in which the alcoholic group is primary and the double bond is at C-2,3. Indeed, such a process may be represented by agathic acid, which is naturally occurring and might have arisen by cycliza- tion followed by oxidation. Similarly, eperuic acid and labdanolic acid may have arisen by cyclization, oxidation, and then reduction of the double bond in the α,β-position to the carboxyl group, but, as in many other areas of isopentenoid metabolism, detailed biochemical studies are much needed to determine the exact sequence of events. An acyclic I_4 acid, for instance, with double bonds at C-6, C-10, and C-14, could be the direct precursor of

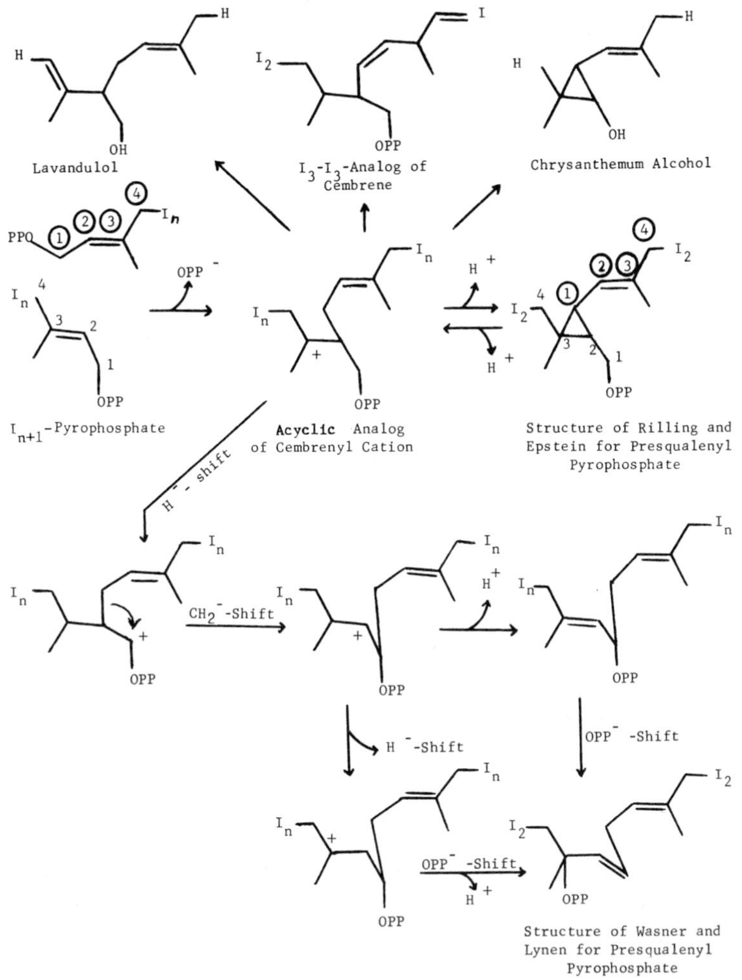

Scheme 8.28. Hypothetical mechanisms relating cembrenyl cation to I_1-I_1- and I_3-I_3-head-to-head dimers.

the bicyclic compounds that possess C-1 oxidized to the acid stage, or, in other words, the bicyclic alcohols and acids may represent a bifurcation in the pathway before rather than after cyclization.

A second group of I_4 compounds, which are tricyclic and appear from their structures to be metabolites of the analogous bicyclic substances, exist in nature. For instance, if manool, or more likely a phosphorylated manool, were to undergo carbon-oxygen cleavage, an ion would be formally produced that, on internal alkylation, would result in closure of a third ring and production of a tricyclic diunsaturated hydrocarbon. Of the three

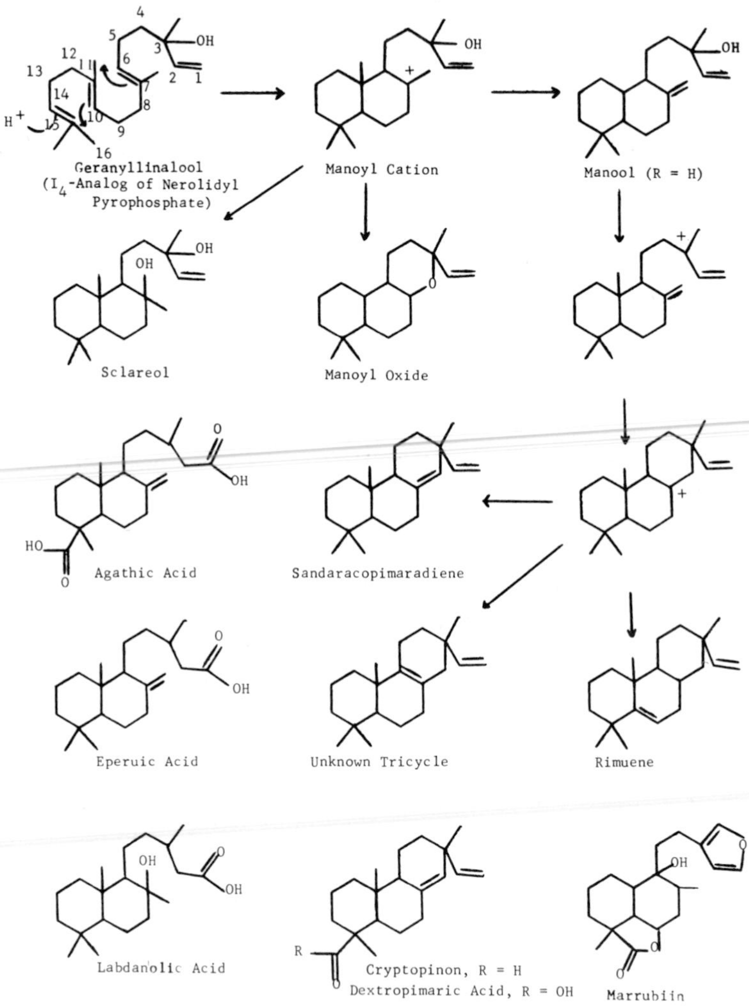

Scheme 8.29. Probable origin of bi- and tricycles at the I₄ stage.

possibilities, one of them, rimuene, is naturally occurring, as are several other compounds, e.g., cryptopinon, dextropimaric acid, and marrubiin, which have the same carbon skeleton and which might be metabolites of the hydrocarbons.

Rimuene by protonation (Scheme 8.30) in the side chain (at C-1) could yield further metabolites. There are two major opportunities for the ion produced (tricyclic ethyl cation) to stabilize itself other than by re-turning to rimuene; these possibilities are addition of OH⁻ and methyl migration. The latter process would be migration of C-3′ to yield the

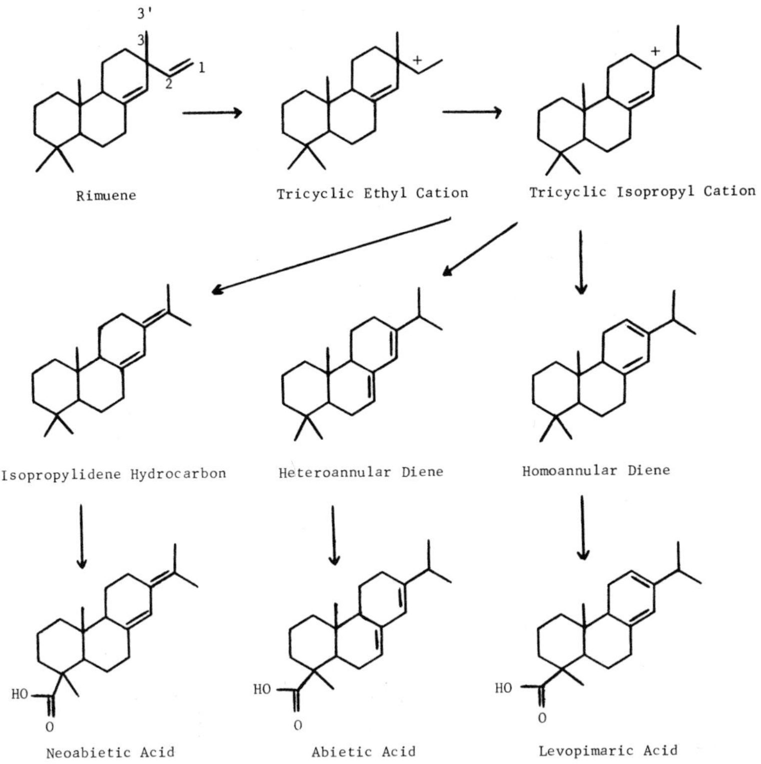

Scheme 8.30. Probable origin of resin acids.

tricyclic isopropyl cation, which now can either add OH⁻ or undergo elimination of a proton at one of three different positions. Of the three possible hydrocarbons that could be produced, all are represented naturally in the corresponding compounds with a *gem*-dimethyl group oxidized to the acid stage (resin acids). Thus, neoabietic acid represents the diene with an isopropylidene group, and levopimaric acid represents the homoannular diene. In addition, abietic acid represents the heteroannular diene, but it is questionable whether abietic acid is really natural. Both neoabietic acid and levopimaric acid are isomerized to abietic acid by acid catalysis, and most (or all?) of the abietic acid that has been isolated is an artifact of one or both of these other two acids. It is, of course, not possible to say at what stage of biosynthesis the *gem*-dimethyl group has been oxidized, and, for instance, an oxidized rimuene rather than rimuene itself may well be the precursor of these acids. Furthermore, it is possible, although it seems less likely, for methyl (C-3′) migration to have occurred before reaching the tricyclic stage rather than afterwards, as shown in Scheme 8.30.

Rimuene should also be amenable to enzymatic protonation at C-7 (Scheme 8.31) instead of at C-1. If protonation at C-7 were to occur, the methyl group (C-3′) could migrate from C-3 to C-7, and an intermediate ion (voucapenyl cation) by stabilization could give a hydrocarbon. A pro-

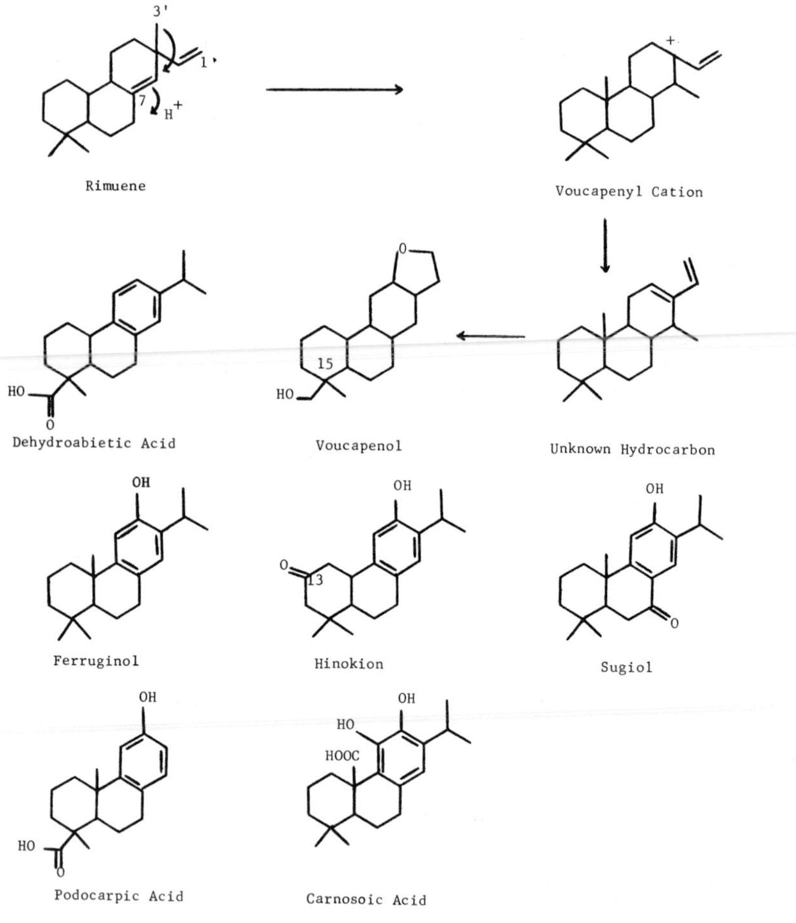

Rimuene

Voucapenyl Cation

Dehydroabietic Acid

Voucapenol

Unknown Hydrocarbon

Ferruginol

Hinokion

Sugiol

Podocarpic Acid

Carnosoic Acid

Scheme 8.31. Apparent metabolites of rimuene.

cess of this sort or one similar to it is presumably represented in the occurrence of voucapenol, which is formally a hydroxyepoxide of the hydrocarbon. The corresponding compound, voucapenic acid, with the primary alcoholic group oxidized to the acid stage, and the C-15 epimer (vinhaticosic acid) of the latter are also natural.

As in the case of other cyclic isopentenoids, aromatization represents a possible metabolic pathway once the rings are formed. Several tricyclic I_4 compounds that are benzenoid are found in plants. Among them are dehydroabietic acid, ferruginol, hinokion, the corresponding alcohol (hinokiol) in which the carbonyl group is reduced, and sugiol. Ferruginol may be an intermediate to carnosoic acid and related quinones (76, 77). Also natural is podocarpic acid, which, however, is missing three carbon atoms. It may be a product of degradation of an I_4 compound, but it might also be a metabolite of an I_3 compound to which two carbons have been added to form ring C.

In addition to the tricyclic I_4 compounds, there are a group of tetracyclic ones, the structures of which indicate that they arise by an extension of the pathways already discussed. A formal ion (prekaurenyl cation, Scheme 8.32) is derivable either directly from the bicyclic system by alkyl-

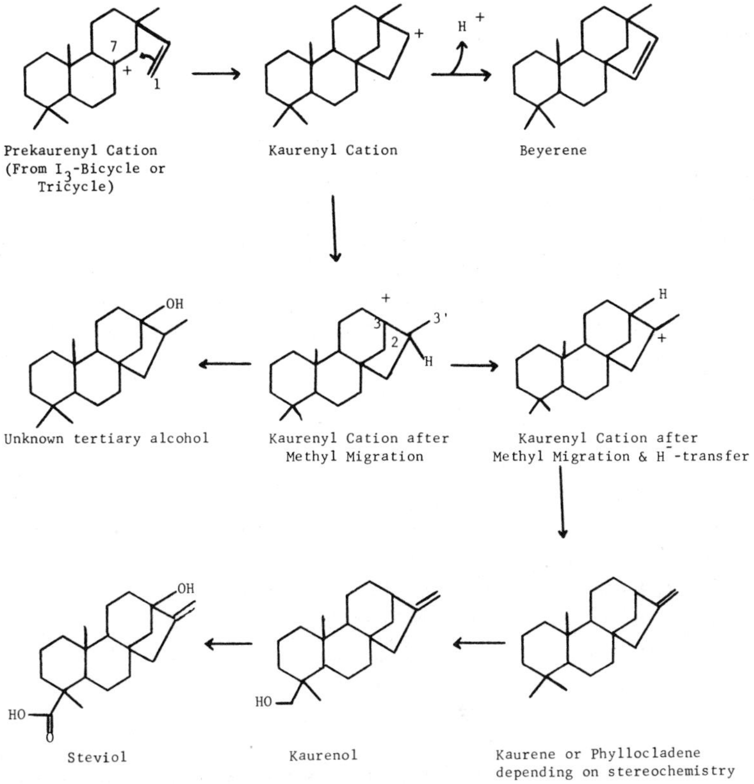

Scheme 8.32. Probable origin of I_4 tetracycles.

oxygen cleavage and ring closure, e.g., from manoyl pyrophosphate, or by protonation of the tricyclic system at C-7', e.g., of rimuene, as shown in Scheme 8.30, but without methyl migration. Closure of a ring from C-7 to C-1 would lead to the kaurenyl cation, which, by elimination, can only give a compound with the structure of the naturally occurring isokaurene or its epimer, isophyllocladene. The kaurenyl cation should also be capable of the migration of a methyl group (C-3'), which would lead to a rearranged ion. This latter ion cannot eliminate a proton directly, because the stereochemistry of the molecule does not allow proper orientation of an sp^2-carbon atom (Bredt's rule). Other alternatives are available, such as addition of OH^- to give a tertiary alcohol or transfer of a hydride ion from C-2 to C-3 and elimination of a proton at C-3; the product of the latter process has the structure of the naturally occurring epimers, kaurene and phyllocladene. The same skeleton is also represented in the naturally occurring steviol (78, 79), presumably derived by oxidation of one of the gem-dimethyl groups at some stage and allylic hydroxylation.

3. Biosynthesis of Gibberellins

The gibberellins are a group of tricyclic I_4 compounds that have attracted wide attention because of their hormonal activity in plants. While their precise physiology remains to be understood, it is known that in both lower and higher plants they regulate many aspects of growth and development (18–20), including the observation of differentiation of flower buds (21). Examination of their structures (Scheme 8.33) reveals a carbon skeleton related to (−)-kaurene. They differ from the latter hydrocarbon, however, in that the angular methyl group between rings A and B has been removed, ring B is five-membered with the sixth carbon atom extruded, and various oxidations have occurred. Three are especially characteristic, viz., hydroxylation in ring A at position 14 of the acyclic precursor, oxidation of two carbon atoms (one of the gem-dimethyl groups on ring A and the C-atom extruded from ring B) to the carboxyl stage, and oxidation of the position lacking the angular methyl group to the alcohol stage. In addition, lactone formation has occurred between the latter and the carboxylic carbon atom on the gem-dimethyl group.

The structural relationship of gibberellins to (−)-kaurene suggests a biosynthetic relationship (80), a suggestion that is supported by the presence of the hormones and the hydrocarbon in the same organism [the molds, Fusarium moniliforme and Gibberella fujikura (81–84), and the photosynthetic plant Echinocystis macrocarpa Greene (85, 86)], by the labeling patterns from [2-^{14}C]mevalonate (84, 87), and by the gibberellin activity of (−)-kaurene and (−)-kaurenol (88, 89). More importantly, (−)-kaurene and (−)-kaurenol biosynthesized from [2-^{14}C]mevalonate in the wild cucumber, Echinocystis macrocarpa Greene, are converted by enzymes from Fusarium moniliforme into gibberellic acid (86, 90), yielding the biosynthetic sequence shown in Scheme 8.33. Steviol (Scheme 8.32) is a possible intermediate following kaurene. It possesses gibberellin activity and has been converted by Fusarium to a substance with the physiological properties of a gibberellin (91), but its place is not yet clear. It must be

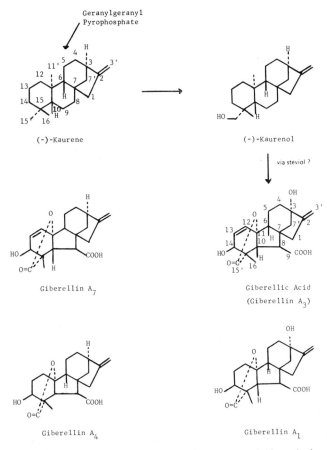

Scheme 8.33. Structures of some gibberellins and demonstrated biosynthetic conversions (numbering system derived from geranylgeranyl pyrophosphate).

pointed out that one could also write a sequence analogous to Schemes 8.29, 8.32, and 8.33 in which hydroxylative ring closure occurs through geranyllinaloyl or geranylgeranyl oxide. The latter compound has been reported in nature (92). Such a sequence would then involve intermediates that are the ring-A-hydroxylated analogs of those shown in Scheme 8.33. Perhaps the demonstration that kaurene, etc., proceeds to gibberellic acid is an artifact of the hydrocarbon's binding to and hydroxylation by the epoxidase. It is also conceivable that one route operates in photosynthetic systems and the other in nonphotosynthetic systems.

The presence of the allylic diol structure in ring A of gibberellic acid may reflect a mechanism of elimination of the angular methyl group analogous to estrogen formation in which the immediate precursor of the desmethyl product is an α,β-unsaturated ketone bearing an aldehydic carbon atom or a carboxyl group at the ring junction. Elimination, respectively, of formic acid or carbon dioxide could then proceed smoothly to give the dienol, which, upon ketonization and allylic hydroxylation before or after reduction of the carbonyl group, would lead to the observed structure (Scheme 8.34). Thus, dihydrogibberellic acid (gibberellin A$_1$) is probably not

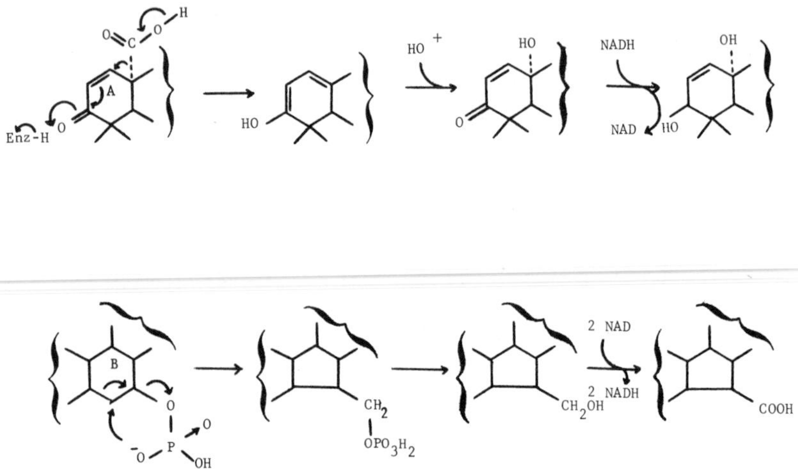

Scheme 8.34. Reasonable mechanisms for changes in the carbon skeleton of (–)-kaurene in proceeding to gibberellins.

a precursor of gibberellic acid. The process of extrusion of a carbon atom in ring B could reasonably occur by hydroxylation, phosphorylation, ring contraction with rearrangement of the phosphoroxy group, hydrolysis to the primary alcohol, and oxidation to the carboxyl group as shown in Scheme 8.34. Driving force for ring contraction is readily discernible in such a series by phosphorylation and elimination of phosphate ion as well as by equilibrium-displacement in the final oxidative steps yielding the carboxyl group.

4. Stereochemistry at the I$_4$ Stage

The great majority of I$_4$ compounds that are presently known have been found to occur in only one of the two enantiomeric forms. However, an example of one that has been isolated in both forms is kaurene, the (–)-enantiomer having been isolated, for instance, from *Agathis australis* (*93*), and the (+)-enantiomer from *Podocarpus ferrugineus* (*94*).

All, or in any event the great majority, of the polycyclic I$_4$ compounds possess a *trans*-fusion of the A/B-decalin system, but these two rings are not always of the same absolute configuration. Indeed, this is most striking in the cases of the otherwise closely related labdanolic acid (*95, 96*) and eperuic acid (*96, 97*), which are antipodal insofar as the juncture of the rings is concerned.

The absolute configurations of additional compounds are shown in Scheme 8.35. For instance, manool (*98*), labdanolic acid (*95*), neoabietic

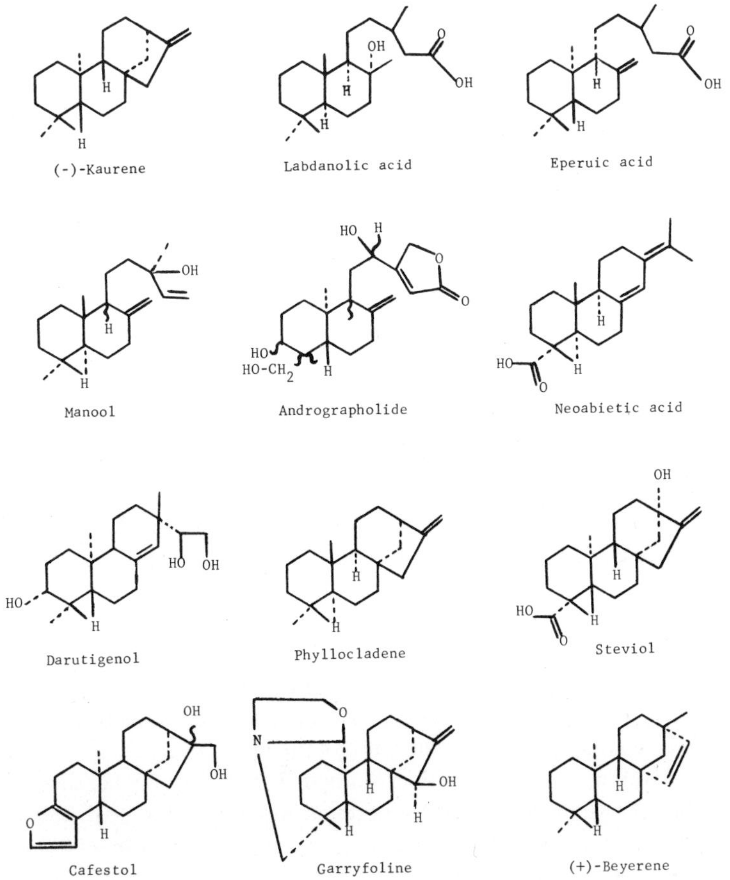

(-)-Kaurene   Labdanolic acid   Eperuic acid

Manool   Andrographolide   Neoabietic acid

Darutigenol   Phyllocladene   Steviol

Cafestol   Garryfoline   (+)-Beyerene

Scheme 8.35. Absolute configurations of some cyclic I₄ compounds.

acid (*99, 100*), phyllocladene (*101, 102*), and (+)-kaurene (*101, 103*) all belong to one series, and eperuic acid (*96, 97*), andrographolide (*104*), darutigenol (*105*), (−)-kaurene (*103, 106*), and steviol (*103*) belong to the enantiomeric series. As a result of various interconversions, it has also been demonstrated that most of the other known I₄ compounds belong to the first of these series in which the methyl group at the ring fusion projects toward the observer. This latter configuration has consequently been referred to as the "normal" one, but the full significance of the apparent biochemical preference for this one remains to be elucidated. It is not the configuration, for instance, of the giberellins.

It is also interesting to observe in this connection that few known compounds at both the I_3 and I_4 stages of biosynthesis that could theoretically have arisen by hydroxylative cyclization and that therefore bear an hydroxyl group possess the absolute configuration of the (−)-kaurene type, in which the angular methyl group (respectively, C-7′ and C-11′) is directed away from the observer. This "generalization" even includes cafestol (107), in which the hydroxyl group has been incorporated into a furan ring. The nitrogen-containing I_4 compounds of the garrya and atisine group, e.g., garryfoline (108), also possess an absolute configuration of the decalin system (positions 6–15) that is the same as that of (−)-kaurene.

It is interesting to note further that (+)-kaurene and phyllocladene, which are epimers at two centers, occur naturally together as a mixture that is separated only with difficulty, and that was formerly known as (+)-mirene (108). In phyllocladene and (+)-kaurene, three (C-6, C-10, and C-11) of the five asymmetric centers have the same absolute configuration and two (C-3 and C-7) have opposite configurations.

In labdanolic and eperuic acids, C-10 and C-11 have opposite absolute configurations, but there is reason to suspect that C-6 has the same absolute configuration in the two compounds, because the corresponding 7-ketones obtained by oxidative removal of C-7′ do not appear to be precise antipodes (96). If C-6 is responsible for this behavior, it means that labdanolic and eperuic acids must possess the same absolute configuration at C-6 but different relative configurations internally, one of them possessing an axial hydrogen atom and the other an equatorial hydrogen atom. The possession of an equatorial hydrogen atom at C-6 is quite unusual when all of the polycyclic isopentenoids are considered, and it seems to be restricted to bicyclic compounds, e.g., the labdanolic-eperuic acid series, although more compounds will have to be examined before a true generalization can be made. The isomerism existing between dextropimaric acid and isodextropimaric acid is an interesting case in point, since arguments have been advanced in favor alternatively of epimerism at C-6 (109) or at C-3 (110). Since the absolute configuration of C-11 and C-15 is believed to be the same in these two acids and of the type found in neoabietic acid, epimerism at C-6 would imply an "antibackbone" in one of them (isodextropimaric acid), while epimerism at C-3 would be consistent with a "normal" backbone.

The relationship of absolute configuration to biological species seems not to offer any obvious generalities. Briggs and his co-workers (106) have called attention to the fact that, while (+)-kaurene co-occurs with I_4 compounds of the same absolute configuration as (+)-kaurene, in at least one species (−)-kaurene co-occurs with agathic acid for which the configuration antipodal to that of (−)-kaurene has been reported (100).

The influence and importance of stereochemistry to the biosynthesis of the polycyclic I_4 compounds has been the subject of much thought and a certain amount of experimentation in model systems. The interested reader should consult Ruzicka (5-7, 111) for additional principles and a key to the literature.

E. CYCLIZATION OF NEUROSPORENE AND LYCOPENE

1. Origin of Acyclic Precursors

The nonreductive coupling of two moles of geranylgeranyl pyrophosphate yields phytoene (112), which is the general precursor (3) of the carotenoid pigments (Schemes 8.36 and 8.37). The biochemistry of these substances

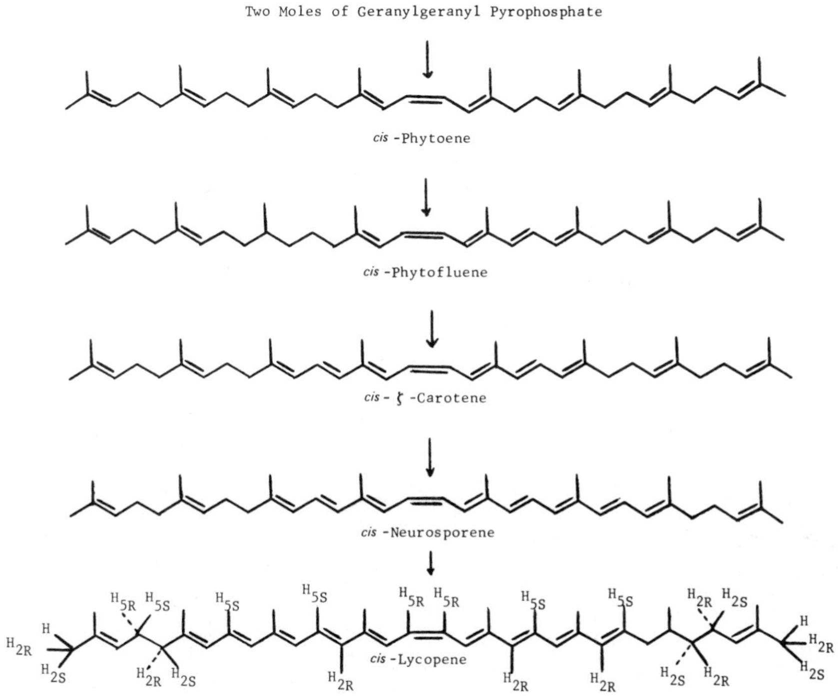

Two Moles of Geranylgeranyl Pyrophosphate

cis-Phytoene

cis-Phytofluene

cis-ζ-Carotene

cis-Neurosporene

cis-Lycopene

Scheme 8.36. Biosynthesis of acyclic carotenoids (origin of H atoms in MVA shown in lycopene).

has been extensively discussed by Goodwin (3). For our present purposes two facts are relevant: (1) many carotenoids possess a six-membered ring at one or both ends of the molecule reminiscent of ambrein (Chapter 7, Section B.10); and (2) cyclization could take place immediately after coupling or at some later stage, i.e., a sequence problem exists. The demonstrated (3) desaturative metabolism of phytoene is shown in Scheme 8.36.

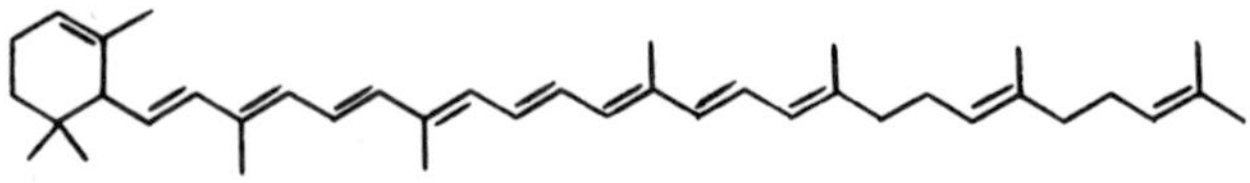

all- *trans* - α -zeacarotene

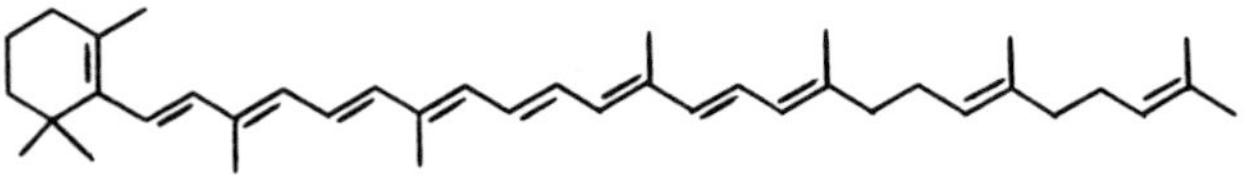

all- *trans* - β -zeacarotene

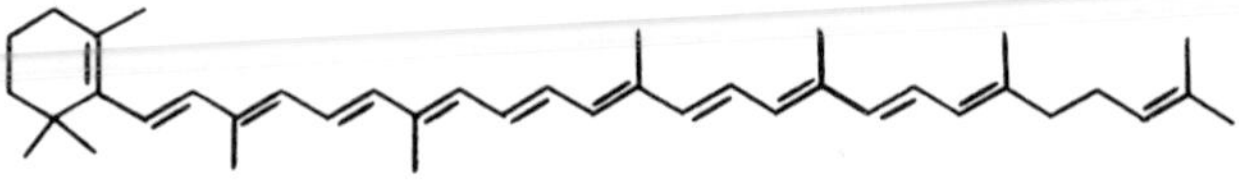

all- *trans* - γ -carotene

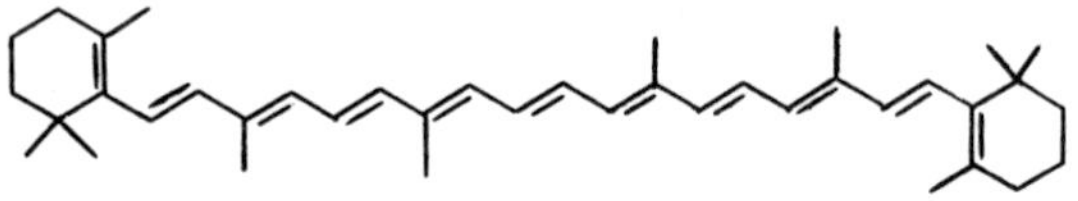

all- *trans* - β -carotene

Scheme 8.37. Structures of some cyclic carotenoids.

Inspection of the structures of phytoene, phytofluene, ζ-carotene, and neurosporene will reveal that at one or both ends of the molecule all possess an I_2 unit of exactly the same sort as in squalene. Consequently, a ring analogous to one of the rings of ambrein or to ring A of tetrahymanol, etc., could be formed. In lycopene the double bond in the second I unit is conjugated with other double bonds which alter its detailed capacity to enter into a ring-forming reaction, but specific sites for protonation-deprotonation on the enzyme could still reasonably induce cyclization. In fact, the present evidence (3) indicates that both neurosporene and lycopene undergo cyclization, while no evidence exists for cyclization before the neurosporene stage of desaturation. Lycopene, the red coloring matter of tomatoes, is the probable precursor, for instance, of β-carotene, which is a widely distributed chloroplastic constituent. Among the experiments that indicate precursor-product relationships and sequencing are the direct conversion of lycopene to cyclic carotenoids in chloroplasts (113–116) and the inhibition of cyclization with nicotine and other substances, which forces neurosporene or lycopene to accumulate in place of β-carotene or other cyclized product (*117–119*).

2. Mechanism

A mechanism similar to the cyclization of squalene can be written in which a proton attacks the terminal double bond of an enzyme-bound conformer of the acyclic molecule with concomitant attack of the π-electrons in the second I unit on the initial positively charged center. This would yield a basic carotenoid cation (Scheme 8.38) that, upon deprotonation at one of

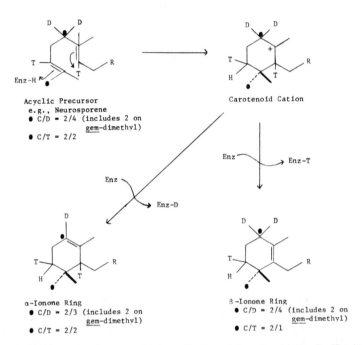

Acyclic Precursor
e.g., Neurosporene
● C/D = 2/4 (includes 2 on gem-dimethyl)
● C/T = 2/2

Carotenoid Cation

Enz ───→ Enz–T

Enz ───→ Enz–D

α-Ionone Ring
● C/D = 2/3 (includes 2 on gem-dimethyl)
● C/T = 2/2

β-Ionone Ring
● C/D = 2/4 (includes 2 on gem-dimethyl)
● C/T = 2/1

Scheme 8.38. Formation of carotenoid rings. R, Remainder of molecule; D, H originating from C-2 of MVA; T, the 4-*pro-R*-H-atom of MVA; ● denotes C atom originating from C-2 of MVA.

the positions adjacent to the positive charge, would yield either the α- or β-ionone ring system. Both of these systems are characteristic of the cyclic products (Scheme 8.37), and the choice of which is produced should depend on the position of a deprotonating group on the enzyme.

Evidence for the essential correctness of the mechanism has been brought forth by Goodwin and his colleagues (*120–122*). Mevalonate labeled at C-2 with ^{14}C and at C-4 or C-2 with tritium has yielded the predicted ^{14}C/^{3}H ratios in the cyclized products. This is shown in Scheme 8.38, where the fate of the H atoms is illustrated in a composite sequence in which D implies an origin in C-2 and T implies one in C-4 of MVA. Since a variety of products has been obtained, only the annular portion of one end of the molecule is shown. Actual values obtained (*120-122*) were as follows. From (4*R*)-[2-¹⁴C, 4-³H]MVA, one ¹⁴C and one ³H atom were introduced in each I unit. Phytoene, with a normalized ¹⁴C/³H ratio of 8:8, was isolated. Lycopene, being acyclic, retained the same ratio, but, in agreement with cyclizative loss of one H atom from each of the annular carbon atoms bearing the acyclic side chain, the ratio was 8:6 in β-carotene, which possesses a β-ionone ring at each end of the molecule. In the analogous α-carotene in which one of the rings has the β-ionone structure and the other has the α-ionone structure, only one of the tritium atoms should be lost. Such was the case. The ratio in α-carotene was 8:7. Similarly, after introduction of two ³H atoms and one ¹⁴C atom into each I unit from [2-¹⁴C, 2-³H₂]MVA, the ratios were 8:16, 8:12, and 8:11 in phytoene, β-carotene, and α-carotene, respectively. These labeling patterns are not only consistent with the proton-initiated mechanism but also prove that the α- and β-ionone rings are each derived directly by cyclization and not by double-bond migration. If the β-ionone ring were derived by isomerization of the α-ionone ring, the former would have to possess one less H atom from C-2 of MVA than is observed. Conversely, if isomerization of the β-ionone to the α-ionone structure occurred, one less H atom from C-4 of MVA should have been incorporated than actually was found.

3. Stereochemistry

There are two major ways in which cyclization could occur, viz., with the carbon atom (C-4, steroid numbering or C-1, carotenoid numbering) bearing the two methyl groups either above ("up conformation") or below ("down conformation") the double bond in the next I unit when the molecule is viewed with the *gem*-dimethyl terminus to the left and toward the bottom of the page as shown in Scheme 8.39. A simple spiral arrangement of the six atoms in the chain will lead in both cases to a conformation approximating the chair-form of the incipient six-membered ring. This conformation and *trans*-reactions then fix all configurations in the products. If the carbon bearing the dimethyl group attacks from above as in the squalene case, then (a) the *trans*-methyl originating in C-2 of MVA must fall away from the observer and become equatorial, (b) elimination of a proton to give the α-ionone ring must be from the axial position below the plane of the ring (which represents the 2-*pro*-S-H-atom of MVA), (c) the configuration at the carbon atom bearing the long side chain must be the same as in position-5 of lanosterol (H atom toward the observer), and (d) elimination of a proton from the carbon atom bearing the side chain to give the β-ionone ring must proceed with the axial proton that points away from the observer and originates in the 4-*pro*-R-H-atom of MVA.

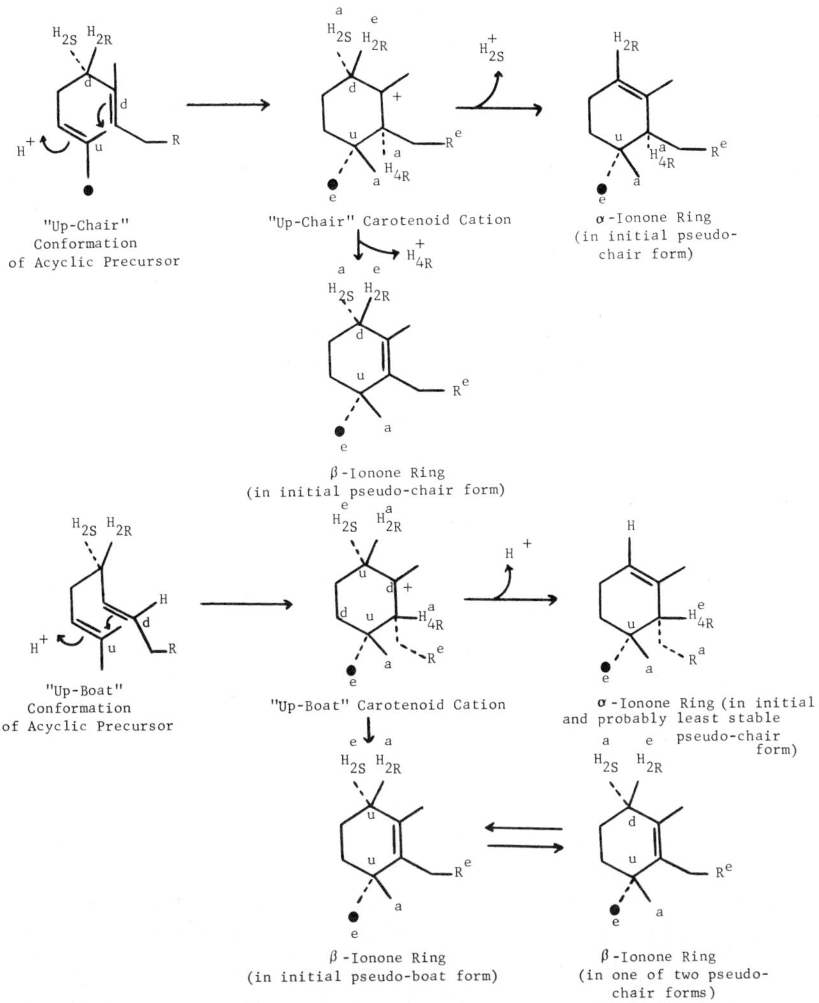

H_{2S} H_{2R}

"Up-Chair"
Conformation
of Acyclic Precursor

H_{2S} H_{2R}

H_{2S}^+

"Up-Chair" Carotenoid Cation

H_{4R}^+

H_{2R}

α-Ionone Ring
(in initial pseudo-
chair form)

H_{2S} H_{2R}

R^e

β-Ionone Ring
(in initial pseudo-chair form)

H_{2S} H_{2R}

"Up-Boat"
Conformation
of Acyclic Precursor

H_{2S} H_{2R}

H^+

"Up-Boat" Carotenoid Cation

H

α-Ionone Ring (in initial
and probably least stable
pseudo-chair
form)

H_{2S} H_{2R}

R^e

β-Ionone Ring
(in initial pseudo-boat form)

H_{2S} H_{2R}

R^e

β-Ionone Ring
(in one of two pseudo-
chair forms)

Scheme 8.39. "Up-chair" and "up-boat" conformations of acyclic presursors and their products of cyclization. R, remainder of molecule, e.g., of neurosporene; u, up; d, down; ●, origin in C-2 of MVA; subscripts refer to *pro*-H atoms of MVA; a, axial; e, equatorial.

A completely enantiomeric condition arises if attack is from below. The methyl bearing C-2 from MVA still becomes the equatorial group but is now on the observer's side, the α-ionone ring arises with elimination of the 2-*pro-R*-H atom from MVA, which is now axial in place of the 2-*pro-S*-atom, and the carbon atom atom bearing the long side chain must possess an axial H atom pointing toward the observer in the α-ionone structure and be eliminated in the β-ionone structure. In both enantiomeric conformations of the acyclic precursor, the proton initiating cyclization must attack axially and become equatorial, on the front side if the terminus of the chain is up and on the back side if the terminus is down. It is worth noting that the carotenoid ring, unlike that in fused polycycles such as steroids, is not rigidly fixed, and can "flip" from one chair-form to the other, which will reverse equatorial and axial characters (but not configurations). However, the direction of attack (from above or below) automatically determines which of the two chair-forms is involved during cyclization, and it is relative to this one that conformations are assigned here. This is also the one that places the large side chain equatorial, and is therefor presumably the more stable.

A subset of conformations is also possible analogous to the condition arising in ring B in the formation of the protosteroid cation (Chapter 7, Section C.3). It is concerned with a conformation resulting from rotation of 180° about the bond joining C-1 to C-10 (steroid numbering) or C-4 to C-5 (carotenoid numbering) as well as smaller rotations about other bonds that then place the two double bonds parallel to each other (Scheme 8.39). Such a conformation approximates the boat-form of the incipient six-membered ring. The 180° rotation involved results in inversion of the configuration produced at the carbon bearing the long side chain. It does not alter the configurational character of the carbon originating in C-2 of mevalonate in the *gem*-dimethyl group, since the terminus of the chain is maintained immobile during the rotations. Although the matter is equivocal, the new conformation probably does reverse the choice for which proton (2-*pro-R*- or 2-*pro-S* of MVA) is removed in forming the α-ionone ring. The resultant of all this is that, in a given series concerned with whether the *gem*-dimethyl terminus is above or below the double bond being attacked, the carbon bearing the side chain in the α-ionone ring has one configuration if derived through the chair-conformation and the opposite configuration if derived through the boat-form. The 2-*pro-S*-H-atom is removed in the first case and may be (depending on the planar character of the cation) the 2-*pro-R*-H-atom in the second, but the labeling of the *gem*-dimethyl group from [2-^{14}C]MVA would be the same in either case.

Obviously, labeling and configurational data can distinguish between the four possible modes of cyclization ("up-chair," "down-chair," "up-boat," and "down-boat"). However, since enantiomeric cyclizations occur among I_2, I_3, and I_4 compounds, it is by no means certain that carotenoid cyclizations will occur in only a single way, and the problem will require investigations of different organisms, etc. These have not yet been done, but preliminary evidence (3) suggests that the 2-*pro-S*-H-atom is removed in Del tomatoes during α-ionone ring formation to give δ-carotene. There are also reasons (3) for believing that the methyl group labeled from [2-^{14}C] MVA in β-carotene is the equatorial one. These two pieces of information would indicate a chair-folding with the terminus up ("up-chair"), as in the cyclization of squalene. Unfortunately, the absolute configuration of the α-ionone ring of α-carotene is reported to be enantiomeric (123) to that expected from the "up-chair" conformation, and a solution to the stereo-chemical problem will have to await further research.

F. ENZYMOLOGY

1. I₂ Stage

No significant studies have yet been made on the cyclase in an enzymological sense, but it is worth noting that soluble plant systems for the biosynthesis of the possible precursors, geraniol and nerol, have been reported (33). It is also of some interest that the pool size of the initial Δ^2- and Δ^3-isopentenyl pyrophosphates is probably not always equal and/or in equilibrium. Thus, the formation of thujone and camphor occurs in some cases with preferential labeling (from [2-¹⁴C]MVA) of the Δ^3-IPP unit (124, 125). Disproportionate labeling at higher stages of polymerization has also been found (126). Occasionally C-2 of MVA is also found to be scrambled (127, 128). Although cyclization at the I₂ level is probably rare in the animal kingdom, it has been reported to occur in the stick insect (*Anisomorpha buprestoides*) from acetate and MVA (129). The product was dolichodial. In addition to studies with CO_2, MVA, etc., in plants, metabolic work of varying degrees of success has been carried out with microorganisms (130–132).

2. I₃ Stage

Enzymology at the I₃ stage is also ill defined. Some biosynthetic work has been done with the molds *Trichothecium roseum* (133), *Ceratocystis timbriata* (134), and *Helminthosporum sativum* (135) and with the gymnosperm *Pinus longifolia* (36), which led to labeling of various cyclic I₃ compounds from [2-¹⁴C]MVA or [1-¹⁴C]acetate. They might then be suitable organisms for further pursuit of enzymology.

3. I₄ Stage

West and his associates have obtained crude enzyme systems from seedlings of *Ricinus communis* (71), seeds of *Echinocystis macrocarpa* (86, 136), and the fungus *Gibberella fujikuroi* (103), which contain cyclases for the formation of (−)-kaurene and other products. Anderson and Moore (137) and Graebe (138) have obtained similar systems from *Pisum sativum*, and Graebe (139) has reported one from *Cucurbita pepo*. Geranylgeranyl pyrophosphate, obtainable in a cell-free system (140a, 140b), serves as precursor (141) in *R. communis* (the castor bean). Partial separation of the various cyclases has been achieved (141), and gel filtration experiments suggest molecular weights of the order of 200,000. Cyclization is stimulated by Mg^{2+} or Mn^{2+}, has an optimal pH range of 7.0–7.2, and is inhibited by sulfhydryl binding agents (141). Plant growth retardants [Amo 1618, 2'-isopropyl-4'-(trimethylammonium chloride)-5-methyl phenyl piperidine-1-

carboxylate, and Phosfon, tributyl-2,4-dichlorobenzylphosphorium chloride, and CCC, β-chloroethyltrimethylammonium chloride] are inhibitory for formation of the tricycles (141). Only phosfon inhibits macrocyclization to give casbene (141). The cyclases were obtained in a soluble condition (supernatant from centrifugation at 78,000 to 105,000 × g) (141).

4. Carotenoid Stage

A cell-free enzyme system from *Phycomyces blakesleeanus* for the formation of phytoene from geranylgeranyl pyrophosphate has been obtained by Chichester and his associates (112), and one has also been obtained from spinach leaves by Porter's group (142) that will convert Δ^3-IPP to phytoene, phytofluene, and lycopene. Geranyllinaloyl pyrophosphate does not appear to be an intermediate (112). Cyclization, presumably of one of the dehydrogenated metabolites, has been achieved in Goodwin's laboratory (120) by the use of slices of ripe tomato fruit and in Porter's laboratory with tomato plastids (143). Disagreement exists on the cofactor requirements for the desaturation and cyclization steps (3, 143, 144).

LITERATURE CITED

1. H. J. Nicholas, *in* P. Bernfeld (ed.), Biogenesis of Natural Products. Pergamon, New York, 1963. p. 829.
2. W. D. Loomis, *in* J. B. Pridham (ed.), Terpenoids in Plants. Academic Press, New York, 1967. p. 59.
3. T. W. Goodwin, *in* O. Isler, H. Gutmann, and U. Solms (eds.), Carotenoids. Birkhauser Verlag, Basel, 1971. p. 577.
4. D. V. Banthorpe and A. Wirtz-Justice, J. Chem. Soc. 541 (1969).
5. L. Ruzicka, Experentia 9:357 (1953).
6. L. Ruzicka, Proc. Chem. Soc. (London) 341 (1959).
7. L. Ruzicka, Pure Appl. Chem. 6:493 (1963).
8. A. R. Battersby, *in* T. W. Goodwin (ed.), Natural Substances Formed Biologically from Mevalonic Acid. Academic Press, New York, 1970. p. 157.
9. L. B. Hendrickson, Tetrahedron 7:82 (1959).
10. J. H. Richards and J. B. Hendrickson, Biosynthesis of Steroids. Terpenes, and Acetogenins. Benjamin, New York, 1964.
11. W. Karrer, Konstitution und Vorkommen der organischer Pflanzenotoffe. Birkhauser Verlag, Basel, 1958.
12. P. de Mayo, The Mono- and Sesquiterpenoids. Vol. II of K. W. Bentley (ed.), The Chemistry of Natural Products. Interscience, New York, 1959.
13. P. de Mayo, The Higher Terpenoids. Vol. III of K. W. Bentley (ed.), The Chemistry of Natural Products. Interscience, New York, 1959.
14. A. J. Haagen-Smit, Fortschr. Chem. Org. Naturstoffe XII:1 (1955).
15. F. Sörm, Fortschr. Chem. Org. Naturstoffe XIX:1 (1961).
16. P. Karrer and E. Jucker, Carotenoids. Elsevier, New York, 1950.
17. T. W. Goodwin, *in* T. W. Goodwin (ed.), Chemistry and Biochemistry of Plant Pigments. Academic Press, New York, 1965. p. 127.
18. B. O. Phinney and C. A. West, Ann. Rev. Plant Physiol. 11:411 (1960).

19. B. O. Phinney and C. A. West, *in* W. Ruhland (ed.), Encyclopedia of Plant Physiology. Vol. XIV. Springer-Verlag, Berlin, 1961. p. 1185.
20. P. W. Brian, J. F. Grove, and J. MacMillan, Fortschr. Chem. Org. Naturstoffe XVIII:350 (1960).
21. R. P. Pharis, M. D. E. Ruddat, C. C. Phillips, and E. Heftmann, Can. J. Bot. 43:924 (1965).
22. J. H. Law and F. E. Regnier, Ann. Rev. Biochem. 40:533 (1971).
23. L. M. Roth and T. Eisner, Ann. Rev. Ent. 7:107 (1962).
24. T. Eisner, Science 148:966 (1965).
25. J. F. McConnell, A. M. Mathieson, and B. P. Schoenborn, Tetrahedron Lett. 445 (1962).
26. M. Kupchan, J. Am. Chem. Soc. 89:465 (1967).
27. M. Kupchan, J. Am. Chem. Soc. 90:3596 (1968).
28. C. P. Whittingham, *in* T. W. Goodwin (ed.), Chemistry and Biochemistry of Plant Pigments. Academic Press, New York, 1965. p. 357.
29. J. H. Burnett, *in* T. W. Goodwin (ed.), Chemistry and Biochemistry of Plant Pigments. Academic Press, New York, 1965. p. 381.
30. G. Wald, J. Gen. Physiol. 19:351 (1935).
31. B. M. Austern and A. M. Gawienowski, Lipids 4:1 (1969).
32. D. L. Naudi and J. W. Porter, Arch. Biochem. Biophys. 105:7 (1964).
33. E. Beytia, P. Valenzuela, and O. Cori, Arch. Biochem. Biophys. 129:346 (1969).
34. P. Valenzuela, A. Yudelevich, and O. Cori, Phytochemistry 5:1005 (1966).
35. S. Winstein, Main Congress Lectures and Lectures in the Sections, 14th International Congress of Pure and Applied Chemitry (Zurich). Birkhäuser Verlag, Basel, 1955. p. 137.
36. W. W. Sandermann and W. Schweers, Tetrahedron Lett. 257 (1962).
37. W. W. Sandermann and W. Schweers, Tetrahedron Lett. 259 (1962).
38. G. W. K. Cavill, Rev. Pure Appl. Chem. 10:169 (1960).
39. E. Ramstad and D. Aqurell, Ann. Rev. Plant Physiol. 15:143 (1964).
40. G. C. Casinovi, J. A. Garbarino, and G. B. Marini, Bettolo, Chem. Ind. (London) 253 (1961).
41. T. Sakan, A. Fujino, F. Murdi, A. Suzui, and Y. Butsugan, Bull. Chem. Soc. (Japan) 33:712 (1960).
42. G. Buchi and R. E. Manning, Tetrahedron Lett. 18:1049 (1959).
43. R. Fusco, R. Trave, and A. Vercellone, Chim. Ind. (Milan) 37:251 (1955).
44. K. J. Clark, G. I. Fray, R. H. Jaeger, and R. Robinson, Tetrahedron 6:217 (1959).
45. A. J. Birch, Ann. Rept. Progr. Chem. (London) 47:192 (1950).
46. R. Thomas, Tetrahedron Lett. 544 (1961).
47. E. Wenkert, J. Am. Chem. Soc. 84:98 (1962).
48. L. Ruzicka and E. Capato, Helv. Chim. Acta 8:259 (1925).
49. B. V. Milborrow, *in* Plant Growth Substances, Proc. Int. Conf. 7th, 1970, 1972, p. 281.
50. B. V. Milborrow and M. Garmstom, Phytochemistry 12:1597 (1973).
51. B. V. Milborrow, Biochem. J. 128:1135 (1972).
52. G. Ourisson, Bull. Soc. Chim. France 895 (1955).
53. W. Sandermann and K. Bruns, Tetrahedron Lett. 261 (1962).
54. G. Buchi, M. S. Wittenaw, and D. M. White, J. Am. Chem. Soc. 81:1968 (1959).
55. J. A. Mills, J. Chem. Soc. 4976 (1952).
56. C. Djerassi and S. Burstein, J. Am. Chem. Soc. 80:2593 (1958).

57. R. Riniker, J. Kalvoda, D. Arigoni, A. Furst, O. Jeger, A. M. Gold, and R. B. Woodward, J. Am. Chem. Soc. 76:313 (1954).
58. C. Djerassi, R. Riniker, and B. Riniker, J. Am. Chem. Soc. 78:6362 (1956).
59. H. Bruderer, D. Arigoni, and O. Jeger, Helv. Chim. Acta 39:858 (1956).
60. L. H. Zalkow, F. X. Markley, and C. Djerassi, J. Am. Chem. Soc. 81:2914 (1959).
61. V. Herout and V. Sykora, Tetrahedron Lett. 4:246 (1958).
62. G. Jacob, G. Ourisson, and A. Rassat, Bull. Soc. Chim. France 475 (1959).
63. C. Djerassi, J. Osiechi, W. Herz, J. Org. Chem. 22:1361 (1957).
64. L. Dolejs, M. Soucek, M. Horak, V. Herout, and F. Sorm, Coll. Czech. Chem. Commun. 23:2195 (1958).
65. J. Caglioti, G. Cainelli, B. Camerino, R. Mondelli, A. Prieto, A. Quilico, T. Salvatori, and A. Salva, Chim. Ind. (Milan) 46:1 (1964).
66. F. Sorm, M. Suchy, and V. Herout, Coll. Czech. Chem. Commun. 16:278 (1951).
67. J. L. Simonsen and D. H. R. Barton, The Terpenes. 2nd Ed. Vol. 3. Cambridge University Press, London, 1952. p. 334.
68. R. L. Rowland, A. Rodgman, J. N. Schumacher, D. L. Roberts, L. C. Cook, and W. E. Walker, J. Org. Chem. 29:16 (1964).
69. W. G. Dauben, W. E. Thiessen, and P. R. Resnick, J. Org. Chem. 30: 1693 (1965).
70. B. Kimland and T. Norin, Acta Chem. Scand. 22:943 (1968).
71. D. R. Robinson and C. A. West, Biochemistry 9:70 (1970).
72. W. W. Epstein and H. C. Rilling, J. Biol. Chem 245:4597 (1970).
73. J. Edmond, G. Popjak, S. Wong, and V. P. Williams, J. Biol. Chem. 246: 6254 (1971).
74. H. Wasner and F. Lynen, Fed. Eur. Biochem. Soc. Lett. 12:54 (1970).
75. R. McCrindle and K. H. Overton, Advan. Org. Chem. 5:47 (1965).
76. C. H. Brieskorn, A. Fuchs, J. B. Bredenberg, J. D. McChesney, and E. Wenkert, J. Org. Chem. 29, 2293 (1964).
77. E. Wenkert, A. Fuchs, and J. D. McChesney, J. Org. Chem. 30:2931 (1965).
78. E. Mosettig and W. R. Nes, J. Org. Chem. 20:884 (1955).
79. E. Mosettig, U. Beglinger, F. Dolder, H. Lichti, P. Quitt, and J. A. Waters, J. Am. Chem. Soc. 85:2305 (1963).
80. B. E. Cross, J. F. Grove, J. MacMillan, and T. P. Mulholland, Chem. Ind. (London), 954 (1956).
81. B. E. Cross, R. H. B. Galt, J. R. Hanson, and W. Klyne, Tetrahedron Lett. 145 (1962).
82. B. E. Cross, R. H. B. Galt, J. R. Hanson, P. J. Curtis, J. F. Grove, and A. Morrison, J. Chem. Soc. 2937 (1963).
83. I. Schechter and C. A. West, J. Biol. Chem. 244:3200 (1969).
84. A. J. Birch and H. Smith, in G. E. W. Wolstenholme (ed.), A Ciba Foundation Symposium on the Biosynthesis of Terpenes and Sterols. Little, Brown, Boston, 1959. p. 245.
85. M. R. Corcoran and B. O. Phinney, Physiol. Planatarum 15:252 (1962).
86. J. E. Graebe, D. T. Dennis, C. U. Upper, and C. A. West, J. Biol. Chem. 240:1847 (1965).
87. A. J. Birch, R. W. Richards, and H. Smith, Proc. Chem. Soc. (London) 192 (1958).
88. M. Katsumi, B. O. Phinney, P. R. Jefferies, and C. A. Henrick, Science 144:849 (1964).
89. B. O. Phinney, P. R. Jefferies, M. Katsumi, and C. A. Henrick, Plant Physiol. 39 (Suppl.): xxvii (1964).

90. B. E. Cross, R. H. B. Galt, and J. R. Hanson, J. Chem. Soc. 295 (1964).
91. M. Ruddat, E. Heftmann, and A. Lang, Arch. Biochem. Biophys. 111:187 (1965).
92. W. B. Mors, M. F. dos Santos, H. J. Monteiro, B. Gilbert, and J. Pellegrino, Science 157:950 (1967).
93. L. H. Briggs and R. W. Cawley, J. Chem. Soc. 1888 (1948).
94. L. H. Briggs, R. W. Cawley, J. A. Loe, and W. I. Taylor, J. Chem. Soc. 955 (1950).
95. J. D. Cocker and T. G. Halsall, J. Chem. Soc. 4262 (1956).
96. C. Djerassi and D. Marshall, Tetrahedron 1:238 (1957).
97. F. E. King and G. Jones, J. Chem. Soc. 658 (1955).
98. E. Kyburz, B. Riniker, H. R. Shenk, H. Heusser, and O. Jeger, Helv. Chim. Acta 36:1891 (1953).
99. D. H. R. Barton, Quart. Rev. 3:36 (1949).
100. W. Klyne, J. Chem. Soc. 3072 (1953).
101. L. H. Briggs, B. F. Cain, and R. C. Cambie, Tetrahedron Lett. 17 (1959).
102. P. K. Grant and R. Hodges, Tetrahedron 8:261 (1960).
103. E. Mosettig, P. Quitt, U. Beglinger, J. A. Waters, H. Vorbrueggen, and C. Djerassi, J. Am. Chem. Soc. 83:3163 (1961).
104. M. P. Cava and B. Weinstein, Chem. and Ind. (London) 851 (1959).
105. J. Pudles, A. Diara, and E. Lederer, Bull. Soc. Chim. France 693 (1959).
106. L. H. Briggs, B. F. Cain, R. C. Cambie, and B. R. Davis, Tetrahedron Lett. 18 (1960).
107. C. Djerassi, M. Cais, and L. Mitschner, J. Am. Chem. Soc. 81:2386 (1959).
108. C. Djerassi, P. Quitt, E. Mosettig, R. C. Cambie, P. S. Rutledge, and L. H. Briggs, J. Am. Chem. Soc. 83:3720 (1960).
109. E. Wenkert, Chem. Ind. (London) 282 (1955).
110. G. C. Harris and T. F. Sanderson, J. Am. Chem. Soc. 70:2081 (1948).
111. L. Ruzicka, in A. Todd (ed.), Perspectives in Organic Chemistry. Interscience, New York, 1956. pp. 265-314.
112. T-C. Lee, T. H. Lee, and C. O. Chichester, Phytochemistry 11:681 (1961).
113. K. Decker and H. Uehleke, Hoppe-Seyler's Z. Physiol. Chem 323:61 (1961).
114. S. C. Kushwaha, C. Subbarayan, D. A. Beeler, and J. W. Porter, J. Biol. Chem. 244:3635 (1969).
115. H. M. Hill and L. J. Rogers, Biochem. J. 113:31P (1969).
116. T. W. Goodwin, Biochem. J. 123:293 (1971).
117. J. S. Knypl, Naturwiss. 56:572 (1969).
118. C. W. Coggins, Jr., G. L. Henning, and H. Yokoyama, Science 168:1589 (1970).
119. C. D. Howes and P. P. Batra, Biochim. Biophys. Acta 222:174 (1970).
120. R. J. H. Williams, G. Britton, and T. W. Goodwin, Biochem. J. 105:99 (1967).
121. T. W. Goodwin and R. J. H. Williams, Biochem. J. 94:5C (1965).
122. T. W. Goodwin and R. J. H. Williams, Biochem. J. 97:28C (1965).
123. C. H. Eugster, R. Buchecker, C. Tscharner, G. Uhde, G. Ohloff, Helv. Chim. Acta 52:1729 (1969).
124. D. V. Banthorpe and D. Baxendale, Chem. Commun. 1553 (1968).
125. D. V. Banthorpe and K. W. Turnbull, Chem. Commun. 177 (1966).
126. M. Biollaz and D. Arigoni, Chem. Commun. 633 (1969).
127. H. Auda, H. R. Juneja, E. J. Eisenbraun, G. R. Waller, W. R. Kays, and H. H. Appel, J. Am. Chem. Soc. 89:2476 (1967).
128. A. Corbella, P. Gariboldi, G. Jommi, and C. Scolastica, Chem. Commun. 634 (1969).

129. J. Meinwald, G. M. Happ, J. Labows, and T. Eisner, Science 151:79 (1966).
130. P. K. Bhattacharyya and K. Ganapathy, Ind. J. Biochem. 2:137 (1965).
131. P. W. Trudgill, R. DuBus, and I. C. Gunsalus, J. Biol. Chem. 241:1194 (1966).
132. P. J. Chapman, G. Meerman, I. C. Gunsalus, R. Srinivasan, and K. L. Rinehart, Jr., J. Am. Chem. Soc. 88:618 (1966).
133. J. Fishman, E. R. H. Jones, G. Lowe, and M. C. Whiting, Proc. Chem. Soc. (London) 127 (1959).
134. T. Akazawa, I. Uritani, and Y. Akazawa, Arch. Biochem. Biophys. 99:52 (1962).
135. P. de Mayo, J. R. Robinson, E. Y. Spencer, and R. W. White, Experientia 18, 359 (1962).
136. C. D. Upper and C. A. West, J. Biol. Chem. 242:3285 (1967).
137. J. D. Anderson and T. C. Moore, Plant Physiol. 42:1527 (1967).
138. J. E. Graebe, Phytochemistry 7:2003 (1968).
139. J. E. Graebe, Planta 85:171 (1969).
140a. M. O. Oster and C. A. West, Arch. Biochem. Biophys. 127:112 (1968).
140b. H. C. Malhotra and W. R. Nes, J. Biol. Chem. 247:6243 (1972).
141. D. R. Robinson and C. A. West, Biochemistry 9:80 (1970).
142. C. Subbarayan, S. C. Kushwaha, G. Suzue, and J. W. Porter, Arch. Biochem. Biophys. 137:547 (1970).
143. S. C. Kushwaha, G. Suzue, C. Subbarayan, and J. W. Porter, J. Biol. Chem. 245:4708 (1970).
144. T-C. Lee and C. O. Chichester, Phytochemistry 8:603 (1969).

Chapter
9

Metabolism
of
Lanosterol
and
Cycloartenol
to
$\triangle^5$ Sterols

A. Basic Pathway 326
B. Lanosterol-Cycloartenol Bifurcation 328
C. Alkylation-Reduction Bifurcation 331
    1. *General Characteristics* 331
    2. *Discovery* 332
    3. *Mechanism of Reduction* 333
    4. *Mechanism of Alkylation* 335
    5. *Variations of Alkylation Mechanism* 344
    6. *Dehydrogenation and Dealkylation at C-24* 346
    7. *Shortening of Side Chain to C_7* 352
D. Removal of Methyl Groups at C-4 and C-14 354
    1. *General Comments* 354
    2. *Elimination from C-4* 355
    3. *Elimination from C-14* 360
E. Origins and Central Role of Δ^7-Sterols 366
F. Introduction of the Δ^5-Bond 367
G. Introduction of the Δ^{22}-Bond 371

H. Sequence 373
  1. *General Comments* 373
  2. *Route in Mammals* 374
  3. *Route in Invertebrates* 377
  4. *Route in Fungi* 383
  5. *Route in Algae* 387
  6. *Route in Tracheophytes* 393
I. Enzymology 394
  1. *General Comments* 394
  2. Δ^{24}-*Reductase and Alkylase* 394
  3. *Enzymes for Removal of Methyl Groups at C-4* 395
  4. Δ^{8}- *to* Δ^{7}-*Isomerase* 397
  5. Δ^{5}-*Dehydrogenase and* Δ^{7}-*Reductase* 398
Literature Cited 398

A. BASIC PATHWAY

In most organisms the dominant steroids possess four structural qualities in common. They are a Δ^5-bond, no carbon substituents on C-4 or C-14, a methyl group at the A/B ring juncture, i.e., no three-membered 9,19-cyclo grouping, and an H atom or a C_1 or C_2 substituent at C-24. Typical examples (Scheme 9.1) are cholesterol and its 24-methyl and 24-ethyl derivatives. The Δ^{22}-derivatives are also common. The detailed distribution of these and other compounds is explored in Chapter 10. With the exception of the presence of a methyl group between rings A and B which is present in lanosterol, neither of the two products of cyclization of squalene oxide (lanosterol and cycloartenol) have the four structural qualities. Since both function as intermediates (Section B), there must be four fundamental biosynthetic processes operating [Δ^5-introduction, demethylation at C-4 and C-14, opening of the 9,19-ring (cycloartenol), and Δ^{24}-metabolism]. The main outline of these transformations is now understood. Two seem to occur quite generally in a definite order. They are removal of the three methyl groups and establishment of Δ^5-unsaturation. This yields a basic sequence (Scheme 9.2) upon which the other two (metabolism at C-24 and opening of the three-membered ring) are superimposed. The superimposition produces major alternative sequences. One, the alkylation-reduction bifurcation (C-24 metabolism), could occur in the beginning, at the end, or at some other point in the pathway. For instance, in proceeding to cholesterol, lanosterol could be reduced to 24,25-dihydrolanosterol, which then undergoes demethylation and double-bond modification; lanosterol could undergo the latter two processes, leading to 24,25-dehydrocholesterol, which is then reduced; or reduction of the Δ^{24}-bond might occur at some intermediate stage, e.g., after removal of one of the three methyl groups. Lanosterol could also undergo alkylation instead of reduction. The other (the lanosterol-cycloartenol bifurcation) involves the analogous superimposition of the ring-opening reaction, which could conceivably occur first, last, or in between. Metabolic experiments and information on the occurrence of sterols indicate that the three-membered ring

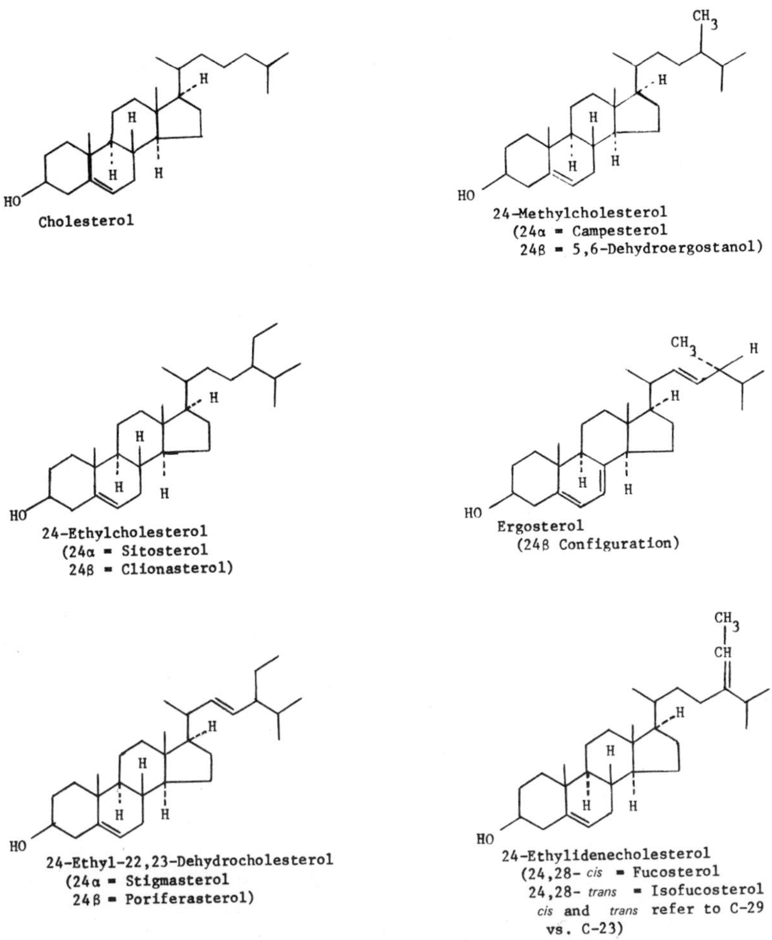

Cholesterol

24-Methylcholesterol
(24α = Campesterol
24β = 5,6-Dehydroergostanol)

24-Ethylcholesterol
(24α = Sitosterol
24β = Clionasterol)

Ergosterol
(24β Configuration)

24-Ethyl-22,23-Dehydrocholesterol
(24α = Stigmasterol
24β = Poriferasterol)

24-Ethylidenecholesterol
(24,28- *cis* = Fucosterol
24,28- *trans* = Isofucosterol
cis and *trans* refer to C-29
vs. C-23)

Scheme 9.1. The dominant sterols of most organisms.

is only rarely opened as the first step, but opening does occur before intro-duction of the Δ^5-bond. Therefore, the lanosterol and cycloartenol routes converge not later than removal of the three methyl groups. Since sequencing of C-24 metabolism and of Δ^{22} introduction adds complications, this does not mean that all routes necessarily have precisely the same common inter-mediates following the convergence. It does mean that if one follows the pathway back from the dominant Δ^5-sterol, ignoring metabolism in the side chain and any specialized metabolism, e.g., hydroxylation, one or more common structural types will be found in most organisms. This common type will bear no methyl groups on C-4 or C-14, will have an angular methyl group between rings A and B, i.e., no three-membered ring, and will possess

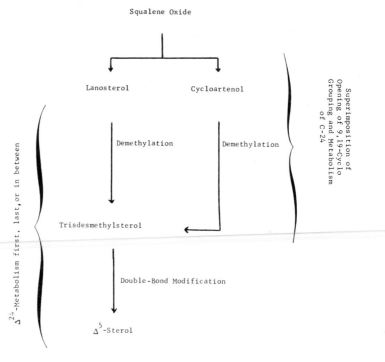

Scheme 9.2. Basic biosynthetic pathways to Δ^5-sterols.

at least one double bond, but not a Δ^5-bond, in the tetracyclic nucleus. This is the "trisdesmethylsterol" of Scheme 9.2. Simple examples are cholest-7-en-3β-ol (lathosterol) and its 24-ethyl derivative (Δ^7-chondrillastenol).

B. LANOSTEROL-CYCLOARTENOL BIFURCATION

The discovery, structure, and biosynthetic intermediacy of lanosterol in the animal kingdom have been discussed elsewhere (Chapter 7, Section A). In fungal biosynthesis the involvement of lanosterol has been demonstrated by the isolation of lanosterol from yeast (1, 2), the conversion of lanosterol (3) or a lanosterol derivative (24-methylene-24,25-dihydrolanosterol) (4, 5) to ergosterol in the same organism, the isolation of 24-methylene-24,25-dihydro-lanosterol from *Phycomyces blakesleeanus* and *Agaricus campestris* (6), and the isolation of a squalene oxide-lanosterol cyclase from *Saccharomyces cerevisiae* (7) as well as from *Phycomyces blakesleeanus* cell-free system (8).

Such information suggests a general plant-animal route of biosynthesis to which added support was given by the conversion of lanosterol to 24-ethylidenecholesterol in a photosynthetic plant (*Pinus pinea*) (9). However, lanosterol has generally been very difficult to find in photosynthetic plants.

Reports of its presence are rare (*10-13*), while positive identification of its 9,19-cyclo derivative, cycloartenol, has been made with relative frequency (e.g., *14-21*). Benveniste, Hirth, and Ourisson (*22, 23*) were particularly impressed with such findings in tobacco plants and postulated that cycloartenol might function as an alternative to lanosterol.

In view of the excellent data showing the involvement of the lanosterol pathway in fungi, it has been pointed out that the alternatives must operate not between animals and plants but rather between nonphotosynthetic and photosynthetic organisms (*21, 24*). Extremely good evidence for this is available. Results from work with cell-free systems have shown that the squalene oxide-lanosterol cyclase occurs in the apparent absence of the squalene oxide-cycloartenol cyclase in both fungi (*8*) and mammals (*25, 26*). The situation is the reverse in both lower and higher photosynthetic systems. In particular, incubations with cell-free systems from the alga, *Ochromonas malhamensis* (*27*), the gymnosperm, *Pinus pinea* (*28*), and the angiosperm, *Phaseolus vulgaris* (*29*), have led to the formation of cycloartenol but not of lanosterol. Tissue cultures of *Nicotiana tabacum* also biosynthesize cycloartenol but not lanosterol (*30*) and the biosynthesis of cycloartenol but not of lanosterol has been recorded in vivo with *Zea mays* (*21*), with tobacco leaf disks (*31*), and with tissue cultures of *Agave toumeyana, Dioscorea composita*, and other plants (*31*). Moreover, a squalene oxide-cycloartenol cyclase has been isolated from *O. malhamensis*. The sole product of this enzyme is cycloartenol (*27*).

Because for steric reasons lanosterol is thermodynamically more stable than cycloartenol, any isomerization of one to the other would be expected to proceed toward lanosterol, and this has been observed chemically (H^+ catalysis) (*32*). Consequently, the formation of cycloartenol in place of lanosterol in photosynthetic systems cannot be an artifact of the lanosterol pathway but must instead represent a truly fundamental route. Conversely, in nonphotosynthetic organisms the lanosterol route cannot be an artifact of the cycloartenol route, because, at least in rat liver, cycloartenol proceeds neither to lanosterol nor cholesterol under conditions readily yielding cholesterol from lanosterol (*21*). Yeast, in addition, lacks the isomerase for cleavage of the cyclopropane ring (*33*). Discrimination is not made by sterol carrier protein, since lanosterol and cycloartenol have essentially the same binding constants (*34*). It is also worthy of note that a cell-free system from nonphotosynthetic tissue (endosperm) of a photosynthetic plant (*Pinus pinea*) forms cycloartenol, not lanosterol, indicating genetic fixation by the presence or absence of photosynthesis in the whole organism. Etiolated *Euglena gracilis* also continues to biosynthesize cycloartenol (*35*) and only 9β,19-cyclo sterols were recovered from the nonphotosynthetic euglenoid, *Astasia longa* (*36*). Finally, labeled cycloartenol has been converted to the normal, dominant Δ^5-sterols of both lower (*24*) and higher (*21, 37*) photosynthetic plants.

In summary, the nature of the squalene oxide cyclase constitutes a

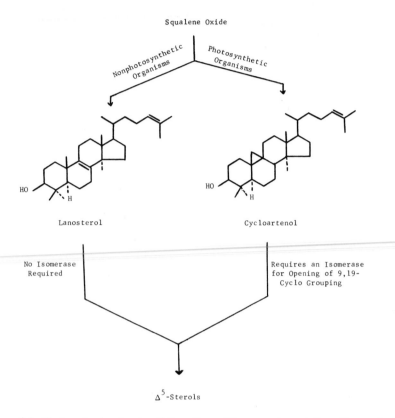

Scheme 9.3. The lanosterol-cycloartenol bifurcation and its apparent association with organismic type.

bifurcation (Scheme 9.3) in the steroid pathway yielding lanosterol as the first cyclized intermediate in nonphotosynthetic organisms and cycloartenol in place of lanosterol in photosynthetic organisms. The existence of the bifurcation is now unequivocal, although the association with organismic types could bear additional definition. At some stage after cyclization into the cycloartenol series, the three-membered ring is opened. The mechanism has not been investigated, but a reasonable hypothesis is that protonation-deprotonation is involved, in which case the enzyme would be an isomerase. An isomerase has been partially purified from blackberry microsomes. While the enzyme is active toward several types of 9β,19-cyclo sterols, 4α-methyl and 4-desmethyl substrates are preferred (38). The substrate specificity is in accord with the frequent occurrence of the 4α-methyl sterols, 31-nor-cycloartenol, cycloeucalenol, and 31-norcyclolaudenol, in higher plants. A clue to the mechanism of isomerization has been provided by Caspi et al. (39), who noted incorporation at C-19 of a hydrogen atom from the medium (water) during sitosterol biosynthesis by *Pisum sativum*. The isomerization can be experimentally bypassed by the administration of lanosterol, which proceeds in about the same yield to Δ^5-sterols as does cycloartenol in *Ochromonas malhamensis* (*24*), *Nicotiana tabacum* (*37*), *Pinus pinea* (*19*), and *Zea mays* (*21*). Exogenous lanosterol also is utilized by *Euphorbia peplus* (*40*).

C. ALKYLATION-REDUCTION BIFURCATION

1. General Characteristics

During cyclization of squalene to either lanosterol or cycloartenol, one of the terminal double bonds remains as the Δ^{24}-bond of the steroid side chain. It has two known routes of metabolism (Scheme 9.4). They are reduction

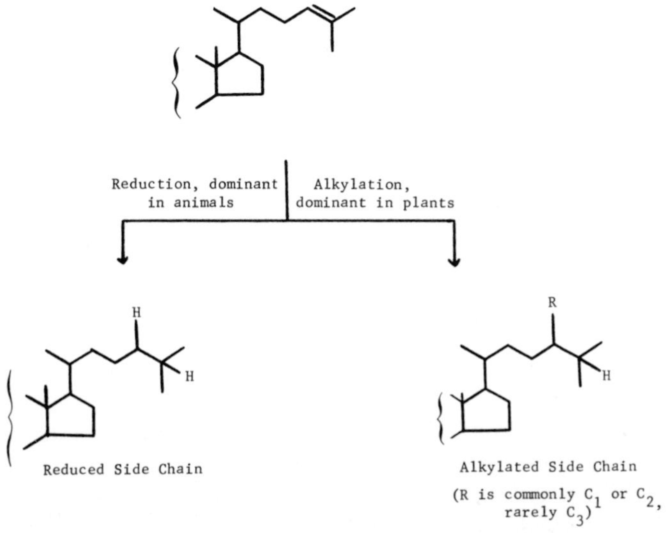

Scheme 9.4. The alkylation-reduction bifurcation and its association with organismic type.

to yield the saturated side chain characteristic of cholesterol and alkylation producing the 24-alkenyl or 24-alkyl sterols, among which sitosterol is probably the most common. Despite the number of studies of the occurrence of squalene in both plants and animals, no dihydro or alkylated derivatives have been found in eukaryots, although 2,3-dihydrosqualene as well as 2,3 22,23-tetrahydrosqualene have been identified in the halophilic bacterium, *Halobacterium cutirubum* (*41*). The integrity of all of the double bonds in squalene in eukaryots together with the occurrence of 24,25-dihydrolanosterol (e.g., *42*), 24,25-dihydrocycloartanol (cycloartanol) (e.g., *21, 43–45*), and 24-methylenecycloartanol (e.g., *21, 43, 46, 47*), indicates that reduction or alkylation occurs usually and perhaps exclusively after, but not before, cyclization. This is corroborated by the experimental reduction of lanosterol (21, 48) and 24-dehydrocholesterol (desmosterol) (49, 50) to 24,25-dihydrolanosterol and cholesterol, respectively, in rats, and by the conversion of lanosterol, cycloartenol, and desmosterol to their respective 24-methylene derivatives in a cell-free system from germinating peas (51). The necessity of the Δ^{24}-double bond has been demonstrated by the failure of 24,25-dihydrolanosterol or cholesterol to undergo alkylation in *Pinus pinea* (51). A cell-free system for Δ^{24}-alkylation has also been reported from yeast (52, 53), *Trebouxia* sp., and *Scenedesmus obliquus* (54).

The steroid pathway possesses a second major bifurcation (Scheme 9.4), which resides in the nature of what we shall call the Δ^{24}-metabolase. The Δ^{24}-metabolase is either an alkylase or a reductase, and both enzymatic types may operate with either lanosterol or cycloartenol as substrates. This is illustrated inter alia by mammalian reduction (21, 48) and plant alkylation (3, 51) of lanosterol on the one hand, and on the other by the presence of the reduced cycloartenol (21, 43–45) and the alkylated 24-methylenecycloartenol (21, 43, 46, 47) in plants as well as the experimental alkylation of cycloartenol by plant enzymes (51). In broad outlines that need much more definition, alkylation is the dominant process in the plant kingdom, and reduction in the animal kingdom. Some overlap exists. Chapter 10 should be consulted for details of the distribution.

2. Discovery

The origin of the saturated side chain from the reduction of the Δ^{24}-bond was first investigated experimentally by Stokes and others after cholesterol and its Δ^{24}-derivative, desmosterol, had been found to accompany each other in rat skin (49, 55) and liver (56), the chick embryo (57), and the barnacle (58). Realizing the possible intermediate role of desmosterol, Stokes and his associates (49) injected a labeled sample intraperitoneally into rats and were able to isolate labeled cholesterol. At about the same time, a report (59) appeared showing the inhibition of cholesterol biosynthesis by the compound triparanol, and shortly thereafter Avigan and Steinberg and their associates (60) proved that it induced the accumulation of desmosterol in place of cholesterol and confirmed the conversion of the former to the latter (50, 61). Lanosterol has also been converted in rats to 24,25-dihydrolanosterol (21, 48), leaving no doubt about reductive metabolism other than the problem of sequence.

Alkylation was first appreciated as a metabolic route for the Δ^{24}-bond by Nes (62), Birch (63), Arigoni (64), and Lederer (65), but the first serious consideration of the origin of the 24-alkyl group was given by Robinson (66) a few years earlier. He suggested that the 24-C_1 group of ergosterol might be derived from utilization of one molecule of propionate instead of acetate at an early biosynthetic stage. It followed that the 24-C_2 group might have an analogous origin in butyrate. However, the hypothesis fails to explain the selective use of an acid other than acetate, the absence of homologs that could arise from the use of higher carboxylic acids (fatty acids in particular), the absence of alkylated squalene derivatives, and, of particular importance, the natural occurrence of 24-methylene and 24-ethylidene sterols. Direct biosynthetic evidence contravening Robinson's hypothesis was soon forthcoming from several laboratories. The carbon atoms of labeled acetate were found not to be the precursor of C-28 in ergosterol (67) or in eburicoic acid (68, 69). Reasoning that the methyl group may be derived from C_1 metabolism, investigators from two laboratories repeated the ergosterol and eburicoic acid experiments using formate instead of acetate. Formate was indeed incorporated selectively into C-28 of both compounds (70, 71). Schwenk and co-workers (72) incubated yeast with labeled acetate, and labeled "methylsqualene" could not be detected by careful examination including degradation. Only squalene was formed. Labeled propionate was not incorporated into ergosterol. Instead, labeled methionine, serine, and formate (methionine being the most efficient) gave rise to C-28 of ergosterol. Further studies with aminopterin (73), which inhibits tetrahydrofolate-linked reduction of formate, led Schwenk and his associates (72, 73) to prove that methionine is an intermediate, and degradation showed that the methyl group of methionine was used exclusively for C-28 (72). The use of the methyl group of methionine as the C_1 source for the 24-C_2 group of sitosterol, etc., was subsequently shown in the laboratories of Nes (62, 74), Arigoni (64), and Lederer (75), and acetyl-CoA and ethionine were excluded (62, 74). Alkylation was thus shown to be a stepwise process (62) of C_1 transfer, the pathway being 24,25-unsaturated sterol to 24-C_1 sterol to 24-C_2 sterol and (in rare cases) to 24-C_3 sterol.

3. Mechanism of Reduction

Reduction of isolated double bonds is not a common biochemical reaction. Although it presumably exists, for instance, in the formation of phytol, it was not well studied until investigations of cholesterol biosynthesis began. With the discovery of desmosterol (Section C.2), it became possible to study the enzymology, which revealed reduced pyridine nucleotide to be the reductant in rat liver (50). Not only was NADPH specifically required, but the H atom on C-4 of the nicotinamide moiety was incorporated into cholesterol, indicating a direct transfer (50). This information suggests (76) a carbonium ion mechanism (Scheme 9.5), which is corroborated by investigations in Akhtar's and Caspi's laboratories (76–80). They showed that a proton originating in water is added to C-24, and a hydride ion from the B side of NADPH is added to C-25 in mammals. The direction of addition agrees with the intermediacy of the tertiary carbonium ion (at C-25). Using 4R-[2-^{14}C, 4-^{3}H]mevalonate as a precursor in rat liver, Caspi and his colleagues (78, 80) demonstrated that cholesterol bearing a 24^{3}H atom had the 24R configuration. Consequently, in the reduction of the Δ^{24}-bond the proton added at C-24 must represent the 24-*pro-S*-H-atom, from which it follows that the proton is on the back side when the planar system comprising the double bond is oriented in the plane of the paper, as shown in Scheme 9.5.

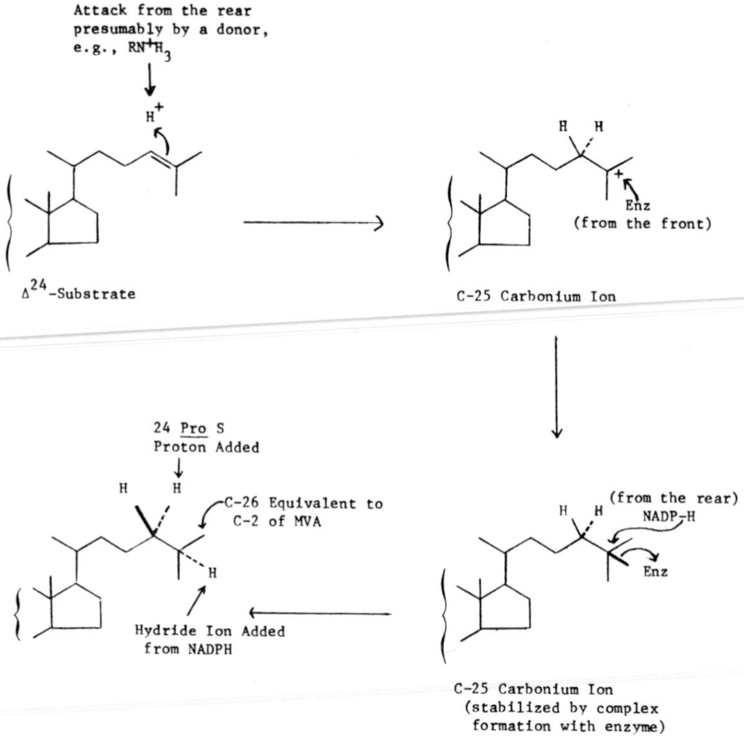

Scheme 9.5. Stereochemistry and probable mechanism of Δ^{24}-reduction in rat liver.

Furthermore, animal cholesterol, biosynthesized from [2-^{14}C]MVA, has been converted in *M. smegmatis* to 26-hydroxycholest-4-en-3-one (*81, 82*). Degradative removal (*82*) of the hydroxylated carbon atom (yielding 26-norcholestenone) entailed loss of ^{14}C, indicating that C-26 is derived from C-2 of MVA. 26-Hydroxycholestenone was then submitted to x-ray crystallography, which proved C-25 to have the S configuration (*82*). In the conformer with C-26 up and in front (Scheme 9.5), the 25-H is then in back. Since C-26 is *trans*-oriented with respect to C-23, the C-25 carbonium ion must have an analogous conformation. Two opposing conclusions can be drawn from this. Either a *cis*-addition of H$^+$ and H$^-$ has occurred, or, as seems much more likely from the chemistry of double bonds, a *trans*-addition of H$^+$ and a donor group from the enzyme proceed to give what is tantamount to a strongly stabilized C-25 carbonium ion that then undergoes H$^-$ attack at C-25 from the opposite side. The final result of the latter process (inversion) would be to place the H^+ and H^- on the same side of the originally planar system, as found experimentally in in vitro systems and recently in in vivo systems (*83*).

4. Mechanism of Alkylation

(*a*) *Orienting Remarks* The actual donor of the C_1 group is *S*-adenosylmethionine (SAM). The first evidence for this came from Parks (*84*), who showed that SAM is a better precursor of the methyl group of ergosterol than is methionine itself. More recently, Gaylor's group (*53*) has succeeded in isolating the yeast *S*-adenosylmethionine: Δ^{24}-sterol methyltransferase (EC 2.1.1.41). Crude enzyme preparations have been reported from the algae *Scenedesmus obliquus* and *Trebouxia* sp. (*54*). The yeast enzyme resides in the mitochondria and promitochondria (*85*), indicating that activity of the enzyme may be linked with energy metabolism. High concentrations of the cations, K^+ and Na^+, are inhibitory (*86*). Mechanistically (*62*), the importance of *S*-adenosylmethionine lies in the presence of a positive charge on the sulfur atom to which the methyl group is attached. Because the Δ^{24}-bond is intrinsically nucleophilic because of the presence of π-electrons, Nes et al. (*62*) pointed out that one can write a reasonable mechanism (Scheme 9.6) that entails transfer of an electron-deficient CH_3 group from

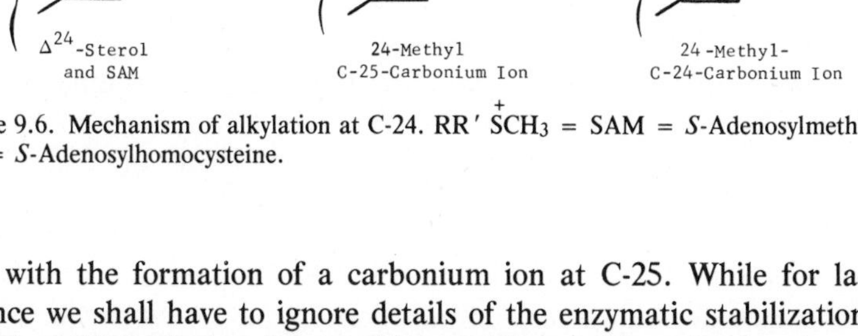

Scheme 9.6. Mechanism of alkylation at C-24. $RR'\overset{+}{S}CH_3 = SAM = S$-Adenosylmethionine, SAH = S-Adenosylhomocysteine.

SAM with the formation of a carbonium ion at C-25. While for lack of evidence we shall have to ignore details of the enzymatic stabilization and half-life of this and related charged intermediates, this carbonium ion mechanism, in contrast to others that have been considered (*65*), best explains the known facts. The mechanism is applicable to fields other than steroids (*87*), Birch (*88, 89*) being the first to call attention to C_1 transfer to double bonds in the case of the nonsteroidal mycophenolic acid.

If the methyl group acting as if it were CH_3^+ were transferred from SAM to the Δ^{24}-bond, the most stable carbonium ion should, as pointed out above, be the one bearing the positive charge on C-25, where it has the opportunity for hyperconjugative interaction with six H atoms on C-26 and C-27. This, together with steric hindrance at C-25 from C-26 and C-27, offers an explanation for the location of the substituent at C-24 and not at C-25. It is entirely analogous to the labeling pattern in Δ^{24} reduction (Section C.3) and to the course of most cyclizations, where the positively charged intermediates usually involve tertiary carbon atoms (Chapters 7 and 8). It may be that the importance of hyperconjugative stabilization and hindrance dictates the final direction of addition only in an evolutionary sense and that enzymes in extant organisms govern the direction exclusively by precise orientation of binding groups for the steroid and SAM. However, the generality of substitution at C-24 strongly indicates that electronic (and steric) factors play or have played some role. Once formed, the C-25 carbonium ion has several fates, depending on the availability and positioning of a deprotonating group or of a source of electrons. The theoretical possibilities are: (1) the immediate addition of hydride ion (62), for which, however, there is no evidence; (2) the direct elimination of a proton from C-24 or C-27, yielding, respectively, $\Delta^{24(25)}$- and $\Delta^{25(27)}$-steroids; and (3) the occurrence of one or more H migrations with elimination of a proton from, for instance, C-28, C-23, or C-22. Because both processes (2) and (3) operate, the common sterols with a saturated side chain arise by reduction of one of several possible double bonds. The configuration at C-24 will therefore be determined by the direction of reduction when C-24 is a part of the double bond, e.g., $\Delta^{24(28)}$, by the direction of alkylation when a $\Delta^{25(27)}$-intermediate is involved, and by the stereochemistry of isomerization if the $\Delta^{24(28)}$-bond is isomerized to the 22,23 position. In what follows we will examine these various alternatives in an order corresponding to the extent of alkylation.

(b) *First C$_1$ Transfer* The most obvious place for deprotonation to occur would be at one of the *gem*-dimethyl C atoms, because this could clearly be a concerted process (Scheme 9.7). In agreement is the occurrence both in tracheophytes (90, 91) and algae (54, 92) of the compound cyclolaudenol, which would result from this process by transfer of a methyl group to cycloartenol, and cyclolaudenol is actually obtained and labeled from S-adenosyl-L-[Me-^{14}C]methionine in *Trebouxia* and *Scenedesmus* species (54). More importantly, administration of 4-tritiomevalonate to the rhizomes of *Polypodium vulgare* leads to cyclolaudenol bearing tritium at C-24 (93). This is consistent with direct introduction of the $\Delta^{25(27)}$-bond and proves that neither a $\Delta^{24(25)}$- nor a $\Delta^{24(28)}$-sterol is an intermediate. Other $\Delta^{25(27)}$-sterols are also known and are discussed in Chapter 10. Other evidence for the route through $\Delta^{25(27)}$-sterols has come from incubations with [^{2}H$_3$]methyl-labeled methionine. In the biosynthesis of the following compounds in various species of green algae, three atoms of deuterium are incorporated: 24β-methyl-cholesterol, its Δ^7-isomer (22-dihydrochondrillasterol), ergosterol, and its 7-dihydro- (brassicasterol) and 5,22-bisdihydro (fungisterol) derivatives

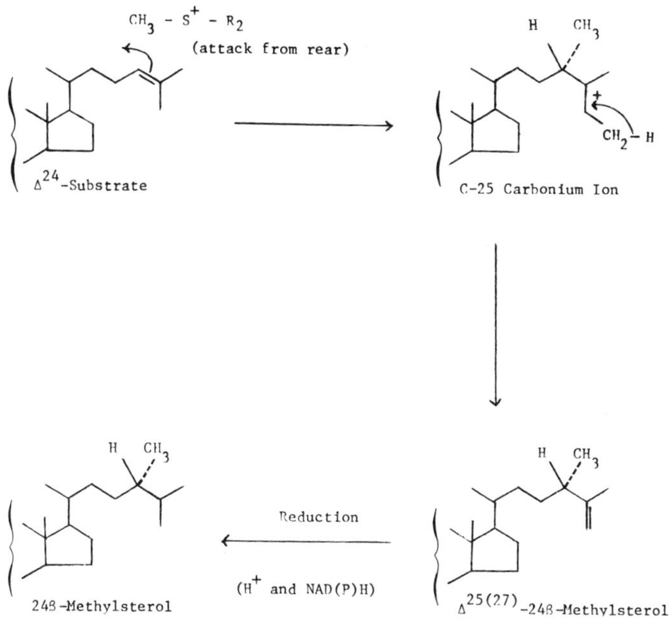

Scheme 9.7. The $\Delta^{25(27)}$-route to 24β-methylsterols in green algae and tracheophytes.

(*92, 94–98*). Furthermore, in *Trebouxia* sp., labeled 31-norcyclolaudenol leads to labeled 24β-methylcholesterol, whereas the labeled 24-methylene derivative (cycloeucalenol) of 31-norcyclolaudenol does not yield labeled 24β-methylcholesterol (*96*). Thus, the $\Delta^{25(27)}$ route clearly is operating, and it is important to note that the configuration at C-24 is therefore established by the direction (β) from which the methyl group attacks C-24 in the alkylation. As is discussed subsequently, this is not the case in other routes.

If elimination from one of the *gem*-dimethyl groups does not occur, only one other H atom (at C-24) can be removed without H migration. No evidence exists for such a process at the 24-C$_1$ level, but there is extensive evidence for elimination from C-28 with H migration from C-24 to C-25 (Scheme 9.8). This leads to a 24-methylenesterol that plays two roles, viz., as a precursor to 24-methylsterols by reduction and as a precursor to 24-ethylidenesterols by a second C$_1$ transfer, which then may proceed by reduction to 24-ethylsterols. Especially in view of its operation in the production of 24-C$_2$ sterols, the route yielding 24-methylenesterols is widely distributed throughout the plant kingdom. The compounds themselves have been found in small quantities in a variety of photosynthetic, nonphotosynthetic, higher, and lower plants, and in a few cases, e.g., pollen (*99*), in large quantities. The predicted (*62*) H migration from C-24 to C-25 has been demonstrated directly at the 24-C$_1$ level with ergosterol in yeast (*100a*), *Mucor pusillus*

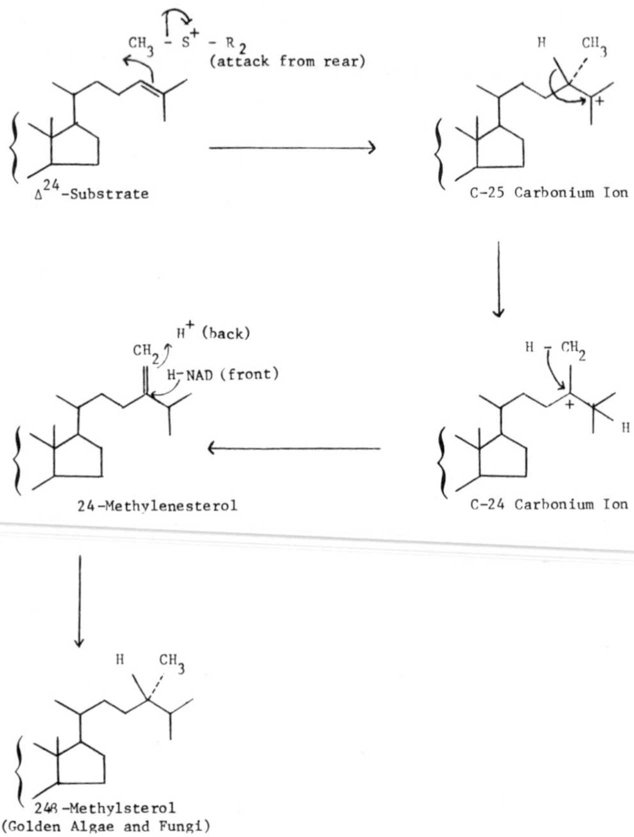

Scheme 9.8. The $\Delta^{24(28)}$-route to 24β-methylsterols in golden algae and fungi.

(*100b*), and *Phycomyces blakesleeanus* (*101*) and by implication from experiments at the 24-C$_2$-level in *Pinus pinea* (*9*) and *Nicotiana tabacum* (*102*) with sitosterol, *Ochromonas malhamensis* with poriferasterol (*103*), *Fucus spiralis* with fucosterol (*104*), and *Monodus subterraneus* with clionasterol (*105*). 4α-Methylergosta-8,24(28)-dien-3β-ol (*106*), ergostatetraenol (*107*), fecosterol (*108*), obtusifoliol (*106*), and episterol (*109*) have also been converted to ergosterol in yeast cultures. Similarly, 24-methylene-24,25-dihydrolanosterol is utilized for the biosynthesis of eburicoic acid (*106*) and ergosterol (*4, 5*) in fungi.

The composite evidence derived from various species of fungi is that: (1) they contain (at the 24-C$_1$ level) only the 24β-configuration (*110a, b*), (2) H migration occurs from C-24 to C-25 (*100a,b, 101*); (3) only two of the H atoms from the methyl group of methionine are found in the sterol (*100b, 101, 111–115*); (4) 24-methylenesterols have been converted to 24β-methylsterols (*4, 5, 106–109*); (5) the $\Delta^{24(28)}$-bond occurs early in the sequence and the Δ^{22}-bond late (6, 108, 109, 116); and (6) mutants of yeast have been obtained lacking the C_1-transferase that still yield sterols with a Δ^{22}-bond (117). The evidence, therefore, is consistent with a pathway via the $\Delta^{24(28)}$-intermediate which is reduced and specifically excludes either a pathway through a $\Delta^{25(27)}$-, $\Delta^{24(25)}$-, or $\Delta^{23(24)}$-intermediate which is reduced or a pathway involving isomerization of the $\Delta^{24(28)}$-bond to the 22-position.

In other organisms reduction of the $\Delta^{24(28)}$-bond may also occur, but the proof for it is equivocal. In *Hordeum vulgare* (barley), 24-methylcholesterol arises with incorporation of only two of the H atoms from methionine (118), and in the pine (*Pinus pinea*) 24-methylenecholesterol proceeds to 24-methylcholesterol (119, 120). While these facts are consistent with direct $\Delta^{24(28)}$-reduction, they are also consistent with isomerization either to a $\Delta^{24(25)}$- or to a Δ^{22}-intermediate, either of which is then reduced. Similarly, in golden algae (*Ochromonas malhamensis* and the diatom *Phaeodactylum tricornutum*) only two H atoms from methionine appear in brassicasterol (97) and its 24-epimer (121), which admits not only of direct reduction of the $\Delta^{24(28)}$-bond but also of the isomerization routes. In the green algae the evidence already discussed (the incorporation of three H atoms from methionine and the presence of cyclolaudenol in them) is best interpreted in terms of a route through a $\Delta^{25(27)}$-sterol. If we assume that all of the information cited at the beginning of this paragraph for various species of fungi applies to each and every species, the configuration of the 24β-methyl group in fungal sterols must be determined by the direction of reduction of the $\Delta^{24(28)}$-bond (Scheme 9.8). If we further assume, by analogy to the known mechanism of reduction of the Δ^{24}- (76, 80), Δ^{7}- (122a), and Δ^{14}- (122b) bonds, that H$^+$ attacks C-28 and that H$^-$ (from reduced pyridine nucleotide) attacks C-24, then hydride ion must attack from the α side of C-24. In the green algae the configuration is apparently determined by the direction of alkylation (Scheme 9.7), since a $\Delta^{25(27)}$-intermediate seems to be involved. In Tracheophytes 24β-methylsterols appear to arise by the $\Delta^{25(27)}$-route, while the 24α-methylsterols are formed through a $\Delta^{24(25)}$-intermediate (via a 24-methylenesterol) (Scheme 9.9) (123).

(c) *Second C_1 Transfer*   In the mechanism first proposed (62) for the second C_1 transfer the π-electrons of a 24-methylene group acted as the acceptor of the electron-deficient methyl group being transferred from *S*-adenosyl methionine. This has been verified in a number of cases, the first

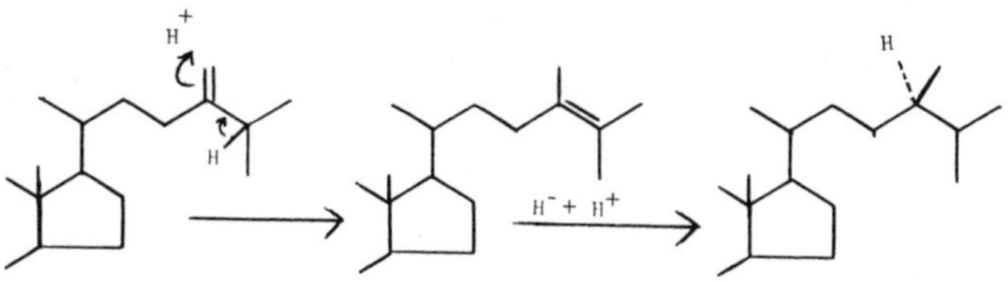

Scheme 9.9. The $\Delta^{24(25)}$-route to 24α-methylsterols in tracheophytes.

of which was the conversion of 24-methylenecholesterol to a 24α-ethylcholesterol (sitosterol) in the tracheophyte *Pinus pinea* (*119, 120*). Subsequently, 24-methylene-24-dihydrolanosterol was found to lead to the Δ^7-analog (spinasterol) of sitosterol in *Spinacea oleracea* (*124*) and to sitosterol itself in *Nicotiana tabacum* (*125*). In the alga *Ochromonas malhamensis*, 24-methylenecycloartanol, 24-methylenelophenol, and obtusifoliol have each yielded the 24β-ethylsterol, poriferasterol (*24, 126, 127*). Furthermore, as mentioned earlier, ethionine and acetyl CoA have been excluded as C_2 sources (*62*), and 24-methylenesterols have been frequently encountered in various plants. Consequently, both for mechanistic and experimental reasons, a 24-methylenesterol is now considered to be an obligatory intermediate to 24-ethylidene- and 24-ethylsterols of both configurations at C-24 and C-28.

A second C_1 transfer to C-28 gives a carbonium ion at C-24, and the 24-H atom of the original $\Delta^{24(25)}$-precursor is at C-25 as a result of the H-migration in the first C_1-transfer (Scheme 9.10). Stabilization of the positively changed intermediate can occur theoretically by elimination of a proton from several positions. The existence of a 24-ethylidenesterol (fucosterol) in brown algae and the possibility that by reduction it could lead to 24-ethylsterols prompted the suggestion (*62*) that the carbonium ion loses a proton from C-28 as in the first C_1 transfer (Scheme 9.10). A 24-ethylidenesterol (isofucosterol) was shortly thereafter discovered in a gymnosperm (*Pinus pinea*) (*120*) and more recently in many other plants. Moreover, 24-methylenecholesterol was experimentally converted to isofucosterol in *Pinus pinea* (*119, 120*) and in the same plant 24-deuteriolanosterol led to 25-deuterioisofucosterol, thereby locating the H atom on the original Δ^{24}-bond (*9*). Retention of this H atom in isofucosterol and its presence at C-25 have also been demonstrated in an angiosperm (*Hordeum vulgare*) (*118*) as well as for fucosterol in the brown alga *Fucus spiralis* (*104*), and 24-ethylidenelophenol in *Hordeum vulgare* contains four atoms of deuterium when biosynthesized with C^2H_3-methionine (*118*). All of this information leaves little doubt that deprotonation can occur from C-28. However, recent evidence shows that deprotonation can occur elsewhere, and although evidence does exist for direct reduction of the $\Delta^{24(28)}$-bond of the 24-ethylidenesterols in golden algae, in tracheophytes the double bond appears first to be isomerized to the $\Delta^{24(25)}$-position (with loss of the H atom originally at C-24) prior to reduction (*123* and Ref. cited therein) (Scheme 9.10).

From a euglenoid (*36*) and from species of the orders Chlorococcales (*128*), Siphonales (*129*), Cucurbitales (*130, 131*), and Verbenales (*132*), 24-ethyl-$\Delta^{25(27)}$-sterols have been isolated, and in all cases (*130–132*) where the asymmetry at C-24 was examined the sterol possessed the β configuration. Furthermore, in a variety of species of the Chlorococcales five H atoms from the methyl group of methionine are incorporated into the 24-ethyl group of the sterol, indicating no intermediacy of a 24-ethylidenesterol (*94–98*), and the H atom originally at C-24 in cycloartenol is found at that position in

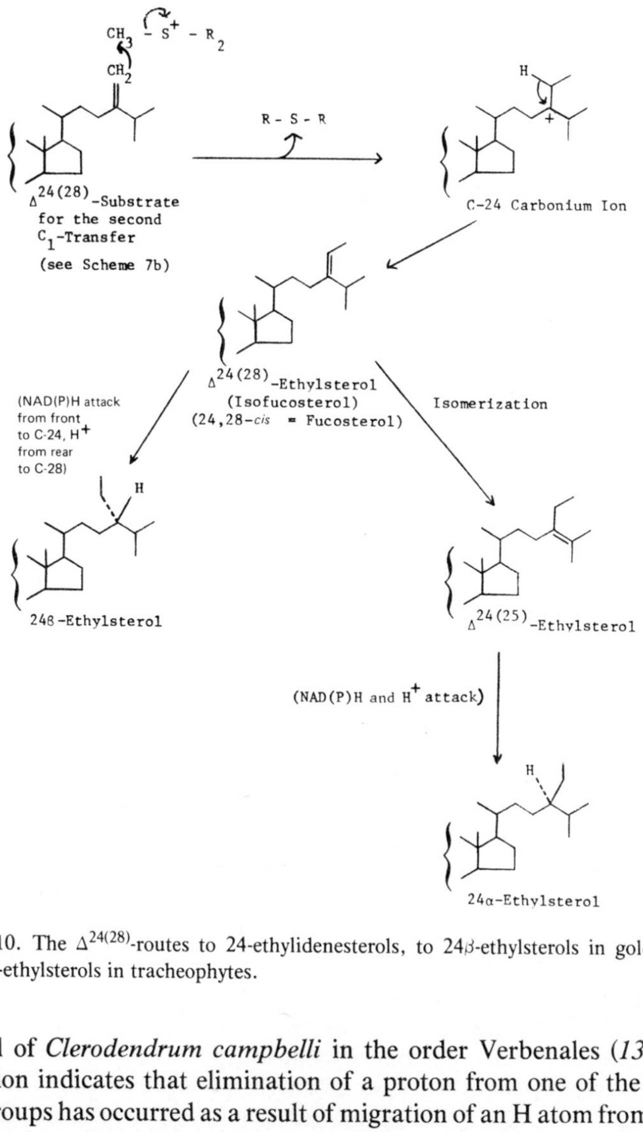

Scheme 9.10. The $\Delta^{24(28)}$-routes to 24-ethylidenesterols, to 24β-ethylsterols in golden algae, and to 24α-ethylsterols in tracheophytes.

the sterol of *Clerodendrum campbelli* in the order Verbenales (*133*). This information indicates that elimination of a proton from one of the *gem*-dimethyl groups has occurred as a result of migration of an H atom from C-25 to C-24 of the 24-ethyl carbonium ion, leaving a positive charge at C-25 (Scheme 9.11). When the *Clerodendrum* sterol was biosynthesized from [2-^{14}C]MVA and the terminal carbon atom of the $\Delta^{25(27)}$-bond was removed by degradation, radioactivity was not lost (*133*). This proved the terminal methylene group is derived from C-3′ of MVA, which we designate C-27 in the sterol.

Of the possible other positions from which a proton could be eliminated after C$_1$ attack on a 24-methylenesterol, there is only experimental work dealing with removal from C-22 with H migration from C-23 to C-24 yielding a Δ^{22}-sterol. This may (*134*) occur in slime molds, but interpretation of the

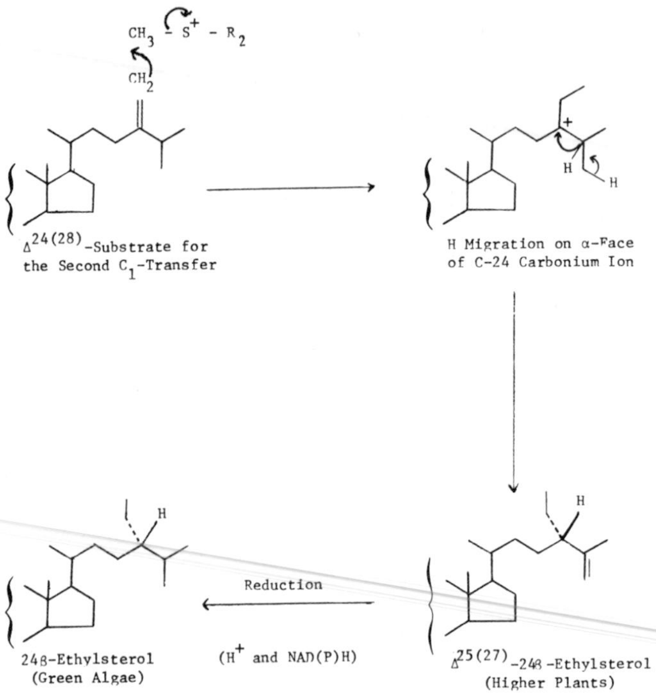

Scheme 9.11. The $\Delta^{25(27)}$-route to 24β-ethylsterols in green algae and to $\Delta^{25(27)}$-24β-ethylsterols in higher plants.

data is equivocal. 24-Ethylcholestanol and its 22-dehydro derivatives are present (135, 136) and both incorporate five H atoms from the methyl group of methionine. However, while this proves that a 24-ethylidenesterol is not an intermediate, attempts (134) to show migration of the H atom from C-23 to C-24 have met with only partial success. When a slime mold was incubated with lanosterol bearing two tritium atoms at C-23, 50% of the label was found at C-24 in the 22-dehydro-24-ethylcholestanol, as the migration process would predict if it were stereospecific, but only 25% was retained at C-23, and in the 24-ethylcholestanol no migration occurred (134). Furthermore, evidence for direct 22-dehydrogenation has been obtained in the conversion of the stanol to the stenol. The equilibrium appears to lie on the side of the Δ^{22}-derivative, since the yield is 4.6% for dehydrogenation and 0.60% for reduction (134).

Direct reduction of the $\Delta^{24(28)}$-bond of 24-ethylidenesterols seems to occur in the golden algae Ochromonas malhamensis and Monodus subterraneus (Scheme 9.10). Only four H atoms from methionine are incorporated into the 24-ethyl group of poriferasterol (97, 137) and clionasterol (105, 135) in which the H atom originally at C-24 has been located at C-25 (103, 105). However, in the tracheophytes, Pinus pinea (123), Larix decidua (138),

Medicago sativa (*139*), *Nicotiana tabacum* (*140*), *Dioscorea tokoro* (*140*), *Spinacea oleracea* (*139*), *Hordeum vulgare* (*118*), *Calendula officinalis* (*141*), and *Cyathula capitata* (*142*), the latter H atom (on C-24) disappears completely in sitosterol, stigmasterol, and spinasterol (depending on the sterol present and studied), but in *H. vulgare* and *C. capitata* it is retained in isofucosterol (*118*) and stigmasta-7, (*trans*)24(28)-dien-3β-ol (*142*). It was located at C-25 as expected. In *H. vulgare*, sitosterol, stigmasterol, and 24-ethylidenelophenol were also found to contain only four H atoms from methionine (*118*). At the present time, the only reasonable interpretation of these various pieces of information is that a 24-ethylidene sterol is formed and subsequently isomerized to a $\Delta^{24(25)}$-sterol by a "push-pull" mechanism in which a proton attacks C-28 and one is eliminated from C-25. The resulting $\Delta^{24(25)}$-sterol is then presumably reduced (Scheme 9.10). Similarly, the $\Delta^{25(27)}$-sterols presumably undergo reduction. The mechanism in the various cases probably is analogous to that demonstrated for the $\Delta^{24(25)}$-bond in mammals (Section C.3). If so, and a proton from water is added to the least substituted carbon atom and a hydride ion from reduced pyridine nucleotide to the most highly substituted one, the source of H atoms at C-28 and C-24 can be predicted for reduction of the $\Delta^{24(28)}$-bond and at C-25 and C-27 for the $\Delta^{25(27)}$-bond. The direction of addition for the symmetrically substituted Δ^{22}- and $\Delta^{24(25)}$-bonds, however, becomes theoretically equivocal. No experimental evidence either for the source or position of H atoms in reduction of any of these double bonds is yet available.

Several reports have appeared showing that sterols, e.g., cholesterol, with a saturated side chain and no 24-alkyl group can lead in *Ochromonas malhamensis* (*143, 144*), *Nicotiana tabacum* (*145*), and invertebrate animals (*146*) to sterols with a 24-C$_1$ or 24-C$_2$ group. Since direct introduction of double bonds has been well documented in both plants and animals, e.g., the Δ^{22}-bond, it seems likely that the saturated side chain is first dehydrogenated at C-24 (*62*) and then alkylated in the normal mechanistic manner (Scheme 9.12). The dehydrogenase is probably the same one operating normally toward reduction. Thus, cycloartenol leads to cholesterol and there is no inherent reason why cholesterol could not lead by the reverse reaction to desmosterol, which then undergoes alkylation in *N. tabacum* or other tracheophytes. In *O. malhamensis*, where the reductase apparently normally operates on the $\Delta^{24(28)}$-bond, if it accepted a conformer of cholesterol in which C-25 is in the place of C-28 (by rotation about the bond between C-23 and C-24), the reductase could catalyze introduction of the $\Delta^{24(25)}$-bond (Scheme 9.12).

In summary, in the tracheophytes a route to 24α-alkysterols seems to occur through isomerization of a $\Delta^{24(28)}$-sterol to a $\Delta^{24(25)}$-sterol that is reduced, but 24β-alkylsterols arise through the intermediacy of $\Delta^{25(27)}$-sterols both in the tracheophytes and in the green algae. In the former case ($\Delta^{24(25)}$-route) the configuration at C-24 presumably is determined by the side (β) from which C-24 is attacked in the reduction. In the latter case ($\Delta^{25(27)}$-route), if

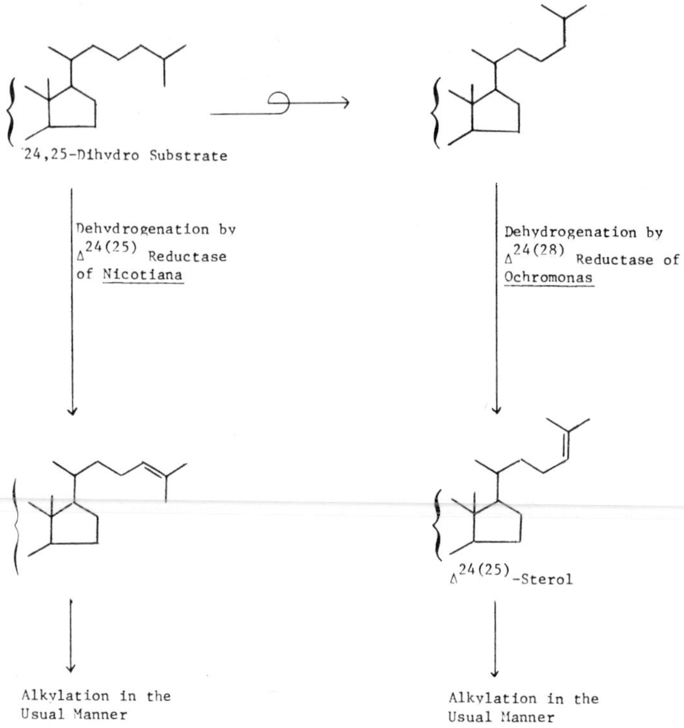

Scheme 9.12. Alkylation of sterols with saturated side chains in *Ochromonas* and *Nicotiana*.

we assume an antiparallel concerted process of C_1 transfer, H migration, and elimination of a proton, the incoming methyl group must attack from the rear (β side) with migration on the α side of the H atom from C-25 to C-24 and elimination of a β-oriented H atom from C-27. β-Side attack of the methyl group also is occurring at the 24-C_1 level in the $\Delta^{25(27)}$-route. In the direct reduction of the $\Delta^{24(28)}$-bond in 24-ethylidenesterols, which appears to occur in the golden algae, the configuration at C-24 is determined by the direction of attack on C-24 (from the α side) in the reduction. It is interesting to note that reduction of a $\Delta^{24(28)}$-bond at the 24-C_1 level in fungi occurs with the same stereochemistry, i.e., 24β-alkyl sterols are produced, as does reduction at the 24-C_2 level in golden algae.

5. Variations of Alkylation Mechanism

If we take the basic character of the mechanism to be reaction between a CH_3^+ donor and the π-electrons of a double bond, a number of possible variations become apparent. They are associated with: (1) the position and origin of the double bond, (2) the direction of addition of the CH_3^+ group, (3) the manner in which the carbonium ion produced is neutralized (loss of

H$^+$ or addition of X$^-$), and (4) the position at which neutralization occurs and whether or not H$^-$ migration occurs. Some of these were discussed in the preceding section (Scheme 9.6). Other variations (Scheme 9.13) are conceivable and some are known.

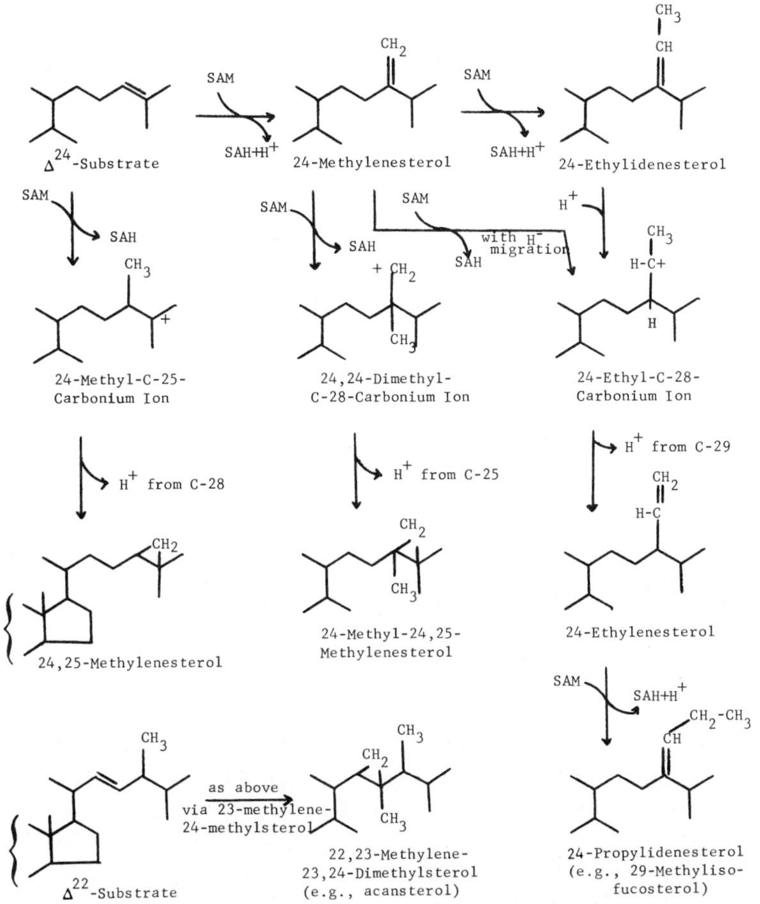

CH$_3$

CH$_2$ CH

SAM   SAM

Δ^{24}-Substrate   SAH+H$^+$ 24-Methylenesterol   SAH+H$^+$ 24-Ethylidenesterol

SAM   SAM   SAM   H$^+$

SAH   SAH   CH$_3$
CH$_3$ with H$^-$ migration   H-C+
                              + CH$_2$ SAH
                                CH$_3$ H

24-Methyl-C-25-   24,24-Dimethyl-   24-Ethyl-C-28-
Carbonium Ion   C-28-Carbonium Ion   Carbonium Ion

H$^+$ from C-28   H$^+$ from C-25   H$^+$ from C-29

                                                CH$_2$
                        CH$_2$ H-C
CH2
                        CH$_3$

24,25-Methylenesterol   24-Methyl-24,25-   24-Ethylenesterol
                        Methylenesterol

                                                SAM
                                                       SAH+H$^+$
                                                        CH$_2$-CH$_3$
CH$_3$ CH$_3$ CH
        CH$_3$ CH$_2$
                              as above
                        via 23-methylene-   CH$_3$
                        24-methylsterol
Δ^{22}-Substrate 22,23-Methylene-   24-Propylidenesterol
                        23,24-Dimethylsterol   (e.g., 29-Methyliso-
                        (e.g., acansterol)   fucosterol)

Scheme 9.13. Some possible variations of alkylation.

While in most cases alkylation stops not later than the second C$_1$ transfer, the 24-ethylidenesterols could undergo two further types of C$_1$ transfer. One would be directly to C-28, yielding, for instance by elimination at C-28 in the usual manner, a 24-isopropylidenesterol. The very crowded environment at C-24 and C-25 might weigh against it, but the existence of such a compound in rare cases would not be surprising. The intermediate carbonium ion would have the favored tertiary structure (at C-24). Although the isopropylidene substituent is so far unknown, a C_3 substituent in the n series has actually been isolated from the scallop *Placopecten magellanicus* (*147*), and more recently from the sponge *Tethya aurantia* (*148*). The compound is *trans*-24-*n*-propylidenecholesterol (29-methylisofucosterol). Also, the *cis* isomer has been isolated from the scallop *Patinopecten yessoensis* (*149*). The origin of these sterols is presumably as usual in a Δ^{24}-substrate, e.g., desmosterol or lanosterol, which is converted to a 24-methylene derivative followed by a second C_1 transfer. The third C_1 transfer must occur, however, in a different way from the normal course of events in that deprotonation ultimately must proceed at C-29 instead of C-28 as a result of H migration or protonation-deprotonation (Scheme 9.7). The resultant olefin, bearing a Δ^{28}-bond instead of a $\Delta^{24(28)}$-bond, can now undergo a third C_1 transfer with elongation of the chain. In view of the lesser stability of secondary (C-28) compared to tertiary (C-24) carbonium ions, this process would be expected to be rare and specialized. Nevertheless, the fact that 29-methylisofucosterol and 29-methylfucosterol occur raises the possibility of the existence of still higher homologs (by further repetition of C_1 transfer with H migration yielding products with a terminal double bond).

The alkylation mechanism also admits of the formation of three-membered rings by elimination of a proton from the attacking methyl group without H migration. Cyclopropyl compounds formed in this way have been well documented in the field of fatty acids (lactobacillic acid, etc.) (*65*), but they have not yet been reported as metabolites of the steroidal Δ^{24}-bond. Nor are they intermediates to the 24-methylsterols, because, while 24-methylenesterols are converted to ergosterol in yeast, the analogous cyclopropyl derivatives (24,25-methylenesterols) fail to yield ergosterol (*135*). On the other hand, analogous cyclopropyl sterols involving C-22 and C-23 have been isolated from marine invertebrates, e.g., (22*R*,23*R*,24*R*)-22,23-methylene-23,24-dimethylcholest-5-en-3β-ol (gorgosterol) and its 23-demethyl derivative (23-demethylgorgosterol) from species of gorgonians of the cnidarian class Anthozoa (*150–155*) and acansterol, the Δ^7-derivative of gorgosterol, from the echinoderm *Acanthaster planci* (*155*). They are presumably formed by alkylation of the Δ^{22}-bond in addition to the Δ^{24}-bond as shown in Scheme 9.7.

Two unusual sterols have been isolated from sponges of the genus *Verongia:* aplysterol (an analog of 24α-methylcholesterol) and 24,28-dehydroaplysterol (an analog of 24-methylenecholesterol) constituting 45% and 25%, respectively, of the total sterol fraction (*156, 157*). These are the only known examples of sterols alkylated at a terminal isopropyl group of the side chain. Such compounds can arise only via alkylation of $\Delta^{25(26)}$- or $\Delta^{25(27)}$-intermediates such as those that are precursors of 24β-methyl and 24β-ethyl sterols in plants (see Section C.4).

6. Dehydrogenation and Dealkylation at C-24

Insects have a nutritional requirement for sterols, and in nearly every case studied cholesterol satisfies this requirement (*158*). In 1959, using the carniverous hide beetle *Dermestes utilpinus* Fabr. (Coleoptera), Clark and Bloch (*159*) found that labeled acetate or fructose fed to the animals failed to yield labeled squalene or sterol, and neither mevalonate nor lanosterol would replace cholesterol as a growth requirement. Clearly, a biosynthetic block was present before the formation of squalene, explaining why cholesterol functions as a growth stimulant. However, many insects are not carniverous and therefore do not have a dietary source of cholesterol. Bergmann (*160*), in fact, had found in the 1930s that the sterol of the silkworm, *Bombyx mori*, is 85% cholesterol despite its feeding exclusively on mulberry leaves. Since it presumably lacks the capacity to biosynthesize cholesterol de novo, it must convert the 24-alkylsterol of the leaves to cholesterol. Other studies also suggested such a conversion. Thus, the nymph of the German cockroach *Blatella germanica* will grow and develop normally on synthetic diets containing ergosterol. This fact provided Clark and Bloch (*161*) with a convenient method of proving dealkylation. Gravid females were placed in a jar with a synthetic diet containing uniformly labeled ergosterol. The resulting nymphs were allowed to feed on the mixture, after which they were killed. Labeled 22,23-dehydrocholesterol was identified as a metabolite, and, when ergosterol labeled at C-28 was present, the metabolite as expected was unlabeled. Subsequently, sitosterol was shown by Robbins and his associates (*162*) to be converted to cholesterol in the cockroach. Sterol biosynthesis in a primitive insect, the firebrat (*Thermobia domestica*), is also known to be blocked (*163*). Many different insect species have been studied subsequently, and all are known to have the ability to dealkylate sitosterol (*158*). To date, the housefly, *Musca domestica*, is the only exception. This insect appears to have lost the ability to dealkylate, because it is unable to convert sitosterol to cholesterol and must rely solely on cholesterol to satisfy its sterol requirement (*164*).

The inability to biosynthesize sterols and the ability to dealkylate exogenous sterol is not confined to insects. Species of free-living and parasitic nematodes require dietary sterol for normal growth and development (*165, 166*). Moreover, it is now known that these nematodes convert plant sterols to cholesterol (*167*). In other invertebrates a dietary sterol requirement has not yet been established, but many organisms are incapable of sterol biosynthesis and dealkylation has been demonstrated in some of these. Both the oyster, *Ostrea gryphea*, and the sea anemone, *Calliactis parasitica*, dealkylate radioactive fucosterol via desmosterol (*168*). At the same time, both animals lack the ability to biosynthesize sterols (*169, 170*). The marine crustaceans *Penaeus japonicus* (prawn) and *Artemia salina* (brine shrimp) cannot biosynthesize sterols de novo; however, sitosterol and 24-methylcholesterol (unknown configuration at C-24) are converted to cholesterol by both animals (*171*). Ergosterol is also utilized by *A. salina* for cholesterol formation (*172*).

The pathway from the 24-alkylsterols to cholesterol has been investigated extensively, especially by Svoboda and Robbins and their associates (*173–179*) using the tobacco hornworm, *Manduca sexta* (Johannson). Stigmasterol yields 22,23-dehydrodesmosterol [cholest-5,22(*trans*), 24-trien-3β-ol] (*176*), and desmosterol itself is a common intermediate from a variety of 24-methyl- or 24-ethylsterols (*173, 175, 178*). 24-Methylenecholesterol (*179*) and *cis*-24-ethylidenecholesterol (fucosterol) (*177*) are also formed, respectively, from 24-methyl- and 24-ethylcholesterol, and labeled fucosterol fed to hornworm larvae is recovered in 80% yield as cholesterol in the pupae (*177*). Evidence for the intermediacy of fucosterol and desmosterol in the conversion of sitosterol to cholesterol in the locust, *Locusta migratoria* L., has similarly been presented (*180*). Clionasterol (labeled at C-25 with tritium and at C-26 with ^{14}C) fed to larvae of the yellow mealworm, *Tenebrio molitor* along with the Δ^{24}-reductase inhibitor, triparanol, resulted in the formation of desmosterol with a ^{3}H/^{14}C atomic ratio of 1:1 (*181*). Acetylation of the recovered desmosterol followed by hydroboration resulted in hydroxylation at C-7 and C-24 with retention of tritium. Tritium was lost when the diol was oxidized to the corresponding C-7 and C-24 dione, demonstrating that the tritium atom was located at C-24 of desmosterol. During dealkylation of the 24-ethylsterol to desmosterol, a migration of the tritium atom from C-25 to C-24 occurred. Previous studies with the same insect had indicated the migration of tritium from C-25 to C-24 during the dealkylation of labeled isofucosterol to cholesterol (*182*). The migration of the C-25 hydrogen atom of [25-^{3}H]sitosterol to C-24 during desmosterol formation has also been observed in larvae of the silkworm, *Bombyx mori* (*183*). Tritium was retained in desmosterol recovered from the incubation. Epoxidation of the benzoate ester of the labeled desmosterol as well as conversion to the 25-methoxy-24-hydroxy derivative resulted in radioactive products. Tritium was lost only when the product was oxidized to the 24-ketone.

It thus seems reasonably certain that the pathway involves dehydrogenation to form the $\Delta^{24(28)}$-bond followed by dealkylation (Scheme 9.14). In the case of 24-methylsterols, exact reversal of the plant alkylation process (Section C.4) would explain the observed facts about intermediates. The dealkylation of 24-ethylsterols probably also occurs by exact reversal. In addition to the common intermediacy of $\Delta^{24(28)}$- and $\Delta^{24(25)}$-sterols is the observation that triparanol inhibits both insect dealkylation of sitosterol (*174*) and plant alkylation of desmosterol (*184*). However, a 24-methylenesterol remains to be demonstrated as an intermediate in removal of the C_2 fragment, and label from sitosterol bearing tritium at C-3 could not be found in 24-methylenecholesterol in the locust (*180*). This could, of course, be a kinetic problem, but protonation of the 24-ethylidenesterol at C-28 followed by transfer of the ethyl group to an acceptor, e.g., *S*-adenosylhomocysteine, cannot yet be absolutely excluded. Finally, it is interesting to note that fucosterol rather than isofucosterol has been reported as the intermediate. These two sterols are difficult to differentiate and the literature does not

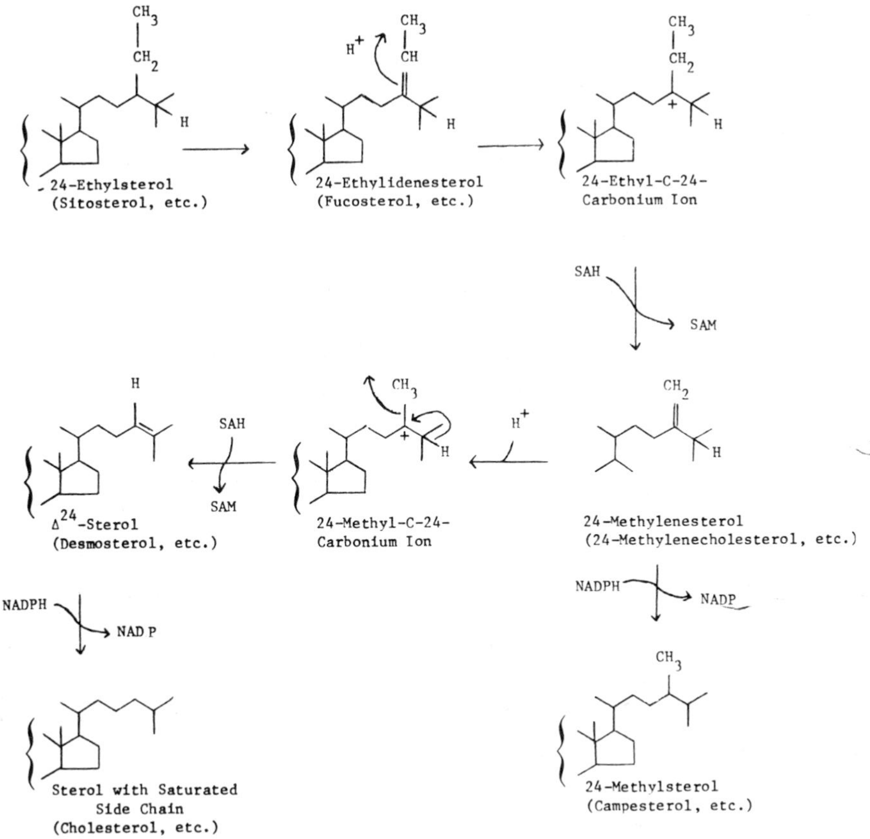

Scheme 9.14. Probable mechanism and pathway of dealkylation at C-24 of sterols in Arthropoda. SAH = S-adenosylhomocysteine, and SAM = adenosylmethionine. If a Δ^{22}-bond is present, a parallel sequence would ensue with or without the addition of Δ^{22}-reduction at some stage.

make it certain that one rather than the other is involved. It will be recalled (Section C.4) that it is the *trans*- rather than the *cis*-ethylidenesterols that seem to be reduced in plants. If fucosterol really is the intermediate in Arthropoda, then the stereochemistry of animal dehydrogenation may be different from the reverse process of reduction in plants; the animal dehydrogenation would also be yielding the isomer expected on stereochemical grounds (Section C.4). Nevertheless, an uncertainty still lies in the nature of the oxidant. The introduction of a double bond into a saturated system would not be expected to be a simple matter, and the origin of the double bond in oleic acid is indeed quite complicated. While one can write a simple reversal of an NADPH-linked reduction, a mixed function oxidase or other complex system may well be involved.

Mechanisms for dealkylation similar to oxidative side chain cleavage of cholesterol to pregnenolone (*185*) or the microbial degradation of pro-gesterone (*186*) have been proposed (*182*). Various intermediates, including 24-keto, 24,28-dihydroxy, 24-hydroxy, 28-hydroxy, 28-keto, and 24-hydroxy, 28-keto sterols, which can be postulated for oxidative cleavage of the C-24 ethyl group of sitosterol, have been considered. Negligible conversion of these steroids to cholesterol was observed in *B. mori* (*187*), *T. molitor* (*182*), or *L. migratoria* (*188*), ruling out any mechanism that mimics known side chain cleavages. However, fucosterol-24,28-epoxide has been implicated as an intermediate in the silkworm (*189*) and the locust (*188*). Fucosterol-24,28-epoxide has been converted to cholesterol by *B. mori* (*189*) in 15% yield and by *L. migratoria* (*188*) in 18% yield. In the same experiment with the silkworm, only 10% conversion of fucosterol to cholesterol was observed. Also, the epoxide supports growth and development of silkworm larvae comparable to cholesterol or sitosterol (*187*). In addition, fucosterol-24,28-epoxide has been tentatively identified after trapping experiments during fucosterol incubations with *B. mori* (*189*). A possible mechanism (*183*) is shown in Scheme 9.15. The intermediacy of the epoxide needs to be inves-tigated more thoroughly and products more rigorously identified because of the instability of fucosterol-24,28-epoxide.

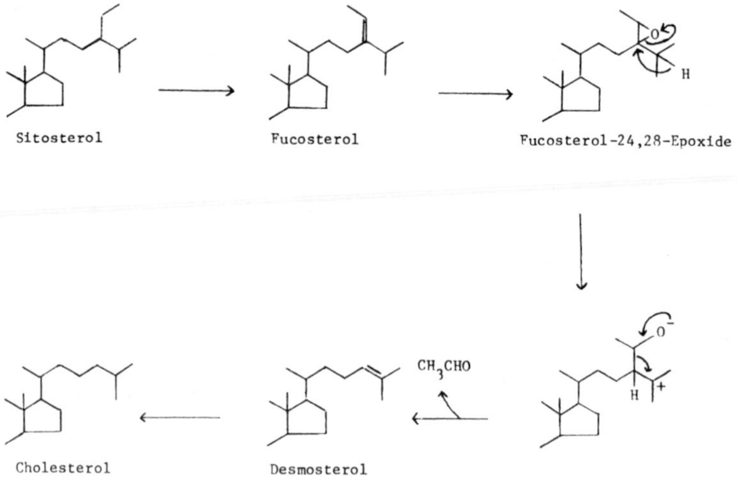

Scheme 9.15. Role of 24(28)-epoxides in dealkylation as proposed by Ikekawa et al. (*183*).

Dealkylation also occurs in the protozoan *Tetrahymena pyriformis* (*190*). However, the mechanism is uncertain. In the first place, unlike insect metabolism, only 24-ethylsterols, and not 24-methylsterols, will dealkylate, and the configuration at C-24 has no effect (*190–194*). Furthermore, neither the *cis*-nor *trans*-isomer of 24-ethylidenecholesterol nor 24-methylenecholesterol will dealkylate, despite efficient incorporation and metabolism by the cells (195). For instance, stigmasterol, cholesterol, sitosterol, and clionasterol yield cholest-5,7,22-trien-3β-ol, but 24-methylenecholesterol and isofucosterol yield only the corresponding 24-methylene and 24-ethylidene derivatives, respectively, of the cholestatriene (Scheme 9.16). A mechanism

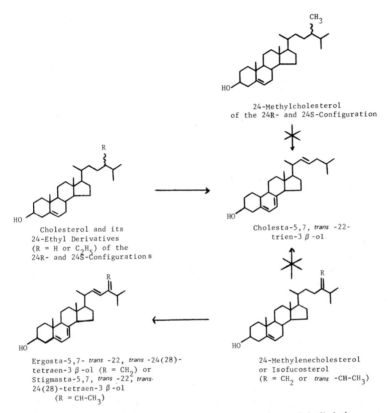

24-Methylcholesterol
of the 24R- and 24S-Configuration

Cholesterol and its
24-Ethyl Derivatives
(R = H or C₂H₅) of the
24R- and 24S-Configurations

Cholesta-5,7, *trans* -22-
trien-3 β -ol

Ergosta-5,7- *trans* -22, *trans* -24(28)-
tetraen-3 β -ol (R = CH₂) or
Stigmasta-5,7, *trans* -22, *trans*-
24(28)-tetraen-3 β -ol
(R = CH-CH₃)

24-Methylenecholesterol
or Isofucosterol
(R = CH₂ or *trans* -CH-CH₃)

Scheme 9.16. Protozoan (*T. pyriformis*) dehydrogenation and dealkylation.

for dealkylation involving oxidation at C-29 and elimination of ethylene with concomitant attack of hydride ion (reduced pyridine nucleotide) at C-24 has been suggested (195). This mechanism implies retention of the C-25 hydrogen atom at C-25. Labeled cholest-5,7,22-trien-3β-ol was isolated from incubations of T. pyriformis with [25-³H, 26-¹⁴C]clionasterol (193). The tritium atom was localized at C-24 according to a method of Akhtar and co-workers (196) by cleavage of the side chain to isovaleric acid and base equilibration of the methyl ester. Dealkylation in T. pyriformis thus involves migration of the C-25 hydrogen atom to C-24 at some point, which is the reverse of what happens in alkylation. These results suggest that a $\Delta^{24(25)}$-bond (analogous to insect dealkylation) may be formed after removal of the C-24 ethyl group. Further work is required to elucidate the exact mechanism, including the degree or type of functionalization of the C-24 ethyl group, cofactors, and the influence, if any of the Δ^{22}-bond.

7. Shortening of Side Chain to C_7

Recently, sterols with less than eight carbon atoms attached to C-17 have been discovered (197–204). The so-called C_{26}-sterols have been observed in marine invertebrates (148, 197, 198, 199–207) and marine phytoplankton (199). The first definitive proof of structure by mass spectroscopy and other means has been obtained for one of them by Idler and his associates (197). The compound, isolated from the scallop *Placopecten magellanicus*, is a 22-dehydrocholesterol lacking the equivalent of C-24. A synthetic sample has the same properties as the natural material (208). It has been given the systematic and equivalent names "22-*trans*-24-norcholest-5,22-dien-3β-ol" (197) and "22-*trans*-26,27-bisnorergosta-5,22-dien-3β-ol" (208), but no evidence exists for the position of the carbon atom(s) actually eliminated. All of the C_{26}-sterols thus far isolated contain a Δ^{22}-bond, with the exception of two sterols from the tunicate *Halocynthia roretzi* (198, 200). The degree of nuclear unsaturation varies, however, and may be Δ^0, Δ^5, Δ^7. As shown in Scheme 9.17, one can arrive theoretically at the C_7 side chain by variations of the alkylation-dealkylation process in which it is not C-24 that is lost but one (or both) of the terminal methyl groups (C-26 or C-27). In mechanism a, protonation of a Δ^{24}-substrate at C-24 and H migration would yield the same C-24 carbonium ion expected in reduction. However, instead of H⁻ addition, C_1 transfer of a terminal methyl group to an acceptor (perhaps S-adenosylhomocysteine) could occur with the production of a 26 (or 27)-desmethyl-Δ^{24}-sterol. Reprotonation to give a desmethyl C-24 carbonium ion and migration of the remaining methyl group to C-24 with concomitant or stepwise reduction would yield the observed side chain. If desmosterol were the Δ^{24}-substrate, "24-norcholesterol" [really a rearranged 26 (or 27)-nor-cholesterol] would result. Superimposition of 22,23-dehydrogenation at some stage would yield Δ^{22}-C-26-sterols. 22-Dehydrocholesterol commonly occurs with the C_{26}-sterols in the same organism (199, 201, 203–207, 209) and could act as substrate by 24,25-dehydrogenation to 22-dehydrodesmosterol, or it may be that the latter is the substrate with the former its alternative metabolite. 24-Methylenecholesterol is another of the sterols in scallops and other molluscs (210, 211), also commonly occurring with C_{26}-sterols, and it could serve as the starting material in mechanism b. This entails protonation at C-28, C_1 transfer of C-26 or C-27 yielding what is tantamount to a rearranged desmosterol, followed by a second protonation at C-25, C_1 transfer of the remaining C-26 or C-27, and reduction of the 26,27-bisdesmethyl-24-methyl-Δ^{24}-sterol to "24-norcholesterol," which in this case would really be a 26,27-bisdesmethyl-24-methylcholesterol. A third mechanism (not shown),

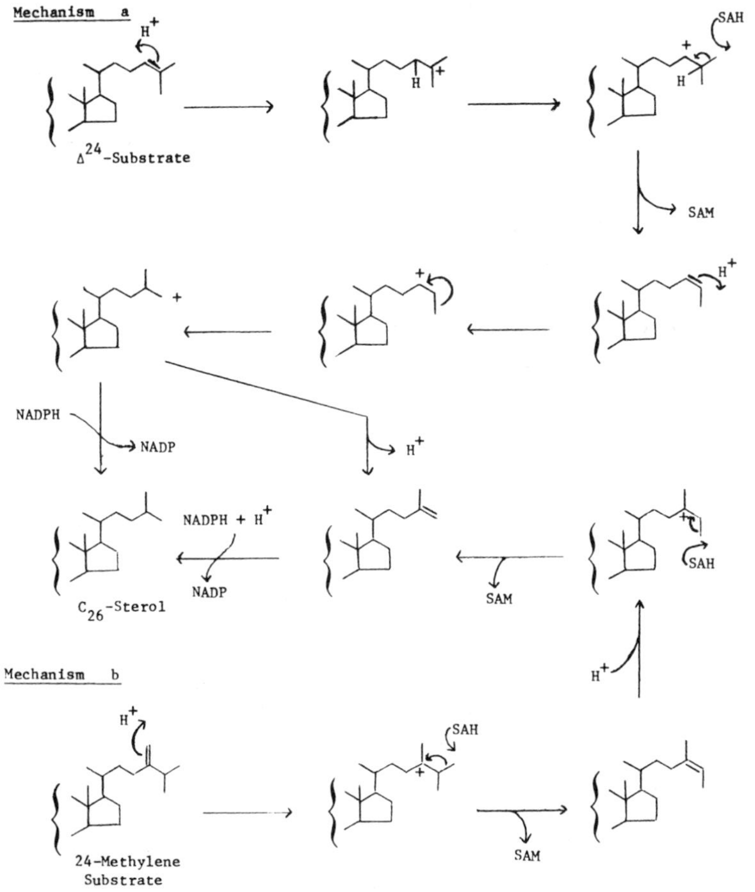

Scheme 9.17. Two possible mechanisms and pathways for the formation of a C_7 side chain.

related to one suggested (*212*) in another connection, is a slight variant of mechanism b in which C-26 (or C-27) and C-28 become scrambled. For instance, after protonation of the 24-methylene group, the C-24 carbonium ion could undergo a rearrangement, with C-26 (or C-27) moving to C-24, and C-28 moving to C-25 to take the place of C-26 (or C-27). The rest of the process as shown in Scheme 9.17 could follow. The only difference is that the added migrations would incorporate C-28 into the final norcholesterol as one of the *gem*-dimethyl groups. The capacity for a process of this sort may also be present in mammals. Aged samples of 24-[28-^{14}C]methylene-cholesterol have been reported to yield labeled cholesterol (*213*). Since freshly prepared samples are not metabolized (*214*), the results may be due to prior rearrangement to 24-[28-^{14}C]methyldesmosterol, which, upon protonation at C-24 and H migration, would give the 24-methyl C-24 carbonium ion of Scheme 9.17.

Results from a recent study by Barbier and co-workers (204) indicate that the C_{26} sterols may not arise by de novo biosynthesis from acetate or mevalonate. The red alga *Rhodymenia palmata* efficiently incorporated these substrates into various C_{27}-, C_{28}-, and C_{29}-sterols. The most heavily labeled of these sterols were 22,23-dehydrocholesterol and 24-methylene cholesterol, but radioactive C_{26}-sterols could not be detected. Seasonal variations in sterol synthesis are not ruled out by these results.

If one or more of the mechanisms suggested here should prove to occur biologically, some heretofore unexpected sterols could exist, e.g., 26-(or 27)-desmethyl sterols and 24-methyl-26(or 27)-desmethyl sterols. It is worthy of note that the latter group would possess 27 carbon atoms in the cholesterol series and might be very difficult to separate and distinquish from the normal *gem*-dimethyl analogs. Chromatographic properties would probably be unaltered, and only slight differences should occur in mass spectra and nuclear magnetic resonance and infrared spectra. It is by no means impossible that they represent or accompany some of the cholesterol already isolated from various sources, e.g., marine invertebrates, where complex mixtures of sterols exist. Indeed, only recently three 27-nor sterols have been recovered from various marine invertebrates differing only in nuclear double bonds (Δ^5, Δ^7, or Δ^0) (149, 215, 216). All possess a *trans*-Δ^{22}-bond and a 24α-methyl group, but lack the C-27 carbon atom.

D. REMOVAL OF METHYL GROUPS AT C-4 AND C-14

1. General Comments

In the absence of appropriate functional groups, it is not theoretically possible to eliminate a methyl group for mechanistic reasons, and no such direct removal is known in biochemistry. In general, it is necessary to have an electron sink in the β-position. The loss of the methyl carbon atom can then ensue with formation of a double bond. However, there must also be an electron source. In the most well-studied case, viz., decarboxylation of a β-keto acid, which occurs, for instance, in the Krebs cycle, the electron sink is a keto group and the electron source is the bond between the acidic proton and the oxygen atom attached to it (or perhaps more properly the negative carboxylate oxygen atom following ionization). In the Krebs cycle, the achievement of functionality appropriate to this mechanism is the reason for the conversion of citrate (a tertiary α-hydroxy acid) to isocitrate (a secondary β-hydroxy acid) to oxalosuccinate (a β-keto acid), which can now lose CO_2. Less well studied but apparently operating in insect dealkylation of 24-alkylsterols, e.g., the conversion of sitosterol to cholesterol (Section C.6), is a process in which an intact methyl could be transferred to an electron source such as S-adenosylhomocysteine. The reverse of the latter process clearly operates in the formation of 24-alkylsterols and branched-chain fatty acids (Section C.4).

2. Elimination from C-4

It was recognized as early as 1957 that the methyl groups on C-4 in mammalian lanosterol are expired quantitatively as carbon dioxide (*217*), suggesting the operation of the β-keto acid route. A few years later Bloch and his associates (*218*) indirectly demonstrated the expected oxidation at C-3 by showing the original 3α-H atom was lost in proceeding to cholesterol. Despite considerable effort, direct proof for the structure of intermediates, especially carboxylic acids, was initially difficult to obtain. Pudles and Bloch (*219*) succeeded in showing that incubation of 4-hydroxymethylenecholest-7-en-3-one aerobically with a liver homogenate led to CO_2 and cholesterol, which was consistent with the β-keto acid route. Furthermore, a variety of polycyclic isopentenoids have been found in nature, particularly plants, which bear an oxidized methyl group at C-4. However, it was the elegant enzymological work in Gaylor's laboratory (*220–229*) that brought forward definitive proof for the principle events in the pathway.

Gaylor was able to study the rates of reaction and to force intermediates to accumulate using purified enzyme preparations, various substrates, and manipulation of cofactor concentrations. Thus, Swindell and Gaylor (*220*) incubated 4,4-dimethyl-5α-cholest-7-en-3β-ol in the absence of exogenous NADPH. Among the products were CO_2 and the corresponding monomethyl-3-ketone, 4-methyl-5α-cholest-7-en-3-one. Similarly, 4α-methyl-5α-cholest-7-en-3β-ol led to CO_2 and 5α-cholest-7-en-3-one. The ketones were then reducible to the 3β-alcohols in the presence of NADPH. While isolation of the ketone products proved a part of the previously assumed pathway, Swindle and Gaylor (*220*) unexpectedly found the 3β-alcohols but not the corresponding ketones would undergo methyl hydroxylation, and only the 3β-alcohols would undergo demethylation by washed microsomes. Simple enzymatic specificity for 3-hydroxy versus 3-keto substrates does not appear to be the entire explanation, for Rahimtula and Gaylor (*224*) demonstrated the substrate in the final step in removal of the carbon atom to be a 3β-alcohol and the reaction NAD^+-dependent. This final substrate had been isolated earlier by Miller and Gaylor (*222*) through an elimination of NAD^+ from the incubate. In the presence of oxygen and an NADPH-generator, 4α-methyl-5α-cholest-7-en-3β-ol led to 3β-hydroxy-5α-cholest-7-en-4α-carboxylic acid. The same acid was isolated independently from incubations of 24,25-dihydrolanosterol with an acetone powder of rat liver microsomes in the absence of NAD (*230*). It was this β-hydroxy acid that underwent the NAD-dependent decarboxylation with formation of the demethylated ketone. As Miller and Gaylor (*221*) point out, 3-ketones must be produced during, not before, decarboxylation. It is not entirely clear what the exact meaning of this is in terms of mechanism. The possibility has been raised that decarboxylation, which occurs ten times faster than the overall demethylation, may actually be nonenzymatic (*224*), implying that the NAD-dependent decarboxylase is essentially or exclusively simply a 3β-ol-dehydrogenase. This is not fully satisfying, since enzymatic separation of the NAD-dependent oxidation of the 3-hydroxy group and NADPH-dependent reduction of the 3-keto group do not then have a logical explanation. However, the facts can be resolved by assuming true, simultaneous, oxidative decarboxylation (mechanism b in Scheme 9.18) to be operating. The single-step mechanism

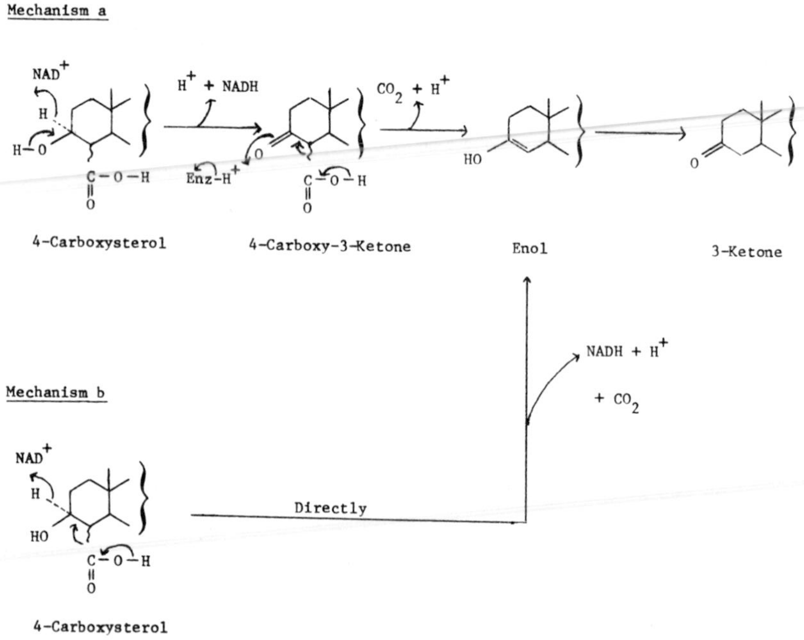

Scheme 9.18. Possible mechanisms for decarboxylation. Mechanism b offers an explanation for the known microsomal sequence. Mechanism a may operate in soluble, more primitive systems.

differs from stepwise oxidation and decarboxylation (mechanism a) in that removal of the 3α-H atom by NAD becomes an integral part of the electron flow in removal of CO_2. In both mechanisms an enol should be produced that then isomerizes to the ketone. The actual intermediacy of the enol is supported by information on the stereochemistry discussed at the end of this section.

The experimental information so far discussed proves the existence of the β-keto acid route either as such or in a modified form and also proves a preferred microsomal sequence exists (in rat liver) in which the methyl group of a 3-hydroxy steroid becomes oxidized to the carboxyl stage prior to oxidation at C-3. The question then arises as to the manner in which the methyl group becomes a carboxyl group. Gaylor (221-223) has demonstrated a requirement for oxygen and NADPH as expected for the initial hydroxylation, but unexpectedly his work shows a similar microsomal requirement for formation of the carboxylic acid (223). A recent investigation of the stoichiometry of the oxidation reaction using sensitive oxygen electrodes to measure oxygen uptake and spectrophotometric monitoring of NADH oxidation reveals that when 4α-hydroxymethyl-5α-cholest-7-en-3β-ol is the substrate for demethylation, two equivalents each of oxygen and NADH are consumed for each methyl group oxidized to the corresponding acid (225). Furthermore, the complete inhibition of oxygen uptake, of oxidation of the methyl groups, and of NADH utilization by cyanide was observed. This inhibition, in addition to the requirement for reduced pyridine nucleotides and the observed stoichiometry of oxygen and NADH utilization, suggests that the oxidizing enzyme is a mixed-function oxidase that catalyzes stepwise oxidation of the C-4 methyl groups to the acid. The intermediacy of a C-4 formyl steroid has been established by Clayton and co-workers (231), who observed that demethylation of 4α-formyl, 4β-methyl-cholestanol occurred at a rate similar to demethylation of the analogous acid.

Isolation and/or properties of the enzymes that catalyze the three steps of C-4 demethylation, 1) oxidation, 2) decarboxylation, and 3) reduction, have been determined. A microsomal mixed-function oxidase, specific only for the 4α-methyl group of 4,4-dimethyl sterols (222), produces the carboxylic acid in the presence of NADPH and O_2 in a stepwise fashion (225). The rate of oxidation increases with each higher oxidation state (223). Further metabolism of the 4α-carboxylic acid occurs only in the presence of a NAD^+-dependent decarboxylase that has been partially purified from rat liver microsomes by chromatography on DEAE-Sephadex A-50 (224). The product is a 4α-methyl-3-ketone. The enzyme has a K_m of 7μm, a V_{max} of 95 nmol/min/mg of protein, a pH optimum of 9.0, and is inhibited by Zn^{++}, but not by CN^-, Fe^{++}, glutathione, Mg^{++}, isocitrate, β-hydroxyglutarate, or various Δ^4-3-keto steroids (224). A NADPH-dependent 3-ketosteroid reductase catalyzes the final step, reduction of the 3-ketone to a 3β-alcohol. This enzyme has been partially purified from rat liver microsomes (228, 229), but its properties have not been established. In the case of the 4,4-dimethyl substrate, the same enzymes presumably catalyze the removal of the remaining methyl group.

The results from a recent study (227) seem to explain the observation that NAD^+ is the only cofactor required for demethylase activity (226). Treatment of rat liver microsomes with snake venom or phospholipase A results in almost complete loss of NAD^+-dependent demethylase activity (227). However, the maximal rates of two of the component reactions, decarboxylation and oxidation, were unaffected. Full demethylase activity is restored by the addition of reduced pyridine nucleotide or the supernatant from snake venom treatment, which appears to be able to supply reducing equivalents. Further investigation revealed that an endogenous NAD^+-dependent cytochrome b_5-reducing system present in the untreated microsomes was solubilized by snake venom. A rat liver microsomal alcohol dehydrogenase, which was partially purified from the snake venom supernatent, appears to supply reducing equivalents to the endogenous NAD^+ reducing system.

The sequence of C-4 demethylation is monohydroxylation of the 4,4-dimethyl substrate, oxidation of the CH_2OH group to the carboxyl stage, oxidative decarboxylation, reduction of the 4-monomethyl-3-ketone to the 4-monomethyl-3β-alcohol and repetition to give the 4-desmethyl-3β-alcohol. What if any preferences are involved in which of the stereochemically different methyl groups at C-4 undergo demethylation first, and what is the stereochemistry of the intermediate 4-monomethyl compound? The answer to both questions is known. The first one is empirical, but the second one has a theoretical basis. After decarboxylation, an enol should be formed (Schemes 9.18 and 9.19). In the sequence for removal of the first methyl group, this enol will retain the second methyl group at C-4, but C-4 is no longer asymmetric. Ketonization, which once again establishes asymmetry, could lead then either to an α- or β-oriented methyl group. On grounds of stability, one would predict the equatorial (α-oriented) configuration. Indeed, nearly all 4-monomethylsterols that have been isolated from either plants or animals possess the 4α configuration. Examples are lophenol (4α-methyl-5α-cholest-7-en-3β-ol) and its 24,25-dehydro, 24-methylene, 24-ethylidene (citrostadienol), 24-methyl, and 24-ethyl derivatives, as well as 4α-methyl-5α-ergosta-8,24(28)-dien-3β-ol, 4α-methyl-5α-cholesta-8,24(25)-dien-3β-ol, 30-norlanosterol, and 30-norcycloartenol. It is the equatorial 4α-methyl group which is lost first in both plants and animals. That is, the 4β-methyl is retained and becomes the 4α-methyl group. This fact, presumably for the reasons given, has been beautifully demonstrated by Clayton and his associates (232) through experiments which depend on the fact that it is the 4α-methyl group which theoretically and demonstrably (233) is derived from C-2 of mevalonate. When [2-^{14}C]MVA labeled also with tritium at C-5 was incubated (232) with a rat liver homogenate, labeled squalene, lanosterol, 4,4,14α-trimethyl-5α-cholest-8-en-3β-ol, 4α-methyl-5α-cholest-7-en-3β-ol, and cholesterol were isolated. From $^3H/^{14}C$ ratios, the extent of ^{14}C labeling of the methyl group in the monomethyl compound could be ascertained. It was found to lack label, proving that it was derived from the 4β-methyl group. Actual values were 10.65 for squalene and 12.83 for the monomethyl sterol. Theory for the latter value would have predicted 12.78. Somewhat simpler but equally decisive evidence (234) is that 4β-methyl-4α-hydroxymethylcholestanol proceeds to cholesterol in 25% yield in a rat liver homogenate, but the epimeric 4α-methyl-4β-hydroxymethylcholestanol is not converted at all. Ubiquity for the process is attested to by evidence (235)

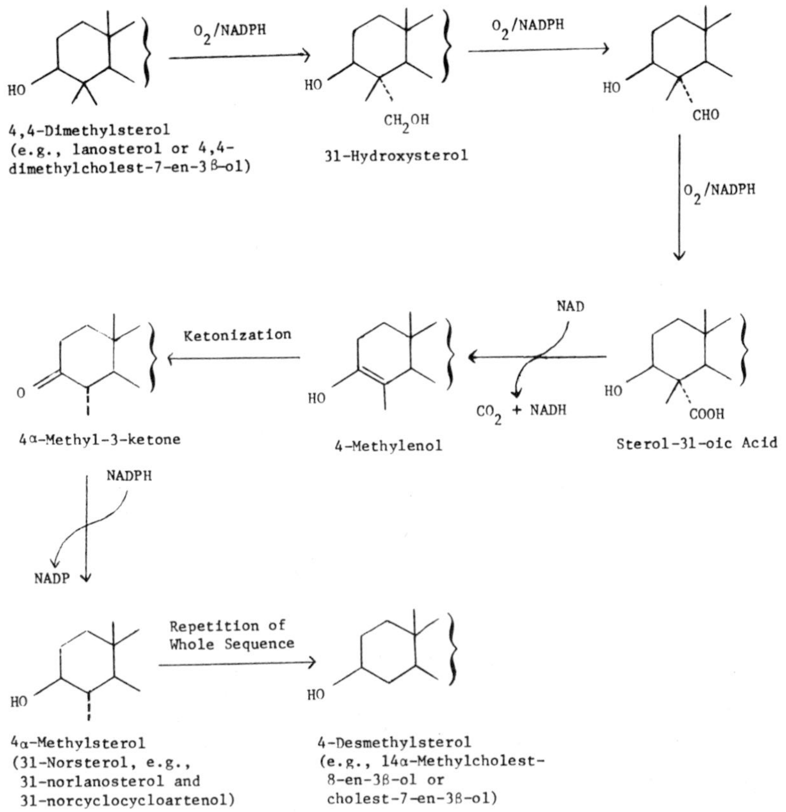

Scheme 9.19. Pathway of demethylation at C-4.

for the loss of the 4α-methyl group of cycloartenol in proceeding to 30-nor-cycloartenol (bearing a 4α-methyl group) in the plant kingdom (*Polypodium vulgare*) and also the 4α-methyl group of 24-methylene cycloartenol or cyclolaudenol in the formation of cycloeucalenol or 30-norcyclolaudenone by banana. However, in fungal (*Fusidium coccineum*) biosynthesis of the 4α-methyl protosteroid, fusidic acid, all six carbon atoms originating in C-2 of MVA are retained (*236*). This suggests strongly that the 4β-methyl group is removed first (*236*). There is, of course, no obvious theoretical reason why one or the other should be removed preferentially except as a result of chance mutations in the evolution of the hydroxylase, which then becomes fixed in a given genetic line. As expected theoretically, however, not only is fusidic acid the more stable 4α-methyl product, but double-labeling experiments have shown (*236*) the original 3α-H atom at C-3 is lost, in keeping with oxidation at C-3 before or during decarboxylation.

Despite the weight of experimental evidence and theoretical argument, there exist in the literature three reports of the isolation of 4β-methyl sterols, i.e., 4β-methyl-5α-cholesta-8,24-dien-3β-ol, from the skins of rats treated with triparanol (237, 238) or from rat liver homogenates incubated with MVA in the presence of cholesta-3β,5α,6β-triol (239). These, however, appear to be incorrect. The infrared spectrum of synthetic 4β-methyl-5α-cholest-8-en-3β-ol revealed marked discrepancies in the 1350–700-cm^{-1} region when compared with the material isolated from rats. Moreover, when the synthetic 4β-methyl steroid was incubated with rat liver homogenate, no cholesterol was detected. These results are in agreement with the previous findings by Clayton and his colleagues (234) of the inability of rat liver to metabolize 4β-methyl-3β-hydroxy steroids.

The loss of the 3α-hydrogen atom during demethylation also appears to be universal. Fucosterol, sitosterol, 30-norcycloartenol, cycloeucalenol, and 30-norcyclolaudenone do not retain a 3α tritium atom when biosynthesized from (4R)-[4-^{3}H$_1$]MVA (104, 141, 235, 241–243) in peas, P. vulgare, Fucus spiralis, marigold, or banana.

The basic demethylation pathway is summarized in Scheme 9.19 without regard to many of the mechanistic problems or to other problems of sequence. Notably ignored is the question of whether the 14α-methyl group is removed preferentially before, during, or after demethylation at C-4. Present evidence indicates removal of the 14α-methyl group frequently occurs first, especially in higher animals and fungi. Also ignored are the lanosterol-cycloartenol and alkylation-reduction bifurcations.

3. Elimination from C-14

Demethylation at C-14 is not as well understood as C-4 demethylation. The C-14 methyl group (C-32 of lanosterol) is expired as CO_2 in animals (217), which suggests oxidation to the carboxyl stage followed by decarboxylation (217, 219). Recent experiments in the laboratories of Akhtar and Barton and their associates (244) indicate, however, that removal of the C-32 carbon atom of lanosterol occurs at the aldehyde stage of oxidation. Radioactive formic acid was isolated from incubations of [32-^{3}H]lanost-7-ene-3β,32-diol with liver microsomes under aerobic conditions in the presence of a NADPH generator. Moreover, in the absence of NADPH (generator), the 32-formyl steroid could be recovered unchanged. 4,4-Dimethylcholesta-7,14-dien-3β-ol was the only steroid product recovered from the demethylation incubations. Absence of formation of 32-formyl steroid (and the $\Delta^{7,14}$-diene product) in the presence of NAD$^+$ or NADP$^+$ (under anaerobic conditions) eliminates oxidation of the C-32 carbon atom via a conventional alcohol dehydrogenase. Cytochrome P-450 may participate, possibly at the level of formation of the 32-hydroxy steroid (245). The exact mechanism of oxidation and cleavage as well as characteristics of the enzyme(s) involved are as yet unknown.

Some sort of involvement of the Δ^8-bond in removal of the 14α-methyl group has been very strongly indicated in rat liver by the complete failure of 4,4,14α-trimethylcholestanol to proceed to cholesterol under conditions in which the 8,9-dehydro derivative (24,25-dihydrolanosterol) yields cholesterol in a 55% yield (*234*). Exactly what assistance is provided remains something of a mystery. The simplest mechanism involving the Δ^8-bond would be protonation at C-9, allowing loss of CO_2 with double-bond migration yielding a $\Delta^{8(14)}$-sterol (Scheme 9.20, mechanism a). Indeed, $\Delta^{8(14)}$-sterols

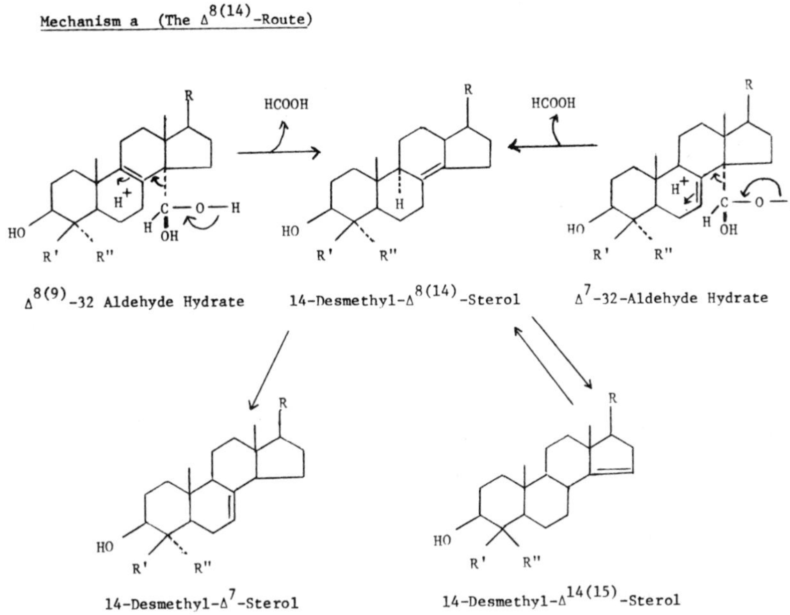

Mechanism a   (The $\Delta^{8(14)}$-Route)

$\Delta^{8(9)}$-32 Aldehyde Hydrate   14-Desmethyl-$\Delta^{8(14)}$-Sterol Δ^7-32-Aldehyde Hydrate

14-Desmethyl-Δ^7-Sterol   14-Desmethyl-$\Delta^{14(15)}$-Sterol

Scheme 9.20. The $\Delta^{8(14)}$-monoene route for removal of the 14α-methyl group. R, side chain; R' and R'' are CH_3 or H.

have been isolated both from rat skin, where 5α-choles-8(14)-en-3β-ol is found (*246, 247*), and from the "rayless goldenrod" (*Aplopappus heterophyllus*), which contains stigmast-8(14),22-dien-3β-ol (*248*). In addition, 4,4-dimethylcholest-8(14)-en-3β-ol has been converted to cholesterol (*249*), as has the 4-desmethyl analog, cholest-8(14)-en-3β-ol (*246*). However, the problem is more complicated than these experiments suggest.

In the course of studies by Goodwin and his colleagues (*250, 251*) on the use of 3R-[2-^{14}C-(2S)-2-^{3}H$_1$]MVA [labeling lanosterol at 1α,7β,15α,22S, 26 (or 27) and 30 (or 31) and its 2R-isomer (labeling lanosterol epimerically) to study the stereochemistry of H elimination at C-7, they observed using rat liver that the 15α-H of lanosterol is missing from cholesterol while the 15β-H is retained. Canonica et al., in Paoletti's laboratory, simultaneously observed the same phenomenon (*252, 253*), as did Akhtar a year later (*254*). The configuration of the 15β hydrogen atom of lanosterol becomes inverted and assumes the 15α orientation during cholesterol biosynthesis (*255*). Inversion of the 15β hydrogen atom to 15α has also been noted in sitosterol and 5α-cholesta-7,24-dien-3β-ol biosynthesized by pea seedlings and by yeast, respectively, from (3RS,2R)-[2-^{14}C, 2-^{3}H]MVA (39, 256). Thus, in some way the 15-position is involved and involved stereospecificity. Although it is generally ignored, Barton and Bruun (257) isolated 14,15-dehydroergosterol from a strain of *Aspergillus niger* as early as 1951.

More recently, the possible role of an 8,14-diene was considered (258), and evidence has been presented for the biosynthesis and metabolic intermediacy of $\Delta^{8,14}$-sterols in cholesterol formation in rat liver (122b, 258–263). In particular, the conjugated dienes, 4,4-dimethylcholesta-8,14-dien-3β-ol (259) and its 4-desmethyl derivative (262) are present. Canonica et al. (258) were the first to obtain conversion of tritiated 4,4-dimethylcholest-8,14-dien-3β-ol to cholesterol by rat liver homogenate (22% conversion of the substrate labeled at C-5, -6, or -7). Substrates labeled at C-2 or C-3 formed cholesterol or ergosterol in much greater yields. Ergosterol was produced in 60% yield by yeast from 5α-ergosta-8,14-dien-3β-ol (260), while similar results were obtained independently by two groups for the metabolism of 5α-cholesta-8,14-dien-3β-ol to cholesterol by rat liver cell-free systems [i.e., 60% (263) and 54% (122b)]. In the latter study, 24,25-dihydrolanosterol, lanosterol, and 4,4-dimethylcholesta-8,14-dien-3β-ol also formed cholesterol in 10%, 24%, and 17% yield, respectively. Furthermore, the $\Delta^{8,14}$-dienes are reduced in rat liver to the $\Delta^{8(9)}$-derivatives (122b). The direction of reduction is H$^+$ to C-15 (15β) and H$^-$ (from NADPH) to C-14 (14α) (122b). These results imply an overall *trans*-reduction of the $\Delta^{14(15)}$-bond coupled with inversion at C-15 of the original 15β hydrogen atom of lanosterol (see discussion). Additional evidence discussed in Section H.3 also supports the intermediacy of 8,14-dienes.

The 8,14-dienes offer a ready explanation for the loss of the 15α-H atom (although alternative explanations are possible, e.g., rapid equilibration of the $\Delta^{8(14)}$-and $\Delta^{14(15)}$-sterols would also lead to the loss of a 15-H atom). In fact, $\Delta^{8,14}$-sterols have been found to occur naturally in *Aspergillus niger* (257) and *Vernonia anthelmintica* (264). It is attractive to believe that the dienes originate concomitantly with elimination of the C-14 methyl group. The $\Delta^{8(9)}$-bond might then function by stabilizing the π-electronic system through conjugation, thus facilitating decarbonylation. Two routes for introduction of the $\Delta^{14(15)}$-bond are immediately conceivable. One is via 15α-hydroxylation followed by elimination of the hydroxyl group and formate. Another is direct oxidative removal (by NAD, etc.) of the 15α-H atom, with elimination of formate (Scheme 9.21, mechanism b). In either event the group attached to or attacking the 15-position would act as the electron sink to allow the bond-breaking reaction at C-14. A 15-hydroxysterol (one of the 15-epimers of 14α-methylcholest-7-en-3β,15-diol) is actually converted to cholesterol by rat liver (265), and an analogy for direct oxidative decarbonylation, bypassing the hydroxy or ketonic derivative, exists in demethyla-

Mechanism b (The Conjugated Diene Route)

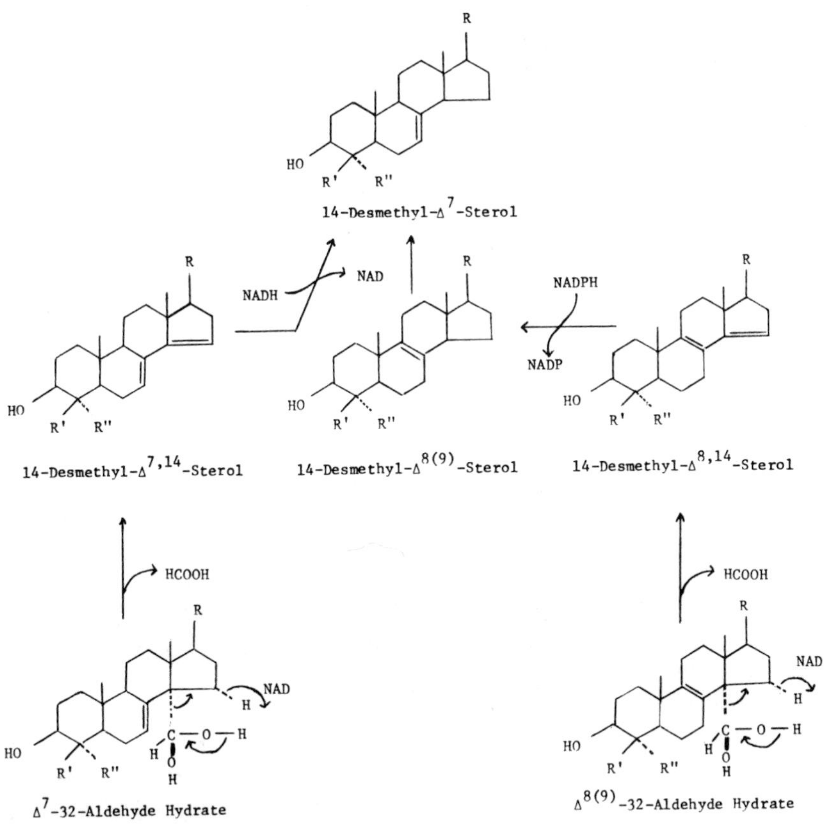

R
HO
R' R''
14-Desmethyl-Δ7-Sterol
NADH
NAD
NADPH
NADP
14-Desmethyl-Δ7,14-Sterol
14-Desmethyl-Δ8(9)-Sterol
14-Desmethyl-Δ8,14-Sterol
HCOOH
NAD
H
C—O—H
O
Δ7-32-Aldehyde Hydrate
Δ8(9)-32-Aldehyde Hydrate

Scheme 9.21. The conjugated diene route for removal of the 14α-methyl group. R, side chain; R′ and R′′ are CH_3 or H.

tion at C-4 (Scheme 9.18 and Section D.2). The direct route is mechanistically and energetically simpler and consequently the more attractive, in which case the observed utilization of the 15-hydroxysterol would be relegated to an artifact of the decarbonylase, probably through nonspecific protonation on the oxygen atom and removal of water. The question could be solved if the decarbonylase accepting a $\Delta^{8(9)}$-32-formyl steroid were found to be NAD dependent without an oxygen requirement.

It has been established, however, that the enzyme produces demethylated product only under aerobic conditions in the presence of NADPH (*244*). This fact does not eliminate the possibility that the various steps of C-14 oxidative demethylation, i.e., C-14 oxidation and decarbonylation, have separate cofactor requirements, analogous to the various steps of C-4 demethylation. The intermediacy of 15-hydroxy sterols has been rendered obscure by the recent finding that only the 15β-hydroxy epimer (14α-methyl-cholest-7-ene-3β,15β-diol) is metabolized to cholesterol by rat liver (266). X-ray analysis unequivocally established the configuration of the metabolically active epimer as 15β. Since the 15α hydrogen atom of lanosterol is lost and the 15β hydrogen is retained at 15α (250–256), enzymatic hydroxylation would involve inversion of configuration at C-15. Hydroxylations of centers in the steroid nucleus usually occur with retention of configuration. Therefore, it is unlikely, but not impossible, that direct hydroxylation at C-15 is occurring with inversion of configuration. Indirect hydroxylation is possible via a $\Delta^{15(16)}$-bond, but this route is also unlikely since it is known that the C-16 hydrogen atoms are not disturbed during cholesterol biosynthesis (254).

In view of the evidence for the $\Delta^{8,14}$-diene route, what role then do the $\Delta^{8(14)}$-monoenes play? The experimental evidence is conflicting. 4,4-Dimethyl-5α-cholest-8(14)-en-3β-ol is not a precursor of the $\Delta^{8,14}$-dienes (267), whereas the conversion of 5α-cholest-8(14)-en-3β-ol to cholesta-8,14-dien-3β-ol has been observed (268). Both the 4,4-dimethyl (249, 267, 269) and 4-desmethyl (269–271) monoene can be metabolized to cholesterol by liver cell-free systems. In trapping experiments, radioactivity from labeled 24,25-dihydrolanosterol could be trapped by unlabeled 4,4-dimethylcholesta-8,14-dien-3β-ol (122b, 259, 272, 273) but not by unlabeled 4,4-dimethylcholest-8(14)-en-3β-ol (272, 274). Even though the 4,4-dimethyl diene cannot trap the 4,4-dimethyl monoene, the formation of cholesterol from the monoene is markedly depressed by the presence of the diene (267, 269). An oxygen-dependent step in the metabolism of the $\Delta^{8(14)}$-monoene is suggested by the lack of conversion of the monoene to cholest-7-en-3β-ol or to cholesterol in the absence of oxygen (275), as well as the accumulation of a mixture of sterols, including the monoene in the absence of oxygen in incubations with cholesta-8,14-dien-3β-ol (263). Both cholest-8(14)-en-3β,15α-diol and -3β,15β-diol are reported to be metabolized to the $\Delta^{8,14}$-diene (275), but rates of conversion of the two sterols are unavailable. Gibbons (276) has compared the substrates, 24,25-dihydrolanosterol, 4,4-dimethylcholesta-8,14-dien-3β-ol, and 4,4-dimethylcholest-8(14)-en-3β-ol under identical incubation conditions with and without the microsomal supernatant fraction (probably sterol carrier protein). In the presence of the supernatant fraction, cholesterol was formed in 15%, 19%, and 4% yield, respectively, and cholest-7-en-3β-ol in 18%, 28%, and 6% yield, respectively. Most of the radioactivity from the monoene incubation is present as cholest-8(14)-en-3β-ol, and no interconversion of either substrate ($\Delta^{8,14} \rightleftharpoons \Delta^{8(14)}$) was observed. In agreement with previous results, the presence of the 4,4-dimethyl diene suppresses monoene metabolism, but the 4-desmethyl diene was not as effective a depressant. The $\Delta^{8(14)}$-monoene is probably not a normal intermediate in cholesterol biosynthesis. Rates of conversion to cholesterol and cholest-7-en-3β-ol are very low, and preference and competition of the enzymes for the actual substrate, i.e., 4,4-dimethylcholesta-8,14-dien-3β-ol or its 4-desmethyl derivative, could reasonably explain the suppression of conversion of the $\Delta^{8(14)}$-sterol by the diene.

More confusing is the possible role of the Δ^7-sterols obtainable by double-bond migration. Cholesta-7,14-dien-3β-ol has been converted to cholesterol (*277*) aerobically. Under anaerobic conditions the Δ^7- and $\Delta^{8(14)}$-monoenes are produced, but not the $\Delta^{8,14}$-dienes (*277*). Is there a pathway Δ^8- to Δ^7- to 14-desmethyl-$\Delta^{8(14)}$-sterol, or perhaps Δ^8- to Δ^7- to 14-desmethyl-$\Delta^{7,14}$-sterol? In liver, the $\Delta^{7,14}$-diene may not be a true intermediate, but it seems to be able to function as a substitute for the $\Delta^{8,14}$-diene (*123*). The C-14 demethylase is insensitive to the presence of the $\Delta^{7 \text{ or } 8}$-bond and can form the $\Delta^{7,14}$- or $\Delta^{8,14}$-diene products (*244, 272*). Furthermore, $\Delta^{7,14}$-sterols apparently can be enzymatically isomerized to $\Delta^{8,14}$-sterols (*278*) even though $\Delta^{8,14}$-sterols are not isomerized to $\Delta^{7,14}$-sterols (*277*). These results suggest the pathway: $\Delta^{8,14} \rightarrow \Delta^8 \rightarrow \Delta^7$.

Obviously, a considerable amount of work needs to be done before these problems will be solved, but it is possible to summarize the present situation in a reasonably coherent if not altogether satisfactory fashion. As discussed in the next two sections, the Δ^7-sterols are definitely on the pathway to Δ^5-sterols, so what has been discussed here simply concerns the conversion of a 14α-methyl-Δ^8-sterol (e.g., lanosterol) to a 14-desmethyl-Δ^7-sterol. 14-Dehydrosterols are isolable from nonphotosynthetic plants (possessing the $\Delta^{5,7,14}$-triene grouping) and from animal tissues (possessing the $\Delta^{8,14}$-diene grouping), and $\Delta^{8(14)}$-sterols have been isolated from both higher animals and higher plants. In rat liver the 15α-H atom is lost, and 14α-methyl sterols bearing a Δ^7-, $\Delta^{8(14)}$- or $\Delta^{8,14}$-grouping are converted to cholesterol. These facts permit two general mechanisms to be considered, on the assumption that a 32-formylsterol is the actual substrate for removal of the carbon atom attached to C-14. (1) Protonation occurs at C-7 of a Δ^7-sterol or at C-8 of a $\Delta^{8(9)}$-sterol and decarbonylation occurs simultaneously with formation of a $\Delta^{8(14)}$-sterol. The latter then isomerizes to a Δ^7-sterol either directly or via a $\Delta^{8(9)}$-sterol. Equilibrium with the $\Delta^{14(15)}$-structure would exchange an H atom at C-15 with water. (2) By analogy to the evidence (Section D.2) consistent with direct microsomal oxidative decarboxylation at C-4, oxidative removal of the 15α-H atom from a Δ^7- or Δ^8-sterol occurs with concomitant loss of formate and formation of a $\Delta^{7,14}$- or $\Delta^{8,14}$-diene, which, upon reduction in the former case, and reduction and double-bond migration in the latter case, yields the Δ^7-sterol (Scheme 9.20). The possibility that the $\Delta^{8(14)}$-route (mechanism a) is a soluble, primitive pathway and the conjugated diene route (mechanism b) an advanced microsomal route should be considered. When the cycloartenol route operates, the three-membered ring is presumably opened before demethylation at C-14.

Finally, it should be noted that, although 14α-methyl-Δ^7-sterols, e.g., lanost-7-en-3β-ol (*279*), are naturally occurring, they are not derived by isomerization of the $\Delta^{8(9)}$-bond (*280*) and may not be derived directly from squalene (*174*), but rather from the demonstrated reduction (*281*) of the $\Delta^{9(11)}$-bond or $\Delta^{7,9(11)}$-sterols, e.g., agnosterol or, as suggested by other evidence, direct deprotonation at C-7 during rearrangement following cyclization of squalene-2,3-oxide (*282*). How the $\Delta^{7,9(11)}$-compounds are formed and what, if any, physiological role they play in providing Δ^{7}- or $\Delta^{8(9)}$-intermediates is unclear. Unfortunately, one can write, for instance, a reasonable pathway, $\Delta^{8} \rightarrow \Delta^{7,9(11)}$- $\rightarrow$14-desmethyl-$\Delta^{8(14),9(11)}$- $\rightarrow$ 14-desmethyl-$\Delta^{8(14)}$- (by reduction) or 14-desmethyl-$\Delta^{8,14}$-sterol (by isomerization), which encompasses the mechanistic approaches of Scheme 9.20 but adds variants. Cholest-7,9-dien-3β-ol and its 4,4,14α-trimethyl derivative (24,25-dihydroagnosterol) have both been converted to cholesterol by an enzyme system prepared from a rat liver homogenate (*281*). Since the isomerization is blocked by the presence of a 14α-methyl group (*280*), the conversion of dihydroagnosterol to cholesterol indicates that demethylation at C-14 can occur with the Δ^{7}-bond intact, either as the $\Delta^{7,9(11)}$-grouping per se or in the reduced Δ^{7} form. Subsequent experiments (*283*) revealed that the conversion of the $\Delta^{7,9(11)}$-sterols to cholesterol may involve initial isomerization to the more stable $\Delta^{8,14}$-diene, which could be initiated by protonation at C-7. The conditions of this incubation (anaerobic and in the absence of NADPH) rule out the possibility of 14α demethylation to the $\Delta^{7,9(11),14}$-triene followed by reduction.

E. ORIGINS AND CENTRAL ROLE OF Δ^{7}-STEROLS

Δ^{7}-Sterols are quite common as minor components of sterol mixtures, and in some cases they comprise the dominant sterol of an organism (Chapter 10). In all investigated systems capable of biosynthesizing sterols de novo, Δ^{7}-sterols are obligatory intermediates. This conclusion rests on the wide occurrence in both the photosynthetic and nonphotosynthetic plant and animal kingdoms of Δ^{7}- and especially $\Delta^{5,7}$-sterols. The latter have been easily and frequently detected in small concentrations, without the use of techniques of separation, through a strong absorption triplet in the ultraviolet spectrum at 280 nm. The conclusion is also supported by extensive work in the animal kingdom showing the operation of the sequence from Δ^{7}- to $\Delta^{5,7}$- to Δ^{5}-sterols (Section F).

The Δ^{7}-sterols have several possible origins. The first and most completely studied is by migration of the $\Delta^{8(9)}$-bond to the Δ^{7}-position. It has been demonstrated in rat liver homogenates under both aerobic and anaerobic conditions (*258, 280, 284, 285*). The anaerobic reaction suggests the occurrence either of an addition-elimination of a proton or of a direct 1,3-transfer of an H atom from C-7 to C-9. Labeling experiments (*285–287*) show the former to be correct, since one H atom from water is incorporated at the 9α position. The reaction does not proceed unless the 14α-methyl group is missing (*280*) and 4α-methylsterols isomerize two or three times as fast as the 4,4-demethyl sterols (*280*). The use of stereospecifically labeled MVA has led to the conclusion that the 7β hydrogen atom is lost in rat liver (*251, 253, 254, 288, 289*), in the alga *Ochromonas malhamensis* (*290*), and in the higher plants, *Calendula officinalis* (*141*), *Camellia sinensis* (*291*), *Larix decidua* (*87*), and *Clerodendrum campbelli* (*87*), but the 7α hydrogen atom is lost in the fungi, yeast (*292, 293*) and *Aspergillus niger* (*87*), and in the alga *Fucus spiralis* (*87*). An addition-elimination mechanism on a C_3 system has the expected stereochemical qualities of double inversion, i.e., a *trans*-process on the first two C atoms followed by a *trans*-process on the second two is tantamount to addition and removal of a proton at the two ends of the system from the same side. Since addition of a proton to C-9 would have to proceed axially from the α side to account for the structure of the known Δ^5-sterols, one would expect loss of the axial 7α-H atom, as found in fungi and some algae. Why there should be a divergence from this in animals and photosynthetic plants is not entirely clear. The most obvious explanation would be as follows. After protonation at C-9, a 1,2-hydride transfer of the 7β-H to C-8 proceeds with stabilization of the C-7 carbonium ion from the α side by the enzyme. This would invert C-7 transforming the original 7α-H into a 7β-H. Elimination of the 8β-H atom and of the 7α-enzyme moiety would then yield the Δ^7-sterol lacking the H atom originally at the 7β position.

Another anomaly is associated with the isomerization of the $\Delta^{8(14)}$-sterols which comprises a second route of formation of Δ^7-sterols. While the cholest-8 (14)-3β-ol yields cholesterol in intact rats (*246*) and cholest-8(14)-3β-ol and its 4,4-dimethyl derivative yield cholesterol and Δ^7-sterols aerobically in liver homogenates (*246, 249*), the former is not metabolized in liver homogenates under anaerobic conditions (*246, 263, 275*). Apparently, an oxidative process is involved (*246, 263, 275*). Possible explanations include allylic hydroxylation at C-7 followed by allylic reduction (H^- to C-14 with elimination of OH^- and double-bond migration) and allylic hydroxylation at C-7 or C-15 followed by allylic dehydration to a $\Delta^{7,14}$-diene and subsequent 14,15-reduction. A third origin of the Δ^7-sterols, which has been demonstrated experimentally, is reduction of a $\Delta^{7,9(11)}$-diene (*281*) (cf. Section D.3). Scheme 9.22 summarizes the various ways by which Δ^7-sterols arise.

Evidence obtained from yeast and liver preparations in three laboratories has shown that the $\Delta^8 \rightarrow \Delta^7$ isomerization is reversible (*108, 293, 294*). During isomerization (of the Δ^7-bond to Δ^8), complete exchange of the 9α hydrogen atom with the medium occurs under anaerobic conditions (*293, 294*). In rat liver incubations of [4-^{14}C,7-^{3}H]cholest-7-en-3β-ol have established that the isomerization occurs with complete retention of the C-7 tritium atom (*294*).

F. INTRODUCTION OF Δ^5-BOND

The presence of a Δ^8-bond in lanosterol and the early experimental conversion

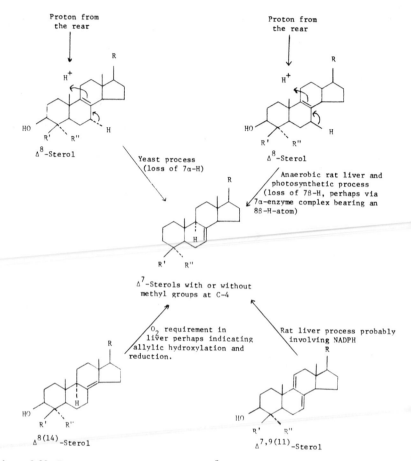

Scheme 9.22. Demonstrated processes yielding Δ^7-sterols. R = side chain; R' and R'' = CH$_3$ or H.

of cholest-7-en-3β-ol (lathosterol) to cholesterol (*295–300*) strongly suggested that a direct isomerization of the double bond occurs from Δ^8 to Δ^5. While this has been verified for the Δ^8- to Δ^7- conversion (Section E), there are both theoretical and experimental reasons for believing the further conversion to a Δ^5-sterol is not an isomerization. If it were, the π system would have to pass through the Δ^6- condition, and, being disubstituted, this double bond is less stable than the trisubstituted Δ^7- or Δ^5- arrangements, making the transformation unlikely. Whether or not the a priori argument is valid, it agrees with the biosynthetic fact. Schroepfer and Frantz (*300*) have experimentally shown that [4-¹⁴C]cholest-6-en-3β-ol is not converted to cholesterol in the rat when injected into the portal vein or fed orally. Furthermore, in 1959 Frantz and his co-workers (*299*) showed that an oxygen requirement existed in the "shift" of the bond to Δ^5. These facts unequivocally eliminated a simple prototropic migration of the double bond.

The common occurrence of $\Delta^{5,7}$-sterols was the key to the problem. If they result from introduction of the Δ^5-bond, then the Δ^7-bond on saturation could produce a Δ^5-sterol by an overall process tantamount to a shift of the double bond in terms of precursor and product, although not in mechanistic terms. In agreement with this pathway, the animal conversion of cholest-5,7-dien-3β-ol (7-dehydrocholesterol) to cholesterol has been amply demonstrated (296, 297, 300–303) and found to proceed anaerobically (300, 303), as is required of a reductive step. This leaves the problem of the introduction of the Δ^5-bond, to which clearly one must now assign the previously mentioned involvement of molecular oxygen. In 1964, Dempsey et al. (304) actually proved the conversion of lathosterol to 7-dehydrocholesterol in a rat liver enzyme system and showed that this step has the oxygen requirement. The further reduction of cholesterol required NADPH (304). The true physiological intermediacy of the $\Delta^{5,7}$-sterols has been proved further by the following facts. 7-Dehydrocholesterol disappears from cell-free liver homogenates incubated anaerobically (303); in the presence of the reductase inhibitors MER-29 and AY-9944, cholest-5,7,24-trien-3β-ol accumulates (305–307); label from tritiated lathosterol is trapped in added 7-dehydrocholesterol (304, 307); and cholest-7,9,24-trien-3β-ol is formed from cholest-8,24-dien-3β-ol (307). The presence or absence of the Δ^{24}-bond is a sequence problem (Section H). Otherwise, the final steps in Δ^5-sterol biosynthesis in higher animals are clearly via the $\Delta^{5,7}$-sterols (Scheme 9.23). None of the steps is reversible in rats (307) or yeast (108), although Tetrahymena pyriformis

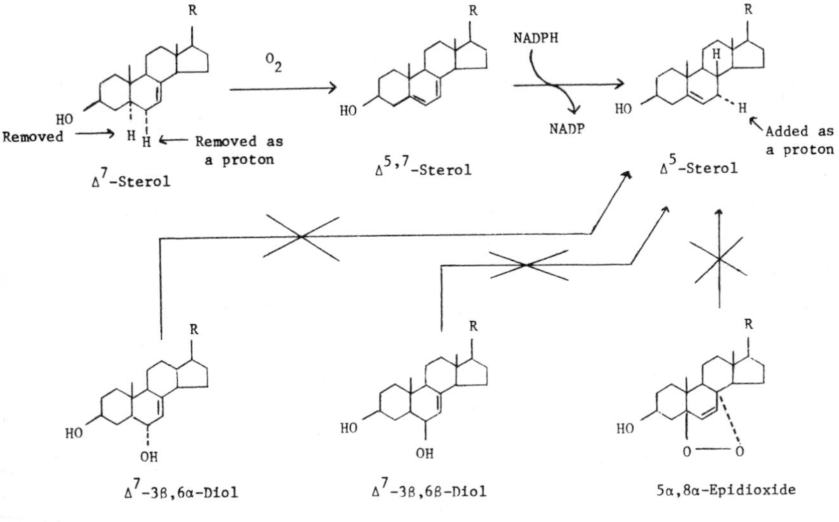

Scheme 9.23. Conversion of Δ^7- to Δ^5-sterols. R, side chain. The reactions marked with an X have been shown not to occur in rats.

(*308*) and some insects can introduce the Δ^7-bond into Δ^5-sterols (*158, 309, 310*). The wide occurrence of $\Delta^{5,7}$-sterols in the plant kingdom is indicative of the ($\Delta^7 \rightarrow \Delta^{5,7} \rightarrow \Delta^5$)-process operating ubiquitously. Direct evidence is unfortunately lacking. Cell-free systems amenable to such experimentation that will perform the final biosynthetic steps have not yet been developed from plants. In yeast, which of course has been well studied, the dominant sterol has the $\Delta^{5,7}$-structure, and so the question of its intermediacy does not arise.

The mechanism of desaturation to form the $\Delta^{5,7}$-system is not yet understood. The oxygen requirement suggests hydroxylation followed by anaerobic dehydroxylation (*311, 312*), but neither cholest-7-en-3β,6α-diol nor its 6β-analog proceeds to cholesterol anaerobically (*313, 314*). Other sterols oxygenated at C-7 and/or C-8, e.g., cholest-7α,8α-epoxy-3β-ol, cholesta-3β,7β,8α-triol, cholest-8-ene-3β,7ξ-diol, cholesta-3β,7α,8α-triol, cholesta-3β,8α-diol-7-one, and cholest-8(14)-ene-3β,7α-diol, also fail to yield cholesterol under anaerobic conditions in the presence of rat liver homogenate (*315*). However, under an oxygen atomsphere, cholesterol was biosynthesized from all except the 3β,7α,8α-triol (*315*). The 5α,8α-epidioxide of ergosterol has been isolated from various fungi (*316–322*), a lichen (*323*), and a sponge (*148*), and a related epidioxide (ascaridole found in several *Chenopodium* species) is known at the I_2 level of isopentenoid polymerization (*324, 325*). However, despite suggestive evidence to the contrary (*326, 327*), the 5α,8α-epidioxide of 7-dehydrocholesterol is not converted to 7-dehydrocholesterol or to cholesterol by rat liver (*328*). On the other hand, yeast enzymes systems are capable of converting 5α,8α-epidioxyergosta-6,22-dien-3β-ol (ergosterol epoxide) to ergosterol (*326, 329*). Another hydroxylated sterol, the Δ^7-3β, 5α-diol, is also metabolized differently by yeast and liver systems, suggesting that alternate pathways for Δ^5-bond introduction may exist. [3α,^{3}H$_1$]Cholest-7-ene-3β,5α-diol is efficiently converted to cholesterol in rat liver in the presence of oxygen; however, no conversion was detected in the absence of oxygen (*311*). In agreement with these results, the analogous [3α,^{3}H$_1$]ergosta-7,22-diene-3β,5α-diol was metabolized to ergosterol by yeast under aerobic conditions with retention of tritium (*312, 330*). In contrast, a purified yeast enzyme (5α-dehydrase) (*331*) efficiently produces ergosterol (with loss of tritium) from the same substrate only under anaerobic conditions (*329*). This is the same enzyme that accepts ergosterol epoxide as a substrate. Some support for the intermediacy of the Δ^7-3β,5α-diol in yeast has been gained by the reported isolation of this compound in small amounts from incubations of yeast with [28,^{14}C]ergosta-7,24(28)-dien-3β-ol (episterol) under aerobic conditions (*330*). In yeast systems the natural C-5 oxygenated intermediate remains unknown. Even less is known about the mechanism of Δ^5-bond introduction in rat liver since little success has been achieved with various substrates and potential intermediate(s) have escaped isolation.

Novel sterols with $\Delta^{5,8}$-double bonds (*115, 332, 333*) have been isolated from several natural sources. The occurrence of this type of sterol is very interesting since isomerization of the Δ^8-bond to Δ^7- and the presence of a Δ^7-bond is generally accepted as a necessary prerequisite for Δ^5-bond introduction. All but one of the species that contain $\Delta^{5,8}$-sterols are lichens. Goodwin and his associates (115) have eliminated the possibility that the Δ^8-bond is a photoinduced isomerization product of the Δ^7-bond by isolation of a $\Delta^{5,8}$-sterol from dark-grown lichen cultures. Analysis of the sterol products of five nystatin-resistant mutants of yeast (334) showed that one mutant lacks the $\Delta^8 \rightarrow \Delta^7$ isomerase since only a mixture of Δ^8-sterols including ergosta-5,8,22-trien-3β-ol accumulates. Formation of the $\Delta^{5,8}$-system from enzyme-induced isomerization of the $\Delta^{5,7}$-system is ruled out in these mutant yeast. Moreover, ergosterol biosynthesis in the mutant yeast strain could only be induced when a Δ^7-sterol was the substrate.

The stereochemistry of the dehydrogenation to produce the Δ^5-bond is such that the 5α and 6α hydrogen atoms (cis elimination) are eliminated in rats (254, 311, 335–337), in Aspergillus fumigatus (338), in yeast (312), in the gymnosperm Larix decidua (339), in the alga O. malhamensis (340), and in the angiosperms Clerodendrum campbelli (87) and Calendula officinalis (141). The 6α hydrogen atom is removed in the rat as a proton (337). It is found in water, not in NADH (337). In the reduction of the Δ^7-bond, a hydride ion is added (from NADPH) to C-7 from the α side and a proton is added from the medium to the 8β position (122a). These results agree with the observed inversion of configuration of the 7α hydrogen atom of lanosterol to the 7β position in cholesterol (251, 288).

G. INTRODUCTION OF Δ^{22}-BOND

Although evidence exists for introduction of the Δ^{22}-bond as a part of the alkylation process at C-24 in the slime molds (134, 136, 341–344), direct 22,23-dehydrogenation seems to be more common and has been demonstrated in both photosynthetic and nonphotosynthetic plants. Thus, 24-methylsterols are converted to ergosterol in yeast (5, 345); stigmastanol proceeds to its 22-dehydro derivative in the slime mold (342, 343); sitosterol is dehydrogenated at C-22,23 to give stigmasterol in Digitalis lanata (346); and spinasterol undergoes the Δ^7- to Δ^5-conversion together with Δ^{22}-introduction, producing stigmasterol in Nicotiana tabacum (347). Only one H atom is involved, as expected, at C-22 or C-23 (345), and in all but a few cases the Δ^{22}-bond is believed to have the trans-configuration relative to C-20 and C-24. The exception is the reports of cholesta-5,cis-22-dien-3β-ol or its 24-methyl analog often occurring with the trans isomer in many marine organisms (201, 348–352). Only two laboratories have achieved spectral identification of the 22-cis sterols (348, 352); the remainder of the reports depend solely on GLC retention times as a basis for characterization.

In the fungus Aspergillus fumigatus, and the verbena Clerodendrum *campbelli*, the 22-*pro-S*- and 23-*pro-S*-H-atoms are removed in proceeding to ergosterol (*338*), or to (24*S*)-24-ethylcholesta-5,22,25-trien-3β-ol (*87*), respectively. In the alga *O. malhamensis* (*340*) and the protozoan *T. pyriformis* (*353*), the 22-*pro-R*- and 23-*pro-R*-H-atoms of 24-alkylsterols are lost (*340*). Identification of one but not both of the hydrogen atoms from C-22 or C-23 has been achieved in several other species. It is reasonable to postulate that, in these organisms, Δ^{22}-bond formation also proceeds via the same overall *cis* elimination observed in the fully characterized species. During ergosterol formation by *Blakeslea trispora* and stigmasterol synthesis by the marigold, the 23-*pro-S* (*87*) and the 22-*pro-S* (*141*) hydrogen atoms are eliminated, respectively. On the other hand the 22-*pro-R* hydrogen atom in *Camellia sinensis* (*291*) and the 23-*pro-R* hydrogen atom in *Ochromonas danica* (*87*) are lost.

In the absence of a substituent at C-24, a nomenclature difficulty arises. While the stereochemistry is the same, the rules for the prochirality at C-23 dictate reversal of the *S* and *R* designations. For instance, during dehydrogenation of cholesterol (as opposed to sitosterol) in *T. pyriformis* the 23-*pro-S*-H-atom is lost, although it is the same atom as is designated 23-*pro-R* in sitosterol. In the actual steric arrangement (Scheme 9.24) the algal, protozoan, and some higher plant dehydrogenations occur from the back side, on the assumption that the *trans*-product arises from an analogous *trans*-conformer in the substrate (*195*). In the fungal case, and in some higher plants, the H atoms are removed from the front.

In all cases, a *cis*-elimination occurs, as is also found for the introduction of the Δ^5-bond (Section F). Direct dehydrogenation at C-7,8 in *T. pyriformis*, yielding the Δ^7-bond, similarly proceeds by *cis*-removal (of the 7β- and 8β-H atoms) (*353*). The reason for the elimination in the side chain occurring from one side in one organism and from the other in another organism is not clear. It may have to do with the substituent at C-24. If dehydrogenation occurs at the $\Delta^{24(28)}$-stage, which is demonstrable in *T. pyriformis* (*195*), where C-24 has no groups protruding on either side, one could argue for less steric hindrance on the back side (due to C-18 and C-19) and hence for preferential enzymatic attack and H elimination from the rear. This would predict the observation (*353*) that in the absence of 24-substitution elimination is indeed from the rear. In view of the known stereochemistry, it would also predict a different sequence for the fungal compared to the algal cases. In the former with the methyl group oriented on the back side, Δ^{22}-introduction would have to follow $\Delta^{24(28)}$-reduction to account for elimination from the front. In the latter, Δ^{22}-introduction would precede reduction, bypassing the problem of steric hindrance at C-24. It will be noticed (Scheme 9.24) that despite the same configuration at C-24 in the Δ^{22}-product in the fungal and algal case, the side of the molecule attacked is not the same. As just described, the hypothesis offered explains this anomaly, although

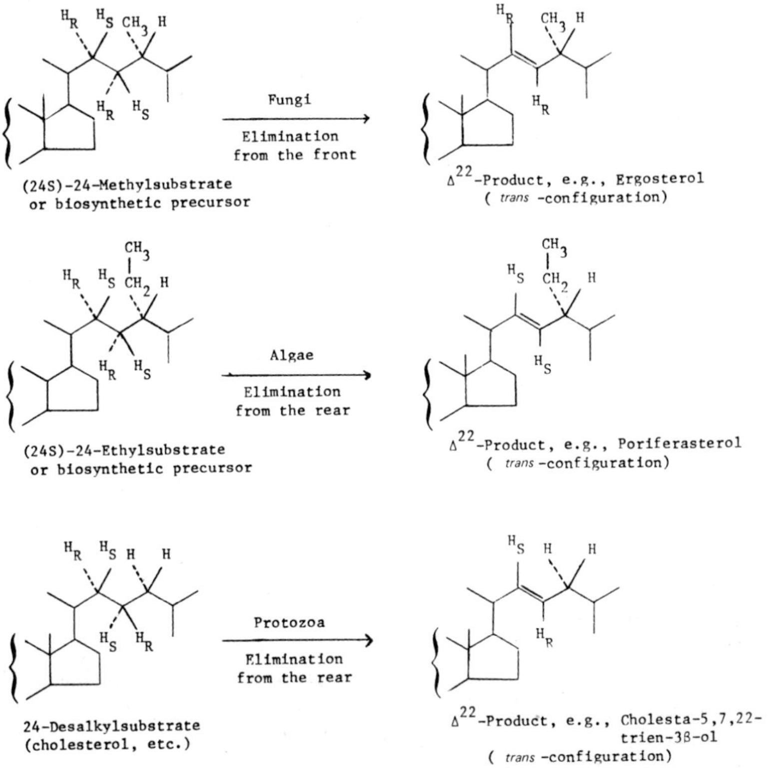

H_R H_S CH_3 H

H_R H_S

Fungi

Elimination
from the front

(24S)-24-Methylsubstrate
or biosynthetic precursor

H_R CH_3 H

H_R

Δ^{22}-Product, e.g., Ergosterol
(*trans* -configuration)

CH_3

H_R H_S CH_2 H

H_R H_S

Algae

Elimination
from the rear

(24S)-24-Ethylsubstrate
or biosynthetic precursor

CH_3

H_S CH_2 H

H_S

Δ^{22}-Product, e.g., Poriferasterol
(*trans* -configuration)

H_R H_S H H

H_S H_R

Protozoa

Elimination
from the rear

24-Desalkylsubstrate
(cholesterol, etc.)

H_S H H

H_R

Δ^{22}-Product, e.g., Cholesta-5,7,22-
trien-3β-ol
(*trans* -configuration)

Scheme 9.24. Stereochemistry of Δ^{22}-introduction. R and S refer to the Cahn-Ingold-Prelog sequence rule. Only in the protozoan case is the actual substrate known. It possessed the unsubstituted side chain of cholesterol. In the other cases the organisms were grown in the presence of stereospecifically labeled MVA, and the Δ^{22}-product was examined.

it of course is equally possible that the side of the molecule attacked is entirely controlled by the enzyme.

H. SEQUENCE

1. General Comments

The sequence of events leading from squalene oxide to functional sterols depends on the ordering of individual reactions, e.g., the point in the pathway at which reduction or alkylation of the Δ^{24}-bond occurs, as well as on the detailed mechanism of a given reaction. In the first case, the determinant presumably lies most commonly in the Michaelis constant of the enzymes involved, while in the second, more complicated enzymological phenomena are implicated. Examples of both types have been well documented. A growing body of evidence also shows a relationship between these sequence phenomena and the type of organism in question. The most dramatic is the association of the cycloartenol-lanosterol bifurcation with the presence and absence of photosynthesis. It represents an example of a mechanistic difference. It is also a major example of a truly alternative pathway. The choice of lanosterol or cycloartenol does not seem to determine the structure of the final sterol. Cholesterol, for instance, is derived by both routes. However, the structural variety of the final sterols is greater in the cycloartenol route, and the variety of known mechanisms in reactions which follow cyclization is also greater in the cycloartenol route. Because of these complexities, it is still not possible to write exact sequences and to say that in a given species A proceeds to B which proceeds to C, etc. In fact, it may well be that no absolute sequence operates in any organism.

2. Route In Mammals

The route in mammals (Scheme 9.25) has been established from work primarily with rats. At least in the dominant sequence, it is characterized by the conversion of squalene to lanosterol, rather than cycloartenol, by reduction rather than alkylation of the Δ^{24}-bond, probably by the removal of the 14α-methyl group before removal of either of the methyl groups at C-4, by introduction of the Δ^5-bond and reduction of the Δ^7-bond as the last biosynthetic process, and by failure to introduce a Δ^{22}-bond. A possible variation is the intermediacy of lanost-7(8),24-dien-3β-ol or lanost-9(11),24-dien-3β-ol in place of lanosterol, but not enough work has been done to assess what if any role these double-bond isomers of lanosterol play. The absence of alkylation at C-24 in normal mammals is assumed from the lack of 24-alkyl or 24-alkenyl sterols other than those that can be ascribed to diet (354–356) as well as from the failure of methyl-labeled methionine to yield sterols labeled only in the side chain (357).

The position in the sequence at which reduction of the Δ^{24}-bond occurs is not known with certainty. The demonstration of the reduction of lanosterol to 24,25-dihydrolanosterol (21, 48), the latter's conversion to cholesterol in a 55% yield (234), together with the natural occurrence of 24,25-dihydrolanosterol, lathosterol, 7-dehydrocholesterol, etc., and the accumulation of 24,25-dihydrosterols in a liver homogenate after treatment with cholestan-3β,-5α,6β-triol (239) lead one to suspect that the main pathway involves early saturation of the Δ^{24}-bond. However, desmosterol is naturally occurring (55–58), is reduced to cholesterol (55), and, if the Δ^{24}-reductase is blocked by inhibitors (triparanol or AY-9944), 4-methylcholesta-8,24-dien-3β-ol, 24,25-dehydrocholesterol (desmosterol) and its 7,8-dehydro derivative accumulate in place of cholesterol (55, 60, 238, 306, 307). These facts prove unequivocally that all the enzymes in the pathway will also accept the Δ^{24}-intermediates. There are thus, in principle, as many pathways as there are steps in the pathway, since one could place reduction between any two of

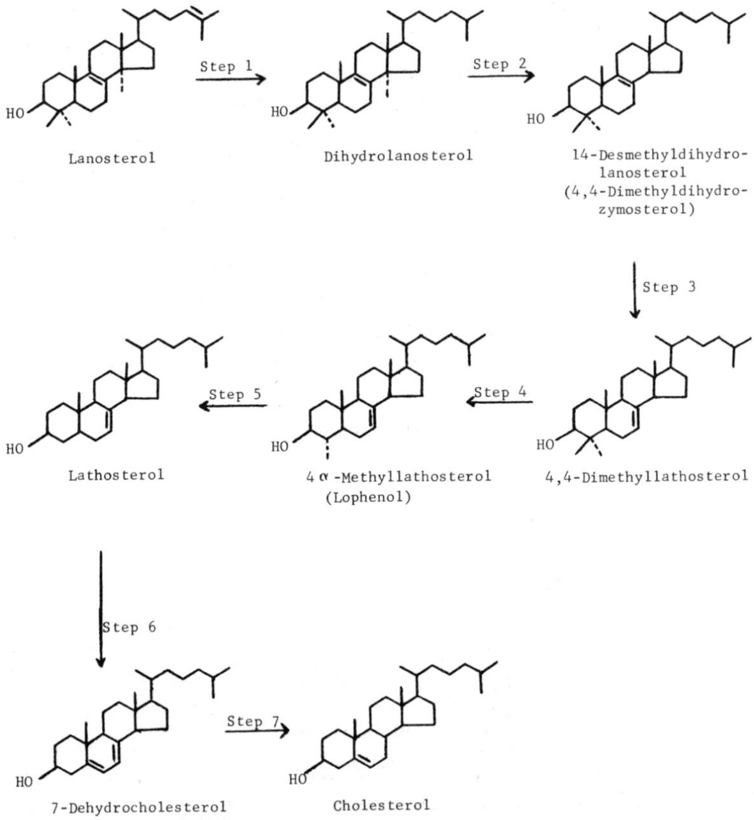

Scheme 9.25. An example of the mammalian route. Major intermediates are shown for what may be the dominant sequence in rats. The text should be consulted for details and alternatives. "Dihydro" refers to C-24,25.

them. For the sake of simplicity we shall tentatively assume reduction to be the first step in the main pathway.

The second step is probably removal of the 14α-methyl group. 14-Desmethyl-4,4-dimethylsterols, e.g., 4,4-dimethylcholest-8-en-3β-ol, have been found in rat liver (*239, 358*) but no 14α-methyl-4,4-desmethylsterols have. Furthermore, 14-desmethyl-4,4-dimethylsterols, e.g., 4,4-dimethylcholest-8-en-3β-ol and 4,4-dimethylcholestanol, will proceed experimentally to cholesterol and cholestanol (*234*), respectively, but 4,4,14α-trimethylcholestanol will not (*234*). These results probably reflect the participation of a Δ^8- or Δ^7-double bond in 14α-demethylation as well as substrate specificity of the C-4 demethylase enzyme system for the absence of the C-14 methyl group. The existence of 4α,14α-dimethyllanost-8-en-3β-ol (24,25-dihydro-30-norlanosterol) (*359*), 4α,14α-dimethyl-9,19-cyclolanost-24-en-3β-ol (30-norcycloartenol) (*360*), 14α-methylcholest-8-ene-3β,6α-diol (macdougallin)

(*361*), pollinastanol (*362*), and 24-methylene pollinastanol (*363*) in the plant kingdom shows that removal of one or two methyl groups at C-4 can, in principle, occur before demethylation at C-14, at least in the cycloartenol route. An absolute answer to the sequence problem will probably have to await better availability of 14α-methyl-4,4-desmethylsterols for use as experimental substrates. The present data, however, would suggest the sequence: lanosterol to 24,25-dihydrolanosterol to 4,4-dimethylcholest-8-en-3β-ol (14-desmethyl-24,25-dihydrolanosterol, 4,4-dimethyl-24,25-dihydrozymosterol) to 4,4-dimethycholest-7-en-3β-ol (4,4-dimethyllathosterol).

4,4-Dimethyllathosterol is probably formed via the corresponding 8,14-diene-14α-formyl sterol, but alternative routes are possible (Section D.3). If the 8,14-diene route operates, an uncertainty remains about the position in the sequence for the isomerization of the Δ^8-bond to the Δ^7-position. The only thing known to be absolutely required (*280*) is that the 14α-methyl group must be absent. Since 4α-methyl- and 4,4-dimethylsterols isomerize at rates within a factor of three of each other (*280*), the possibility of a dual route arises. The 4α-methylsterols isomerize faster, from which one is tempted to believe that removal of one methyl group at C-4 prior to double bond migration is the dominant route, but, if the absolute rate at the 4,4-dimethyl stage is sufficient, all the newly biosynthesized Δ^8-sterol would isomerize immediately after removal of the 14α-methyl group, regardless of the relative rate. For this reason the simplest view at the moment is that 4,4-dimethylathosterol is the dominant intermediate formed by isomerization (step 3) of 4,4-dimethylcholest-8-en-3β-ol. The alternative would be to proceed from the latter to 4α-methylcholest-8-en-3β-ol, from which two further alternatives are admissable. One is to form 4α-methyllathosterol and the other to yield 4,4-desmethylcholest-8-en-3β-ol (24,25-dihydrozymosterol). Step 4 is the sequence for removal of the two methyl groups at C-4. Evidence for the ordering of events is described in Section D.2. The sequence is comprised by hydroxylation of the 4α-methyl group, oxidation to the carboxyl stage, oxidative decarboxylation yielding the enol, ketonization, and reduction to give the 4α-methylsterol, which undergoes (step 5) the same sequence of reactions to produce lathosterol. Finally, steps 6 and 7 are the formation of cholesterol through Δ^5-introduction to give 7-dehydrocholesterol followed by Δ^7-reduction.

The conversion of lanosterol to cholesterol by the sequence given (steps 1–7, Scheme 9.25) would involve one reaction in step 1, possibly as many as five or six reactions in step 2, one in step 3, five or six in step 4, five or six in step 5, probably one in step 6, and one in step 7 for a total of 19–22 reactions. This means there are about 20 intermediates in a single route. Because several routes may exist, the actual number of different sterols that could exist between squalene and cholesterol is of the order of magnitude of 10^2.

3. Route in Invertebrates

Sterol biosynthesis is not detectable in most invertebrates. These organisms depend for the most part on dietary sources of sterols, which may be suitably modified by dealkylation or nuclear double-bond migration. Alkylation and Δ^{22}-introduction is observable in molluscs, but the source of these activities, possibly some associated algae, remains to be discovered. Substrate administration and adequate uptake present problems of incorporation, especially in the less complex invertebrates. In several phyla, lack of experimentally observed sterol biosynthesis has been corroborated by the requirement for exogenous sterol, either cholesterol or the 24-alkysterols, for the maintenance of growth and reproduction, as well as the accumulation of label from radioactive substrates in farnesol, squalene, squalene-2,3-oxide, or lanosterol, rather than in sterol.

Little is known of sterol synthesis or metabolism in the phylum Porifera. Several attempts have been made to investigate sterol biosynthesis in these organisms using the substrates [1-^{14}C]acetate or [2-^{14}C]MVA—with little success. The apparent absence of active sterol synthesis may have resulted from low uptake of the precursors. Because of their multicellular, colonial structure, there is no easy route for substrate administration; i.e., substrate was added to the aquarium water or substrate solution was dropped on moist animals outside of the aquarium (*170, 367*). Low viability of the animals during the incubation period has been another obstacle. Of three species that have been examined, only *Grantia compressa* was able to biosynthesize sterols from [2-^{14}C]MVA (*170*). The crude 4-desmethylsterol fraction was not further identified. In the same study, another species, *Suberites domuncula*, accumulated radioactivity from [2-^{14}C]MVA only in farnesol and geranylgeraniol and no radioactivity was found in squalene. Both species formed significant amounts of ubiquinone and dolichol. The third species, *Verongia aerophoba*, failed to utilize either of the sterol precursors as well as [*Me-*^{14}C] methionine (*367*).

The sterol content of various species of sponges is more well known. Bergmann has provided a detailed examination of the sterol composition of more than 50 species of sponges, which is reviewed in Ref. 368. Each of the families and orders appears to have a characteristic major sterol component. Marked variation in the distribution of sterols between species was noted. More recent reports of sponge-sterol composition have benefited from modern techniques and instrumentation (*148, 156, 201, 369, 370*) (see Chapter 10). Without correlation of incorporation of label from sterol precursors into any specific known sponge sterol, it is not possible to derive a biosynthetic route for sterol biosynthesis in Porifera. Some species may be incapable of de novo sterol biosynthesis. The remainder of the Porifera probably depend on dietary sources.

Similarly to Porifera, little is known of sterol metabolism in the Coelenterates, but there is extensive information about sterol occurrence (see Chapter 10). In five species examined, four sea anemones [*Metridium senile* (*170, 351*), *Anemonia sulcata* (*351*), *Calliactis parasitica* (*169*), and *Cerianthus membranaceus* (*351*)] and one jellyfish [*Rhizostoma* sp. (*371*)], little or no incorporation of acetate or MVA into squalene and sterols was observed. Coelenterates may depend entirely on exogenous sterol sources, which explains the occurrence of a variety of sterols, including cholesterol (widely distributed among marine organisms). Cholesterol could be derived via the dealkylation of one or several 24-alkylsterols. At least one of the Coelenterates, the sea anemone *C. parasitica*, in which cholesterol is the major sterol, can dealkylate [³H]fucosteryl propionate via desmosterol in the formation of cholesterol (*168*). The absence of label in the C_{28} sterols indicates that the C-24 ethyl group may be removed in one step similar to dealkylation in insects (*183*) (see Section C.6).

Sterol biosynthesis from MVA or acetate has not been observed in parasitic or free-living members of the phylum Platyhelminthes (*372–379*) or in free-living members of the class Nematoda of the phylum Aschelminthes (*167, 380, 381*). Cholesterol appears to be the major sterol in all of the forms studied, but the major sterols of *Turbatrix aceti* are cholesterol and 7-dehydrocholesterol (*167*). Among the Platyhelminthes, the parasitic forms and the carnivorous free-living planarian *Dugesia dorotocephala* probably depend on their hosts or diet for a direct cholesterol source. Direct absorption of cholesterol from the host through the wall of the hydatid cyst (*377*) as well as hydrolysis of cholesterol esters (*375*) occurs in the cat tapeworm *Echinococcus granulosus*. Moreover, sterol biosynthesis is blocked in *E. granulosus* and *Taenia hydatigena* at the level of farnesol, which appears to have the *cis, trans* rather than the all-*trans* configuration (*382*). Two species of the free-living nematodes require exogenous sterols in axenic culture. The block in the biosynthesis of sterols in *Panagrellus redivivus* occurs after lanosterol, which is the sole metabolite of [4-³H]squalene-2,3-oxide (*383*). Moreover, lanosterol is a normal constituent of this species (*384*). Growth and reproduction of *Caenorhabditis briggsae* can be maintained by the addition to the medium of ergosterol, 7-dehydrocholesterol, sitosterol, or stigmasterol. Cholesterol is not as effective in maintaining normal levels of growth and reproduction (*380*). The possibility of dealkylation of the 24-alkylsterols to an analog of cholesterol in this species was not examined. Dealkylation of sitosterol and fucosterol is found in the vinegar eel *Turbatrix aceti* (*167*). Desmosterol accumulates in the presence of triparanol succinate. Moreover, rapid formation of a $\Delta^{5,7}$-sterol (7-dehydrocholesterol) from cholesterol also occurs.

Very slight incorporation of acetate into a complex sterol mixture (90% cholesterol) by carnivorous nemertinean *Cerebratulus marginatus* (phylum Rhynchocoela) has been noted (*385*). Members of this genus of marine organisms are known to feed on molluscs, presumably the source of cholesterol as well as of the trace sterols not found in nematodes or flatworms.

Annelids differ in their ability to biosynthesize sterols. Uptake and metabolism of [1-^{14}C]MVA with evolution of $^{14}CO_2$ by the polychaetes *Nereis diversicolor* and *Arenicola marina* (marine annelids) (*386*) are indicative of sterol biosynthesis. The results of this early study are supported by a more recent report of the incorporation of [2-^{14}C]MVA into squalene and un-identified 4,4-dimethyl-, 4-methyl-, and 4-desmethylsterols by *Nereis pelagica* (*170*). On the other hand, a representative oligochaete, *Lumbricus terrestris*, failed to evolve $^{14}CO_2$ from [1-^{14}C]MVA (*386*), indicating an inability to biosynthesize sterols or at least squalene and other isoprenoids. In a more recent study, this species also failed to utilize [^{14}C]squalene for sterol bio-synthesis (*387*).

The inability to biosynthesize sterols from MVA or acetate seems to be a general condition of members of the phylum Arthropoda. Two classes, Insecta and Crustacea, of the subphylum Mandibulata have been extensively studied, and all require exogenous sterol in the form of cholesterol itself or 24-alkylsterols which are dealkylated to cholesterol. Much is known about the mechanism of dealkylation and the intermediates involved especially in insects (Scheme 9.26) (see Section C.6). The same pathway (Scheme 9.26) is probably utilized by crustaceans. Sterols containing an unsaturation in the side chain at C-22,23 are also satisfactory substrates in addition to the substrates shown in Scheme 9.25. After introduction of the $\Delta^{24(28)}$-bond in 24-methyl- and 24-ethylsterols, dealkylation probably proceeds by reversal of alkylation yielding a $\Delta^{24(25)}$-sterol (desmosterol) which is reduced to cho-lesterol. The 24(28)-epoxide of fucosterol has been implicated (*188, 189*) as an activated oxygenated intermediate that could give rise directly to desmo-sterol via the removal of acetaldehyde (*183*). There is no evidence for an analogous epoxide in the dealkylation of the 24-methylsterols.

Insects readily carry out transformations of nuclear double bonds of the B ring of cholesterol, forming a $\Delta^{5,7}$-sterol (7-dehydrocholesterol) impli-cated as a precursor of ecdysone (*388*). Four transformations have been documented: 1) $\Delta^5 \rightarrow \Delta^{5,7}$ (*309, 389, 390*), 2) $\Delta^5 \rightarrow \Delta^0 \rightarrow \Delta^7$ (*392, 393*), and 4) $\Delta^7 \rightarrow \Delta^{5,7}$ (*394*) (see Scheme 9.27). The first two of these are reversible (*161, 395*). Introduction of the Δ^7-bond into cholesterol by *Calliphora eryth-rocephala* proceeds by *cis*-removal of the 7β- and 8β-H atoms (*309*). This is the same stereochemistry found in *Polypodium vulgare* (*396*) during ecdysone biosynthesis from cholesterol and in *Tetrahymena pyriformis* (*353*).

The phylum Mollusca is divided in sterol-synthesizing ability. The primitive mollusc, the chiton *Liolophura japonica* (class Amphineura) readily labels squalene and lathosterol from the substrate [2-^{14}C]MVA (*397*). Sim-ilarly, with the exception of the whelk, *Buccineum undatum* (order Stenoglosa) (*398*), all Gastropoda that have been studied are able to synthesize sterols

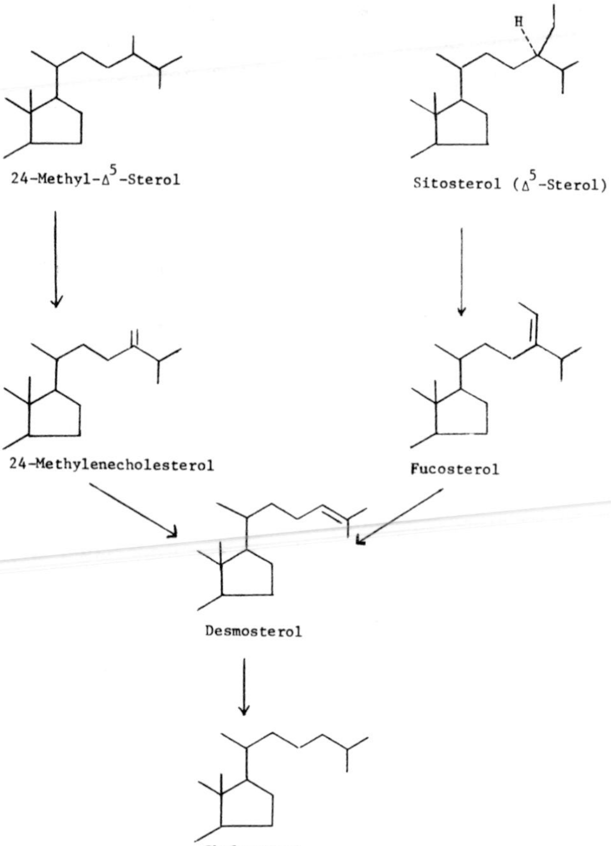

Scheme 9.26. Route for the dealkylation of 24-methyl and 24α-ethylsterols in arthropods.

from radioactive acetate or MVA (*170, 205, 399-403*). Labeled sterols were not identified in any of these studies. Data on members of the orders Anisomyaria and Eulamellibranchia of the class Pelecypoda are conflicting. *Ostrea* sp. (*168, 404*) and *Atrina fragilis* (*404*) of the former order cannot biosynthesize squalene or sterols from labeled acetate or MVA; however, the presence and absence of sterol biosynthesis in *Mytilus edulis* of the same order have been reported (*170, 205, 404*), and labeled digitonin-precipitable substances were recovered from incubation of *Mytilus californianus* with [^{14}C]acetate or [^{14}C]squalene (*405*). Sterol biosynthesis was observed in all Eulamellibranchia studied (*405, 406*), but incorporation of acetate or MVA was very low in four out of the five species examined (*406*). The sole representative member of the class Cephalopoda, *Sepia officinales* (cuttlefish), cannot utilize acetate for cholesterol biosynthesis (*407*).

Alkylation, dealkylation, and the introduction of the Δ^{22}-bond have

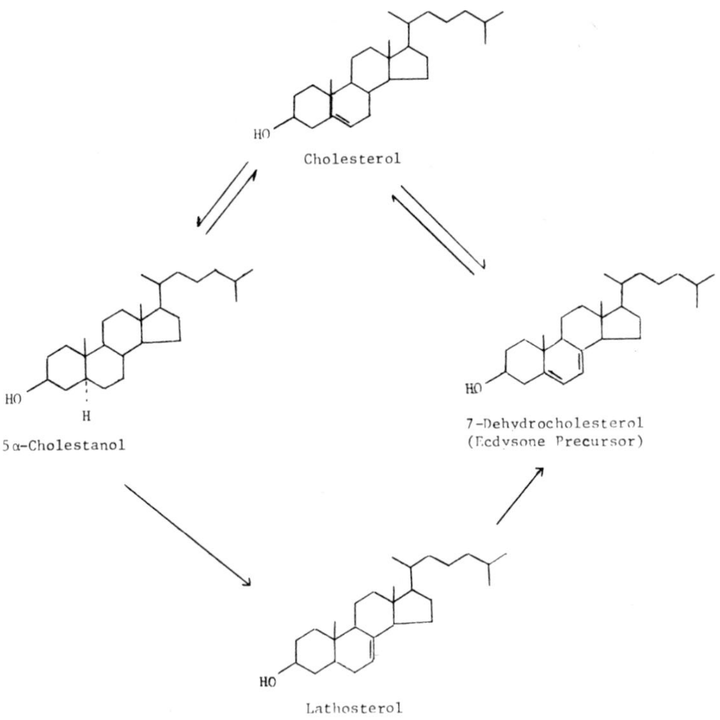

Cholesterol

5α-Cholestanol

7-Dehydrocholesterol
(Ecdysone Precursor)

Lathosterol

Scheme 9.27. Nuclear double-bond transformations by insects.

been observed in several mollusc species. *Ostrea grypha* dealkylates ^{3}H-fucosterol via desmosterol in the formation of cholesterol (*168*). This route is similar to insect dealkylation. In *Mytilus edulis*, 22-dehydrocholesterol and 24-methylenecholesterol were formed from [2-^{14}C]MVA (*205*), and in *Saxidomus gigantea* labeled cholesterol gave rise to 24-methylenecholesterol and other sterols with Δ^{22}- or Δ^{25}-bonds (*146, 408*).

Recent studies have shown that Echinoderms are able to biosynthesize sterols. Among the well-characterized Asteroids (representative species, *Asterias rubens* and *Laister leachii*), lathosterol rather than cholesterol is the end product of the pathway (*409, 410*). After cyclization of squalene, presumably as the epoxide, the resultant lanosterol undergoes removal of the 14α-methyl group, followed by Δ^8 to Δ^7 migration in *A. rubens* and *Henricia sanguinolenta*. Subsequent removal of the 4,4-dimethyl groups and Δ^{24}-bond reduction leads to lathosterol (*411*) (Scheme 9.28). The sequencing of Δ^{24}-bond reduction may vary within orders and may depend on the activity of the Δ^{24}-reductase. Labeled dihydrolanosterol was found in *H. sanguinolenta* incubated with [2-^{14}C]MVA (*410*) but not in *A. rubens* (*410, 411*). The pathway in Scheme 9.28 is the same as the sequence from

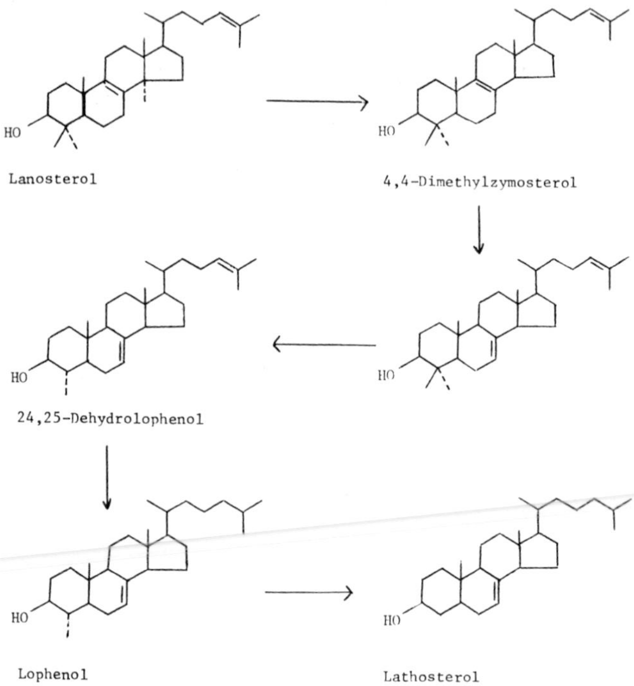

Lanosterol

4,4-Dimethylzymosterol

24,25-Dehydrolophenol

Lophenol

Lathosterol

Scheme 9.28. Sequence of sterol biosynthesis in asteroids.

lanosterol to lathosterol in mammals with the exception of Δ^{24}-reduction, which presumably occurs first in mammals (see Section H.2). Label from [2-^{14}C]MVA accumulates predominantly in squalene and the 4,4-dimethylsterols in A. rubens (411), indicating a rate-limiting step after lanosterol. In mammals the 4-desmethylsterols are the most heavily labeled from the same substrate. The various C_{28}- and C_{29}-sterols that have been isolated from A. rubens were not labeled from [2-^{14}C]MVA (411). The 9β,19-cyclopropylsterols [cycloartenol, cycloartanol, and 30-norcycloartanol (412)] were also not labeled from MVA (411). Interconversions among these three sterols are possible, such as the reduction of the Δ^{24}-bond similar to rat liver (21) or C-4 demethylation similar yeast (33) to yield cycloartanol or 30-norcycloartanol, respectively.

The other Echinoderm classes, Echinoids, Holothuroids, and Ophiuroids, have not been examined as extensively as the Asteroids. Members of all three classes biosynthesize only C_{27}-sterols from MVA (199, 413). In the Holothuroid, Cucumaria elongata, lathosterol is the end product of the pathway (199); however, in the Echinoids, the final product is cholesterol (the major sterol) (413). Most of the label from [2-^{14}C]MVA accumulates in desmosterol in these organismisms and only a small amount reaches cholesterol. Dihydrolanosterol is readily converted to cholesterol, indicating that the Δ^{24}-reductase is rate limiting. Echinoids cannot dealkylate sitosterol. Transformations of nuclear double bonds (Δ^5 to Δ^7) have been documented in the Asteroids, *A. rubens* and *Solaster papposus* (*414*). These carnivorous starfish feed primarily on molluscs in which cholesterol is the major sterol. Only minor amounts of cholesterol are found in *A. rubens* (*412*). Cholesterol is converted to a mixture of 5α-cholestanol and lathosterol, and 5α-cholestanol yields lathosterol (*414*). Cholest-4-en-3-one has been implicated as an intermediate in *A. rubens* by the conversion of the ketone to 5α-cholestanone, 5α-cholestanol, and lathosterol (*414*). A probable pathway is shown in Scheme 9.29.

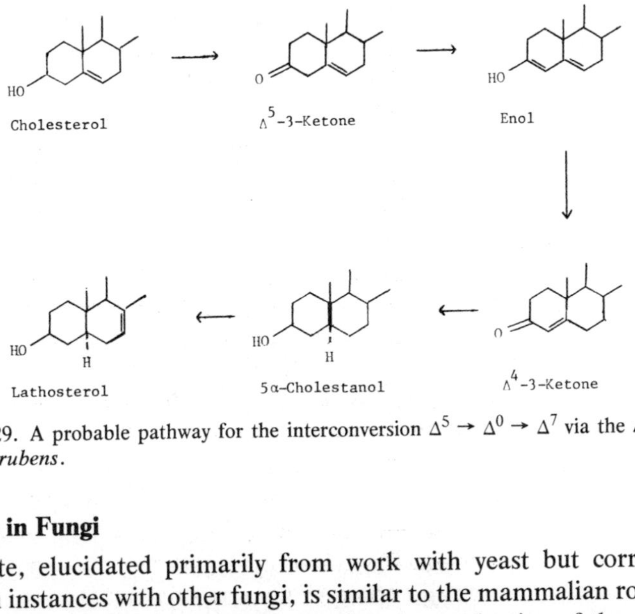

Scheme 9.29. A probable pathway for the interconversion $\Delta^5 \rightarrow \Delta^0 \rightarrow \Delta^7$ via the Δ^4-3-ketone in *Asterias rubens*.

4. Route in Fungi

This route, elucidated primarily from work with yeast but corroborated in certain instances with other fungi, is similar to the mammalian route, with three notable exceptions. Alkylation, rather than reduction of the Δ^{24}-bond, usually dominates, Δ^7-reduction is commonly absent, and Δ^{22}-introduction is present. The resultant is the conversion of squalene via lanosterol to 24β-methyl-7,22-bisdehydrocholesterol (ergosterol) instead of to cholesterol. The fungal route is further characterized by two points that distinquish it from pathways in other plants. The first is that in fungi only a single C_1 transfer usually occurs to C-24, while in both lower and higher types of photosynthetic plants two C_1 transfers are common. The second characteristic that differentiates the fungal route from the higher plant route (but not from the algal route) is the configuration produced at C-24. In Ascomycetes and Basidiomycetes, in which ergosterol is the dominant sterol, ergosterol has been shown by degradation (*110*a) and nuclear magnetic resonance spectroscopy (*110*b, *194*) to have the 24β configuration.

Much less work has been done to elucidate the sequence in fungi than has been accomplished with rats. Little is known directly about the mechanism of removing the three methyl groups at C-4 and C-14, and we can only assume tentatively that reactions of the mammalian type occur. Since there is an apparent block in Δ^7-reduction, there remains only to consider the sequence of removal of the methyl groups in relation to metabolism in the side chain. Yeast (*Saccharomyces*) sterol metabolism differs from the other species of fungi, *Phycomyces blakesleeanus*, *Agaricus campestris*, and *Candida* sp., at several points. After demethylation and C-24 alkylation, each species seems to have a preferred route, although the enzymes are nonspecific and will accept a wide variety of substrates for ergosterol biosynthesis.

The first step after lanosterol formation in all of the fungal species, with the exception of *Saccharomyces*, is C-24 alkylation. Relatively large amounts of 24-methylene and 24-methyl derivatives of lanosterol have been isolated from cultures of *Candida* sp. (*116*). In additon, labeled 24-methylene-24,25-dihydrolanosterol has been recovered from incubations of *P. blakesleeanus* with [*Me*-^{14}C]methionine, and the same sterol has been found in control cultures as well as in *A. campestris* (*6*). For these reasons, C_1 transfer may be the first step in the fungal route taking the same place in the major sequence as reduction appears to take in the mammalian route. If we then proceed sequentially with 24-methylene-24,25-dihydrolanosterol as we did with mammalian 24,25-dihydrolanosterol through demethylation at C-14, isomerization of the Δ^8- to the Δ^7-bond, and demethylation at C-4, we would pass through 24-methylene analogs of the mammalian intermediates. This may well precisely occur (Scheme 9.30).

Several lines of evidence indicate that, unlike higher plants, and the other fungi in which C-24 alkylation is the first step in the metabolism of cycloartenol to the phytosterols, C-24 alkylation in *Saccharomyces* is delayed until some or all of the 4,4,14-methyl groups are removed. Substrate specificity of *S*-adenosylmethionine Δ^{24}-sterol methyltransferase (EC 2.1.1.41) has been determined with the aid of purified enzyme preparations. Parks and Gaylor and their associates (*53, 86, 364*) found that zymosterol is the most efficient substrate, and addition of zymosterol to a *Saccharomyces* cell-free preparation stimulates methyltransferase activity sixfold. In addition, there is evidence for more than one yeast methyltransferase, each with different K_m values for zymosterol. One of these has a K_m of 55 μM zymosterol. Earlier, Katsuki and Bloch (*52*) had observed inhibition of *S*-adenosylmethionine-dependent alkylation by zymosterol. Inhibition of C-24 alkylation by breakdown products of unstable zymosterol preparations (*86*) may account for the results obtained by Katsuki and Bloch (*52*). Oxygen-starved yeast (*Saccharomyces*) rapidly synthesizes lanosterol, 4,4-dimethylzymosterol, and 4α-methyl zymosterol during the initial phases of aerobic growth, and 24-methylene sterols are not detectable during this phase of rapid onset of sterol biosynthesis (*108*). Moreover, labeled 4,4-dimethyl sterols were not

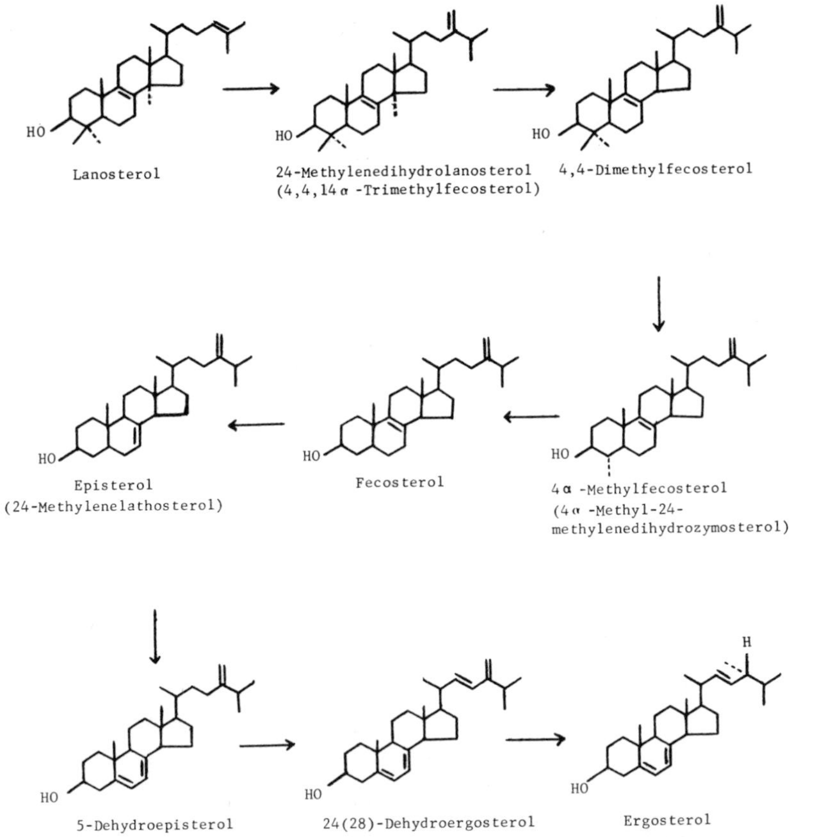

Lanosterol → 24-Methylenedihydrolanosterol
(4,4,14α-Trimethylfecosterol) → 4,4-Dimethylfecosterol

Episterol
(24-Methylenelathosterol) ← Fecosterol ← 4α-Methylfecosterol
(4α-Methyl-24-
methylenedihydrozymosterol)

5-Dehydroepisterol → 24(28)-Dehydroergosterol → Ergosterol

Scheme 9.30. An example of the fungal route (*A. campestris* and *P. blakesleeanus*). Only major intermediates are shown. The text should be consulted for details and alternatives. "Dihydro" refers to C-24,25.

isolated in aerobic incubations of oxygen-starved yeast with [*Me*-^{14}C]methionine and only trace amounts of radioactive 4α-methylsterols were detected (*365*). Incubation of a mixture of [26,27-^{14}C]lanosterol and [2,4-^{3}H]zymosterol with yeast and analysis of the ^{14}C/^{3}H atomic ratio of the products showed that during initial sterol biosynthesis, alkylation does not occur until zymosterol. Later, when large amounts of zymosterol have accumulated, 4α-methyl zymosterol will be alkylated (*366*). The major early pathway of *Saccharomyces* sterol biosynthesis is thus lanosterol → 4,4-dimethyl zymosterol → 4α-methyl zymosterol → fecosterol (Scheme 9.31). The pathway 4,4-dimethyl zymosterol → 4α-methyl zymosterol → 4α-methyl fecosterol → fecosterol, probably assumes minor importance.

The Δ^{7}-analog of fecosterol is episterol, which is a minor yeast sterol and is also converted to ergosterol by enzymes from *Phycomyces blakesleeanus*

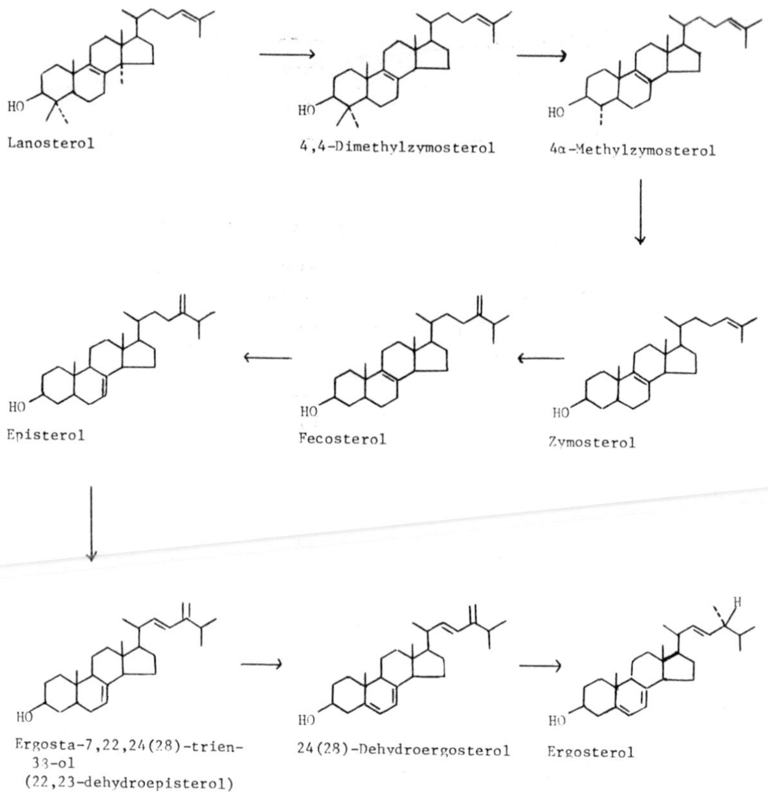

Lanosterol   4,4-Dimethylzymosterol   4α-Methylzymosterol

Episterol   Fecosterol   Zymosterol

Ergosta-7,22,24(28)-trien-   24(28)-Dehydroergosterol   Ergosterol
3β-ol
(22,23-dehydroepisterol)

Scheme 9.31. Saccharomyces—major route of sterol biosynthesis.

(415), Saccharomyces (108), and Candida (116). However, somewhat more
Δ⁸- than Δ⁷-sterols have been isolated from fungi. For this reason, in the
route shown in Schemes 9.30 and 9.31, isomerization of the Δ⁸-bond has
been placed after removal of the methyl groups at C-4. This ordering is no
more secure than the alternative sequence (isomerization after demethylation
at C-14) suggested tentatively for the mammalian route. The sequence of
Scheme 9.30 has the advantage of incorporating known fungal steroids,
viz., 4α-methyl fecosterol (415), which has also been converted to ergosterol
(415), fecosterol (416, 417), and episterol (416, 418), on a reasonable pathway. Recent experimental evidence supports the Δ⁸ to Δ⁷-isomerization
(fecosterol to episterol) as the next step. Incubations of labeled fecosterol
with Saccharomyces cells resulted in 46% incorporation, which was trapped
as episterol, ergosta-5,7,22,24(28)-tetraen-3β-ol, and ergosterol (108). During
similar incubations with episterol, some fecosterol was isolated, indicating
reversal of the isomerization in agreement with mammalian systems (see
Section E.).

Episterol then leads logically and experimentally in *P. blakesleeanus* (*419*) to 5-dehydroepisterol, a known fungal steroid (*419*), by Δ^5-introduction. For the same reasons, the introduction of the Δ^{22}-bond and the reduction of the $\Delta^{24(28)}$-bond are placed in that order as the last two steps (Scheme 9.30). The tetraene, 24(28)-dehydroergosterol, is a companion of ergosterol (*420*), and by judicious selection of growth conditions can be made to be the dominant sterol by baker's yeast (*421*). Furthermore, it has been converted to ergosterol (*422*). Yeast (*Saccharomyces*) may utilize a slightly different route than *P. blakesleeanus* in the later stages of ergosterol synthesis. Labeling and trapping experiments have shown that the major route in yeast is: episterol $\rightarrow$ ergosta-7,22,24(28)-trien-3β-ol $\rightarrow$ ergosta-5,7,22,24(28)-tetraen-3β-ol $\rightarrow$ ergosterol (*108, 109*) (Scheme 9.31). The route via 5-dehydroepisterol (ergosta-5,7,24(28)-trien-3β-ol) to the tetraene, as well as a route involving the sequence $\Delta^{24(28)}$-reduction, Δ^{22}-introduction, and Δ^5-introduction, assumes minor importance. In *Candida*, the quantitatively important route is episterol $\rightarrow$ 24(28)-dihydroepisterol $\rightarrow$ ergosta-5,7-diene-3β-ol $\rightarrow$ ergosterol (*116*).

5. Route in Algae

Algae are photosynthetic plants, and their sterol biosynthesis differs from the nonphotosynthetic mammalian and fungal routes in the utilization of cycloartenol rather than lanosterol as the first cyclized intermediate (Section B). Also, the algal route frequently (but not always) possesses the enzymatic apparatus for introduction of the Δ^5-bond as well as reduction of the Δ^7-bond. This is similar to what is found in the mammalian and higher plant routes but contrasts with the common fungal route. This and other differences in algae lead to the formation of cholesterol, 24-methylenecholesterol, 24-ethylidenecholesterol, (24*S*)-24-methylcholesterol, (24*S*)-24-ethylcholesterol (clionasterol), and *trans*-22,23-dehydroclionasterol (poriferasterol) as common products of metabolism. In some species that lack the final steps, Δ^7-analogs of the latter sterols are found. An important example is the Δ^7-analog of poriferasterol, chondrillasterol [(24*R*)-24-ethylcholesta-7,22-*trans*-dien-3β-ol, (24*R*)-24-ethyl-22,23-dehydrolathosterol], found in some *Chlorella* (*128*) and *Oocystis polymorpha* (*423*). For reasons that are mysterious, those *Chlorella* species that accumulate $\Delta^{5,7}$-sterols and therefore apparently lack the Δ^7-reductase do not carry out the second C_1 transfer. Ergosterol is their dominant sterol, as it is in fungi (*92*).

Little is known directly about the origin of cholesterol in either algae or higher plants beyond the fact that in the red alga *Rhodymenia palmata* acetate proceeds to 22-dehydrocholesterol (*204*) and that cholesterol itself is derivable experimentally from pollinastanol in *Nicotiana tabacum* (*424*). Its biosynthesis presumably occurs by the least complicated of the plant pathways, differing from the mammalian route primarily in the intermediacy of cycloartenol, together with the additional step of opening of the 9,19-cyclo grouping. Cycloartenol and 30-norcycloartenol have actually been identified in *R.*

palmata (*204*). On the assumption that the Δ^8-bond aids removal of the 14α-methyl group (Section D.3), opening of the ring must occur before the latter step. However, this does not necessarily imply its occurrence before removal of one or both of the methyl groups at C-4, and 9,19-cyclosterols bearing a 14α-methyl group but only one or no methyl group has actually been isolated from green algae (*128*). One possible route is through 14α-methyl-9β,19-cyclocholestanol (pollinastanol). This would probably mean a sequence of cycloartenol to cycloartanol to pollinastanol to 14α-methyl-24,25-dihydrozymosterol to 24,25-dihydrozymosterol to lathosterol to cholesterol (Scheme 9.32). It is supported by the frequent occurrence of cycloartanol in higher plants, the isolation of pollinastanol from pollen (*362*), and the above-mentioned conversion of pollinastanol to cholesterol in tobacco plants (*424*). 24-Methylenepollinastanol was not detected in normal *Chlorella emersonii* cells, but was isolated in appreciable amounts from triparanol-treated cells (*128*). The amounts of other 9β,19-cyclopropyl sterols were also elevated, indicating a probable inhibition of the 9β,19-isomerase. The occurrence of 30-norcycloartenol in the pollen of the cactus *Garnegiea gigantea* (*360*), of 30-norcycloartanol in the pollen of the dandelion *Taraxacum dens leonis* (*425*), and of 24,25-dihydro-30-norlanosterol in the pollen of the latter plant (*359*) attest, however, to the operation of an alternative route (Scheme 9.31). The substrate specificity of the enzyme that opens the 9β,19-cyclopropane ring has been determined (*38*). This enzyme is from the blackberry, but the algal enzyme may well have the same substrate preference. Substrates lacking a 4β-methyl group, i.e., cycloeucalenol and 24-methylene pollinastanol, were converted at similar rates to the corresponding Δ^8-sterols, but 4,4-dimethyl sterols (cycloartenol and 24-methylenecycloartanol) were poor substrates. Since the isomerase is nonspecific once the 4β-methyl group is removed, the quantitatively important route may depend on the substrate requirements of the enzyme system catalyzing the removal of the methyl group from the 4α-methylsterols.

The route to 24-alkylsterols is more complicated. The multistep alkylation process is superimposed on the problem of opening the 9β,19-ring, and more than one pathway of alkylation exists. Three algae have been the primary subject of study. They are *Ochromonas malhamensis* (*127, 137*), *Chlorella emersonii* (formerly *Chlorella vulgaris*) (*128*), and *Chlorella ellipsoidea* (*426*). 24-Methylenecycloartanol has been found in the first two (*128, 427*) as well as in *O. dancia* (*427*), *Enteromorpha linea* (*428*), *Ulva lactuca* (*428*), *Fucus spiralis* (*104*), *Euglena gracilis* (*35*), *Porphyridium cruentum* (*429*), and *Astasia longa* (*36*). It has also been converted in *O. malhamensis* to the dominant sterol (poriferasterol, 24R-stigmasta-5,22-*trans*-dien-3β-ol) (*127*). In triparanol-treated cultures of *Chlorella emersonii* there is a 65% decrease in the content of chondrillasterol (24R-stigmasta-7,22-*trans*-dien-3β-ol), one of three dominant sterols, and a 20-fold increase in 24-methylenecycloartanol (*128*). The latter increases from 3 to 59 μg/g dry weight. Other 24-methylene-

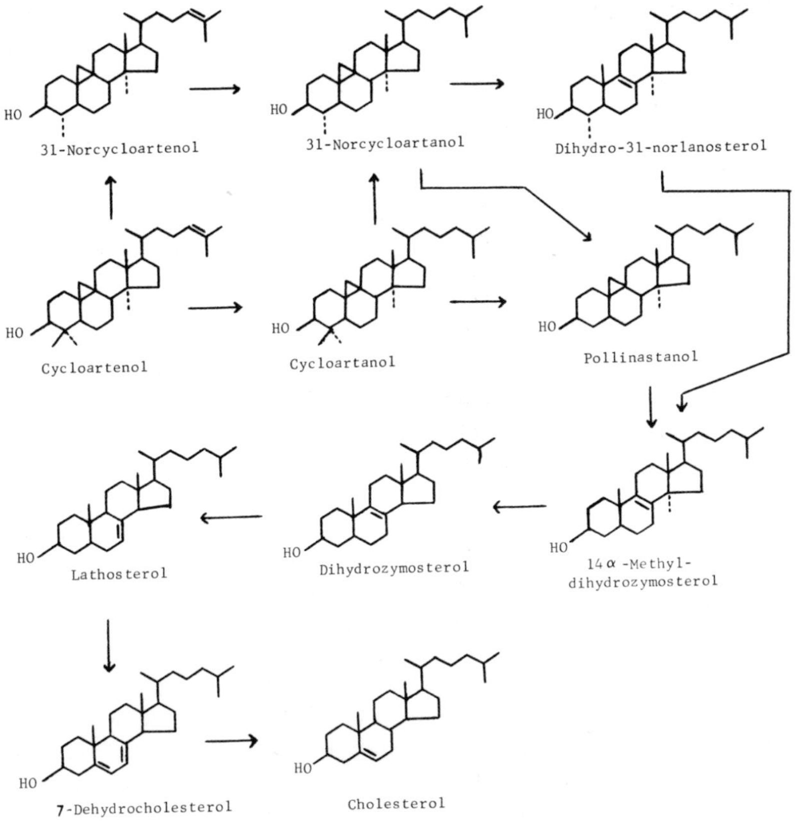

Scheme 9.32. Possible sequences to cholesterol in algae and tracheophytes. The sequences are based on analogy to the mammalian route of cholesterol biosynthesis and the documented occurrence in plants of most of the compounds shown. "Dihydro" refers to C-24,25.

sterols also accumulate dramatically. These include particularly cycloeucalenol (4α,14α-dimethyl-24-methylene-9,19-cyclocholestan-3β-ol), 24-methylenepollinastanol (14α-methyl-24-methylene-9,19-cyclocholestanol), obtusifoliol (4α,14α-dimethyl-24-methylenecholest-8-en-3β-ol), and 24-methylene-24,25-dihydrozymosterol. It thus seems almost certain that C$_1$ transfer yielding 24-methylenecycloartanol is, or at least can be, the first step leading to 24-ethylsterols (*127, 128, 362, 424, 425*). Because cycloeucalenol is converted to poriferasterol in *O. malhamensis* (*127*) and accumulates in triparanol-treated *Chlorella emersonii* cultures (*128*), the next step is believed to be removal of one methyl group at C-4 (*127, 128*). The data from the triparanol experiments indicating accumulation of obtusifoliol, which is the Δ^8-analog of cycloeucalenol, must mean (*127, 128*) that opening of the 9β,19-ring can occur next, but this sequence does not appear to operate always. The isolation of 24-methylenepollinastanol and of $4\alpha,14\alpha$-dimethyl-($24S$)-stigmast-8-en-3β-ol in the *Chlorella* experiments (*128*) shows in the first instance that both methyl groups can be removed before opening of the ring, and in the second that other changes (the second C_1 transfer and reduction) can take place in the presence of the 4α-methyl group. Despite this uncertainty, no sterols bearing a 4-methyl group without an accompanying 14-methyl group were found in the *Chlorella* studies. A 14α-methylsterol lacking a methyl group at C-4 was found, which implies (*128*) that both substituents at C-4 are removed before elimination of the 14α-methyl group. This is at variance with the sequence suggested (*127*) for *O. malhamensis* based on the incorporation of label into poriferasterol from 4α-methyl-14-desmethylsterols (24-methylene- and 24-ethylidenelophenol). The fact that an organism will utilize an exogenous substrate does not necessarily require its physiological intermediacy, but the conflicting data raise the possibility of dual routes, which can be resolved only by further work.

  Chlorella ellipsoidea, which normally biosynthesizes 24-methyl- and 24-ethyl-Δ^5-sterols, accumulates the corresponding 24-methyl- and 24-ethyl-8,14-dienes, ($24S$)-ergosta-8,14-dien-3β-ol and ($24S$)-stigmasta-8,14-dien-3β-ol, in the presence of AY-9944, indicating the operation of the 8,14-diene route for the removal of the 14α-methyl group (*426*). It also indicates complete elaboration of the saturated ethyl group in *Chlorella* prior to completion of the demethylations. The latter is further attested to by the isolation of 14α-methyl-($24S$)-stigmast-8-en-3β-ol and its 4α-methyl derivative from *Chlorella emersonii* (*128*). The tentative conclusions (*128*) from these data are that (a) the second C_1 transfer occurs before elimination of the 14α-methyl group and can occur even before elimination of the second 4-methyl group, and (b) isomerization of the Δ^8-bond to the Δ^7-position occurs after removal of the methyl groups at C-4. Again, the sequence suggested (*127*) in *O. malhamensis*, based on the conversion of 24-methylene- and 24-ethylidenelophenol to poriferasterol, is at variance with the *Chlorella* work. Both in *Chlorella* and in *O. malhamensis* there is, however, a unanimity of opinion concerning the introduction of the Δ^{22}-bond. It seems to occur at a late stage, because no Δ^{22}-sterols are found in *Chlorella* other than the final products, and in *O. malhamensis* 24-ethylidenelophenol will proceed to poriferasterol (*127*). The preceding discussion of the sequencing of alkylation, demethylation, and double-bond migration in algae is summarized in Scheme 9.33.

  The sequence of events leading to 24-methyl- and 24-ethylsterols depends on several factors having to do with the stereochemistry and site of deprotonation in the mechanism of alkylation, whether or not the first or second C_1 transfer is involved, whether or not isomerization occurs, and whether, when reduction occurs, the reduction proceeds on C-24, and, if so, whether from the α or from the β side. Our present understanding of this subject in algae depends on determinations of the nature and configuration of the substituent

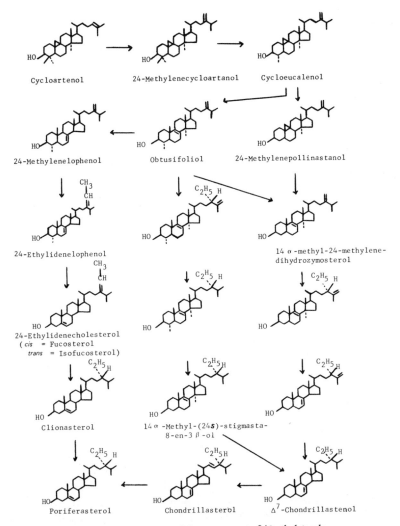

Scheme 9.33. Some possible sequences to 24β-ethylsterols.

at C-24, assessment of the number of H atoms transferred from the methyl group of methionine, and investigations of the presence and position of the H atom originally at C-24 in cycloartenol. All three of these parameters are necessary to make a clear interpretation of the sequence of events, and unfortunately they have not all been studied in each algal group. In the red algal species that biosynthesize 24-alkylsterols, e.g., *Rhodymenia palmata*, nothing of the three parameters is known except that alkylation occurs (*204*). Conversely, in the brown algae the route through the $\Delta^{24(28)}$-sterols must clearly proceed (Scheme 9.33), because 24-methylene- and *cis*-24-ethylidenecholesterol are the well-investigated dominant sterols. A $\Delta^{24(28)}$-reductase is presumably lacking, as was suggested earlier (Section C.4).

In the golden algae the problem becomes more complicated. *Ochromonas* species biosynthesize both 24β-methyl- and 24β-ethylsterols (*97, 135, 211*). In both cases one H atom from methionine is lost at each C_1 transfer (*97, 135*), i.e., two and four, respectively, are incorporated, which implies beyond doubt a $\Delta^{24(28)}$-intermediate (Scheme 9.33). Since the 24-H atom is retained (presumably at C-25) in the 24β-ethyl case (*103*), α-side-reduction of a 24-ethylidene intermediate must occur. α-Side reduction of the 24-methylene intermediate may also occur, but such a conclusion must await knowledge of the fate of the 24-H atom. In the diatoms that usually biosynthesize only a 24-methylsterol, the configuration at C-24 is α and only two H atoms from methionine are incorporated (*121*). This implies the same route as in *Ochromonas* except that the second C_1 transfer is blocked and the reduction appears to occur from the opposite, or β, side. The direction of reduction must, however, remain, as in the genus *Ochromonas*, uncertain until we know whether or not the 24-H atom is retained at C-25. The latter piece of information would eliminate the route through a $\Delta^{24(25)}$-intermediate, which could occur by isomerization of the 24-methylene derivative.

The green algae (Chlorophyta) are still more complicated. Both cyclolaudenol and several $\Delta^{25(27)}$-sterols are known to be present in one or more species of the orders Chlorococcales and Siphonales, which produce 24β-methyl- and 24β-ethylsterols, and in a number of cases that have been examined among the Chlorococcales, three and five H atoms from methionine are incorporated into the 24β-methyl- and 24β-ethylsterols, respectively. These facts indicate the $\Delta^{25(27)}$-route (Scheme 9.33), but other green algae also biosynthesizing 24β-alkylsterols are known to contain substantial amounts of 24-ethylidenesterols. Thus, in some species of the order Ulvales, isofucosterol is essentially the only sterol present (*428*), and in species of the order Cladophorales it is a major sterol, accompanied by 24-methylenecholesterol and 24-methyl- and 24-ethylcholesterol and the latter's Δ^{22}-derivatives (*430*). This distribution suggests the $\Delta^{24(28)}$-sterols are reduced to the saturated 24-alkyl side chains that are dehydrogenated to the 24-alkyl-Δ^{22}-sterols, but the configuration at C-24, the number of H atoms incorporated into the saturated alkyl group, and the fate of the 24-H atom remain uninvestigated, leaving the pathway equivocal. Similarly, two species of the order Charales in the phylum Charophyta may utilize 24-ethylidene intermediates, since isofucosterol is definitely present (*431*), along with 24-ethylcholesterol, the configuration of which is known to be β. The problem that remains is whether there are actually two routes operating in the order Charales of the phylum Charophyta and in the orders Ulvales and Cladophorales of the phylum Chlorophyta, one to 24-ethylidenesterols, which are not reduced, and the other through 24β-ethyl-$\Delta^{25(27)}$-sterols, which are reduced (Scheme 9.33).

Two species of Euglenophyta have been investigated, one, *Euglena gracilis*, which will operate either photosynthetically or nonphotosynthetically, and one, *Astasia longa*, a naturally white euglenoid. A variety of 24-alkylsterols of uncertain configuration has been identified in both species (*432, 433*) and only four H atoms from methionine are incorporated into the ethyl group in *E. gracilis* (*97*). While this as well as the presence of isofucosterol in *A. longa* indicates the $\Delta^{24(28)}$-route (Scheme 9.33), *A. longa* also contains some 14α-methyl-24β-ethylcholesta-8,25(27)-dien-3β-ol (the 14α-methyl-Δ^8-analog of clerosterol) (*432*). Thus, the problem with respect to routes among the Euglenophyta is similar to that discussed for the Chlorophyta and Charophyta.

6. Route in Tracheophytes

Several important structural features distinguish Tracheophyte sterols from those found in algae. Sterols with a Δ^5-bond predominate in the former and the major tracheophyte sterol (sitosterol) lacks the Δ^{22}-bond, in contrast to poriferasterol, the common algal sterol. Tracheophyte and algal sterols also differ in most organisms by the orientation of the 24-alkyl group, which is predominantly α in the former and β in the latter. The configuration of the common 24-ethylsterols, stigmasterol and sitosterol, is α, but the common 24-methylsterol is a mixture of α and β forms (campesterol and dihydrobrassicasterol), in which the former predominates as a general rule (*194*). A few 24β-alkylsterols have been reported in several species, but all contain a $\Delta^{25(27)}$-bond, e.g., cyclolaudenol from *Polypodium vulgare* (*91*), cyclolaudenone from *Musa sapientum* (*242*), and the various 24β-ethyl-$\Delta^{25(27)}$-sterols from the Cucurbitales (*130, 131*) and a species of Verbenales (*132*). All of the current evidence is consistent with the isomerization-reduction route ($\Delta^{24(28)}$ to $\Delta^{24(25)}$) followed by reduction of the latter (Scheme 9.34) to the 24α-alkylsterols at both the 24-C_1 and 24-C_2 levels. Section C.4 should be consulted for a discussion of the detailed evidence. The 24β-alkylsterols that are known to possess the $\Delta^{25(27)}$-bond clearly are derived by the $\Delta^{25(27)}$-route, and labeling data confirm this conclusion (Section C.4). The 24β-alkylsterols that do not contain the $\Delta^{25(27)}$-bond e.g., the important compound dihydrobrassicasterol, also seem to arise by the $\Delta^{25(27)}$-route (*123*) (Scheme 9.35). This allows the simple generality that all the 24β-alkylsterols probably are derived by the $\Delta^{25(27)}$-route.

The problem of sequencing is essentially the same as discussed for the algae. In fact, some of the algal intermediates described, e.g., obtusifoliol, cycloeucalenol, and 24-methylenelophenol, were first isolated from Tracheophytes. Based on occurrence, the Tracheophyte sequence, for which little else is known directly, is presumably much the same as for the algal sequence (Scheme 9.33) to 24α-alkylsterol. The Tracheophyte sequence to 24α-alkylsterols presumably differs primarily only at some unknown stage at which the isomerization ($\Delta^{24(28)}$- to $\Delta^{24(25)}$) (Scheme 9.34) is interposed. A reasonable route is shown in Schemes 9.36 and 9.37.

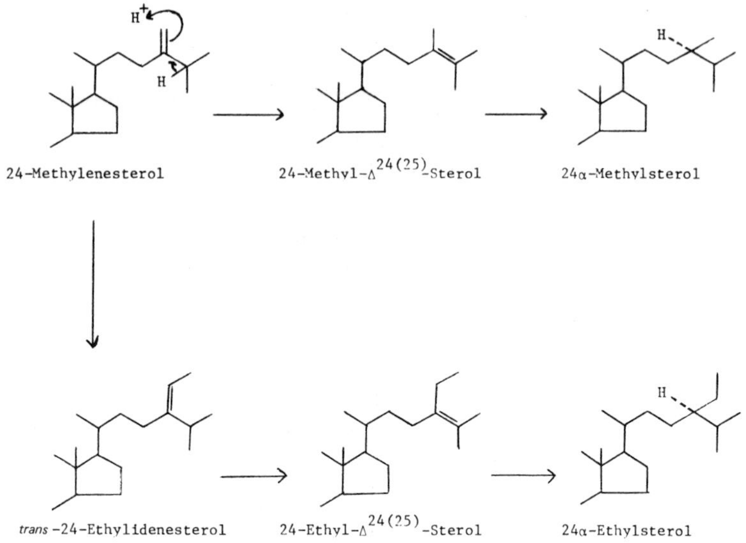

Scheme 9.34. The isomerization route to 24α-alkylsterols.

I. ENZYMOLOGY

1. General Comments

All the enzymes necessary to convert mevalonate via lanosterol to cholesterol have been obtained in a single preparation from mammalian liver (*434a,b*). None of the reactions appear to be reversible (*307*), with the exception of Δ^8- to Δ^7-isomerization (*108, 293, 294*). Similarly, a cell-free system has been prepared from yeast that will convert acetate via lanosterol to ergosterol (*3*), but it has not been possible so far to convert cycloartenol to a Δ^5-sterol in a photosynthetic plant except in the presence of intact cells. The most extensive enzymatic mixture isolated from a photosynthetic plant (*Pinus pinea*) will transform mevalonate only as far as 24-methylenecycloartanol (*28*). In mammalian systems all the enzymes on the pathway between lanosterol and cholesterol are microsomal, but a soluble carrier protein (squalene and sterol carrier protein, SCP) is also required (*434c, 435–437*) (Chapter 7, Section D.3).

2. Δ^{24}-Reductase and Alkylase

The reduction of the Δ^{24}-bond of lanosterol, desmosterol, and cycloartenol can be achieved in a cell-free system from rat liver (*21, 48, 76*), but no detailed enzymology is available. A cell-free system has also been obtained from peas (*51*) and pines (*28*) that will convert cycloartenol to 24-methylenecycloartanol. Lanosterol and desmosterol similarly yield (*51*) their respective

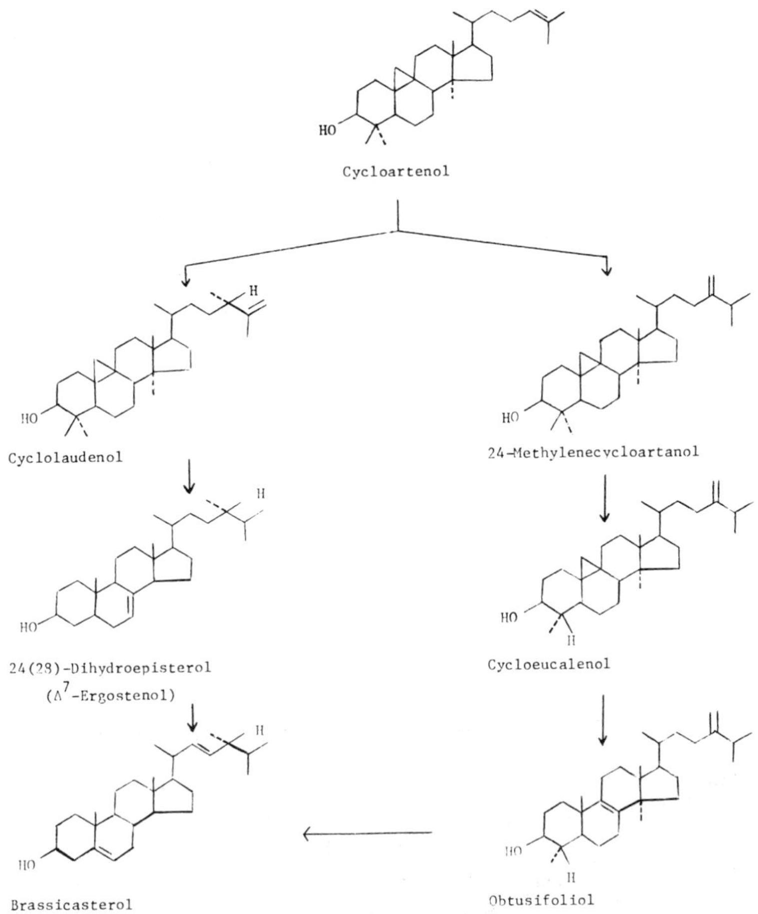

HO
Cycloartenol
H
HO
Cyclolaudenol
HO
24-Methylenecycloartanol
H
HO
24(28)-Dihydroepisterol
(Δ7-Ergostenol)
HO
H
Cycloeucalenol
H
HO
Brassicasterol
HO
H
Obtusifoliol

Scheme 9.35. An example of the $\Delta^{24(28)}$-$\Delta^{25(27)}$-bifurcation at the first C_1 transfer and possible subsequent events.

24-methylene derivatives, indicating, as for the Δ^{24}-reductase, marked lack of substrate specificity. The alkylase (*S*-adenosylmethionine:Δ^{24}-sterol methyltransferase) has been extensively purified from the microsomal fraction of yeast (*52, 53*). Maximal activity requires glutathione, Mg^{++}, and a pH of 7.5. As an ammonium sulfate precipitate, the enzyme is stable during storage at $-25°$. K_m for zymosterol has the value 6.2×10^{-5} M (*53*).

3. Enzymes for Removal of Methyl Groups at C-4

These enzymes have been found in rat liver microsomes (*222–224, 232*) and yeast (*438*). The conversion of the 4α-methyl group to the carboxylic acid stage requires NADPH and oxygen and therefore involves a mixed-function

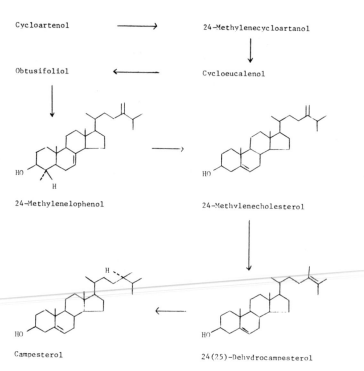

Scheme 9.36. A reasonable sequence in tracheophytes to 24α-methylsterols.

oxidase (223). For each equivalent of 4-hydroxymethylsterol oxidized to the acid, two equivalents each of O_2 and NADH(PH) are consumed (225). The properties of the oxidase for the formation of the 4α-hydroxymethyl group are substantially the same as those for the further conversion to the acid (223), and the same enzyme system may be involved in the entire transformation (222, 224). Cytochrome P-450 is not present. Only 3β-hydroxysterols, not 3-ketones, undergo the reaction. The 4α-hydroxymethyl-Δ^7-sterols are oxidized somewhat faster than the 4α-methyl-Δ^7-sterols. K_m values for the former are about 1.0×10^{-5} and, for the latter, 3.5×10^{-5} M. While the mixed-function oxidase has been obtained only in the form of Triton-treated microsomes, the 4α-carboxylic acid decarboxylase has been solubilized by treatment with sodium deoxycholate and separated from other enzymes of the pathway by chromatography on diethylaminoethyl-Sephadex A-50 (224). The enzyme operates anaerobically and selectively utilizes NAD. NADP is only 5% as effective. The pH optimum is 9.0 and the enzyme is completely inactive in acidic media. It is inhibited by Zn^{++} but not by EDTA, CN^-, Fe^{++}, glutathione, Mg^{++}, isocitrate, or β-hydroxybutyrate. For 3β-hydroxy-4β-methylcholest-7-en-4α-oic acid, K_m is 7 μM and V_{max} is 95 nmol/min/mg of protein. The corresponding 3-ketone is the product. Reduction

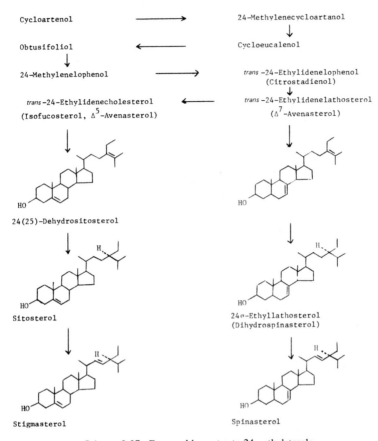

Scheme 9.37. Reasonable routes to 24α-ethylsterols.

to the 3β-alcohol occurs under the influence of an NADPH-dependent reductase, which also is bound to microsomes (*220, 224*).

4. Δ⁸- to Δ⁷-Isomerase

The isomerase is present in rat liver microsomes (*280*). It requires neither
oxygen nor cofactors (*304*) and is not inhibited by triparanol. The relative
rates of isomerization (*280*) are 54 for cholesta-8,24-dien-3β-ol, 47 for cholest-
8-en-3β-ol, 38 for 4α-methylcholesta-8-en-3β-ol, 36 for 4α-methylcholesta-
8,24-dien-3β-ol, 14 for 4,4-dimethylcholest-8-en-3β-ol. No isomerization
occurs with three 14α-methylsterols examined (14α-methylcholest-8-en-3β-
ol, its 4,4-dimethyl and Δ²⁴-4,4-dimethyl derivatives) and 4,4-dimethyl-
cholest-8-en-3-one as well as a variety of Δ⁷-sterols, e.g., 4α-methylcholest-
7-en-3β-ol, are unchanged. The isomerization is reversible. Independent
evidence of reverse isomerization in 4,4,14-desmethylsterols has been achieved
in three laboratories with the aid of yeast and liver preparations (*108, 293,*

294). Under anaerobic conditions which prevent further metabolism of the Δ^7-intermediate, almost 100% exchange of the 9α-hydrogen atom of lathosterol is observed (*294*). On the other hand, in the presence of oxygen, only 34% change is observed, indicating rapid turnover of the Δ^7-sterols once they are formed.

5. Δ^5-Dehydrogenase and Δ^7-Reductase

Both of these enzymes obtainable from rat liver are microsomal (*304, 307*). They have not been significantly solubilized, although treatment with Sephadex G-25 may release some enzyme. The Δ^5-dehydrogenase requires (*304, 439*) molecular oxygen and no reduced pyridine, yielding a $\Delta^{5,7}$-sterol from a Δ^7-sterol. The Δ^7-reductase requires NADPH but no oxygen (*304*), yielding a Δ^5-sterol from a $\Delta^{5,7}$-sterol. Both Δ^{24}- and 24,25-dihydrosterols are accepted by the two enzymes. The reactions, e.g., of lathosterol to cholesterol, are not reversible. The microsomal preparation retains activity at $-20\,°C$ for 4 weeks and is contaminated with the Δ^{24}-reductase. Since sterols lacking nuclear unsaturation, e.g., 4,4-dimethylcholestanol, yield cholestanol rather than cholesterol in liver preparations containing the Δ^5-dehydrogenase and Δ^7-reductase (*234*), Δ^5-introduction must require the presence of a Δ^7-bond in the mammalian system.

LITERATURE CITED

1. H. Wieland, H. Pasedach, and A. Ballauf, Justus Liebigs Ann. Chem. 529: 68 (1937).
2. L. Ruzicka, R. Deuss, and O. Jeger, Helv. Chim. Acta 29:204 (1946).
3. E. Schwenk and G. J. Alexander, Arch. Biochem. Biophys. 76:65 (1958).
4. D. H. R. Barton, D. M. Harrison, and G. P. Moss, Chem. Commun. 595 (1966).
5. M. Akhtar, M. A. Parvez, and P. F. Hunt, Biochem. J. 113:727 (1969).
6. G. Goulston, E. I. Mercer, and L. J. Goad, Phytochemistry 14:457 (1975).
7. I. Schechter, F. W. Sweat, and K. Bloch, Biochim. Biophys. Acta 220:463 (1970).
8. E. I. Mercer and M. W. Johnson, Phytochemistry 8:2329 (1969).
9. K. H. Raab, N. J. de Souza, and W. R. Nes, Biochim. Biophys. Acta 152: 742 (1968).
10. A. G. Gonzalez and M. C. G. Mora, An. R. Soc. Esp. Fis. Quim., Ser. B 48:475 (1952).
11. A. G. Gonzalez and A. H. Toste, An. R. Soc. Esp. Fis. Quim., Ser. B 48: 487 (1952).
12. G. Ponsinet and G. Ourisson, Phytochemistry 7:89 (1968).
13. B. L. Williams and T. W. Goodwin, Phytochemistry 4:81 (1965).
14. K. Schreiber and G. Osske, Kulturpflanze 10:372 (1962).
15. M. von Ardenne, G. Osske, K. Schreiber, K. Steinfelder, and R. Tummler, Kulturpflanze 13:115 (1965).
16. P. Benveniste, L. Hirth, and G. Ourisson, C. R. Hebd. Séances Acad. Sci. 259:2284 (1964).
17. C. Djerassi and R. McCrindle, J. Chem. Soc. 4034 (1962).

18. J. Bergman, B. O. Lindgren, and C. M. Svahn, Acta Chem. Scand. 19:1661 (1965).
19. B. L. Williams, L. J. Goad, and E. I. Mercer, Biochem. J. 96:31P (1965).
20. B. A. Nagasampagi, J. W. Rowe, R. Simpson, and L. J. Goad, Phytochemistry 10:1101 (1971).
21. G. F. Gibbons, L. J. Goad, T. W. Goodwin, and W. R. Nes, J. Biol. Chem. 246:3967 (1971).
22. P. Benveniste, L. Hirth, and G. Ourisson, Phytochemistry 5:45 (1966).
23. P. Benveniste, L. Hirth, and G. Ourisson, Phytochemistry 5:31 (1966).
24. J. Hall, A. R. H. Smith, L. J. Goad, and T. W. Goodwin, Biochem. J. 112:129 (1969).
25. P. D. G. Dean, P. R. Ortiz de Montellano, K. Bloch, and E. J. Corey, J. Biol. Chem. 242:3014 (1967).
26. S. Yamamoto, K. Lin, and K. Bloch, Proc. Natl. Acad. Sci. U.S.A. 63: 110 (1969).
27. H. H. Rees, L. J. Goad, and T. W. Goodwin, Biochim. Biophys. Acta 176: 892 (1969).
28. H. C. Malhotra and W. R. Nes, J. Biol. Chem. 247:6243 (1972).
29. H. H. Rees, L. J. Goad, and T. W. Goodwin, Tetrahedron Lett. 723 (1968).
30. U. Eppenberger, L. Hirth, and G. Ourisson, Eur. J. Biochem. 8:180 (1969).
31. J. D. Ehrhardt, L. Hirth, and G. Ourisson, Phytochemistry 6:815 (1967).
32. H. H. Rees, L. J. Goad, and T. W. Goodwin, Biochem. J. 107:417 (1968).
33. C. Anding, L. W. Parks, and G. Ourisson, Eur. J. Biochem. 43:459 (1974).
34. M. E. Dempsey and W. R. Nes, unpublished observations.
35. C. Anding, R. D. Brandt, and G. Ourisson, Eur. J. Biochem. 24:259 (1971).
36. M. Rohmer and R. D. Brandt, Eur. J. Biochem. 36:446 (1973).
37. M. J. E. Hewlins, J. D. Ehrhardt, L. Hirth, and G. Ourisson, Eur. J. Biochem. 8:184 (1969).
38. R. Heintz and P. Benveniste, J. Biol. Chem. 249:4267 (1974).
39. E. Caspi, J. Sliwowski, and C. S. Robichaud, J. Am. Chem. Soc. 97:3820 (1975).
40. D. J. Baisted, R. L. Gardner, and L. A. McReynolds, Phytochemistry 7: 945 (1968).
41. J. K. G. Kramer, S. C. Kushwaha, and M. Kates, Biochim. Biophys. Acta 270:103 (1972).
42. L. Ruzicka, E. Rey, and A. C. Muhr, Helv. Chim. Acta 27:472 (1944).
43. L. J. Goad and T. W. Goodwin, Eur. J. Biochem. 1:357 (1967).
44. D. H. R. Barton, J. Chem. Soc. 1444 (1951).
45. H. R. Bentley, J. A. Henry, D. S. Irvine, and F. S. Spring, J. Chem. Soc. 3673 (1953).
46. G. Ohta and M. Shimuzu, Chem. Pharm. Bull. 6:325 (1958).
47. E. Rotchie and W. C. Taylor, Aust. J. Chem. 14:473 (1961).
48. J. Avigan, D. S. Goodman, and D. Steinberg, J. Biol. Chem. 238:1283 (1963).
49. W. M. Stokes, F. C. Hickey, and W. A. Fish, J. Biol. Chem. 232:247 (1958).
50. J. Avigan and D. Steinberg, J. Biol. Chem. 236:2898 (1961).
51. P. T. Russell, R. T. van Aller, and W. R. Nes, J. Biol. Chem. 242:5802 (1967).
52. H. Katsuki and K. Bloch, J. Biol. Chem. 242:222 (1967).
53. J. T. Moore, Jr. and J. L. Gaylor, J. Biol. Chem. 244:6334 (1969).
54. Z. A. Wojciechowski, L. J. Goad, and T. W. Goodwin, Biochem. J. 136: 405 (1973).

55. R. B. Clayton, A. N. Nelson, and I. D. Frantz, Jr., J. Lipid Res. 4:166 (1963).
56. W. M. Stokes and W. A. Fish, J. Biol. Chem. 235:2604 (1960).
57. W. M. Stokes, W. A. Fish, and F. C. Hickey, J. Biol. Chem. 220:415 (1956).
58. U. H. M. Fagerlund and D. R. Idler, J. Am. Chem. Soc. 79:6473 (1957).
59. T. R. Blohm and R. D. McKenzie, Arch. Biochem. Biophys. 85:245 (1959).
60. J. Avigan, D. Steinberg, H. E. Vroman, M. J. Thompson, and E. Mosettig, J. Biol. Chem. 235:3123 (1960).
61. D. Steinberg and J. Avigan, J. Biol. Chem. 235:3127 (1960).
62. M. Castle, G. Blondin, and W. R. Nes, J. Am. Chem. Soc. 85:3306 (1963).
63. A. J. Birch, in T. Swain (ed.), Chemical Plant Taxonomy. Academic Press, New York, 1963. p. 112.
64. S. Bader, L. Guglielmetti, and D. Arigoni, Proc. Chem. Soc., London 16 (1964).
65. E. Lederer, Biochem. J. 93:449 (1964).
66. R. Robinson, Structural Relations of Natural Products. Claredon, Oxford, 1955. pp. 19-20.
67. D. G. Hanahan and S. J. Wakil, J. Am. Chem. Soc. 75:273 (1953).
68. W. G. Dauben and J. H. Richards, J. Am. Chem. Soc. 78:5329 (1956).
69. W. G. Dauben, Y. Ban, and J. H. Richards, J. Am. Chem. Soc. 79:968 (1957).
70. W. G. Dauben, G. J. Fonken, and G. A. Boswell, J. Am. Chem. Soc. 79: 1000 (1957).
71. H. Danielsson and K. Bloch, J. Am. Chem. Soc. 79:500 (1957).
72. G. J. Alexander, A. M. Gold, and E. Schwenk, J. Biol. Chem. 232:599 (1958).
73. G. J. Alexander and E. Schwenk, J. Biol. Chem. 232:611 (1958).
74. M. Castle, G. A. Blondin, and W. R. Nes, J. Biol. Chem. 242:5796 (1967).
75. V. R. Villanueva, M. Barbier, and E. Lederer, Bull. Soc. Chim. Fr. 1423 (1964).
76. D. C. Wilton, I. A. Watkinson, and M. Akhtar, Biochem. J. 119:673 (1970).
77. M. Akhtar, K. A. Munday, A. D. Rahimtula, I. A. Watkinson, and D. C. Wilton, J. Chem. Soc. D 1287 (1969).
78. E. Caspi, K. R. Varma and J. B. Greig, J. Chem. Soc. D 45 (1969).
79. E. Caspi, M. Galli-Kienle, K. R. Varma, and L. J. Mulheirn, J. Am. Chem. Soc. 92:2161 (1970).
80. J. B. Greig, K. R. Varma, and E. Caspi, J. Am. Chem. Soc. 93:760 (1971).
81. K. Schubert, G. Kaufman, and G. Horhold, Biochim. Biophys. Acta 176: 170 (1969).
82. D. J. Duchamp, C. G. Chichester, J. A. F. Wickramasinghe, E. Caspi, and B. Yagen, J. Am. Chem. Soc. 93:6283 (1971).
83. B. Yagen, J. S. O'Grodnick, and E. Caspi, J. Chem. Soc. Perkin 1:1994 (1974).
84. L. W. Parks, J. Am. Chem. Soc. 80:2023 (1958).
85. E. D. Thompson, R. B. Bailey, and L. W. Parks, Biochim. Biophys. Acta 334:116 (1974
86. R. B. Bailey, E. D. Thompson, and L. W. Parks, Biochim. Biophys. Acta 334:127 (1974).
87. L. J. Goad and T. W. Goodwin, in L. Reinhold and Y. Liwschitz (ed.), Progress in Phytochemistry. Vol. 3. Interscience, New York, 1972. pp. 113-198.
88. A. J. Birch, D. Elliott, and A. R. Penfold, Aust. J. Chem. 7:169 (1954).

89. A. J. Birch, R. J. English, R. A. Massey-Westropp, M. Slaytor, and H. Smith, Proc. Chem. Soc., London 204 (1957).

90. H. R. Bentley, J. A. Henry, D. S. Irvine, D. Mukerji, and F. S. Spring, J. Chem. Soc. 596 (1965).

91. G. Berti, F. Bottari, B. Macchia, A. Marsili, G. Ourisson, and F. Piotrowska, Bull. Soc. Chim. Fr. 2359 (1964).

92. J. T. Chan, G. W. Patterson, S. R. Dutky, and C. F. Cohen, Plant Physiol. 53:244 (1974).

93. E. L. Ghisalberti, N. J. de Souza, H. H. Rees, L. J. Goad, and T. W. Goodwin, J. Chem. Soc. D 1401 (1969).

94. Y. Tomita, A. Uomori, and E. Sakuri, Phytochemistry 10:573 (1971).

95. Y. Tomita, A. Uomori, and H. Minato, Phytochemistry 9:555 (1970).

96. L. J. Goad, F. F. Knapp, J. R. Lenton, and T. W. Goodwin, Biochem. J. 129:219 (1972).

97. L. J. Goad, J. R. Lenton, F. F. Knapp, and T. W. Goodwin, Lipids 9:582 (1974).

98. J. H. Adler and G. W. Patterson, unpublished.

99. L. N. Standifer, M. Devys, and M. Barbier, Phytochemistry 7:1361 (1968).

100. (a) M. Akhtar, P. F. Hunt, and M. A. Parvez, Biochem. J. 103:616 (1967). (b) E. I. Mercer and D. J. R. Carrier, Phytochemistry 15:283 (1976).

101. E. I. Mercer and S. M. Russell, Phytochemistry 14:451 (1975).

102. Y. Tomita and A. Uomori, J. Chem. Soc. D 1416 (1970).

103. A. R. H. Smith, L. J. Goad, and T. W. Goodwin, Phytochemistry 11:2775 (1972).

104. L. J. Goad and T. W. Goodwin, Eur. J. Biochem. 7:502 (1969).

105. E. I. Mercer and W. B. Harries, Phytochemistry 14:439 (1975).

106. D. H. R. Barton, D. M. Harrison, G. P. Moss, and D. A. Widdowson, J. Chem. Soc. C 775 (1970).

107. D. H. R. Barton, T. Shioiri, and D. A. Widdowson, J. Chem. Soc. D 939 (1970).

108. M. Fryberg, A. C. Oehlschlager, and A. M. Unrau, J. Am. Chem. Soc. 95:5747 (1973).

109. M. Fryberg, A. Oehlschlager, and A. M. Unrau, Biochem. Biophys. Res. Commun. 48:593 (1972).

110. (a) K. Tsuda, Y. Kishida, and R. Hayatsu, J. Am. Chem. Soc. 82:3396 (1960). (b) J. H. Adler, M. Young, and W. R. Nes, Lipids. 12:364 (1977).

111. G. Jaurequiberry, J. H. Law, J. A. McCloskey, and E. Lederer, C. R. Hebd. Seances Acad. Sci. 258:3587 (1964).

112. M. Lenfant, G. Farrugia, and E. Lederer, C. R. Hebd. Séances Acad. Sci. 268:1986 (1969).

113. J. Vareune, J. Polonsky, N. Cagnoli-Bellavista, and P. Ceccherelli, Biochimie 53:261 (1971).

114. J. R. Lenton, L. J. Goad, and T. W. Goodwin, Phytochemistry 12:2249 (1973).

115. J. R. Lenton, L. J. Goad, and T. W. Goodwin, Phytochemistry 12:1135 (1973).

116. M. Fryberg, A. C. Oehlschlager, and A. M. Unrau, Arch. Biochem. Biophys. 173:171 (1975).

117. D. H. R. Barton, J. E. T. Corrie, D. A. Widdowson, M. Bard, and R. A. Woods, J. Chem. Soc., Chem. Commun. 30 (1974).

118. J. R. Lenton, L. J. Goad, and T. W. Goodwin, Phytochemistry 14:1523 (1975).

119. R. T. van Aller, H. Chikamatsu, N. J. de Souza, J. P. John, and W. R. Nes, Biochem. Biophys. Res. Commun. 31:842 (1968).

120. R. T. van Aller, H. Chikamatsu, N. J. de Souza, J. P. John, and W. R. Nes, J. Biol. Chem. 244:6645 (1969).

121. I. Rubinstein and L. J. Goad, Phytochemistry 13:485 (1974).

122a. D. C. Wilton, K. A. Munday, S. J. M. Skinner, and M. Akhtar, Biochem. J. 106:803 (1968).

122b. I. A. Watkinson, D. C. Wilton, K. A. Munday, and M. Akhtar, Biochem. J. 121:131 (1971).

123. M. L. McKean and W. R. Nes, Phytochemistry. In press (1977).

124. M. Devys, A. Alcaide, and E. Lederer, Phytochemistry 7:613 (1968).

125. A. Alcaide, M. Devys, J. Bottin, M. Fetizon, M. Barbier, and E. Lederer, Phytochemistry 7:1773 (1968).

126. F. F. Knapp, L. J. Goad, and T. W. Goodwin, J. Chem. Soc., Chem. Commun. 149 (1973).

127. J. R. Lenton, J. Hall, A. R. H. Smith, E. L. Ghisalberti, H. H. Rees, L. J. Goad, and T. W. Goodwin, Arch. Biochem. Biophys. 143:664 (1971).

128. P. J. Doyle, G. W. Patterson, S. R. Dutky, and M. J. Thompson, Phytochemistry 11:1951 (1972).

129. I. Rubinstein and L. J. Goad, Phytochemistry 13:481 (1974).

130. W. Sucrow and B. Girgensohn, Chem. Ber. 103:750 (1970).

131. W. Sucrow, B. Schubert, W. Richter, and M. Slopianka, Chem. Ber. 104: 3689 (1971).

132. L. M. Bolger, H. H. Rees, E. L. Ghisalberti, L. J. Goad, and T. W. Goodwin, Tetrahedron Lett. 3043 (1970).

133. L. M. Bolger, H. H. Rees, E. L. Ghisalberti, L. J. Goad, and T. W. Goodwin, Biochem. J. 118:197 (1970).

134. R. Ellouz and M. Lenfant, Eur. J. Biochem. 23:544 (1971).

135. E. Lederer, Quart. Rev. Chem. Soc. 23:453 (1969).

136. M. Lenfant, R. Ellouz, B. C. Das, E. Zissman, and E. Lederer, Eur. J. Biochem. 7:159 (1969).

137. A. R. H. Smith, L. J. Goad, T. W. Goodwin, and E. Lederer, Biochem. J. 104:56C (1967).

138. P. J. Randall, H. H. Rees, and T. W. Goodwin, J. Chem. Soc., Chem. Commun. 1295 (1972).

139. W. L. F. Amarego, L. J. Goad, and T. W. Goodwin, Phytochemistry 12: 2181 (1973).

140. Y. Tomita and A. Uomori, J. Chem. Soc., Perkin 1:2656 (1973).

141. S. Sliwowski and A. Kasprzyk, Phytochemistry 13:1451 (1974).

142. R. Boid, H. H. Rees, and T. W. Goodwin, Biochem. Physiol. Pflanz. 168:27 (1975).

143. G. H. Beastall, H. H. Rees, and T. W. Goodwin, Biochem. J. 128:179 (1972).

144. L. B. Tsai, J. H. Adler, and G. W. Patterson, Phytochemistry 14:2599 (1975).

145. T. C. Tso and A. L. S. Cheng, Phytochemistry 10:2133 (1971).

146. U. H. M. Fagerlund and D. R. Idler, Can. J. Biochem. Physiol. 39:1347 (1961).

147. D. R. Idler, L. M. Safe, and E. F. MacDonald, Steroids 18:545 (1971).

148. Y. M. Sheikh and C. Djerassi, Tetrahedron 30:4095 (1974).

149. M. Kobayashi, and H. Mitsuhashi, Steroids 26:605 (1975).

150. W. Bergmann, M. J. McLean, and D. Lester, J. Org. Chem. 8:271 (1943).

151. N. C. Ling, R. L. Hale, and C. Djerassi, J. Am. Chem. Soc. 92:5281 (1970).
152. R. L. Hale, J. Leclercq, B. Tursch, C. Djerassi, R. A. Gross, Jr., A. J. Weinheimer, K. Gupta, and P. J. Scheuer, J. Am. Chem. Soc. 92:2179 (1970).
153. F. J. Schmitz and T. Pattabhiruman, J. Am. Chem. Soc. 92:6073 (1970).
154. J. H. Block, Steroids 23, 421 (1974).
155. Y. M. Sheikh, C. Djerassi, and B. M. Tursch, J. Chem. Soc. D 217 (1971).
156. P. DeLuca, M. DeRosa, L. Minale, and G. Sodano, J. Chem. Soc., Perkin 1:2132 (1972).
157. P. DeLuca, M. DeRosa, L. Minale, R. Puliti, G. Sodano, F. Giordano, and L. Mazzarella, J. Chem. Soc., Chem. Commun. 825 (1973).
158. J. A. Svobada, J. N. Kaplanis, W. E. Robbins, and M. J. Thompson, Ann. Rev. Entomol. 20:205 (1975).
159. A. J. Clark and K. Bloch, J. Biol. Chem. 234:2578 (1959).
160. W. Bergmann, J. Biol. Chem. 107:527 (1934).
161. A. J. Clark and K. Bloch, J. Biol. Chem 234:2589 (1959).
162. W. E. Robbins, R. C. Dutky, R. E. Monroe, and J. N. Kaplanis, Ann. Entomol. Soc. 55:102 (1962).
163. J. N. Kaplanis, W. E. Robbins, H. E. Vroman, and B. M. Bryce, Steroids 2:547 (1963).
164. J. N. Kaplanis, W. E. Robbins, R. C. Monroe, T. J. Shortino, and M. J. Thompson, J. Insect Physiol. 11:251 (1965).
165. S. R. Dutky, W. E. Robbins, and J. V. Thompson, Nematologica 13:140 (1967).
166. R. J. Cole and S. R. Dutky, J. Nematol. 1:72 (1969).
167. R. J. Cole and L. R. Krusberg, Life Sci. 7:713 (1968).
168. A. Saliot and M. Barbier, J. Exp. Mar. Biol. Ecol. B:207 (1973).
169. J. P. Ferezou, M. Devys, and M. Barbier, Experientia 28:153 (1972).
170. M. J. Walton and J. F. Pennock, Biochem. J. 127:471 (1972).
171. S. Teshima, Comp. Biochem. Physiol. B 39:815 (1971).
172. S. Teshima and A. Kanazawa, Comp. Biochem. Physiol. B 38:603 (1971).
173. J. A. Svoboda, M. J. Thompson, and W. E. Robbins, Life Sci. 6:395 (1967).
174. J. A. Svoboda and W. E. Robbins, Science 156:1637 (1967).
175. J. A. Svoboda and W. E. Robbins, Experientia 24:1131 (1968).
176. J. A. Svoboda, R. F. N. Hutchins, M. J. Thompson, and W. E. Robbins, Steroids 14:469 (1969).
177. J. A. Svoboda, M. J. Thompson, and W. E. Robbins, Nature New Biol. (London) 230:57 (1971).
178. J. A. Svoboda and W. E. Robbins, Lipids 6:113 (1971).
179. J. A. Svoboda, M. J. Thompson, and W. E. Robbins, Lipids 7:156 (1972).
180. J. P. Allais and M. Barbier, Experientia 27:506 (1971).
181. P. J. Pettler, W. J. S. Lockley, H. H. Rees, and T. W. Goodwin, J. Chem. Soc., Chem. Commun. 844 (1974).
182. P. J. Randall, J. G. Lloyd-Jones, I. F. Cook, H. H. Rees, and T. W. Goodwin, J. Chem. Soc., Chem. Commun. 1296 (1972).
183. Y. Fujimoto, A. Awata, M. Morisaki, and N. Ikekawa, Tetrahedron Lett. 4335 (1974).
184. H. C. Malhotra and W. R. Nes, J. Biol. Chem. 246:4934 (1971).
185. S. Burstein and M. Gut, Advan. Lipid Res. 9:291 (1971).
186. L. Tan and L. L. Smith, Biochim. Biophys. Acta 152:758 (1968).
187. M. Morisaki, H. Ohotake, N. Awata, and N. Ikekawa, Steroids 24:165 (1974).

188. J. P. Allais, A. Alcaide, and M. Barbier, Experientia 29:944 (1973).
189. M. Morisaki, H. Ohtaka, M. Okubayashi, and N. Ikekawa, J. Chem. Soc., Chem. Commun. 1275 (1972).
190. F. B. Mallory and R. L. Conner, Lipids 6:149 (1971).
191. R. L. Conner, F. B. Mallory, and W. R. Nes, unpublished observations.
192. W. R. Nes, A. Alcaide, F. B. Mallory, J. R. Landrey, and R. L. Conner, Lipids 10:140 (1975).
193. A. S. Beedle, P. J. Pettler, H. H. Rees, and T. W. Goodwin, FEBS Lett. 55:88 (1975).
194. W. R. Nes, K. Krevitz, and S. Behzadan, Lipids 11:118 (1976).
195. W. R. Nes, P. A. G. Malya, F. B. Mallory, K. A. Ferguson, J. R. Landrey, and R. L. Conner, J. Biol. Chem. 246:561 (1971).
196. I. A. Watkinson, D. C. Wilton, A. D. Rahimtula, and M. M. Akhtar, Eur. J. Biochem. 23:1 (1971).
197. D. R. Idler, P. M. Wiseman, and L. M. Safe, Steroids 16:451 (1970).
198. A. Alcaide, J. Viala, F. Pinte, M. Itoh, T. Nomura, and M. Barbier, C. R. Hebd. Séances Acad. Sci. 273:1386 (1971).
199. (a) J. L. Boutry, A. Alcaide, and M. Barbier, C. R. Hebd. Séances Acad. Sci. 272:1022 (1971). (b) L. J. Goad, I. Rubinstein, and A. G. Smith, Proc. Roy. Soc. (London), Ser. B 180:223 (1972).
200. J. Viala, M. Devys, and M. Barbier, Bull. Soc. Chim. Fr. 3626 (1972).
201. T. R. Erdman and R. H. Thomson, Tetrahedron 28:5163 (1972).
202. M. Kobayashi, R. Tsuru, K. Todo, and H. Mitsuhashi, Tetrahedron Lett. 2935 (1972).
203. J. P. Ferezou, M. Devys, and M. Barbier, Experientia 28:407 (1972).
204. J. P. Ferezou, M. Devys, J. P. Allais, and M. Barbier, Phytochemistry 13: 593 (1974).
205. S. Teshima and A. Kanazawa, Comp. Biochem. Physiol. B 47:555 (1974).
206. S. Teshima, A. Kanazawa, and T. Ando, Comp. Biochem. Physiol. B 41: 121 (1972).
207. S. Yasuda, Comp. Biochem. Physiol. B 48:225 (1974).
208. M. Fryberg, A. C. Oehlschlager, and A. M. Unrau, J. Chem. Soc. D 1194 (1971).
209. T. Tamura, T. Wainai, B. Truscott, and D. R. Idler, Can. J. Biochem. 42:1331 (1964).
210. D. R. Idler and U. H. M. Fagerlund, J. Am. Chem. Soc. 77:4142 (1955).
211. U. H. M. Fagerlund and D. R. Idler, J. Org. Chem. 21:372 (1956).
212. W. R. Nes, Lipids 6:219 (1971).
213. W. R. Nes, N. S. Thampi, and J. W. Cannon, Fed. Proc. 29:911 (1970).
214. W. R. Nes, J. W. Cannon, N. S. Thampi, and P. A. G. Malya, J. Biol. Chem. 248:484 (1973).
215. M. Kobayashi and H. Mitsuhashi, Steroids 24:399 (1974).
216. M. Kobayashi and H. Mitsuhashi, Tetrahedron 30:2147 (1974).
217. J. A. Olson, M. Lindberg, and K. Bloch, J. Biol. Chem. 226:941 (1957).
218. M. Lindberg, F. Gautschi, and K. Bloch, J. Biol. Chem. 238:1661 (1963).
219. J. Pudles and K. Bloch, J. Biol. Chem. 235:3417 (1960).
220. A. C. Swindell and J. L. Gaylor, J. Biol. Chem. 243:5546 (1968).
221. W. L. Miller and J. L. Gaylor, J. Biol. Chem. 245:5369 (1970).
222. W. L. Miller and J. L. Gaylor, J. Biol. Chem. 245:5375 (1970).
223. W. L. Miller, D. R. Brady, and J. L. Gaylor, J. Biol. Chem. 246:5147 (1971).
224. A. D. Rahimtula and J. L. Gaylor, J. Biol. Chem. 247:9 (1972).
225. J. L. Gaylor, Y. Miyake, and T. Yamano, J. Biol. Chem. 250:7159 (1975).

226. W. L. Miller, M. E. Kalafer, J. L. Gaylor, and C. V. Delwiche, Biochemistry 6:2673 (1967).
227. M. M. Bechtold, C. V. Delwiche, K. Comai, and J. L. Gaylor, J. Biol. Chem. 247:7650 (1972).
228. J. L. Gaylor, Advan. Lipid Res. 10:89 (1972).
229. J. L. Gaylor and C. V. Delwiche, Ann. N. Y. Acad. Sci. 212:122 (1973).
230. G. M. Hornby and G. S. Boyd, Biochem. Biophys. Res. Commun. 40:1452 (1970).
231. J. A. Nelson, S. Kahn, T. A. Spencer, K. B. Sharpless, and R. B. Clayton, Bioorg. Chem. 4:363 (1975).
232. R. Rahman, K. B. Sharpless, T. A. Spencer, and R. B. Clayton, J. Biol. Chem. 245:2667 (1970).
233. K. J. Stone, W. R. Roeske, R. B. Clayton, and E. E. van Tamelen, J. Chem. Soc. D 530 (1969).
234. K. B. Sharpless, T. E. Snyder, T. A. Spencer, K. K. Maheshwari, G. Guhn, and R. B. Clayton, J. Am. Chem. Soc. 90:6874 (1968).
235. E. L. Ghisalberti, N. J. de Souza, H. H. Rees, L. J. Goad, and T. W. Goodwin, J. Chem. Soc. D 1403 (1969).
236. L. J. Mulheirn and E. Caspi, J. Biol. Chem. 246:2494 (1971).
237. A. Sanghvi, D. Balasubramanian, and A. Moskowitz, Biochemistry 6:869 (1967).
238. A. Sanghvi, J. Lipid Res. 11:124 (1970).
239. T. J. Scallen, A. K. Dhar, and E. D. Loughron, J. Biol. Chem. 246:3168 (1971).
240. F. F. Knapp, S. T. Trowbridge, and G. J. Schroepfer, Jr., J. Am. Chem. Soc. 97:3522. (1975).
241. F. F. Knapp and H. J. Nicholas, J. Chem. Soc. D 399 (1970).
242. F. F. Knapp and H. J. Nicholas, Phytochemistry 10:97 (1971).
243. H. H. Rees, E. I. Mercer, and T. W. Goodwin, Biochem. J. 99:726 (1966).
244. K. Alexander, M. Akhtar, R. B. Boar, J. F. McGhie, and D. H. R. Barton, J. Chem. Soc., Chem. Commun. 383 (1972).
245. G. F. Gibbons and K. A. Mitropoulis, Eur. J. Biochem. 40:267 (1973).
246. W. H. Lee, B. N. Lutsky, and G. J. Schroepfer, Jr., J. Biol. Chem. 246: 2494 (1971).
247. B. N. Lutsky and G. J. Schroepfer, Jr., Biochem. Biophys. Res. Commun. 35:288 (1969).
248. L. H. Zalkow, G. A. Cabat, G. L. Ghetty, M. Ghosal, and G. Keen, Tetrahedron Lett. 5727 (1968).
249. J. Fried, A. Dudowitz, and J. W. Brown, Biochem. Biophys. Res. Commun. 32:568 (1968).
250. G. F. Gibbons, L. J. Goad, and T. W. Goodwin, Chem. Commun. 1458 (1968).
251. G. F. Gibbons, L. J. Goad, and T. W. Goodwin, Chem. Commun. 1212 (1968).
252. L. Canonica, A. Fiecchi, M. Galli-Kienle, A. Scala, G. Galli, E. Grossi-Paoletti, and R. Paoletti, J. Am. Chem. Soc. 90:3597 (1968).
253. L. Canonica, A. Fiecchi, M. Galli-Kienle, A. Scala, G. Galli, E. Grossi-Paoletti, and R. Paoletti, Steroids 12:445 (1968).
254. M. Akhtar, A. D. Rahimtula, I. A. Watkinson, D. C. Wilton, and K. A. Munday, Eur. J. Biochem. 9:107 (1969).
255. E. Caspi, P. J. Ramm, and R. E. Gain, J. Am. Chem. Soc. 91:4012 (1969).
256. E. Caspi, J. P. Moreau, and P. J. Ramm, J. Am. Chem. Soc. 96:8107 (1974).

257. D. H. R. Barton and T. Bruun, J. Chem. Soc. 2728 (1951).
258. L. Canonica, A. Fiecchi, M. Galli-Kienle, A. Scala, G. Galli, E. Grossi-Paoletti, and R. Paoletti, J. Am. Chem. Soc. 90:6532 (1968).
259. I. A. Watkinson and M. Akhtar, J. Chem. Soc. D 206 (1969).
260. M. Akhtar, W. A. Brooks, and I. A. Watkinson, Biochem. J. 115:135 (1969).
261. M. Akhtar, I. A. Watkinson, A. D. Rahimtula, D. C. Wilton, and K. A. Munday, Biochem. J. 111:757 (1969).
262. D. C. Wilton, Biochem. J. 125:1153 (1971).
263. B. N. Lutsky and G. J. Schroepfer, Jr., J. Biol. Chem. 245:6449 (1970).
264. D. J. Frost and J. P. Ward, Rec. Trav. Chim. 89:1054 (1970).
265. J. A. Martin, S. Huntoon, and G. J. Schroepfer, Jr., Biochem. Biophys. Res. Commun. 39:1170 (1970).
266. T. E. Spike, A. H. Wang, I. C. Paul, and G. J. Schroepfer, Jr., J. Chem. Soc., Chem. Commun. 477 (1974).
267. A. Fiecchi, A. Scala, F. Cattabeni, and E. Grossi-Paoletti, Life Sci. 9:1201 (1970).
268. B. N. Lutsky and G. J. Schroepfer, Jr., Lipids 6:957 (1971).
269. R. Paoletti, G. Galli, E. Grossi-Paoletti, A. Fiecchi, and A. Scala, Lipids 6:134 (1971).
270. W. H. Lee, B. N. Lutsky, and G. J. Schroepfer, Jr., J. Biol. Chem. 244:5440 (1969).
271. W. H. Lee and G. J. Schroepfer, Jr., Biochem. Biophys. Res. Commun. 32:635 (1968).
272. K. T. W. Alexander, M. Akhtar, R. B. Boar, J. F. McGhie, and D. H. R. Barton, J. Chem. Soc. D 1479 (1971).
273. A. Fiecchi, L. Canonica, A. Scala, F. Cattabeni, E. Grossi-Paoletti, and R. Paoletti, Life Sci. 8:629 (1969).
274. A. Fiecchi, M. Galli-Kienle, A. Scala, G. Galli, E. Grossi-Paoletti, F. Cattabeni, and R. Paoletti, Proc. Roy. Soc. (London), Ser. B 180:147 (1972).
275. G. J. Schroepfer, Jr., B. Fourcans, S. Huntoon, B. N. Lutsky, and J. Vermilion, Fed. Proc. 30:1105 (1971).
276. G. F. Gibbons, Biochem. J. 144:59 (1974).
277. B. N. Lutsky, J. A. Martin, and G. J. Schroepfer, Jr., J. Biol. Chem. 246:6737 (1971).
278. H. M. Hsiung, T. E. Spike, and G. J. Schroepfer, Jr., Lipids 10:623 (1975).
279. J. L. Gaylor, J. Biol. Chem. 238:1649 (1963).
280. J. L. Gaylor, C. V. Delwiche, and A. C. Swindell, Steroids 8:353 (1966).
281. A. D. Rahimtula, D. C. Wilton, and M. Akhtar, Biochem. J. 112:545 (1969).
282. G. M. Hornby and G. S. Boyd, Biochem. J. 124:831 (1971).
283. M. Akhtar, C. W. Freeman, A. D. Rahimtula, and D. C. Wilton, Biochem. J. 129:225 (1972).
284. I. F. Frantz, Jr., T. J. Scallen, A. W. Nelson, and G. J. Schroepfer, Jr., J. Biol. Chem. 241:3818 (1966).
285. W. H. Lee, R. Kammereck, B. N. Lutsky, J. A. McCloskey, and G. J. Schroepfer, Jr., J. Biol. Chem. 244:2033 (1969).
286. M. Akhtar and A. D. Rahimtula, Chem. Commun. 259 (1968).
287. L. Canonica, A. Fiecchi, M. Galli-Kienle, A. Scala, G. Galli, E. Grossi-Paoletti, and R. Paoletti, Steroids 11:287 (1968).
288. E. Caspi, J. B. Grieg, P. J. Ramm, and K. R. Varma, Tetrahedron Lett. 3829 (1968).
289. L. Canonica, A. Fiecchi, M. Galli-Kienle, A. Scala, G. Galli, E. Grossi-Paoletti, and R. Paoletti, Steroids 11:749 (1968).

290. A. R. H. Smith, L. J. Goad, and T. W. Goodwin, Chem. Commun. 926 (1968).
291. R. K. Sharma, J. Chem. Soc. D 543 (1970).
292. E. Caspi and P. J. Ramm, Tetrahedron Lett. 181 (1969).
293. (a) D. C. Wilton, A. D. Rahimtula, and M. Akhtar, Biochem. J. 114:71 (1969). (b) M. Akhtar, A. D. Rahimtula, and D. C. Wilton, Biochem. J. 117:539 (1970).
294. A. Scala, M. Galli-Kienle, M. Anastasia, and G. Galli, Eur. J. Biochem. 48:263 (1974).
295. R. M. Lemmon, F. T. Pierce, Jr., M. W. Biggs, M. A. Parsons, and D. Kritchevsky, Arch. Biochem. Biophys. 51:161 (1954).
296. R. P. Cook, A. Kliman, and L. F. Fieser, Arch. Biochem. Biophys. 52:439 (1954).
297. A. A. Kandutsch and A. E. Russell, J. Biol. Chem. 235:2256 (1960).
298. M. W. Biggs, R. M. Lemmon, and F. T. Pierce, Jr., Arch. Biochem. Biophys. 51:155 (1954).
299. I. D. Frantz, Jr., A. G. Davidson, E. Dulit, and M. L. Moberley, J. Biol. Chem. 234:2290 (1959).
300. G. J. Schroepfer, Jr. and I. D. Frantz, Jr., J. Biol. Chem 236:3137 (1961).
301. M. Glover, J. Glover, and R. A. Morton, Biochem. J. 51:1 (1952).
302. E. I. Mercer and J. Glover, Biochem. J. 73:5 P (1959).
303. A. A. Kandutsch, Fed. Proc. 20:232 (1961).
304. M. E. Dempsey, J. D. Seaton, G. J. Schroepfer, Jr., and R. W. Trockman, J. Biol. Chem. 239:1381 (1964).
305. I. D. Frantz, Jr., A. T. Sanghvi, and R. B. Clayton, J. Biol. Chem. 237: 3381 (1962).
306. D. Dvornik, M. Kraml, and J. F. Bagli, J. Am. Chem. Soc. 86:2739 (1964).
307. M. E. Dempsey, J. Biol. Chem. 240:4176 (1965).
308. R. L. Conner, F. B. Mallory, J. R. Landrey, and C. W. L. Iyenger, J. Biol. Chem. 244:2325 (1969).
309. P. Johnson, I. F. Cook, H. H. Rees, and T. W. Goodwin, Biochem. J. 152: 303 (1975).
310. M. J. Thompson, J. A. Svoboda, J. N. Kaplanis, and W. E. Robbins, Proc. Roy. Soc. (London), Ser. B 180:203 (1972).
311. S. M. Dewhurst and M. Akhtar, Biochem. J. 105:1187 (1967).
312. M. Akhtar and M. A. Parvez, Biochem. J. 108:527 (1968).
313. W. E. Harvey and K. Bloch, Chem. Ind. (London) 595 (1961).
314. M. Slator and K. Bloch, J. Biol. Chem. 240:4598 (1965).
315. A. Fiecchi, M. Galli-Kienle, A. Scala, G. Galli, R. Paoletti, and E. Grossi-Paoletti, J. Biol. Chem. 247:5898 (1972).
316. P. Wieland and V. Prelog, Helv. Chim. Acta 30:1028 (1947).
317. M. Endo, M. Kajiwara, and K. Nakanishi, J. Chem. Soc. D 309 (1970).
318. J. D. White and S. I. Taylor, J. Am. Chem. Soc. 92:5811 (1970).
319. E. P. Serebryakov, A. V. Simolon, V. F. Kicherov, and B. V. Rosynov, Tetrahedron 26:5215 (1970).
320. Y. Tanahashi and T. Takahashi, Bull. Chem. Soc. Jap. 39:8118 (1966).
321. J. Arditti, R. Ernst, M. H. Fisch, and B. H. Flick, J. Chem. Soc., Chem. Commun. 1217 (1972).
322. G. Bauslaugh, G. Just, and F. Blank, Nature (London) 202:1218 (1964).
323. Z. A. Wojciechowski, L. J. Goad, and T. W. Goodwin, Phytochemistry 12: 1433 (1970).
324. E. K. Nelson, J. Am. Chem. Soc. 33:1404 (1911).
325. H. H. Szmant and A. Halpaern, J. Am. Chem. Soc. 71:1133 (1949).
326. J. G. Hamilton and R. N. Castrejon, Fed. Proc. 25:221 (1966).

327. G. Blondin, B. D. Kulkarni, and W. R. Nes, J. Am. Chem. Soc. 86:2528 (1964).
328. A. M. Paliokas and G. J. Schroepfer, Jr., Biochim. Biophys. Acta 144:167 (1967).
329. R. W. Topham and J. L. Gaylor, Biochem. Biophys. Res. Commun. 47:180 (1972).
330. M. Fryberg, A. C. Oehlschlager, and A. M. Unrau, Biochem. Biophys. Res. Commun. 51:219 (1973).
331. R. W. Topham and J. L. Gaylor, J. Biol. Chem. 245:2319 (1970).
332. S. Safe, L. M. Safe, and W. S. G. Maass, Phytochemistry 14:1821 (1975).
333. G. W. Patterson, M. J. Thompson, and S. R. Dutky, Phytochemistry 13:191 (1974).
334. D. H. R. Barton, J. E. T. Corrie, D. A. Widdowson, M. Bard, and R. A. Woods, J. Chem. Soc., Perkin 1:1326 (1974).
335. A. M. Paliokas and G. J. Schroepfer, Jr., J. Biol. Chem. 243:453 (1968).
336. M. Akhtar and S. Marsh, Biochem. J. 102:462 (1967).
337. D. J. Alberhart and E. Caspi, J. Biol. Chem. 246:1387 (1971).
338. T. Bimpson, L. J. Goad, and T. W. Goodwin, J. Chem. Soc. D 297 (1969).
339. L. J. Goad, G. F. Gibbons, L. M. Bolger, H. H. Rees, and T. W. Goodwin, Biochem. J. 114:885 (1969).
340. A. R. H. Smith, L. J. Goad, and T. W. Goodwin, Chem. Commun. 1259 (1968).
341. M. Lenfant, E. Zissman, and E. Lederer, Tetrahedron Lett. 1049 (1967).
342. R. Ellouz and M. Lenfant, Tetrahedron Lett. 3967 (1970).
343. R. Ellouz and M. Lenfant, Tetrahedron Lett. 609 (1969).
344. R. Ellouz and M. Lenfant, Tetrahedron Lett. 2655 (1969).
345. M. Akhtar, M. A. Parvez and P. F. Hunt, Biochem. J. 106:623 (1968).
346. R. D. Bennett and E. Heftmann, Steroids 14:403 (1969).
347. A. Alcaide, M. Devys, and M. Barbier, Phytochemistry 9:1553 (1970).
348. D. R. Idler and P. Wiseman, Comp. Biochem. Physiol. A 38:581 (1971).
349. P. A. Voogt, Comp. Biochem. Physiol. B 41:831 (1972).
350. P. A. Voogt and J. W. A. Van Rheenen, Experientia 29:1070 (1973).
351. P. A. Voogt, J. M. van DeRuit, and J. W. A. Van Rheenen, Comp. Biochem. Physiol. B 48:47 (1974).
352. S. Teshima, A. Kanazawa, and T. Ando, Comp. Biochem. Physiol. B 47: 507 (1974).
353. T. Bimpson, L. J. Goad, and T. W. Goodwin, Biochem. J. 115:857 (1969).
354. W. R. Nes, N. S. Thampi, and J. T. Lin, Cancer Res. 32:1264 (1972).
355. N. McIntyre, K. Kirsch, J. C. Orr, and K. J. Isselbacher, J. Lipid Res. 12: 336 (1971).
356. G. Salen, E. H. Ahrens, and S. M. Brundy, J. Clin. Invest. 49:952 (1970).
357. E. Caspi, J. G. L. Jones, P. Heidel, G. H. Friedell, A. J. Tiltman, and S. Yalciner, J. Chem. Soc. D 1201 (1971).
358. F. Gautschi and K. Bloch, J. Biol. Chem. 233:1343 (1958).
359. A. M. Atallah and H. J. Nicholas, Steroids 17:611 (1971).
360. M. Devys, A. Alcaide, F. Pinte, and M. Barbier, Tetrahedron Lett. 4621 (1970).
361. C. Djerassi, J. G. Knights, and D. I. Wilkinson, J. Am. Chem. Soc. 85: 835 (1961).
362. M. F. Hugel, M. Barbier, and E. Lederer, Bull. Soc. Chim. Fr. 81:2012 (1964).
363. F. F. Knapp, D. O. Phillips, L. J. Goad, and T. W. Goodwin, Phytochemistry 11:3497 (1972).

364. J. T. Moore and J. L. Gaylor, J. Biol. Chem. 245:4684 (1970).
365. L. W. Parks, C. Anding, and G. Ourisson, Eur. J. Biochem. 43:451 (1974).
366. M. Fryberg, L. Avruch, A. C. Oehlschlager, and A. M. Unrau, Can. J. Biochem. 53:881 (1975).
367. M. DeRosa, L. Minale, and G. Sodano, Comp. Biochem. Physiol. B 45:883 (1973).
368. W. Bergmann, in M. Florkin and H. S. Mason (eds.), Comparative Biochemistry. Vol. 3. Academic Press, New York, 1962. p. 103.
369. L. Minale and G. Sodano, J. Chem. Soc., Perkin 1:2380 (1974).
370. L. Minale and G. Sodano, J. Chem. Soc., Perkin 1:1888 (1974).
371. H. E. Van Aarem, H. J. Vonk, and D. I. Zandee, Arch. Int. Physiol. Biochim. 72:606 (1964).
372. F. Meyer, H. Meyer, and E. Bueding, Biochim. Biophys. Acta 210:257 (1970).
373. C. Ginger and D. Fairbairn, J. Parasitol. 52:1097 (1966).
374. N. Jacobsen and D. Fairbairn, J. Parasitol. 53:355 (1967).
375. G. A. Digenis, R. E. Thorson, and J. Konyalian, J. Pharm. Soc. 59:676 (1970).
376. F. Meyer, S. Kimura, and J. F. Mueller, J. Biol. Chem. 241:4224 (1966).
377. G. J. Frayha, Comp. Biochem. Physiol. 27:875 (1968).
378. G. J. Frayha, Comp. Biochem. Physiol. B 39:167 (1971).
379. T. M. Smith, T. J. Brooks, and V. G. Lockard, Lipids 5:854 (1970).
380. W. F. Hieb and M. Rothstein, Science 160:778 (1968).
381. M. Rothstein, Comp. Biochem. Physiol. 27:309 (1968).
382. G. J. Frayha, Comp. Biochem. Physiol. B 49:93 (1974).
383. J. D. Willett and W. L. Downey, Biochem. J. 138:233 (1974).
384. J. D. Willett and W. L. Downey, Comp. Biochem. Physiol. B 45:139 (1973).
385. P. A. Voogt, Arch. Int. Physiol. Biochim. 81:871 (1973).
386. J. A. M. Wootton and L. D. Wright, Comp. Biochem. Physiol. 5:253 (1962).
387. P. A. Voogt, J. W. A. Van Rheenen, and D. I. Zandee, Comp. Biochem. Physiol. B 50:511 (1975).
388. M. N. Galbraith, D. H. S. Horn, E. J. Middleton, and J. A. Thomson, J. Chem. Soc. D 179 (1970).
389. W. E. Robbins, M. J. Thompson, J. N. Kaplanis, and T. J. Shortino, Steroids 4:635 (1964).
390. R. E. Monroe, J. L. Hopkins, and S. A. Walder, J. Insect Physiol. 13:219 (1967).
391. J. A. Svoboda, M. J. Thompson, T. C. Elden, and W. E. Robbins, Lipids 9:752 (1974).
392. S. J. Louloudes, M. J. Thompson, R. E. Monroe, and W. E. Robbins, Biochem. Biophys. Res. Commun. 8:104 (1962).
393. R. B. Clayton and A. M. Edwards, J. Biol. Chem. 238:1966 (1963).
394. K. C. Goodnight and H. W. Kircher, Lipids 6:166 (1971).
395. M. J. Thompson, J. N. Kaplanis, W. E. Robbins, and J. A. Svoboda, Advan. Lipid Res. 11:219 (1973).
396. I. F. Cook, J. G. Lloyd-Jones, H. H. Rees, and T. W. Goodwin, Biochem. J. 136:135 (1973).
397. S. Teshima and A. Kanazawa, Comp. Biochem. Physiol. B 44:881 (1973).
398. P. A. Voogt, Arch. Int. Physiol. Biochim. 75:809 (1967).
399. P. A. Voogt, Comp. Biochem. Physiol. B 39:139 (1971).
400. P. A. Voogt, Comp. Biochem. Physiol. B 31:37 (1969).
401. P. A. Voogt, Arch. Int. Physiol. Biochim. 75:492 (1967).
402. P. A. Voogt, Comp. Biochem. Physiol. 25:943 (1968).

403. P. A. Voogt, Arch. Int. Physiol. Biochim. 76:721 (1968).
404. P. A. Voogt, Comp. Biochem. Physiol. B 56:499 (1975).
405. U. H. M. Fagerlund and D. R. Idler, Can. J. Biochem. Physiol. 38:997 (1960).
406. P. A. Voogt, Comp. Biochem. Physiol. B 50:505 (1975).
407. D. I. Zandee, Arch. Int. Physiol. Biochim. 75:487 (1967).
408. U. H. M. Fagerlund and D. R. Idler, Can. J. Biochem. Physiol. 39:505 (1961).
409. S. Teshima and A. Kanazawa, Comp. Biochem. Physiol. B 52:437 (1975).
410. A. G. Smith and L. J. Goad, Biochem. J. 123:671 (1971).
411. A. G. Smith and L. J. Goad, Biochem. J. 146:25 (1975).
412. A. G. Smith, I. Rubinstein, and L. J. Goad, Biochem. J. 135:443 (1973).
413. A. G. Smith and L. J. Goad, Biochem. J. 142:421 (1974).
414. A. G. Smith and L. J. Goad, Biochem. J. 146:35 (1975).
415. D. H. R. Barton, D. M. Harrison, and D. A. Widdowson, Chem. Commun. 17 (1968).
416. H. Wieland, F. Rath, and H. Hesse, Justus Liebigs Ann. Chem. 548:34 (1941).
417. D. H. R. Barton and J. D. Cox, J. Chem. Soc. 214 (1949).
418. D. H. R. Barton and J. D. Cox, J. Chem. Soc. 1354 (1948).
419. G. Goulston and E. I. Mercer, Phytochemistry 8:1945 (1969).
420. O. N. Breivik, J. L. Owades, and R. F. Light, J. Org. Chem. 19:1734 (1954).
421. K. Petzoldt, M. Kuhne, E. Blanke, K. Kieslich, and E. Kasper, Justus Liebigs Ann. Chem. 709:203 (1967).
422. D. H. R. Barton, T. Shiori, and D. A. Widdowson, J. Chem. Soc. C 1968 (1971).
423. D. M. Orcutt and B. Richardson, Steroids 16:429 (1970).
424. M. Devys, A. Alcaide, and M. Barbier, Phytochemistry 8:1441 (1969).
425. M. Devys, D. Andre, and M. Barbier, C. R. Hebd. Seances Acad. Sci. 269:798 (1969).
426. L. G. Dickson, G. W. Patterson, C. F. Cohen, and S. R. Dutky, Phytochemistry 11:3473 (1972).
427. M. C. Gershengorn, A. R. H. Smith, G. Goulsten, L. J. Goad, T. W. Goodwin, and T. H. Haines, Biochemistry 7:1698 (1968).
428. G. F. Gibbons, L. J. Goad, and T. W. Goodwin, Phytochemistry 7:983 (1968).
429. G. H. Beastall, H. H. Rees, and T. W. Goodwin, Tetrahedron Lett. 4935 (1971).
430. G. W. Patterson, Comp. Biochem. Physiol. B 47:453 (1974).
431. G. W. Patterson, Phytochemistry 11:3841 (1972).
432. M. Rohmer and R. D. Brandt, Eur. J. Biochem. 36:446 (1973).
433. R. D. Brandt, R. J. Pryce, C. Anding, and G. Ourisson, Eur. J. Biochem. 17:344 (1970).
434. (a) N. L. R. Bucher, J. Am. Chem. Soc. 75:498 (1953). (b) N. L. R. Bucher and J. McGarrahan, J. Biol. Chem. 221:1 (1956). (c) M. E. Dempsey, Ann. N. Y. Acad. Sci. 148:631 (1968).
435. M. C. Ritter and M. E. Dempsey, Biochem. Biophys. Res. Commun. 38:921 (1970).
436. M. C. Ritter and M. E. Dempsey, J. Biol. Chem. 246:1536 (1971).
437. T. J. Scallen, W. W. Schuster, and A. K. Dhar, J. Biol. Chem. 246:224 (1971).
438. J. T. Moore, Jr. and J. L. Gaylor, Arch. Biochem. Biophys. 124:167 (1968).
439. T. J. Scallen and M. W. Schuster, Steroids 12:684 (1968).

Chapter 10

Occurrence, Physiology, and Ecology of Sterols

A. Orienting Remarks 412
B. Less Advanced Nonphotosynthetic Organisms 415
    1. *Viruses, Mycoplasmas, and Bacteria* 415
    2. *Protozoa* 419
    3. *Slime Molds* 421
    4. *Fungi*. 421
    5. *Sponges*. 425
    6. *Coelenterates and Other Less Advanced Animals* 428
C. More Advanced Nonphotosynthetic Organisms (Eucoelomate Animals) 432
    1. *Invertebrate Animals* 432
    2. *Vertebrate Animals*. 442
D. Less Advanced Photosynthetic Organisms. 458
    1. *Prokaryotic Organisms* 458
    2. *Eukaryotic Algae*. 461
    3. *Lichens* 478
E. More Advanced Photosynthetic Organisms 479
    1. *Bryophyta* 479
    2. *Tracheophyta* 480
Literature Cited. 518

A. ORIENTING REMARKS

Sterols have been found in all major groups of organisms, from blue-green algae to man, but not in all species. For instance, some species of mycoplasmas require sterols, while others do not. In all cases that have been adequately investigated, however, the absence of biosynthesis or of a requirement for sterols correlates with the biosynthesis of an isopentenoid that takes the place of the sterol. This has been especially well documented with the mycoplasmas and protozoa. In fact, of the sterol-less species, only the bacteria and the vegetative phase of certain fungi remain to be fully studied in this regard. The known sterol-less species are also confined to the less advanced nonphotosynthetic organisms, and even among these groups sterol-less species do not seem to be common. All slime molds, for instance, and the vast majority of fungi that have been studied, have sterols in all their parts and at all stages of development. Even the few fungi that lack sterols in the vegetative phase require sterols for reproduction. With the possible exception of the photosynthetic bacteria, which have not been investigated yet, all examined photosynthetic organisms biosynthesize sterols. Similarly, all animals either biosynthesize or require sterols. It is, therefore, obvious that sterols, or in rare cases isopentenoids that mimic sterols, are found in all eukaryotic organisms as well as in many of the prokaryotic ones. One can conclude from this that the sterol structure, if not essential to the very nature of life, is at least essential to the finely balanced sophistication found in advanced forms. While more work needs to be done to make a precise evaluation, it appears from the information presently at our command that there is minimally a correlation between the development of cellular differentiation (and especially sexual phenomena) in nonphotosynthetic organisms and an absolute requirement for sterols. In photosynthetic organisms, regardless of cellular differentiation, there seems to be a sterol requirement that is fulfilled by biosynthesis. The distribution of sterols among these organisms is rather a complicated matter in terms of the relationship between structure and occurrence, even with the dominant sterols (the ones that comprise the bulk of the sterols present), which presumably are, in most cases, the functional sterols. When one adds intermediates, which happen to be present at identifiable levels, still greater diversity arises, further complicated by interorganismic dependencies that develop from the inability of some organisms to biosynthesize their own sterol.

In heterotrophic systems, as is true for other biochemical components, a needed sterol can be supplied exogenously preformed or as some biosynthetic precursor. Under these circumstances an ecological relationship can develop between the receiver and the giver of the sterol. In the simplest case, represented by those species of mycoplasma and protozoa that lack the machinery for the biosynthesis of sterols, the sterol can be nonorganismically present in and directly absorbed from the medium. If, in addition, biosynthetic pathways are present for modification of the sterol to the receiving organism's preferred structure, the organism will not have great dependence on a single type of donator. *Tetrahymena pyriformis*, for instance, which can utilize both cholesterol or 24α-ethylcholesterol, both sterols being converted to 7,22-bisdehydrocholesterol, can accept sterols from a variety of plant and animal sources, since 24α-ethylcholesterol is the common dominant sterol of vascular plants and cholesterol the common one of animals. On the other hand, a species of fruit fly (*Drosophila pachea*) cannot reproduce on a standard fruit fly medium, and in the wild breeds exclusively in the rotting stems of a single species of giant cereus cactus, the senita cactus (*Lophocereus schottii*). *D. pachea* has been found, quite unusually for an animal, to be unable to utilize cholesterol for growth and development. When axenic cultures are placed on a cholesterol-containing medium, larval death occurs in the second and third instars. However, on 24-alkyl-$\Delta^{5,7}$-sterols, or lathosterol, or on 7-dehydrolathosterol, which is formed in vivo in *D. pachea* from lathosterol, normal life ensues. *D. pachea* obviously then requires $\Delta^{5,7}$-sterols for its existence, lacks a Δ^{7}-dehydrogenase, but has a Δ^{5}-dehydrogenase. Since, as other insects do, it also lacks the capability for de novo biosynthesis of sterols, it must develop an ecological relationship with an organism rich in either Δ^{7}- or $\Delta^{5,7}$-sterols. Not many organisms can fulfill this role, since most biosynthesize Δ^{5}-sterols and manintain Δ^{7}-, $\Delta^{5,7}$- and other intermediates at a very low steady-state level. Furthermore, in the Sonoran Desert of northern Mexico where the fly lives, the organismic choice of a donator is highly limited. It so happens, though, that the senita cactus, living on the same desert, is biochemically complementary to the fly. It contains unusually high levels of 24α-ethyl-lathosterol (named schottenol because it was isolated from this species), which serves both theoretically and experimentally as the needed sterol for the fly, and the fly, rewarded with life, submits to a specific ecological dependence on the cactus.

The known ecological relationships demonstrate two further points: (1) the biological role of a given sterol molecule can be manifested sequentially in two different organisms, e.g., cholesterol in an animal, passing to a choleplasma where it is necessary and not metabolized, and (2) a biosynthetic pathway, e.g., cycloartenol to 24α-ethylcholesterol to 7,22-bisdehydrocholesterol, can take place with the early part occurring in one organism (a plant in the example given) and the later part in a second organism (a protozoan in this example).

It follows from the foregoing remarks that the distribution of sterols among organisms has a number of complicating parameters. If we next examine the distribution in different tissues of a given organism, similar complicating features arise. If cholesterol is not the only important sterol of all animals, perhaps it is not the only important sterol of all tissues within an individual. Such is indeed the case. Rat skin, for instance, is high in lathosterol and the wool of sheep is rich in lanosterol, the very name lanosterol being derived from this. Sterols are also passed from one cell to the other to play the same function in both, e.g., the biosynthesis and membraneous role of cholesterol in liver, from which it passes via the blood to erythrocytes and other tissues, where it also acts in membranes. Finally, blood cholesterol, originating principally in liver and gut, can be used for adrenal cortical hormone production, which exemplifies the role of two different tissues in a total biosynthetic pathway.

It is not now possible to give as simple and as satisfying an explanation for most of these phenomena as is possible with the *D. pachea*-cactus relationship, but a great deal of information on both the inter- and intraorganismic distributions is known at levels of structure and, to a lesser extent, of amount. This information could be arranged in a variety of ways. Function appears at first sight to be one of them, but there are reasons to believe the function is always primarily in membranes (Chapter 11), and little at the requisite level of detail is known about other functions, aside from that of being precursors to hormones, etc., a subject that is treated in Chapter 11. Another possibility is to catalog the distribution according to structure, but it does not seem to be terribly meaningful, for instance, to place red algae and people together under the heading "cholesterol," even though in both this sterol is the major one. What, among other things, does one do with ferns, in which cholesterol is not a major sterol but is still present, or with some species of red algae, where it is not the major sterol? We have actually chosen to arrange the distribution according to a phylogenetic scale. This choice was made in deference to two major divisions of biology that are correlatable with sterol structure and suggest a true biochemical relationship with organismic type. They are the association of the cycloartenol-lanosterol bifurcation with the presence and absence, respectively, of photosynthesis (for which no exceptions exist phylogenetically) and the association in a more complicated way of the configuration at C-24 with evolutionary level. As a first approximation, the less advanced organisms have β-oriented alkyl groups and the more advanced ones have α-oriented groups. The primary complication (but not the only one) lies in the definition of more and less advanced, which is much more diffuse than a definition of photosynthesis. However, if one takes classic morphological characteristics, which have been used for taxonomic and phylogenetic purposes, the two generally being interdependent, one arrives at the approximation stated above. It is likely, as a result of further examination of the configurational problem, that greater insights into the evolutionary process and the differences between organisms will emerge. We have, consequently, divided biology into the organisms with and without present or phylogenetic photosynthesis, with subdivisions into more or less advancement. We have taken the more advanced nonphotosynthetic systems to be the animals, owing to their common feature of a nervous system. This means we have placed the sponges among the less advanced organisms because at best they have poorly defined nervous tissue. In the photosynthetic category the main subdivisions are into Thallophytes and Embryophytes, in keeping with common practice. Both the detail of occurrence and of the known ecological relationships, together with biosynthetic explanations where possible, are presented under the organism concerned. Thus, the influence of sterol structure on the life of *D. pachea* is discussed in the section on invertebrate animals. The fact that the senita cactus has Δ^7-sterols and serves as a donator of sterol to the fly is pointed out, but a detailed discussion of the cactus and its relationship to other plants that biosynthesize Δ^7-sterols is found in the section on vascular plants.

B. LESS ADVANCED NONPHOTOSYNTHETIC ORGANISMS

1. Viruses, Mycoplasmas, and Bacteria

a. Viruses   Viruses are a polymolecular complex lacking membranes and independent metabolism, and consequently are not living organisms in a dynamic sense. The simplest ones, e.g., tobacco mosaic virus, not surprisingly lack sterols and other lipids. However, more complicated ones exist that do contain lipids, and several have been found to contain cholesterol as well as other membraneous components. These include avian BAI strain A (myeloblastosis) virus (*1*), influenza virus (PR8) (*2*), and fowlpox virus (*3*). In the first two, cholesterol amounts to 34–35% by weight of the lipid, and no steryl ester was detected. In fowlpox virus, cholesterol amounts to less (5%), but cholesteryl esters (18%) are present, as is squalene (17%). The suggestion (*4*) has been made that the presence of membraneous lipids (sterol and phospholipid) in these viruses indicates an interaction of the virus with cellular membrane. In the cases of the avian tumor virus just mentioned and of the example given from the influenza group of myxoviruses, it is in fact known that they mature at the surface of the host cell by passage through and envelopment with the membrane (*4*). The fowlpox virus, however, was isolated from inclusions without contact with the cell membrane (*3*).

b. Mycoplasmas   Mycoplasmas are a group of prokaryotic organisms that are very similar to bacteria except that the former lack a cell wall. More precisely, they resemble the bacterial L phase in which the cell wall has been discarded, leaving only the cytoplasmic membrane. Two sorts of mycoplasma exist (*5*). In neither is sterol biosynthesized, but one of them requires sterol. The other does not. The former has been classified (*6*) in the genus *Mycoplasma* (sometimes called choleplasma) and the latter in the genus *Acholeplasma*. *Acholeplasmas* biosynthesize carotenoids (so-called carotenols) bearing a hydroxyl group. Both the sterol in the choleplasmas, e.g., *Mycoplasma gallinarum,* and the carotenols in the *Achole-*

plasmas, e.g., *Acholeplasma laidlawii,* are distributed completely into the cytoplasmic membrane. The relationship between sterol structure and function in these organisms is discussed in Chapter 11. Both genera will accept sterols, and absolute specificity for cholesterol does not exist.

c. *Bacteria*   Bacteria, which belong to the phylum Schizomycophyta and are prokaryotic, can be divided into three groups: those with and those without (obligate anaerobes) the capacity to utilize molecular oxygen and, third, the photosynthetic bacteria. Since the cyclization of squalene to lanosterol, cycloartenol, or other possible intermediates, e.g., parkeol, to 4-desmethylsterols requires molecular oxygen, obligate anaerobes and aerobic bacteria functioning anaerobically (facultative anaerobes) could not operate the sterol pathway beyond squalene, and no sterols could be biosynthesized. Before our ability to make such a theoretical analysis, von Behring (7) in 1930 and much earlier Hammarschlag (8) empirically investigated a number of bacterial species and came to the conclusion that they lacked sterols. The problem of sterols in bacteria, however, is more complicated than either of these restricted theoretical and empirical analyses suggests. In the first place, it has been known sine the 1930s that feces contain saturated sterol (notably coprostanol), which Dam (9) showed is actually produced in the feces. Then in the 1950s work by Dam and his co-workers (*10a, 10b*) explained the source of saturated sterol by demonstrating the reduction of cholesterol by anaerobic bacteria from human feces. Sitosterol is also reduced (*10c*). More recently, Eubacterium ATTC 21408 has been shown to reduce cholesterol to coprostanol with an H shift from C-4 to C-6, in agreement with the intermediacy of cholestenone (*11a, 11b*). Thus, sterol can actually be present in bacteria. The sterol in the fecal organism does not, of course, originate de novo. However, the existence of the isopentenoid pathway per se in bacteria is well documented. It first came to light in the very discovery of mevalonic acid, which served in the form of a yeast extract ("distillers' solubles") as a nutritional replacement of acetate in the anaerobe, *Lactobacillus acidophilus,* as discussed in detail in Chapter 4. *L. acidophilus* (and many other bacteria) uses MVA to make a polyisopentenoid functioning as a carbohydrate-carrier in cell-wall biosynthesis. The question then arises as to whether the isopentenoid pathway is used only to make an acyclic, head-to-tail polymer or whether at least in some cases dimerization at the I_3 stage can occur to give squalene, whether squalene can be cyclized and, if so, how, i.e., to give sterols, tetracyclic or pentacyclic or pentacyclic triterpenoid alcohols, or triterpenoid hydrocarbons.

In relation to the sterols, this problem has been unequivocally resolved by several investigators who grew bacteria on totally synthetic media and found squalene, sterols, or both (Table 10.1). Schubert and his associates (*12-14*) were the first to use such culturing methods, coupled with modern chromatographic and mass spectral techniques for the identification of the compounds. They examined bacteria that had already been reported by

Table 10.1. Occurence of squalene and sterols in bacteria

Species	Substance Reported	Ref.
Escherichia coli	Cholesterol (major component)	12
	Coprostanol	10,11
Streptomyces olivaceus	Cholesterol alone	13
Azotobacter chroococcum	Δ^7-, $\Delta^{7,22}$-, and $\Delta^{5,7,22}$-24ξ-Methylsterol and sterols with two (major component) and three methyl groups	
Micromonospora sp.	Sterol mixture	14
Methylococcus capsulatus	Squalene, 4,4-dimethyl-Δ^8- and 4,4-dimethyl-$\Delta^{8,24}$-sterol, their respective 4-monomethyl derivatives, zymosterol, a triterpenoid hydrocarbon (m/e 410), and farnesol	21
Halobacterium cutirubrum	Squalene, dihydrosqualene, and tetrahydrosqualene	18
Staphylococcus sp.	Squalene and no sterol	22a,22b
Rhodospirillum rubrum	Squalene and no sterol	23
Rhodomicrobium vannielli	Squalene	24
Aerobacter cloacae	No sterol or squalene but a C_{16}-hydroxyketone	24
Bacillis subtilis	No sterol	14
Lactobacillus vulgaricus	No sterol	14
Corynebacterium pseudodiphtheri-ticum	No sterol	14
Mycobacterium smegmatis	No sterol	14
Mycobacterium tuberculosis	No sterol	14
Mycobacterium bovis	No squalene	14

Siefferd and Anderson (*15*) and Dauchy et al. (*16, 17*) to contain sterols. Carefully growing the organisms on fully synthetic media through five subcultures before analyzing them, they were able to demonstrate that the sterols isolated really originated de novo in, for instance, *Azotobacter chroococcum* (*14*). Moreover, in the latter organism the sterol composition (Table 10.1), including substantial amounts of di- and trimethylsterols as well as of a $\Delta^{5,7}$-sterol, indicated a primitive kinetic control of the pathway which was not likely to have been derived from a host. Much the same phenomenon was subsequently discovered by Bird et al. (*18*) in *Methylococcus capsulatus*, which was grown on a synthetic medium with methane as the sole carbon source. A whole biosynthetic array of intermediates was identified (Table 10.1) from farnesol, through squalene, 4,4-dimethyl-, 4-monomethyl-, as well as 4-desmethylsterols. The unusual (verifying origin in the bacterium) and primitive kinetic control was illustrated by quantitative dominance of the intermediates compared to the end product (8,22-dehydrocholestanol, zymosterol), and further primitive character was apparent in the inability of the organism to proceed beyond the Δ^8-stage of sterol formation. No known eukaryotic organism biosynthesizes only Δ^8-sterols. The pathway always proceeds at least to the Δ^7-stage and most commonly to the Δ^5-stage. However, some bacteria also apparently do this, since cholesterol has been isolated both from *Escherichia coli* (*12*) and *Streptomyces olivaceus* (*13*), and it is noteworthy that completion of the pathway is apparently accompanied in these organisms, as it is in higher ones, by the accumulation of few, if any, intermediates. It is interesting further that the genera *Escherichia* and *Streptomyces* are ones that infect animals. Although there can now be no doubt that bacteria as a group can biosynthesize sterols, this does not mean all must do so. Indeed, careful, recent investigations of several species have failed to reveal any above the 0.0001% level of dry cell weight (*14*) (Table 10.1).

The absence of sterols in some bacterial species raises the question as to whether they may biosynthesize a pentacyclic triterpenoid or other substance which can mimic a sterol as is the case with tetrahymanol in some protozoa. Both pentacyclic triterpenoid alcohols and the related hydrocarbons of the hopane family have in fact now been found, and the hydrocarbons are common constituents of sedimentary organic matter (*19*). Moreover, the ability of bacteria to carry out biosynthesis rather than just assimilation has been demonstrated (*20*) by proof of the existence of a squalene cyclase in a cell-free system from *Acetobacter rancens* that yields hop-22(29)-ene and hopan-22-ol from squalene and the corresponding 3-hydroxy derivatives from squalene oxide (Scheme 10.1). Because the 3-hydroxy triterpenes do not occur naturally in this organism, a biosynthetic block must occur at the epoxidation. Primitive character was also demonstrated by the ability of the cyclase to utilize either enantiomer of squalene oxide, generating epimeric hydroxy products at C-3 in the two cases.

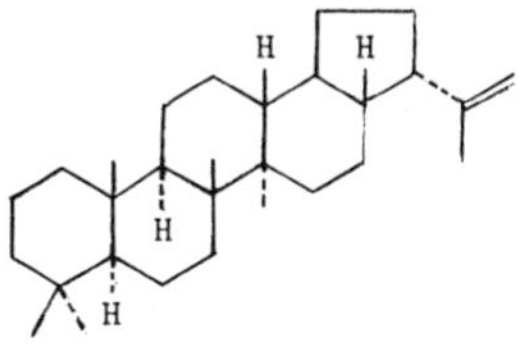

Hop-22(29)-ene

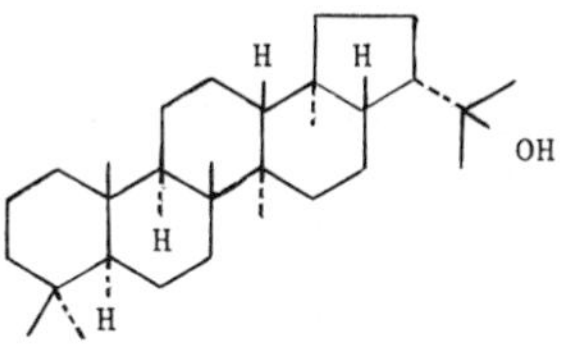

Hopan-22-ol
(Diplopterol)

Scheme 10.1. Triterpenoids of *Acetobacter rancens*.

2. Protozoa

Protozoa are a highly diverse group of unicellular organisms comprising a phylum. Classically they included nonphotosynthetic cells with self-locomotion, and many of the species engulf their food by phagocytosis. These properties reminded the early classifiers of simplified animal characteristics (beings moving around eating), from which the idea of "first animals" (protozoa) arose. In a more modern context such an evolutionary relationship is not supposed, but the character of locomotion remains a dominant feature of classification. The class Ciliata have cilia; Flagellata have flagella; Sarcodonia move by cytoplasmic flowing (amoeba); and Sporozoa lack these forms of locomotion. If the possession of flagella implies that the organism is a protozoan, does the genus *Ochromonas* with flagellated, phagocytosing cells belong to the phylum protozoa in the animal kingdom? Since it is photosynthetic, a real problem arises. Many classifiers include it in the phylum, while others consider it an alga in the plant kingdom. Since there is a strict correlation between photosynthesis and the cycloartenol pathway (known to be operative in *Ochromonas,*), we have chosen not to include the photosynthetic organisms under this phylum.

A nutritional requirement for sterols has often been encountered with protozoa, indicating that the sterol-requiring species lack all or a part of the biosynthetic pathway. *Paramecium aurelia* was the first ciliate shown to have such a requirement, and it must have not only sterol (*25*) but also fatty acid (*26*) supplied in the medium. Both stigmasterol and cholesterol pass into the cells and both are metabolized to their 7-dehydro derivatives, but of the two only stigmasterol will support (*27*) growth (see also Chapter 11). Some but not all species of the genus *Tetrahymena* also require sterols (*28–30*). Among the species lacking a sterol requirement is *Tetrahymena pyriformis,* which is perhaps the best studied of the protozoa in terms of sterols and related isopentenoids. As with *P. aurelia, T. pyriformis* will absorb sterols without regard for their ability to stimulate growth and will convert them to their 7-dehydro derivatives (*31–35*). In addition, *T. pyriformis* introduces a Δ^{22}-bond (*31–34*) and dealkylates 24-ethylsterols (*34*) but not 24-methylsterols (*35*). 24α-Ethyl- and 24α-ethyl-22-dehydrocho-

lesterol are both converted to 7,22-bisdehydrocholesterol (*34*), as is cholesterol (*31*), while 24α-methylcholesterol is converted (*35*) to 24α-methyl-7,
22-bisdehydrocholesterol (epiergosterol). The mechanism of the dealkylation has been studied (*33, 36*) but not resolved. $\Delta^{24(28)}$-Sterols fail to undergo dealkylation and are presumed not to be on the pathway (*33*). *T. pyriformis* also contains and biosynthesizes tetrahymanol and diplopterol
anaerobically from squalene (*37–42*). The inability of *T. pyriformis* to
convert squalene to sterols is supported by a number of facts (*43, 44*),
including the failure of [2-^{14}C]MVA to proceed to labeled material in an
appropriate sterol chromatographic fraction (*33, 45*) under conditions (in
vivo) in which the substrate leads to tetrahymanol. Chapters 7 and 11
should be consulted for a further discussion of the mechanism of biosynthesis of tetrahymanol, structure-function relations of sterols in protozoa,
and the inhibition of tetrahymanol biosynthesis by sterol. The nonrequire-
ment for sterol by *T. pyriformis* is thought to relate to the ability of tetrahymanol (Scheme 10.2) to mimic the sterol structure. (*46*).

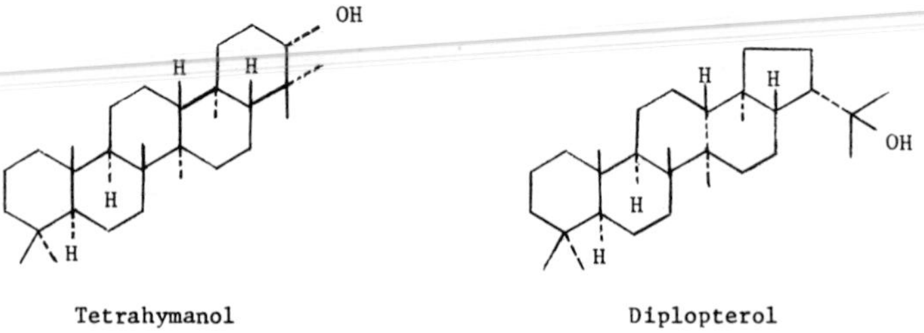

Tetrahymanol   Diplopterol

Scheme 10.2. Pentacycles in *Tetrahymena pyriformis*.

Another group of protozoa which has been the subject of some study
are the Tripanosomatidae. Some species are disease-causing in animals,
e.g., *Trypanosoma gambiense* (mid-African sleeping sickness in human
beings) and *T. evansi* (surra in horses and cattle). The monogenetic species
in the genera *Leptomonas, Herpetomonas, Crithidia,* and *Blastocrithidia*
contain ergosterol as the dominant sterol, together with lesser amounts
of others. In the digenetic trypanosomes, ergosterol is also found, but only
when the organism is grown on a medium containing no animal serum. In
the presence of the serum, or when growth occurs in the animal host,
cholesterol is absorbed. It is thought that cholesterol is not metabolized
and plays an architectural role, while ergosterol plays a multiple role. For
a key to the literature see Dixon et al. (*47a*) and von Brand et al. (*47b*).
Soil amoebas of the genera *Mayorella, Acanthamoeba,* and *Hartmannella*
are another example of protozoa that contain sterols (*47c*). Ergosterol and
24ξ-ethyl-22-dehydrocholesterol are dominant.

3. Slime Molds

Two species of slime mold (phylum Myxomycophyta) have been investigated, *Dictyostelium discoideum* and *Physarum polycephalum*. The former contains 24-ethyl-22-dehydrocholestanol and its saturated analog (*48a*). They are thought, without rigorous proof, to be in the 24α-series. Only the fully saturated 24-methyl- and 24-ethylcholestanols have been found in *P. polycephalum* (*48b*), and the configuration at C-24 is uncertain. The absence of unsaturation in ring B is a unique feature of the sterols of slime molds. All other organisms have Δ^5-, Δ^7-, or $\Delta^{5,7}$-sterols.

4. Fungi

More than 150 species of fungi (phylum Eumycophyta) have been examined (*49, 50*), and in all but a very few cases sterols have been found. In the vegetative phase of *Pythium* and *Phytopthora* genera, sterols are absent (*51, 52*), but in the reproductive phase sterols are required (*52-57*), indicating the absence of biosynthesis at all stages. The possible presence of substances that mimic sterols, e.g., pentacycles, has not been studied. Interestingly, sterols enhance vegative growth (*58-60*). The spores of the primitive parasitic *Plasmodiophora brassicae* also appear to lack sterol biosynthesis (*61*). In the remaining fungi, ergosterol is the sterol most often encountered, at least in Ascomycetes, Basidiomycetes, and Deuteromycetes. The configuration at C-24 has been demonstrated (*62*) to be of the β series through a comparison of the PMR spectra of the fungal sterol with that of authentic 24-epiergosterol (*35*) in two Ascomycetes, *Saccharomyces cerevisiae* and *Neurospora crassa*, and one Homobasidiomycete, *Agaricus* sp. Ergosterol is sometimes accompanied by small amounts of its dihydro derivatives in which the Δ^5- and/or Δ^{22}-bonds are absent, as in *Agaricus bisporus* sporophores (*63*). The absence of both double bonds gives fungisterol, and in the Basidiomycetous bracket fungus, *Fomes applanatus*, fungisterol and 22-dehydrofungisterol actually take the place of ergosterol as the dominant sterol (accompanied by a 16-dehydrosterol) (*64*). Fungisterol is also the major sterol in spores of the Phycomycete, *Linderina pennispora*, and the Deuteromycete, *Penicillium claviforme* (*65*).

In all examined cases of Ascomycetes and Homobasidiomycetes, the dominant sterol bears a 24-methyl group. Minor sterols, e.g., zymosterol, lacking this group, are encountered at times, e.g., in *Saccharomyces*, but 24-ethylsterols have only rarely been detected and not with absolute certainty. Extracts of the Ascomycete *Pullularia pullulous* contain ergosterol and a substance with the gas-liquid chromatographic retention time of stigmasterol (*65a*), and, from *Leptosphaeria typhae*, ergosterol has been isolated principally, with traces (a few percent) of 24ξ-methyl- and 24ξ-ethyl-, cholesterol (*65b*). The latter two were primarily esterified. The identification, primarily by M^+ in the mass spectrum, leaves some doubt about the structures. It is not clear that the compounds were not methylated in the nucleus. When the fungi were grown on "oak water," cholesterol was also reported present. Cholesterol, however, is reported not only to be present but to be the only sterol of the Deuteromycete *Penicillium funiculosum* (*66*), although ergosterol is found in *Asperigillus flavers* (*67*) and most of the other Deuteromycetes, e.g., four species of the genus *Microsporum*, *Epidermophyton floccosum*, and six species of *Tricophyton* (*68*). Cholesterol has also been reported as a minor component of the spores of the Hetero-basidiomycetous smut fungus, *Ustilago maydis* (*65*), and is present in some species of the Mucorales, Saprolegniales, and Leptomitales orders of the Phycomycetes (*69, 70*). The presence of cholesterol raises two interesting points: some fungi appear to reduce the Δ^{24}-bond as well as to reduce the Δ^7-bond, which are functions absent in others.

Fungal diversity is made greater by the isolation of C_{29}-sterols from several groups. Thus, spores of the Deuteromycete *Penicillium claviforme* contain small amounts of 24-ethyllathosterol, which becomes the dominant sterol in spores of the rust fungi (Heterobasidiomycetes) *Puccinia grammis* and *P. striiformis* (*65*), and 24-ethyllathosterol and 24-ethylidenelathosterol are the major sterols of flax rust (*Melampsora lini*) (*71*). From the Phyco-mycetes 24-dehydro-, 24-methylene-, 24-methyl-, 24-ethylidene-, and 24-ethylcholesterol as well as 22-dehydrocholesterol and its 24-methyl and ethyl derivatives have been isolated (*69, 70*). These sterols occur in various com-binations in species of the Saprolegniales and Leptomitales orders, while, with the exception of two species, only ergosterol and its 22-dihydroderiva-tive are found in the Phycomycete order Mucorales (*50*).

From a biosynthetic point of view it would appear that as a phylum the fungi have the ability to carry carbon through the entire pathway to Δ^5-24-ethylsterols. Partial and complete blocks at various biosynthetic stages then explain the differences observed in the sterol compositions. The As-comycetes and Homobasidiomycetes presumably fail to possess an active Δ^7-reductase for the $\Delta^{5,7}$-system (*72*), and also lack both a second C_1-trans-ferase and a $\Delta^{24(25)}$-reductase. The Phycomycetes, Deuteromycetes, and Heterobasidiomycetes, however, seem to contain some species in which these enzymes are present. The absence of the reductive enzymes in the Ascomycetes is attested to not only in the sterol structures of the organism grown in a normal way but also by the facts that *Saccharomyces cerevisiae* can be manipulated so as to produce the $\Delta^{5,7,22,24(28)}$-tetraene as the dom-inant sterol (*73–75*), that reduction of ergosterol does not occur in *S. cerevisiae* under anaerobic conditions (*76*), and that zymosterol, with a $\Delta^{24(25)}$-bond, occurs naturally in *S. cerevisiae*. The di- and tetrahydroderivatives of ergosterol that occur naturally are then readily explained as intermediates to, rather then metabolites of, ergosterol. In the cases where they are the only sterol, the organism must lack the desaturase(s); where they are not present, the enzyme(s) must be very active; and where they occur along with ergosterol, the activities must be intermediate. Although the presence of cholesterol in plant extracts can often be suspect, since the isolations involve human hands, the reality of the C_{27}-sterols in the Phycomycetes is given considerable credence by the biosynthetic array that was reported from Δ^{24}- through 24-ethylidene- to 24-ethylsterols. The only question remaining about their presence is whether or not they were biosynthesized or assimilated. From *Phycomyces blakesleeanus* the biosynthetic intermediate 24-methylene-24-dihydrolanosterol was isolated and [^{14}C]methionine and [2-^{14}C]mevalonate were incorporated, demonstrating biosynthetic capability in Phycomycetes (*77a*), but this organism does not make C_{29}-sterols. Similarly, the Phycomycete *Mucor pusillus* biosynthesizes ergosterol from mevalonate and methionine (*77b*). The problem of assimilation is especially acute with the smut and rust fungi, which grow on higher plants possessing 24-ethylsterols, but again the structural feature of a Δ^{7}- rather than a Δ^{5}-bond (found, for instance, in the genus *Puccinia*) weighs heavily in favor of biosynthesis. Furthermore, the major sterol of bean rust uredospores (*Uromyces phaseoli*) is *trans*-24-ethylidenelathosterol (*78*), and plants of the legume family have dominant sterols not only in the Δ^{5}-series but with a saturated $\Delta^{24(28)}$-bond. It therefore seems likely that the C_{29}-sterols really are of fungal origin, but determination of the configuration at C-24 would be of further value in discriminating between biosynthesis and assimilation. Incidentally, words such as stigmasterol or Δ^{7}-stigmastenol, which are used in the literature to describe the 24-ethylsterols of fungi, erroneously imply that the configuration was elucidated and found to be of the 24α-series. Configurational information was not presented by the time of the present writing.

Fungi contain a tetracyclic group of metabolites of squalene oxide other than the usual monohydroxysterols. They are oxygenated at C-21, and among them is eburicoic acid, its C-21 alcohol (eburicodiol) and aldehyde (eburical), its $\Delta^{7,9(11)}$-derivative, its 16α-hydroxy derivative (tumulonic acid), and the latter's $\Delta^{7,9(11)}$-3-ketone (polyporenic acid C) (Scheme 10.3). They occur in various species of the genera *Fomes, Lentinus, Porio,* and *Polyporous.* For a key to the literature on occurrence and biosynthesis, see Ourisson et al. (*79*) and Anderson and Epstein (*80*). The presence of the oxygen at C-21 is quite unusual, but the $\Delta^{7,9(11)}$-grouping is found in agnosterol, which accompanies lanosterol in sheep's wool. Fungi also contain the protosterol, fusidic acid, and its derivatives, which occur, for instance, in the genera *Cephalosporum* and *Fusidium.* For a key to the literature, see Kulshreshtha et al. (*81*). In the Basidiomycete, *Scleroderma aurantium,* 23-hydroxylanosterol is found (*82*). It has the 23(*S*)-configuration. The filamentous water mold of the genus *Achyla* contains an oxygenated derivative of a 24-ethylsterol with a lactone grouping forming a five-membered ring between C-23 and C-24. It is known as antheridiol (Scheme 10.3) be-

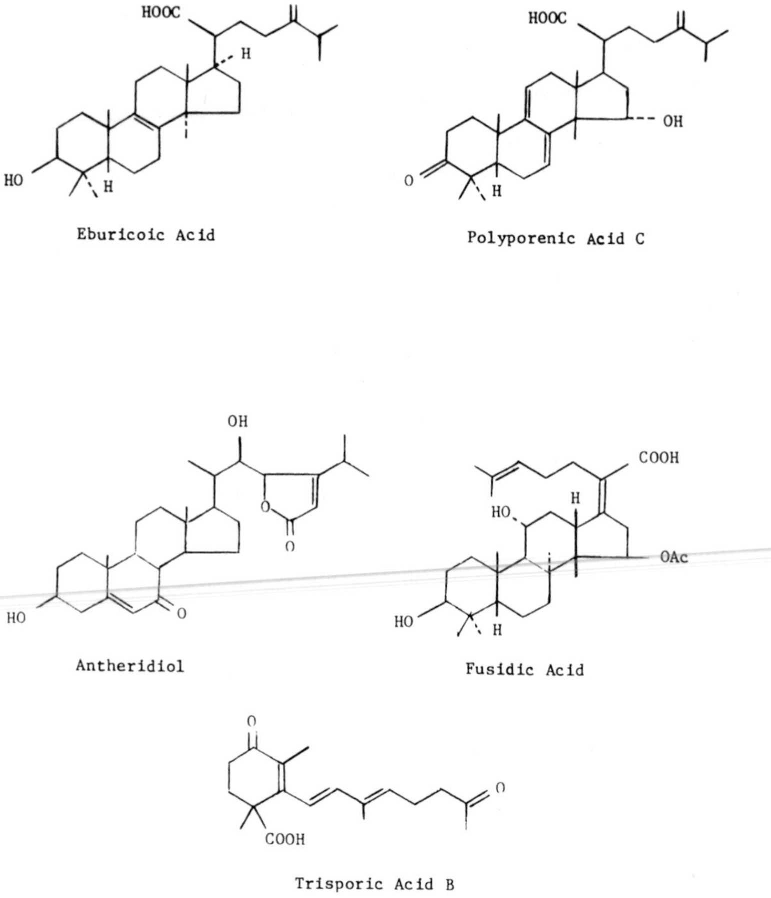

Eburicoic Acid

Polyporenic Acid C

Antheridiol

Fusidic Acid

Trisporic Acid B

Scheme 10.3. Fungal steroids and protosterols oxygenated at C-21 and fungal reproductive hormones.

cause of its hormone-like ability to induce the formation of the male sex organ (antheridium) at the tip of a lateral branch. For a key to the litera-ture, see Barksdale et al. (*83*). Sexual reproduction in other fungi is thought also to be under hormonal control, but not necessarily by hormonal steroids. The trisporic acids in species of the Phycomycete order Mucorales, for in-stance, in *Blakeslea trispora*, are isolable from plus-minus cultures (but not either alone) and are monocyclic keto-carboxylic acids with three iso-pentenoid units and an extra C_3 group at the terminus that appears to have been derived from a fourth C_5 unit. They induce zygophores, and influence carotenoid and steroid biosynthesis, among other things. For a key to the literature see Barksdale (*84*). Interestingly, all the substances involved come out of the isopentenoid pathway.

5. Sponges

Sponges belong to the phylum Porifera ("pore bearers"), frequently placed under Animalia (a kingdom) in the subkingdom Metazoa. They include about 5,000 extant species. Their exact place in the evolutionary hierarchy, however, is uncertain, since, while they are cellularly differentiated, there are no true tissues as such, and little, if any, formal nervous system. Certain characteristics resemble those of colonial protozoa. In view of these difficulties, the organisms are sometimes placed in a subkingdom known as Parazoa.

As early as 1904, Henze (*85*) isolated a sterol from the Mediterranean sponge, *Suberites domuncula*, and called it spongesterol. A few years later, Dorée (*86*) made a study of sterols in the animal kingdom and from the cosmopolitan sponge, *Cliona celata*, isolated still another sterol, which he named clionasterol. Neither of these sterols was the same as cholesterol. While both subsequently proved to be mixtures, from extensive work of Bergmann (*87, 88*), the very early work was interpreted to mean that cholesterol did not have to be the only sterol of animals. Henze's spongesterol was actually a mixture including cholestanol and its 24ξ-methyl-22-de-hydro derivative (*89*). Dorée's clionasterol was a mixture of 24β-ethylcholesterol (now referred to as clionasterol) and its *trans*-22-dehydro derivative, which Bergmann named poriferasterol (*90*).

Bergmann's pioneering studies (*87, 88*) encompassed more than 50 species (collected off the North American Atlantic coast) in 21 families of eight orders of the class Demospongia and one species in the class Calcispongia. Because he lacked modern analytical techniques, which meant some of his samples were mixtures (*91*), a detailed analysis of his findings is inappropriate here. What is important is that he showed that all sponges contain sterols and that many contain cholesterol, some cholestanol, many 24β-ethylsterols, some 24-methylenesterols, most Δ^5-sterols, and a few Δ^7-sterols. In the case of the Δ^7-sterols, incidentally, the name chondrillasterol for the Δ^7-analog of poriferasterol is derived from its first isolation from the genus *Chondrilla* in the family Chondrillidae, order Carnosa. The name chalinasterol for 24-methylenecholesterol (better known as ostreasterol from its presence in oysters) is derived from its first isolation from *Haliclona* (*Chalina*) *oculata* in the family Haliclonidae (order Haposclerina). Unfortunately, though, the relation of structure to zoological classification is not apparent, since, for instance, from *Haliclona rubens* cholesterol "and others" were isolated, and from *Haliclona coerulescens* clionasterol and poriferasterol were obtained. Thus, the family does not appear to be homogeneous in sterol content, nor are others. Bergmann reports various species in the genus *Halichondria* of the family Halichondridae to contain cholestanol while others contain cholesterol. The differences could have their origins in varying relative amounts, the luck of isolations, and the absence of gas-liquid chromatographic and other analytical techniques, but the problem is further complicated by the food (algae, etc.) ingested by sponges. If some or all of the sterols are of exogenous origin, the composition in the mixture could vary from time to time.

Some recent isolation studies have confirmed and expanded the earlier work. The original English species (*C. celata*) of Dorée has been shown (*92*) to contain cholesterol with lesser amounts of its *cis*- and *trans*-22-dehydro-, 24-methylene-, 24β-methyl-, 24β-methyl-22-dehydro-, 24β-ethyl-, and 24β-ethyl-22-dehydroderivatives as well as the fascinating C_{26}-analog of 22-dehydrocholesterol (lacking a CH_2 group in the side chain). The C_{26} sterols are also found in other invertebrates and certain algae. In the same study (*92*), *Hymeniacidon perleve* was shown to have cholestanol, with lesser amounts of its *trans*-22-dehydro-, 24-methylene-, 24-ethylidene-, and 24β-methyl-22-dehydro-derivatives, along with the Δ^5-sterols, 24β-methyl-22-dehydro- and 24α-ethylcholesterol and the Δ^{22}-norsterol (C_{26}) lacking both a CH_2 group in the side chain and a Δ^5-bond. In another recent study (*93*), *Axinella cannabina* was reported to contain 7-dehydro- and 7,22-bisdehydrocholesterol and their 24ξ-methyl derivatives along with six 5,8-epidioxy derivatives, of which those from 7,22-bisdehydrocholesterol and its 24ξ-methyl derivative were identified. A species of the same genus, *A. polypoides*, was found by Minale and Sodano (*94a*) to have an even more remarkable sterol composition. It contains C_{25}-, C_{26}-, C_{27}-, and C_{28}-sterols either in the Δ^0-series or in the Δ^{22}-series. All of these compounds lack the angular methyl group (C-19) between rings A and B, and represent a series of 19-norcholestanol, its 24ξ-methyl-, 24-methylene, 24ξ-ethyl and *trans*-22-dehydroderivatives in the 24-H and 24-methyl cases as well as *cis*-22-dehydrocholestanol (*94a*). Another species of this genus, *A. verrucosa*, contains only 3β-hydroxymethylsterols with a five-membered ring A (C-3 having been extruded) and conventional C_8, C_9, and C_{10} side chains (*94b*) (Scheme 10.4). On the other hand, Sheikh and Djerassi (*94c*) found that some sponges contain a great variety of common and uncommon sterols. *Stella clarella* has at least 20 identifiable steroids, of which 24-methylenecholest-4-en-3-one is the major (23%) one, followed by 24-methylenecholesterol (14%), (E)-24-ethylidenecholest-4-en-3-one (13%), and (E)- and (Z)-24-ethylidenecholesterol (11%). 24-Methylenecholesterol was also the major sterol of *Tethya aurantia, Lissodendoryx noxiosa,* and *Haliclona permollis.* All four of the latter sponges also contained traces of C_{26} sterols, and all four contained C_{27}-, C_{28}-, and C_{29}-sterols in the Δ^5-series. In addition, *Tethya aurantia* contained (Z)-24-propylidenecholesterol (placosterol; see the section on molluscs) and various 5,8-peroxides. Still another unusual type of sterol has been isolated from sponges of the *Verongia* (*Aplysina*) genus. It has an

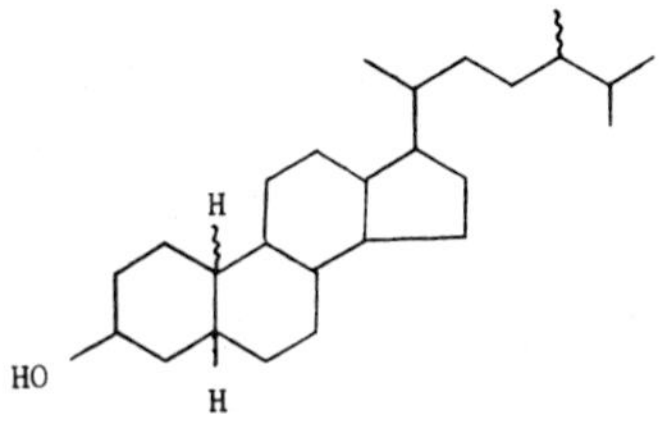

24-Methyl-19-norcholestanol

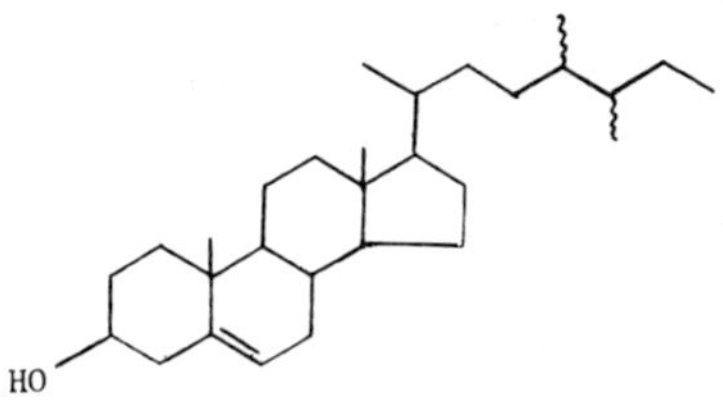

24,26 (or 27)-Dimethylcholesterol

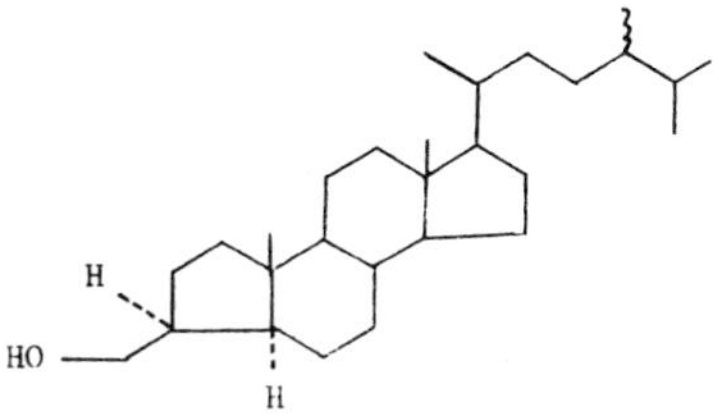

Rearranged 3β -hydroxymethyl sterol
of *Axinella polypoides*

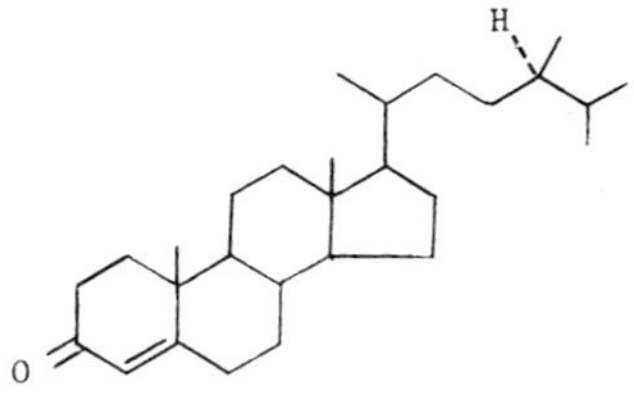

24 α-Methylcholest-4-en-3-one

Scheme 10.4. Some steroids of sponges.

extra methyl on C-26 (or C-27). Two known are 24,26-dimethylcholesterol (aplysterol) and its 24(28)-dehydroderivative. They are found in *Verongia aerophoba* (*94d*). Some structures of sponge sterols are given in Scheme 10.4. *Verongia aerophoba,* in which aplysterol accounts for 45% of the sterol, did not incorporate label from [1-^{14}C]acetate, [2-^{14}C]MVA, or methionine labeled with ^{14}C in the methyl group (*95a*). Biosynthesis also did not occur, either of squalene or of any 4,4-desmethyl-, 4-monomethyl-, or 4,4-dimethylsterols, in the sponge *Suberites domuncula,* but all of them were biosynthesized in *Grantia compressa* (*95b*). The precise structures of the sterols were not determined.

In summary, sponges are highly complex and variable in their sterol structures. Cholesterol is present in some but not in others. 24-Methylene-cholesterol and 24-methyl- and 24-ethylsterols are frequently encountered. Most remarkable is that some sponges contain sterols with a five-membered ring A, with a carbon lacking in the side chain (C$_{26}$-sterols), with C-19 missing, with a carbon added to C-26 (or C-27), and with an oxidized C-3 (to Δ^4-3-keto), as well as Δ^{5,7}-sterols and their 5,8-peroxides. Some sponges do, and some apparently do not, biosynthesize sterols.

6. Coelenterates and Other Less Advanced Animals

a. Phylum Coelenterata   Unlike the sponges, the coelenterates (jelly-fish, sea anemones, corals, etc.) and the related ctenophores (sea walnuts and other organisms with comb plates) have well-defined tissues. Their body wall is constructed of epidermis, mesoglea, and gastrodermis, al-though there is no definite organ system as in higher animals, and the coelenterate body either has radial, bilateral, or no symmetry. The animals do not possess a coelom. About 10,000 species of coelenterates are known and about 1% of that number of ctenophores. Bergmann (*88*) is primarily responsible for their early investigation. He found cholesterol most fre-quently, but also reported 24-methylenecholesterol (*96 a, b*) and what he considered to be brassicasterol (*88*), and others reported sitosterol (*97*). No relationship between classification and sterol was apparent. Out of ten species, for instance, of the sea anemones (order Actiniaria), Bergmann isolated cholesterol, from one species 24-methylenecholesterol, from one sitosterol, and from one a mixture called "actiniasterol." These organisms, commonly regarded from their morphology as animals, thus clearly contain at least in some cases sterols bearing extra carbon at C-24. Especially interesting was his discovery of an entirely new kind of sterol. From *Plexaura flexuosa,* one of the so-called gorgonians (or horny corals) in the order Gorgonacae (class Anthozoa), he and his colleagues (*98*) isolated a C_{30}-sterol (gorgosterol), which has since been shown to occur more widely among Anthozoa in the Gorgoniacea and Zoanthidea (*99*). The three extra carbon atoms in gorgosterol are not on the nucleus but rather at C-24 (CH_3), C-23 (CH_3), and a bridge between C-22 and C-23. The structure, including stereochemistry, has been precisely determined (*100*) (Scheme 10.4), and 23-desmethylgorgosterol has been isolated from *Gorgonia flabellum* and *G. ventitian* (*101a*). The seco-derivative of gorgosterol in which the 9(11)-bond is broken (9-keto,11-ol) also occurs along with 23-desmethylgorgosterol in *Pseudopterogorgia americana* and the absolute configurations (22R, 23R, and 24R) were determined (*101b*). Recent examination of the gorgonians *Muricea appressa, Plexaura* sp., and *Eugoria ampla* has shown cholesterol as the major sterol and gorgosterol, when present, the next most abundant (*102*). However, also present were a C_{26}-sterol, 22-dehydrocholesterol, 24ξ-methylcholesterol, 24ξ-ethylcholesterol and its 22-dehydroderivative, 24-methylenecholesterol, and 24ξ-methyl-22-dehydrocholesterol. It has been suggested (*99*) that gorgosterol and related sterols are derived from or associated with the symbiotic flagellates (zooanthellae, yellowish photo-synthetic algae that inhabit the gastrodermis of polyps). However, while this may be so for the gorgonians, the zooanthellae from the anemone *Anthopleura elegantirsima* do not appear to contain gorgosterol.

The jellyfish (orders Hydrozoa and Scyphozoa) were first investigated by Haurowitz and Waelsch in 1926 (*103*). They found cholesterol in *Velella spirans.* More recently *Physalia physalis* (Portuguese Man-of-War) (*104*), and the Scyphozoa, *Rhizostoma* sp. (*105*), also yielded cholesterol, but the jellyfish *Cassiopea xamachana* has been shown to have a sterol mixture comprised more than 50% of alkylated sterols (*99*). Alkylsterols have also been shown by modern methods to comprise several percent of the mixture in the Anthomedasae, *Spirocodon saltatrix,* in the class Hydrozoa, the Semaeostomae, *Aurelia aurita* (moon jelly) in the class Scyphozoa, and in *Stomolophus* sp. in the order Rhizostomas (*106*). However, as in most of the other jellyfish, cholesterol was the principal sterol (72–88% in the three species quoted). The minor sterols were 24-methylene-, 24ξ-methyl-, 24-ethylidene-, and 24ξ-ethylcholesterol, along with 24ξ-methyl-22-dehydrocholesterol, desmosterol, 22-dehydrocholesterol, and a C_{26}-sterol. No C_{30}-sterol was detected.

Species of the Zoanthidea in recent examination have yielded cholesterol, 24-methylene-, 24ξ-methyl-, and 24β-methyl-22-dehydrocholesterol in *Zoanthus convertus* from Hawaii (*107*). The $\Delta^{5,22}$-24β-methylsterol was the principal component. Cholesterol, 24β-methyl-, 24β-methyl-22-dehydro-, and 24ξ-ethylcholesterol were found, in addition to a "gorgosterol" in *Palythoa tuberculosa* from Eniwetok. The 24β-methylcholesterol was the principal component. This latter mixture was probably related to the "palysterol" isolated by Bergmann, Feeney, and Swift (*96a*) from Atlantic *Palythoa maminilosa.* From Atlantic *Zoanthus proteus* Bergmann and Dusza (*96b*) had reported 24-methylenecholesterol, and in a *Palythoa* species from Tahiti that sterol is reported to occur alone (*107*). From an alcyonaria (soft corals) cholesterol, 24α-methylcholesterol, gorgosterol, and 25-hydroxy-24ξ-methylcholesterol are reported (*108*).

The Actinaria (sea anemones) in recent examination have yielded cholesterol as the main sterol (61–74%), accompanied by its *cis-* and *trans-*22-dehydro-, 24-dehydro-, 24-methylene-, 24-ethylidene-, 24ξ-methyl-, 24ξ-ethyl-, 24ξ-methyl-22-dehydro-, 24ξ-methyl-7,22-bisdehydro-, and 24ξ-ethyl-22-dehydroderivatives in *Metridium senile* and *Anemonia sulcata* (both Actinaria) and *Cerianthus membranaceus* (order Ceriantharia (*109*)). In *Calliactis parasitica* cholesterol is also dominant, accompanied by its fully saturated derivative (cholestanol), 22-dehydrocholesterol, 24-methylenecholesterol, "brassicasterol," and a C_{26}-sterol (*110*). The Madreporaria (corals) require more investigation. Bergmann's work (*88*) indicated a complex mixture, including cholesterol.

In summary, the coelenterates as a group contain Δ^5-sterols, with cholesterol most often the principal component, accompanied by a biosynthetic array in terms of alkylation and dehydrogenation of the side chain. Rarely, a saturated stanol is encountered. Often a C_{26}-sterol is found, and in the Anthozoa the 22,23-cyclopropylsterols, e.g., gorgosterol, are present. The ctenophores seem to be unexplored. Very little is known about biosynthesis. In a sea anemone (A. sulcata), radioactivity from [2-^{14}C]mevalonate highly labeled phospholipids and fatty acids but gave very little label in sterols (109). The results suggest conversion of MVA to acetate. In two other species (M. senile and C. membranaceus), [1-^{14}C]acetate gave much the same results (109, 95b) in that only little label went into sterols. In other studies (110a,b), [1-^{14}C]acetate failed to label either squalene or sterols in the sea anemone Calliactis parasitica. On balance, it seems likely that the coelenterates cannot biosynthesize sterols de novo, leaving the origin of the frequently complex mixture of sterols enigmatic. Perhaps they absorb sterols and further metabolize them.

   b. Phylum Platyhelminthes The phylum Platyhelminthes (flatworms and flukes), with about 7,000 species, are more complex than the coelenterates. They have definite organs and organ systems, bilateral symmetry, and one end is different from the other. A typical flatworm possesses a nerve and, at the head, ganglia and eye spots. Organs reside in the merenchyme and the animals are acoelomate, while in higher animals there is a true body cavity, the coelom or, more precisely, eucoelom. Three classes of this phylum exist, the Turbellaria, Trematoda (flukes), and Cestoda (tapeworms).

   Some species are parasitic and some not ("free-living" forms). Only the former, due to their ability to cause disease in vertebrates, have been well investigated. The liver fluke, Fasciola hepatica, was found in 1928 to contain cholesterol (111) and the cestodes, Botriocephalus latum (Diphyllobotrium latum, the fish tapeworm), and Taenia taeniaeformis and T. saginata (cat and cattle tapeworms), also yielded cholesterol in the early work (112-114). The latter genus (Taenia) is spread worldwide, infecting both man and animals. Recently, the work of Frayha and others has expanded our knowledge of these organisms. The larval stage (hydatid cysts) of T. hydatigena was shown to contain (115) but not to biosynthesize cholesterol from labeled acetate (116), the sterol being derived from the host's pool by absorption through the hydatid cyst wall (117). A related tapeworm is Echinoccoccus granulosus, also worldwide and infecting the liver and other organs of man and many other mammals. The cysts formed can be enormous. As with Taenia, cholesterol is derived, perhaps partly from esters (118), from the host (115) in G. granulosus and E. multilocularis, both of which also incorporate acetate and mevalonate into lipids other than cholesterol (115). These lipids were shown to include an alcohol with a mobility in thin-layer chromatography similar to that of the configurational isomer of farnesol with a cis- double bond, a C-2 (2-cis-6-trans-farnesol) and different from that of farnesol (116). The isomer was also identified in the cestode Hymenolopsis diminuta (119), which, as in the other cases, absorbs cholesterol from the host (120). This inability to biosynthesize sterols seems to occur also in the Trematoda. The blood fluke, Schistosoma mansoni, does not convert either acetate or mevalonate to cholesterol, contains sterol which is at least 90% cholesterol, and absorbs exogenous cholesterol, which was demonstrated using the latter in radioactive form (121).

In summary, the Platyhelminthes appear not to have the ability to synthesize sterols, and cholesterol, always found in the organisms, is demonstrably absorbed from an exogenous source. At least in the tapeworms, the biosynthetic block occurs in the conversion of geranyl pyrophosphate to the all-*trans*-isomer of squalene.

   c. **Phylum Nemathelminthes** Unsegmented round worms with triploblastic embryos, bilateral symmetry, and a body cavity in which the wall and gut are not lined with peritoneum (a pseudocoelom) are known as the phylum Nemathelminthes (formerly a part of the phylum Aschelminthes). They include the class Nematoda (sometimes considered a phylum), among which is a common parasite of man and the pig, *Ascaris lumbricoides*. Cholesterol is its dominant sterol (122), accompanied (when isolated from pigs) by substantial amounts of cholestanol, by 24ξ-methylcholestanol and its Δ^5-derivative, and by 24ξ-ethylcholestanol, and the latters' Δ^5-derivative, giving an array of Δ^0- and Δ^5-sterols in the 24-H, 24-CH$_3$-, and 24-C$_2$H$_5$-series (123). Some quantitative differences occurred between the free and esterified pools, notably in terms of the 24-ethyl components, which were mostly esterified in both sexes. Differences between sexes also occurred, but not dramatically. Three nonparasitic ("free-living") nematodes have also been studied. *Caenorhabditis briggsae* has an absolute requirement for exogenous cholesterol or other sterols for growth and reproduction (124) and neither it (125), *Turbatrix aceti* (125), nor *Panagrellus redivivus* (125) can convert [2-^{14}C]MVA or [2-^{14}C]acetate to cholesterol. However, when the substrate was [4-^{3}H]squalene 2,3-oxide-labeled lanosterol (but no C$_{27}$-sterol) was reported in the latter organism (126). It has also been identified in the organism lacking exogenous squalene oxide (127), and growth of *Nippostrongyllus brasiliensis* larvae is minimally supported by squalene and lanosterol (128). The inability of nematodes to biosynthesize sterols is corroborated by several reports of a cholesterol requirement (124, 129–131). While [4-^{14}C]cholesterol does not yield labeled CO$_2$ (125) in *C. briggsae* or *T. aceti,* other metabolites have been found, of which 7-dehydrocholesterol has been identified (125). 7-Dehydrocholesterol is one of the sterols supporting growth and reproduction in *C. briggsae* (124).

   In summary, animals in this phylum contain cholesterol (and, in some cases, also 7-dehydrocholesterol, 24-alkylsterols, and Δ^0-sterols) that is demonstrably absorbed from an exogenous source. The biosynthetic pathway proceeds, at least in some cases, as far as lanosterol (unlike the Platyhelminthes), after which a block occurs at an unknown step. The ability of one species to metabolize cholesterol to its $\Delta^{5,7}$-derivative has been reported, but C-4 does not appear as CO$_2$, indicating that severe catabolic metabolism does not occur.

C. MORE ADVANCED
NONPHOTOSYNTHETIC ORGANISMS (EUCOELOMATE ANIMALS)

1. Invertebrate Animals

a. Phylum Annelida   The annelids (13,500 species) differ from other worms in that the body is constructed from similar parts arranged in segments (somites or metameres) following each other linearly. They possess a true body cavity (eucoelom), as do the remaining animal phyla to be discussed. In the annelids the coelom is quite developed.

Marine annelids (polychaetes), e.g., *Nereis diversicolor,* have been found to convert MVA to sterols (*132a, 95b*), while MVA proceeds only as far as squalene in a terrestrial species, *Lumbricus terrestris* (*132a,b*). In *N. diversicolor,* one of the sterols was identified as cholesterol. Cholesterol has also been reported to be present in all other annelids studied (genera *Amphitrite, Arenicola, Lumbricus,* and *Pseudopotamilla,* comprising both marine and terrestrial forms). For a key to the literature, see Wooton and Wright (*132a*). Reports of "ergosterol" in *L. terrestris* (*133*) and of "brassicasterol" in *L. spencer* (*134*) are not supported by adequate data. However, an excellent recent study of the marine annelid *Pseudopotamilla occelata* by Kobayashi and Mitsuhashi (*135*) has shown the presence of no less than 10 sterols. Cholesterol (50%), 24-dehydrocholesterol (18%), and 22-*trans*-dehydrocholesterol (6%) comprised three-fourths of the mixture. The remaining fourth was primarily 24-alkyl-Δ^5-sterols (20%, 24-methylene-, 24ξ-methyl-, 24ξ-ethyl-, 24-methyl-22-*trans*-dehydro-, and 24-ethyl-22-dehydrocholesterol). The last 5% was composed of two quite different C_{26}-sterols. The main one (4.4%, 22-dehydrohalosterol) was 24,24-dimethylchola-5,22-*trans*-dien-3β-ol (nomenclature parent: cholane, a C_{24}-hydrocarbon) in which a carbon atom is missing between C-20 and the terminal isopropyl group. The other one is a homolog and is formally 26(or 27)-nor-24α-methyl-22-dehydrocholesterol, named occelasterol (Scheme 10.5). Both C_{26}-sterols are found in other marine invertebrates, and both are reasonably,

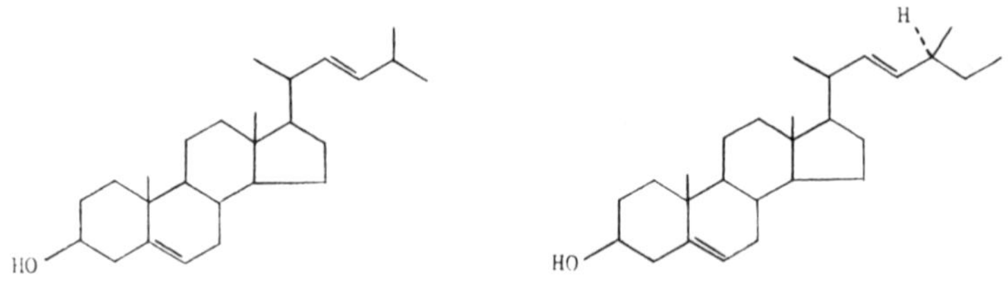

24,24-Dimethylchola-5,22-*trans*-dien-3β-ol
(22-Dehydrohalosterol)

24α-Methyl-22-*trans*-dehydro-26(or 27)-norcholesterol
(Occelasterol)

Scheme 10.5. C_{26}-Sterols of a marine annelid.

though not yet experimentally, derived from 24α-methylsterols. Epibrassi-casterol (diatomsterol) of the diatoms, which are believed to represent the major biomass of the oceans, is an especially good candidate for the precursor (*135*).

b. Arthropods   The phylum Arthropoda includes three-quarters of all known animal species. While considerably varied, all have the following body plan: bilateral symmetry, segments, an exoskeleton of chitin, a nervous system of the annelid type, and a small coelom filled with a sort of blood called hemolymph. In several ways they are related to the annelids more than are, say, the echinoderms, which have radial symmetry as adults and no segmentation. This relationship leads us to choose the arthropods for discussion immediately after the annelids. The possible precursor character of the annelids in an evolutionary sense, which has been suggested by some zoologists, is not, however, clarified by the sterol story.

It will be recalled from the previous section that some annelids (marine) are reported to biosynthesize sterols while others (terrestrial) carry carbon from mevalonate only as far as squalene. A number of arthropoda have now been studied and (with exceptions to be discussed) none have the ability even to synthesize squalene. This was first demonstrated in 1959 by Clark and Bloch (*136*) with an insect, the hide beetle (*Dermestes vulpinus*). It was known that all insects examined by that time had a nutritional requirement that was satisfied by cholesterol (*137*). That this was due to the absence of the biosynthetic machinery was demonstrated by the failure of mevalonic acid, squalene, lanosterol, or 4,4-dimethycholest-8-en-3β-ol to replace the sterol requirement of larvae and by the failure of labeled acetate to give labeled sterol despite the appearance of label in other lipids (hydrocarbons and fatty alcohols) (*136*). When less than the minimal amount of cholesterol was provided, the precursors still did not allow growth, i.e., there was not even a "sparing" activity. Such results have since been verified more generally among the higher orders of insects. However, a report of a very small incorporation of label from acetate into cholesterol in the more primitive German cockroach (*138*) raised aseptically, and a high incorporation into a silverfish of the genus *Ctenolepisma* (*139*) raised under nonaseptic conditions, led Kaplanis et al. (*140*) to study the very primitive insect *Thermobia domestica* (the firebrat) under nonaseptic conditions. Even without rigid exclusion of microbiological contaminants, only 0.001% of the label appearing in lipids resided in cholesterol. This (3.5 cpm/mg or 39 cpm) was barely above background, and one-fourth of that found in the cockroach. As the authors (*140*) concluded, one should be reluctant to ascribe cholesterol synthesis to these insects without further study, and the high incorporation (1,000 times that in the firebrat) in the case of the silverfish certainly remains worthy of reexamination before assessment. One possible problem that could explain the latter results is microbial biosynthesis.

Others of the arthropods besides insects have also failed to yield sterols by de novo biosynthesis. Thus, the crayfish *Astacus astacus,* on injection with labeled acetate, gave neither labeled squalene nor sterols, and there was no seasonal variation (*141, 142*). The lobsters *Homarus grammarus* (*143*) and *Panulirus japonicus* (*144*), the prawn *Penaeus japonicus* (*144*), and the crabs *Portunus trituberculatus* (*144*) and *Cancer pagurus* (*145*) also all failed to biosynthesize sterols (or squalene in several cases where it was examined) from acetate or in some cases studied from mevalonate. In some of the studies the radioactive acetate was shown to provide label for fatty acids, which demonstrated that the precursor was absorbed into active enzymatic sites. As with insects and consistent with lack of sterol biosynthesis, the prawn (*P. japonicus*) has a nutritional requirement for sterol that is satisfied by cholesterol (*144*). Sterol biosynthesis also could not be demonstrated from acetate in a spider (*Avicularia avicularia*) (*143*) or in a millepede, *Graphidostreptus tumuliporus* (*143*).

The sterols of insects very early became the subject of controversy. In the period 1907–1910, Lewkowitsch (*146*) reported the isolation of cholesterol from the chrysalis oil of the silk moth, *Bombyx mori,* but Tsujimoto thought sitosterol was present (*147*), and Menozzi and Moreschi (*148*) believed the moth had an entirely new sterol they called "bombicesterol." It was not until 1934 that Bergmann (*149*) clarified the subject by showing "bombicesterol" to be a mixture of cholesterol and a 24-alkylsterol. A few years later Wieland and Kotzschmar (*150*) showed cholesterol unequivocally to be the major and perhaps only sterol of a butterfly (*Pieris brassica*). These investigations, together with nutritional studies (*151*) showing that insects in the orders Orthoptera, Coleoptera, Lepidoptera, and Diptera required dietary sterols, made it clear, especially to Bergmann (*88*), that insects are variable in their sterol composition and that there is an ecological relationship with their food source. Carniverous insects would have, seemingly, cholesterol, while phytophagous ones would have 24-alkylsterols. Unfortunately, this idea was too simple, as Bergmann himself showed. The amount of cholesterol (85%) in the silk worm did not correlate with its diet of 24-alkylsterols in mulberry leaves (*149*). Furthermore, larvae of the fly *Musca vicina* were grown by another group (*152*) on a diet containing 24-ethylsterol. The pupae were then fed to the hide beetles *Dermestes vulpinus* and *D. cadaverinus,* which then grew normally. Since the latter had a nutritional C_{27}-sterol requirement, dealkylation presumably occurred in the fly. In 1959 Clark and Bloch (*153*) more precisely and directly demonstrated dealkylation in an insect. Using the cockroach *Blattella germanica,* they showed that ergosterol proceeds to 22-dehydrocholesterol. Subsequently, Robbins et al. (*154*) showed the same beetle converted sitosterol to cholesterol. Still more recently, dealkylation in *Eurycotic floridana* (*155*), *Bombyx mori* (*156*), and *Neodiprion pratti* (*157*), has been reported, and extensive studies in *Manduca sexta* (the tobacco hornworm) by Svoboda and Robbins and their associates, which have been reviewed (*157*), began in 1967 (*158*). The hornworm was shown to dealkylate 24α-ethyl, 24-*cis*-ethylidene, 24α-methyl, and 24-methylene groups from Δ^5-sterols. Desmosterol proved to be an intermediate and cholesterol the product. The hornworm and the cockroach both, therefore, are able to remove both C_1 and C_2 groups. The housefly, *Musca domestica*, however, does not dealkylate ingested sterols (*159*). When pupae were reared on 24α-methyl- or 24α-ethylcholesterol, the sterol found subsequently in the animals was unchanged in structure. Despite this, the pupae clearly prefer the unalkylated side chain. When sterol mixtures were presented to the pupae, the order of selective absorption was 24-H- before 24α-methyl- , before 24α-ethyl-cholesterol (*159*).

The foregoing studies indicated that: (1) insects may prefer but do not necessarily have to possess cholesterol; (2) what preferences there are are achieved either by selective absorption of, at least in some cases, cholesterol or of a sterol most closely resembling it; or (3) the preference is achieved or approximated by metabolism. Actually, not enough precise studies have been made to state whether or not most insects do or do not primarily possess or prefer cholesterol itself. In the carniverous cases where the diet consists of material from higher animals, cholesterol would be expected to be dominant, but if the animal eaten is an invertebrate or a plant, such may or may not be the case. This is further verified by studies of the honey bee *Apis mellifica*. Queen larvae contain 24-methylenecholesterol as a major sterol (*160*). The same is true for mature queens (*161*), royal jelly (*161, 162*), workers (*161*), and honey (*163*). When bees and honey were taken from the same hive, 24-methylenecholesterol and sitosterol were found in the bees, and these, together with cholesterol, were in the honey (*163*). The source of the sterol has been shown to be pollen (*164, 165*). The termite *Nasutitermes rippertii* contains a sterol mixture composed of only 56% cholesterol (*166*). Most of the rest is primarily 24-alkylsterol, but, surprisingly, sterols with drastically reduced side chains were also reported, e.g., pregnenolone with a C_2 side chain, androst-5-en-3β-ol with no side chain at all, and its 17-isopropyl derivative with a C_3 side chain. The honey-bee is also known to metabolize, while not normally containing, progesterone (*167*).

The absence of an absolute necessity for unalkylated sterols in the Insecta is matched by the absence of a rigid requirement for sterols with a Δ^5-bond. This has been demonstrated unequivocally by studies with the fruit fly *Drosophila pachea*, which will not utilize cholesterol for growth and development (*168*). Larvae grown on a medium containing only this sterol die in the second and third instars, but 7-dehydrocholesterol is nutritionally satisfactory, indicating a requirement for a $\Delta^{5,7}$-sterol (*169*). Proof was obtained by the use of lathosterol, which supports growth (*169*) and is converted to 7-dehydrocholesterol (*168*). Similarly, the beetle *Xylaborus ferrugineus* requires $\Delta^{5,7}$-sterols for pupation (*170*). The beetle will accept either ergosterol or 7-dehydrocholesterol, suggesting that dealkylation of the C_1 group can occur, but in the case of the fruit fly it cannot. 24β-Methyllathosterol does not serve nutritionally (*169*). 24α-Ethyl-7-dehydrocholesterol is also satisfactory, but female adults are infertile. Fertility can be restored when they are placed on a diet of senita cactus (*Lophocereus schotti*). This cactus constitutes the fly's exclusive breeding site in the wild, and 24α-ethyllathosterol (schottenol) is present in the cactus in unusually high quantities (*171*). Schottenol when used nutritionally was found to allow normal development (*169*). These experiments clearly show a complex requirement for Δ^7- and $\Delta^{5,7}$-sterols (with and without 24-ethyl groups) that is not met by Δ^5-sterols, and it explains the ecological dependence that the fly has for the senita cactus.

In summary, arthropods belonging to the classes Crustacea, Insecta, Arachnida, and Myriapoda fail to biosynthesize sterols de novo except in one or two cases that probably should be reinvestigated. Sterols, which are always present and required, are provided by the diet and are usually in the Δ^5- but occasionally in the Δ^7- and $\Delta^{5,7}$-series. The side chain is often of the cholesterol type. Cholesterol itself is frequently found and usually acts as a sufficient nutritional requirement. 24-Alkylsterols are also frequently encountered, and in at least some cases they alone are present, and will support normal function. Some of the animals can remove a C_1 or a C_2 group at C-24, while others cannot, and some can introduce a Δ^5-bond into a Δ^7-sterol. The sterol composition is a variable function of the diet of the organism's control of absorption from the diet, of the organism's capacity to metabolize ingested sterols by alterations in ring B and the side chain, and of the detailed role the sterols play in the organism. These variables can and in some cases demonstrably do impose either (or both) a variation of the sterol composition in a given insect with variations in its environment or an ecological dependence of the organism on a particular environment.

c. Molluscs Animals of the phylum Mollusca, with about 80,000 species, are bilateral in symmetry, unsegmented, eucoelomate, and develop from a triploblastic embryo. They are extensively examined by early investigators, whose work has been surveyed by Bergmann (*88*). Cholesterol and its 24-methylene-, 24α-ethyl-24β-methyl-22-dehydro-, 7-dehydro-, 22-dehydro-, 24α-methyl-7-dehydro-, 24α-ethyl-7-dehydro-, 24β-ethyl-7-dehydro-, 24α-ethyl-7,22-bisdehydro- derivatives were found, along with lathosterol and others, including many mixtures of unidentified components.

The conclusion of Bergmann (*88*) that the molluscs contain generally complex mixtures has been verified and extended by investigations with modern methodology. Idler and his associates (*172–175*) have been especially painstaking in these studies, using the scallop *Placopecten magellanicus*. It contains no less than 17 4,4,14-trisdesmethylsterols, all of which have been

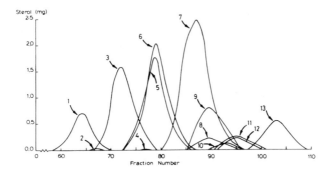

Figure 10.1. Sterols of *Placopecten magellanicus* as they distribute themselves on Lipophilic Sephadex. 1, 22-*trans*-dehydrohalosterol; 2, 22-*trans*-dehydrohalostanol; 3, 22-*cis*- and 22-*trans*-dehydrocholesterol and 22-dehydrocholestanol; 4, halosterol; 5, 24-methylenecholesterol; 6, 24ξ-methyl-22-dehydrocholesterol; 7, cholesterol and cholestanol; 8, 24ξ-ethyl-22-dehydrocholesterol; 9, fucosterol and isofucosterol; 10, placosterol; 11, 24ξ-methylcholesterol; 12, (Z)-24-propylidenecholesterol; 13, 24ξ-ethylcholesterol. From Idler et al. (*174*).

identified (*174, 175*), and their relative amounts can be determined from the manner in which the separations (*174*) were obtained (Figure 10.1). Cholesterol was present as an important constituent, but neither it nor any other single sterol constituted more than half of the mixture, which was composed (Figure 10.1) entirely of Δ^5-sterols except for some cholestanol. The sterols varied by alterations at C-24 [methyl, ethyl, methylene, (E)- and (Z)-ethylidene, and (E)-propylidene] and C-22 (desaturation), and by removal of a carbon atom from the backbone of the side chain. Four of these sterols, the (E)-24-propylidenecholesterol, which we shall call placosterol, 24,24-dimethylchola-5-en-3β-ol, which we shall call halosterol from its first isolation from a tunicate, *Halocynthia roretzi* (*176*), 22-*trans*-dehydrohalosterol, and 22-*trans*-dehydrohalostanol have not been found either in mammals or tracheophytes, and they constitute new and fascinating types. Placosterol has so far been found only in this scallop, but 22-*trans*-dehydrohalostanol and halosterol have recently been isolated from other animals below the chordates. Another scallop, *Patinopecten yessoensis,* has been shown to contain more than 20 sterols, including placosterol, 22-*trans*-dehydrohalosterol, the 26(or 27)-norsterols, and occelasterol and its 5,6-dihydroderivative, patinosterol (Scheme 10.6) (*177*). The possibility of the presence of the 22-*cis*-isomer of brassicasterol (or 24-epibrassicasterol) in the edible parts of the shortnecked clam *Tapes philippinarum* is another interesting example of the diversity of mollusc sterols (*178*).

In other recent studies of molluscs, much the same results have been obtained. Voogt (*179–184*) surveyed 27 species of Gastropoda, Bivaliva, and Cephalopoda using gas-liquid chromatography and found C_{26}-sterols (traces to 8%), cholesterol (19–95%, average: 63%), cholestadienols ($\Delta^{5,22}$, $\Delta^{5,24}$,

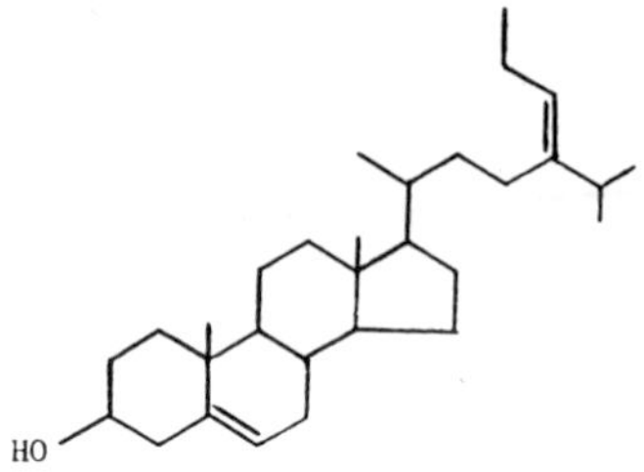

Placosterol

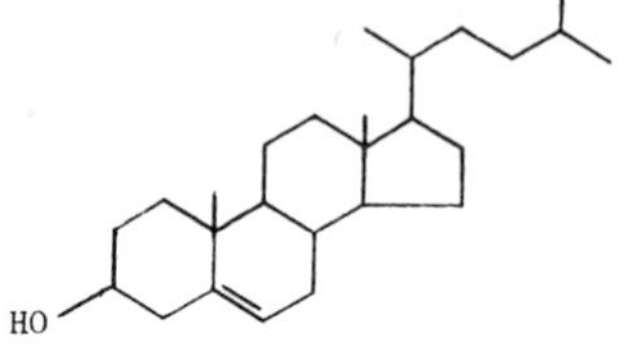

Halosterol

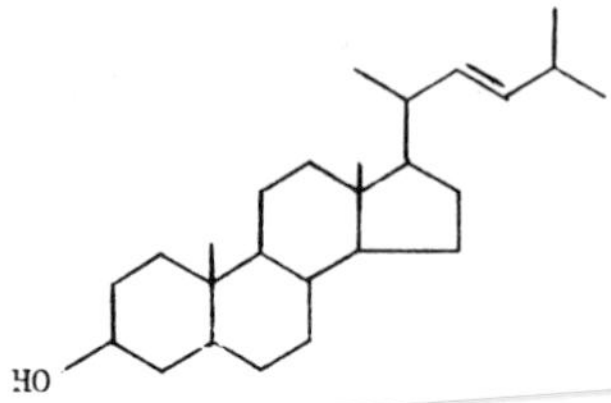

22-*trans*-Dehydrohalostanol

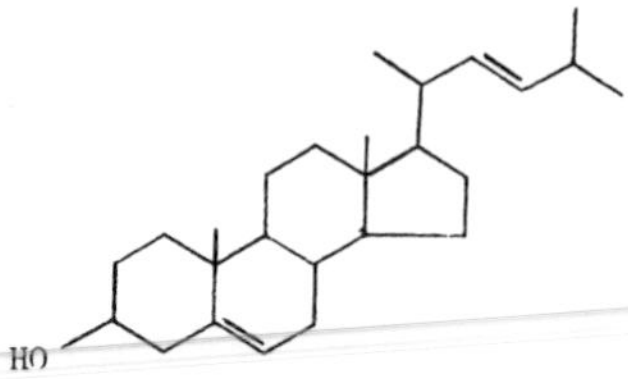

22-*trans*-Dehydrohalosterol

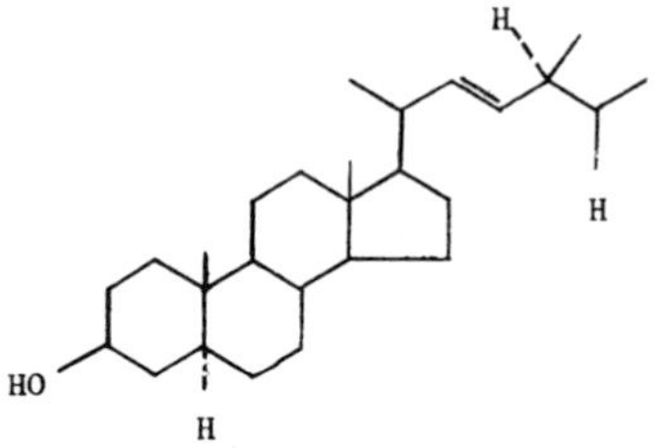

5,6-Dihydrooccelasterol
(Patinosterol)

Scheme 10.6. Some sterols of scallops.

and $\Delta^{5,7}$; traces to 42%), 24-methylcholesterol and $\Delta^{5,22}$- and $\Delta^{5,24(28)}$-dienols (1-63%), and 24-ethylcholesterol and $\Delta^{5,22}$- and $\Delta^{5,24(28)}$-dienols (1-19%). *Sepia officinalis, Octopus vulgaris, Eledone aldrovandi, Lymnaea stagnalis, Planobarius corneus, Succinea putris,* and *Monodonta turbinata* had cholesterol contents of 80% or greater (percentage of sterol mixture). Except for *Lepidochitona cinerea,* which is thought to possess principally Δ^7-sterols, and the primitive mollusc *Liolophura japonica*, which has 97% lathosterol and 3% cholesterol (*185*), all mollusc sterols have primarily Δ^5-bonds occasionally mixed with lesser amounts of Δ^0-sterols and dienols.

Mesogastropods tend to have more complicated mixtures including more $\Delta^{5,7}$-sterols than do archeogastropods.

Voogt (*179–184*) and Teshima and Kanazama (*185, 186*) have made extensive analyses of the ability of many molluscs to biosynthesize sterols. It appears that de novo biosynthesis is a common property of all of them, with more intense capacity in the herbiverous than in the carniverous species. This may relate to the need for an unalkylated side chain, but dealkylation has not been well studied. Acetate will proceed in most species to sterols, but in some cases, e.g., *Natica cataena,* only mevalonate will. It is especially interesting that the mussel *Mytilus edulis* is tentatively believed to convert mevalonate not only to cholesterol but to 24-methylenecholesterol. The ability of molluscs to convert cholesterol to its 24-methylene derivative was shown much earlier in the clam *Saxidomus giganteus,* by Fagerlund and Idler (*187*), who also demonstrated the conversion of cholesterol to its Δ^{22}- and Δ^{25}-derivatives in the same clam (*188*).

In summary, molluscs contain C_{26}-, C_{27}-, C_{28}-, C_{29}-, and C_{30}-sterols in complex and varied mixtures. Biosynthesis from mevalonate occurs in all species investigated, with one exception (*95b*), and the C_{27}- and 24-methyl-enesterols are believed to arise at least in part by this route. Whether the other sterols are derived by biosynthesis or by ingestion is not clear, but there are suggestive reasons for believing that dietary habit is an important factor.

d. Echinoderms The phylum Echinodermata consists of marine spiny-skinned sea stars, brittle stars, sea urchins, sea cucumbers, and sea lilies. The larvae have bilateral symmetry, which changes to biradial symmetry in the adult, and they possess internal, calcareous skeletons.

Starfish were shown in 1944 by Bergmann and Stansbury (*189*) to contain sterol mixtures, following earlier work by Dorée (*86*) and by Kossell and Edlbacher (*190*). Subsequent work in Bergmann's and other investigators' laboratories, which Bergmann has reviewed (*88*), showed that cholesterol (and other Δ^5-sterols) could be isolated from many echinoderms, while in others lathosterol (and other Δ^7-sterols) were dominant. Much of the data depended on optical rotation of unpure sterols, but the work did show unequivocally that cholesterol was not necessarily the only sterol of these animals. His information suggested that Δ^5-sterols were present in sea lilies (Crinoidea), brittle stars (Ophiuroidea), and especially in sea urchins (Echinoidea), and Δ^7-sterols in starfish (Asteroides) and sea cucumbers (Holothuroidea).

As with other studies of marine invertebrates, recent studies have shown the sterols present in echinoderms to be even more complex than earlier imagined, and sterols with structures not found outside the marine environment occur (Scheme 10.7). From *Asterias amurensis,* among other Δ^7-sterols, Kobayashi et al. (*191–193*) have isolated 24α-methyl-22-*trans*-dehydro-26(or 27)-norlathosterol (amurensterol) lacking the terminal *gem-*

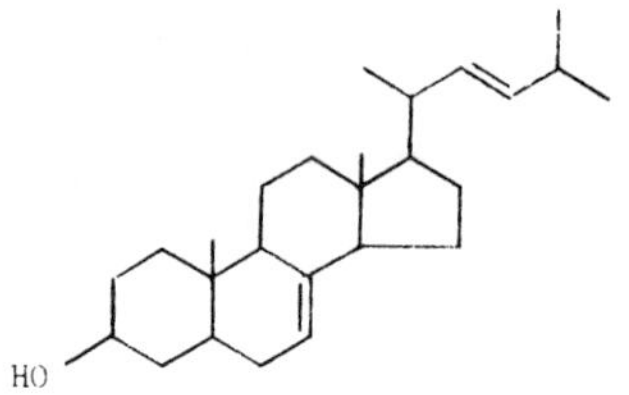

Asterosterol

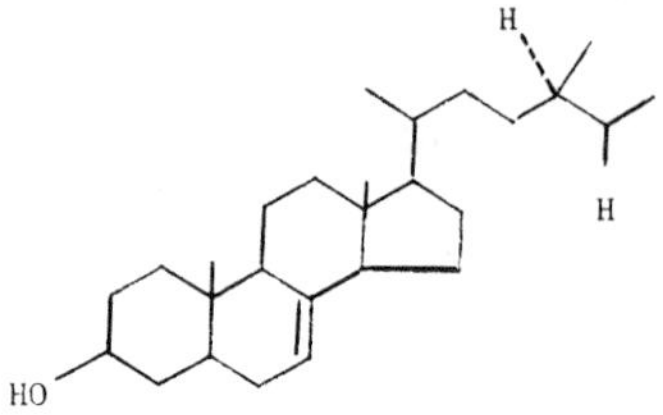

Amurensterol

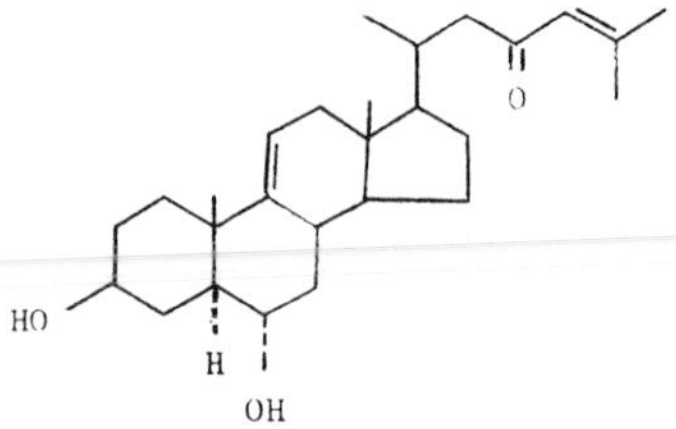

Marathasterone

Scheme 10.7. Some unusual sterols in starfish.

dimethyl groups (*191*) as well as the C_{26}-sterol (asterosterol) that is the Δ^7-analog of 22-*trans*-dehydrohalosterol lacking a C-atom between C-20 and the terminal isopropyl group (*192*). The latter has also been found in *Distolaterias sticantha, Asterias pectiuifera, Certonardoa semiregularis,* and *Lysastrosoma anthostictha,* and in the holothurian *Stichopus japonicum* (*193*). Goad and his associates (*194, 195*) identified as many as 22 sterols in *Asterias rubens.* The major ones had a Δ^7-bond, and lathosterol predominated over other mono- and diunsaturated sterols which belonged not only to the C_{27}- but also to the C_{26}-, C_{28}- and C_{29}-series. The latter two types were 24-methylene-, 24-methyl-, (E)- and (Z)-24-ethylidene, and 24-ethyl-lathosterols. The C_{26}-sterol was asterosterol. This Δ^7-C_{26}-sterol has also been described as "26,27-dinorergosta-7,22-dien-3β-ol" (*194*). Since this implies biosynthetic removal of C-26 and C-27, which remains to be demonstrated, the systematic name 24,24-dimethylchola-7,22-*trans*-dien-3β-ol is preferable unless the trivial name is used. *A. rubens* also yielded small amounts of cholesterol, cholestanol, and sterols methylated at C-4 including cycloartenol. The starfish *Acanthaster planci* contains 5α-cholesta-9(11),-20(22)-diene-3β,6α-diol,23-one and its 20(22)-dihydroderivative in addition to cholestanol and Δ^7-C_{27}- to C_{30}-mono- and diunsaturated sterols (*196*).

Asterosterol could not be detected in *A. planci* or in *Linckia multiflora*, *Protoreaster nodosus*, *Protoreaster lincki*, *Culcita schmideliana*, or *Nardoa varilata*, but otherwise the sterol compositions were all similar (*196*). The 23-ketones have been suggested (*196*) as deriving from gorgosterol and its relatives, which would be ingested from the diet. Starfish feed on corals, but there is another possibility discussed at the end of this section.

Reinvestigation (*197*) of the sea urchin *Echinus esculentus* has also confirmed and extended the earlier ideas. This animal contains an array of Δ^5-sterols that mimic the Δ^7-sterols of the asteroids. Thus, cholesterol replaces lathosterol, 22-*trans*-dehydrohalosterol replaces asterosterol, and the 24-methylene-, 24-methyl-, and 24-ethylidene-, and 24-ethylcholesterols are found instead of the corresponding lathosterol derivatives.

Two groups of investigators (*198a,b 199*) have examined biosynthesis in starfish and both agree that mevalonate proceeds to squalene, lanosterol, and lathosterol in *A. rubens* and *Henricia sanguinolenta* (*198a,b*) and in *Laister leachii* (*199*). Both groups also agree that alkylation at C-24 does not occur, nor did either 9,19-cyclosterols or Δ^{22}-sterols arise from mevalonate. A third investigator (*200*) using *Marthasterias glacialis*, *Astropecten aurantianus*, and *Euchinaster sepositers* similarly demonstrated biosynthesis and also found it in the holothurians, *Cucumaria planci*, *Holothuria tubulosa*, *Stichopus regalis*, and *Cucumaria elongata* (*201*). Δ^5-Sterols are converted to Δ^7-sterols in asteroids (*202*) as well as Δ^5- to Δ^0-sterols (*203*).

Asteroids also contain steroidal glycosides (*196, 204–207*). They are thought to play a role in inhibiting unfavorable spawning early in the breeding season (*208*). The alglycones are all oxygenated at C-23 and C-26 and bear a $\Delta^{9(11)}$-group. They are known as asterosaponins, and they differ in whether the 23-oxygen atom is ketonic or hydroxylic and whether or not another double bond is present. The only other known organism to contain a 23-oxygenated sterol is the fungus *Scleroderma aurantium*, which contains 23-hydroxylanosterol (*82*). Label from mevalonate appears in higher quantity in squalene and 4,4-dimethylsterols than it does in lathosterol in asteroids. The suggestion has been made (*198*) that these precursors are also used for biosynthesis of the asterosaponins, which is a divergent idea from the one suggested (*196*) in the discussion of *Acanthaster planci*.

In summary, early work indicated echinoderms were divisible into Δ^5- and Δ^7-sterol-containing classes (*88*, also see *209*). Recent work has clearly demonstrated that the starfish (Asteroidea) do indeed belong to the latter, and the sea urchins (Echinoidea) to the former. Both the starfish and the sea urchins contain sterols with and without one or two extra carbon atoms at C-24, but they biosynthesize only the 24-desalkylsterols that are dominant (cholesterol and lathosterol), and they do so through squalene and lanosterol. Cycloartenol is found, but, along with the 24-alkylsterols, is presumably of dietary origin. Cholestanol is also found, along with 23-

oxygenated sterols, the latter being present frequently as glyosides (aster-osaponins). In asteroids Δ^5-sterols can serve as precursors for Δ^7- and Δ^0-sterols, but the 23-oxygenated sterols are thought to be derived from 22,23-cyclopropylsterols in the diet. Echinoderms frequently include in their lipids sterols that have side chains modified by shortening of the side chain in two ways so that they give sterols with a carbon missing from the un-branched or from the terminal isopropyl portions. They are presently thought to be of dietary origin. The former are found in other marine organisms.

2. Vertebrate Animals

a. Organismic and Tissue Occurrence, Biosynthesis, and Turnover Cholesterol was first isolated from a human being in the form of gall stones. In many subsequent investigations too numerous to mention it was found to be the dominant sterol of all higher vertebrates. Except for the gastrointestinal tract, mammalian sterol is nearly but not completely pure cholesterol. Considering the possibility that changes might occur in lower vertebrates, Nes and his associates (*210*) investigated fish and showed here too that nearly pure cholesterol was present and arose through squalene, lanosterol, and 7-dehydrocholesterol from mevalonate in the livers of fresh salt water bass (*Micropterus salmoides* and *Roccus saxtilis*). Carp (*Scarelinius erythrophthalmus*) similarly biosynthesizes sterols (*211*). Nes et al. (*212*) also demonstrated the inability of mammalian (rat) liver to reduce or alkylate 24-methylenecholesterol to give 24-methyl-, 24-ethylidene-, or 24-ethyl-cholesterol, which supports the contention that mammals and presumably other vertebrates do not have a pathway to 24-alkylsterols. Furthermore, human beings and other mammals investigated usually do not absorb enough dietary sterol (other than cholesterol) for it to appear consequentially in their tissues. There is a strong suggestion that this discrimination against sterols with modified side chains begins with the vertebrates, because the tunicate *Halocynthia roretzi*, which is a primitive chordate but not a verte-brate, has been shown by Barbier and others (*176, 213a,b*) to have a com-plex sterol mixture. While its principle sterols include cholesterol (29%), desmosterol (1%), lathosterol (4%), and cholestanol (9%), it also contains 24-methylenecholesterol (19%), 24-ethylidenecholesterol, other 24-alkyl-sterols, and significant amounts (7%) of the C_{26} sterols, halosterol, its 22-*trans*-dehydroderivative, and the latter's 5-dihydroderivative and Δ^7-analog. Halosterol was first isolated from this tunicate (*213a,b*) and subsequently found in molluscs. Its origin is uncertain.

Unlike tunicates and still lower animals, vertebrate tissues usually (see below for exceptions) not only contain no sterols with side chains which have been alkylated, shortened, or enlarged, but also no Δ^{22}-sterols. How-ever, the sterol of vertebrates is by no means always absolutely pure choles-terol. The most outstanding (and questionable) example is "γ-sitosterol," which is believed to be the only sterol in the venom of toads (mixed with cholesterol in the skin) of the genus *Bufo* and to be biosynthesized in the animal (*214*). "γ-Sitosterol" has also been isolated from soybeans and corn. It was thought to be clionasterol. The problem with this is that the plant "γ-sitosterol" is not a pure sterol. It has unequivocally been shown to be a 1/1 mixture of 24ξ-methyl- and 24α-ethylcholesterol (*215*). Since no modern chromatographic work, e.g., gas-liquid chromatography, or structural elucidation has been done with toad "γ-sitosterol," its nature remains uncertain. Nevertheless, common animal sterol does unquestionably include along with cholesterol small amounts of the Δ^0- and Δ^7-analogs, (cholestanol and lathosterol), the Δ^{24}-derivative (desmosterol), and $\Delta^{5,7}$-derivative (7-dehydrocholesterol), and others. Windaus (*216*) was the first to recognize the $\Delta^{5,7}$-diene in animals. He identified it spectroscopically as a 0.2% component of the sterols in Chinese dried egg yolk, cow placenta, and hog pancreas, and a 4% component in pigskin, from which the sterol was then isolated. Cholestanol was suspected by Schoenheimer (*217*) to be a companion of cholesterol, and its isolation was accomplished by Fieser (*218a,b*) from commercial cholesterol. Cholesterol will proceed to cholestanol apparently via cholest-4-en-3-one (*219, 220*) in rat liver microsomes (*221*). Lathosterol was first isolated by Fieser (*218a,b*) as well as by Idler and Baumann (*222*). It is present in many human tissues at levels of 0.3–3% and in dog and rat skins in much higher quantities (9–19%). Stokes, Fish, and Hickey (*223*) discovered desmosterol in the chicken embryo and subsequently found it as a 5–8% component of rat skin (*224*). Some mammalian cholesterol also has 4,4-dimethylsterols as significant companions. As long ago as 1872, Shulze (*225*) isolated "isocholesterol" from wool fat (known as "degras"). Fifty-seven years later, Drummond and Baker (*226*) obtained 9 pounds of "isocholesterol" as a waxy mixture along with 4 pounds of cholesterol from 53 pounds of degras, and shortly afterwards Windaus and Tschesche (*227*) obtained "isocholesterol" in a purer condition, named it lanosterol, and found that it was accompanied by its $\Delta^{7,9(11)}$-derivative, which they named agnosterol. Ruzicka et al. (*228*) in 1944 discovered that degras also contained 24-dihydrolanosterol as well as 24-dihydroagnosterol. Analysis by modern gas-liquid chromatographic techniques shows that commercial "lanosterol" from degras contains slightly more 24-dihydrolanosterol than lanosterol, and ultraviolet analysis indicates about 16% of the $\Delta^{7,9(11)}$-dienes. Serum sterols in the normal human have been shown (*229*) by mass spectroscopy and other means to include lanosterol, with lesser amounts of dihydrolansterol and several other sterols methylated at C-4. The total amount is 1 μg/mg of cholesterol or 0.1%. Other sterols that have been isolated from mammalian tissues are 26ξ-hydroxycholesterol from the human aorta (*230, 231*) and from commerical cholesterol derived from bovine brain and spinal cord (*232*), and 24β-hydroxycholesterol (cerebrosterol) from the horse and human brain (*233*). The configuration at C-

24 (S by the sequence rule), originally deduced (234) from rotations, has been confirmed by other methods (235). Cerebrosterol also occurs in bovine, rabbit, and rat brain. Its biosynthesis in the latter tissue from cholesterol has been reported (236).

Nervous tissue, and especially brain, is extremely rich in cholesterol. Of the dry weight, some 10% is this sterol, contrasted to perhaps 1% in other tissues. The sterol composition of the normal human brain has been shown (237a) to be 99.1% cholesterol, 0.3% cholestanol, 0.1% 24-dihydrozymosterol, and 0.003–0.02% each of the following types of sterol: C_{30}-Δ^8, C_{29}-Δ^8, C_{28}-Δ^8, C_{30}-$\Delta^{8,24}$ (lanosterol), C_{29}-$\Delta^{8,24}$, C_{28}-$\Delta^{8,24}$, C_{27}-$\Delta^{8,24}$ (zymosterol), C_{27}-$\Delta^{5,24}$ (0.02%, desmosterol), and C_{27}-Δ^{14}. Adult rat brain has a similar but not identical composition (237b). Only 98.0% of the sterol is cholesterol. The 0.9% difference from the human case is derived primarily from a greater amount (0.80%) of desmosterol in the rat brain. In another study (238) of human brain, 24-hydroxycholesterol (major trace substance), 25-hydroxycholesterol, 7-ketocholesterol, cholesta-3,5-dien-7-one, 7α-hydroxycholesterol, 7β-hydroxycholesterol, and 5α-cholestane-3β,5,6β-triol were reported and from a formalin-preserved brain (but not fresh brain) 3β-hydroxy-5α-cholest-6-ene-5-hydroperoxide. Some of these may be artifacts. The distribution of cholesterol in the white and gray matter of brains of man and a variety of domestic mammals is not the same (239–242). White matter is the richer, the white/gray ratio varying from a low of 2.9 in the rabbit to 5.1 in the ox; in man it is 3.9. Brain biosynthesizes sterols de novo from mevalonate through lanosterol (243).

The sterols of feces and intestinal contents of germ-free and control rats beautifully document the importance of microorganisms (244). Germ-free feces contain mostly cholesterol. Minor components include lathosterol, 24ξ-methylcholesterol, 24ξ-ethylcholesterol (presumably sitosterol), and the latter's Δ^{22}-derivative (presumably stigmasterol). The same sterols are also present in the small intestine and the cecum. No coprostanol is present, but it becomes the major sterol in feces and cecum of control rats that also contain cholesterol, lathosterol, 24ξ-ethylcoprostanol, and 24ξ-ethylcholesterol (presumably sitosterol). Small intestines of controls have little coprostanol. The reduced products, as deduced earlier, are clearly derived by microbial metabolism. Both sitosterol and cholesterol when labeled and incubated with human feces give the corresponding labeled stanol in the same proportions (245). Reduction of Δ^5-sterols has been observed in several other mammalian species, and there is little structural specificity, as the foregoing sentence suggests. With Eubacterium 21,408 isolated from the rat cecum, sterols proceeding to their 5β-H-derivatives include campesterol, stigmasterol, and 7-dehydrocholesterol (246). The 7(8)-bond was not reduced in either 7-dehydrocholesterol or lathosterol, but the bacterium did reduce cholest-4-en-3-one to coprostanol. The cholestenone is believed to be an intermediate from cholesterol in which the 4-H atom has shifted to C-6 (247). The intestinal mucosa of rat, guinea pig, and rabbit also contain substantial amounts of sterols other than cholesterol (249).

Although the solubility of sterols in water would lead one at first sight to believe that urine would be sterol-free, cholesterol has been identified there by chromatographic (gas-liquid chromotography) and spectroscopic (IR) methods as well as by x-ray diffraction analysis (249). Evidence exists for its being protein-bound (250).

Sterol mixtures on the surface of animals, as noted earlier in this section for wool, is a common phenomenon. Lanosterol has been found in the sebum (secretion of sebaceous glands that is believed to be the primary source of lipids) of sheep, llama, goat, and dromedary (251). From the sebum of human skin a great variety of lipids have been isolated, including 12% squalene, but only traces of sterol (252). On the other hand, the epidermis lipids are composed of little squalene and 30% sterols and steryl esters (252). Surface lipids (10% squalene and 4% sterol and sterylesters) derive from both sources as well as environmental contamination (253–255). The structures identified in the human case include cholesterol, with several percent of lathosterol, lanosterol, 24-dihydrolanosterol, squalene, and in some cases 24-alkylsterols (253, 254).

All animal tissues that have been investigated have the capacity to synthesize sterols de novo, but the relative rates vary greatly. In rats, monkeys, and man, the liver and intestines appear to have the highest rates, but in the pig the intestine contributes only 4% to the total sterol synthesis, in contrast to liver and adipose tissue, which account for 67% and 29%, respectively. For a key to the literature see Romsos et al. (256a). Circulating (blood) cholesterol is derived from these sources as well as from the diet, and to greater or lesser extents is transferred to and between tissues in a very dynamic and complex fashion. This distribution has been assessed by Avigan, Steinberg, and Berman (256b), who administered [4-^{14}C]cholesterol orally to rats followed by an examination of label in serum and various tissues. After about 1 day the tissue:serum ratio of specific activities of cholesterol was near 1.0 in liver, small intestine, heart, lung, and spleen. In the first two tissues it remained approximately constant for 7 weeks, indicating a tissue-to-serum equilibrium, but it rose to about 1.5 in the latter three tissues. The ratio in kidney and muscle did not attain a value of 1.0 until about a week, and then did not remain constant. It continued to rise to 6 and 3, respectively, at the end of 7 weeks. Brain exhibited a still slower absorption of blood cholesterol. The ratio failed to reach 1.0 until 5 weeks had elapsed, and then continued to rise sharply thereafter. The specific activity of rat cholesterol both in the whole animal and in various tissues began to fall after a day or so, reaching very low levels by the end of 7 weeks. The half-time for the whole animal was about 16 days. Qualitatively similar results were obtained with the rabbit.

The rapid turnover in the rat described in the foregoing paragraph is paralleled in man. It has been examined by a number of investigators using a variety of methods. For a detailed review see Dietschy and Wilson (257). All authors agree that the rate of production of cholesterol is near 1.0 g/day. The values range from 0.72 to 1.87 and depend on various factors. The absorption of dietary sterol is about 0.2 g/day. Sterol is removed primarily in the feces and appears roughly in a 5:4 ratio as neutral sterols and bile acids, respectively. The sterol content of practically all human tissues and fluids has been determined, and much is known about other animals. For detailed reviews see the books by Kritchevsky (258) and Cook (259). Some of the data are summarized in Table 10.2. A person contains 300-600 mg of sterol per 100 g wet weight or about 4.59/kg. This means that for an individual of 150 lbs (68 kg) there are about 306 g of cholesterol. In a steady state with a production rate of 1 g/day there is

Table 10.2. Approximate cholesterol content in animals (exact values vary with age, sex, species, etc.)

	Amount (mg/100 g wet weight)
Intact Animal	
Earthworm	100
Crab	48
Fish	75
Frog	40
Snake	80
Rabbit	117
Rat	460
Human being	450
Human Tissues	
Hair	5,000
Adrenals	5,000
Spinal cord	4,000
Brain	3,000
Nerves	1,500
Nails	500
Duodenum	430
Aortas	400
Muscle	360
Liver	300
Kidneys	300
Spleen	300
Lung	200
Uterus	200
Ovary	200
Fat	200
Blood	200
Milk	25

Adapted from Kritchevsky (258) and Cook (259).

something like a total turnover of sterol every year. Of course, this calculation, which implies a half-time of a month or two, is highly simplified and ignores specific tissues, diet, age, health, cholesterol pools, etc., but it does give us an approximation of what is happening. The turnover of cholesterol in myelin (which contains roughly half of brain cholesterol) is believed to be much slower than in other parts of the body. Davison and Wajda (260) have shown that labeled cholesterol has been found to reside primarily in myelin and mitochondria (261–264). Cerebral cholesterol, including myelin, of the adult rat derives from the plasma as well as from biosynthesis in situ, and cerebral capillary walls are labeled rapidly (in one day) from plasma-tritiated cholesterol while cerebral structures incorporate label more slowly. This information has been interpreted (268) to mean that the "blood-brain" barrier does not exist at the level of the cerebral capillaries. Davison (265), Kabara (266), and Paoletti et al. (267) have reviewed brain sterols and their metabolism in greater depth.

   b. Serum Cholesterol, Absorption, and Diet   Measurement of serum cholesterol has an important function in clinical medicine. Although in normal human beings there is a considerable variation (nearly 100%) even when the people are of the same age and sex (Table 10.3), the mean

Table 10.3. Normal serum cholesterol levels in human beings (mg/100 ml)

	Age							
	Under 35		35–44		45–54		55 and over	
	Male	Female	Male	Female	Male	Female	Male	Female
Low	148	138	158	153	174	168	173	189
Mean	216	205	239	226	249	256	243	268
High	283	270	320	300	324	343	314	347

From Metropolitan Life Statistical Bulletin, 52:4 (1971). Data are for a healthy employee population.

values are statistically different for men and women. Below age 45, males tend to have lower values than females, but the reverse is true above age 45. Elevated levels have been found in such disease states as arteriosclerosis and hypothyroidism. The age profile is especially dramatic. In both sexes the mean serum level advances after age 35. It reaches a maximum at about 50 years old in men and declines slightly thereafter. In women there is a continuing rise at least to age 65. The phenomenon of age dependence was elegantly demonstrated in 1950–1952 by Keys and his associates (269, 270), although it had been known as early as 1935 (271–272). The results of Keys are shown in Figure 10.2. In the horse a recent study has reported little or no difference by sex, despite a slight decline (5%) in geldings, but as in the human being there is an individual and age dependence (273).

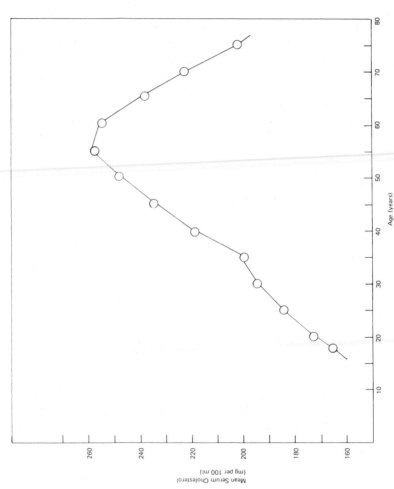

Figure 10.2 Age dependence of serum cholesterol in healthy male human beings. Adapted from the early work of Keys (270) on 1,492 urban, "white-collar" men in Minnesota. A number of variables are not included. For precise modern values see, for instance, Table 10.3.

Highest levels (132 mg%) were found during the first 6 months (perhaps due to suckling), then they declined to 92 mg% by about 2 years of age, reached a maximum 102 at age 4-6 years, and declined to 95 by age 8 and remained there to old age (13 years). The individual variation in horses (range of 102-216 during the first 8 weeks) was as high as in people, but the average value reported for adult horses is only about half as much as is well documented for men and women. Serum cholesterol levels of many different animals (from the horseshoe crab and caterpillar to monkeys) were measured many years ago. Man, with levels reaching above 200 mg%, is among those with the highest values. The serum of the horse is much more representative of the animal kingdom, which has typically a value ranging from about 50 to 150 mg%. For greater detail see Kritchevsky (258) and Cook (259). With increasing interest in an experimental animal evolutionarily near man, investigators have closely studied other primates during recent years. The baboon, for instance, has been shown to have a whole-body rate of cholesterol biosynthesis comparable with that in man. However, the serum cholesterol is near 102 mg%, roughly divided evenly between α- and β-lipoproteins. Cholesterol levels in the baboon, cynomolo-gus, and rhesus monkeys, as well as in man, show seasonal fluctuations. For more detail see Kritchevsky (274). The effect of weaning on blood cholesterol in various mammals has been well studied. In man serum cholesterol is low at birth and increases rapidly during the first few weeks of life, apparently as a result of diet. The newly elevated level is then maintained (and actually increases; see Figure 10.2) but not in rats and rabbits, in which it drops after weaning. This elevation after birth followed by a drop after weaning is observable also in calves, lambs, and pigs. See Carroll and Hamilton (275) for a key to the literature.

The relationship of diet, etc., to serum cholesterol in the adult human being as well as other adult animals has been the subject of particularly extensive study. One of the more complete investigations was that of a large (5,128 people) sample of the citizens, ages 30-59, of Framingham, Mass., begun in 1949 and carried on for eight years (known as the "Framing-ham Study") (276, 278). For one-fifth of this group, whose diet was moni-tored, the average intake of cholesterol was 704 mg/day for men and 492 mg/day for women (277). The procedures for calculating cholesterol intake have been published (276). It was concluded (277) that "the evidence linking the diet and serum cholesterol is still problematical, especially in free populations in highly developed countries." The problem is very complicated, as seen in other studies. Increased absorption of cholesterol from the diet evokes at least two compensatory mechanisms: (1) decrease in synthesis, and (2) increase in excretion; and these, at least in the case of the first, are quantitatively dependent on the individual (279). These compensatory mechanisms usually prevent accumulation of excess cho-lesterol in body pools, but not in all people. Among those individuals with high cholesterol diets, some do in fact accumulate cholesterol, but this is not necessarily reflected by increased serum cholesterol (*279, 280*). Keys (*280*), for instance, was unable a quarter of a century ago to observe significant correlations with serum cholesterol over a range of about 250–800 mg/day of cholesterol in the diet of men, a conclusion essentially the same as that of the more recent Framingham Study, which went on to say there was "no significant correlation between various dietary components and the serum cholesterol level" (*277*). What probably needs to be done is to examine more closely the various parameters (absorption, feedback on biosynthesis, tissue storage, serum levels, etc.) in individual cases, because the report of the Framingham study also concluded that the "evidence linking serum cholesterol and coronary heart disease is, we believe, incontrovertible" (*277*). People with the higher values have a greater risk of the disease.

Absorption of sterols from the diet is quantitatively limited, concentration-dependent, structurally dependent, probably species-dependent, and in man perhaps individually dependent. For instance, in the rat, as measured by transfer of dietary sterol to the lymph, 3–6% of sitosterol was estimated to be absorbed in 24 hours as a linear function of the amount (over a 70-fold range), while 30% of cholesterol administered together with the sitosterol was absorbed (*281*). In man, a 50-mg oral dose of sitosterol resulted in 0.015 mg% of this sterol in blood (*282*). The disappearance rate from blood was higher than for cholesterol, and 0.5% of a 258-mg dose remained in blood and visceral organs after 5 days (*282*). In another study of human beings, 50% of oral cholesterol was absorbed and 5% less of oral sitosterol (*283*). About 20% of the sitosterol was excreted as bile acid, the rest as neutral material, and sitosterol was esterified more slowly and excreted more quickly than cholesterol (*283*). In worms (*Ascaris suum*) the structural discrimination is much less. Movement of cholesterol across the intestine is only twice that of sitosterol (*284*). The specificity is believed to relate to the epithelial cells, which accumulate only cholesterol (*284*).

c. Carrier Proteins   Two types of proteins carrying sterols have been identified. They are "sterol carrier protein" (SCP) in cells functioning in the biosynthetic pathway and "lipoproteins" of several sorts functioning in blood.

SCP was discovered by Ritter and Dempsey (*285–287*) in the soluble fraction of liver homogenates and further investigated by them, by Scallen et al. (*288*), and others. For a key to the literature see Dempsey (*289*) and Scallen et al. (*290*). It is essential for the conversion of water-insoluble precursors (including squalene) to cholesterol by microsomal enzymes, and a functionally similar protein has been identified in human placenta and liver, other mammalian tissues, protozoa, and yeast. The protein with a protomer molecular weight of 16,000 has a marked tendency to aggregate, which is facilitated by phospholipids and sterols. The aggregate has a molecular weight range of 2.5×10^5 to 2.0×10^6.

The first lipoprotein from blood was isolated from horse serum by Macheboeuf (*291*) as early as 1929. It has been extensively studied in the intervening years. See Skipski (*292*) for a review. The lipid-to-protein ratio varies widely and in part is reflected in the density of the lipoprotein. Very low-density lipoproteins (VLDL) have a density less than 1.006 g/ml; the density of low-density lipoproteins (LDL) is between 1.006 and 1.063 g/ml; and high-density lipoproteins have a density greater than 1.063 g/ml. The classes and subclasses are also designated by negative sedimentation Svedberg units (10^{-13} cm/sec.-dyne-g), which is the "flotation rate," designated as S_f. One VLDL subclass (density 1.006–0.97 g/ml), for instance, is S_f 20–400. Large particles at the end of the VLDL spectrum, which are nearly pure lipid, are called chylomicrons. Their cholesterol (and ester) content is low (a few percent) and variable. The VLDL fraction (93% lipid) has the next highest cholesterol (and ester) content (15–20% of the lipids present), while the lipid in the LDL fraction ("β-lipoprotein") is about 40% cholesterol and its esters. The alcohol/ester ratio is about ⅓. The LDL fraction is 80% lipid. Most of the blood cholesterol is believed to be present in this fraction in human beings. The lipids of the HDL fraction (α-lipoprotein, 45% lipid) are composed of about 30% cholesterol, which is thought to be esterified even to a higher degree (approximately ⅕) than in the LDL fraction. The most abundant fatty acids esterifying cholesterol are linoleic, oleic, and palmitic acids. The amount of "total cholesterol," i.e., alcohol and ester, in blood is determined in part by the amount of lipoprotein, which in turn is determined genetically and by other means (pregnancy, disease, medication, age, etc.).

d. Sterols in Development and Aging   While there has been little investigation of the influence of ontogeny on sterol patterns, several pioneering studies of brain development suggest that this subject may be a fruitful one to examine. Three things have now been well established. During development of the brain, the total amount of cholesterol increases dramatically (200–400%), apparently by biosynthesis in situ, the proportion of the cholesterol present as ester decreases from several percent essentially to zero, and the structural distribution in cholesterol (versus other sterols) increases to approximately 99%. Qualitatively, these changes occur in a variety of animals, including birds, mammals below primates, and man; they are associated with myelination. The principal sterol other than cholesterol in the early phases of development is desmosterol. Its amount varies from a few percent in late gestation in humans to as much as one-fourth of the total sterol in rodents at birth. When myelination is complete, which occurs only after birth in rodents, e.g., the rat, the amount of desmosterol approaches zero. More exact numbers can be found in Table

10.4. The desmosterol/cholesterol ratio is greatest in the thalamus and hypothalamus and lowest in the cerebellum (*293*). For greater detail see the reviews by Kabara (*266*) and Paoletti et al. (*267*). The fatty acids esterify-

Table 10.4 Desmosterol in developing brains

Species	% of Total Sterol				
	Developmental Stage				
	Gestation (weeks)				
	2	4	25	At Birth	Adult
Man			6	2	None
Rabbit				18	None
Guinea pig		18		Traces	None
Rat	20			26	0.8
Mouse				22	—
Chicken	11			1	—

Adapted from Paoletti et al. (*267*).

ing cholesterol have principally C_{16}, C_{18}, and C_{20} chain lengths (*294a*). The dominant one is oleate, and the ester profile of developing adult human brains is much the same (*294*).

As described in Section C.2.b, in man there is a marked influence of age on serum cholesterol. This was first observed in adults. More recently, the serum levels of newborn infants has been measured and found to be below 100 mg/100 ml. This level then rapidly increases and is thought to be correlated with the development of intestinal flora. The bacteria dehydroxylate bile acids at C-7. For a key to the literature see Samuel et al. (*294b*). The reasons why there should be a correlation are not clear in detail, but, because much of cholesterol is excreted as bile acids that have some sort of a feedback effect on the liver, there is a rough principle relating bile acids to serum cholesterol. The suggestion from the elevation of serum cholesterol and increased 7α-desoxybile acids is that the latter fail to inhibit cholesterol synthesis and/or decrease passage of the sterol into the bile. The reasons why serum cholesterol should continue to rise after microbial colonization, however, remain obscure, although it may well be associated with the balance between synthesis, bile acid formation, and fecal metabolism. Rat liver preparations have shown decreased oxidation of C-26 to CO_2 and decreased 7α-hydroxylation as a function of age. These are important steps in bile acid formation. Decreased conversion of acetate to cholesterol also occurs. Thus, there appears to be a general retardation of metabolism with time. For a key to the literature see Story and Kritchevsky (*294*).

e. Sterols and Disease   A lipidosis is a condition in which lipids are abnormal in some way and produce undesirable affects. Lipidoses have not been as well studied as, say, malfunction of the endocrine system. Obesity is an important, long-standing, and still poorly understood example. The fact of excess deposition of triglycerides is simple enough to see, but the regulatory factors governing it are more elusive. In the case of sterols, only a few lipidoses are even well described. One that has been known for many years and in which excess cholesterol deposits in a highly localized area is gallstones. Little has been discovered about the causes of it, although there is some suggestion of a genetic factor. The deposition results from a complicated function of the biosynthetic rate and the composition of the bile. American Indian women have an unusually high prevalence of gallstones. The lithogenic (stone-producing) bile results from decreased output of bile acids and increased output of cholesterol, which in turn is associated with a high rate of total body cholesterol formation and diminished amounts of bile acid in the stools. For a key to the literature see Adler et al. (*295*).

Cholestanol and cholesterol accumulate in the familial disease known as cerebrotendinous xanthomatosis. While rare, this genetic condition can be fatal at middle age. All tissues accumulate sterols, with the brain, lung, and Achilles tendon xanthomas being especially involved. Greatly increased proportions of cholesterol are especially obvious, and may appear in skin deposits. Lanosterol, lathosterol, and cholesterol appear in excessive quantities in the bile (*296*). These facts suggest aberrations in the relative rates of various biosynthetic steps, especially increased total biosynthesis and increased Δ^5-reduction. Evidence does in fact exist for hyperactive biosynthesis (*297*) as well as for the conversion of cholesterol to cholestanol in these patients (*298*).

Tumors (glioblastoma) of the brain are associated with increased quantities of desmosterol, as shown in Paoletti's laboratory (*299, 300*). The cholesterol content falls from 99.1% of the sterols to 95.6% and the desmosterol content rises from 0.02% to 1.2%. There is also 2.5% increase in unidentified sterols. When the tumor is incubated with [2-^{14}C] MVA, there is massive incorporation of label into desmosterol and only little into cholesterol. Δ^8-Precursors also accumulate great quantities of label, while incubation of a normal brain produces mostly labeled cholesterol. The biosynthetic data are summarized in Table 10.5. The tumor, interestingly, is suggestive of the undeveloped brain. When patients with brain tumors are treated with a Δ^{24}-reductase inhibitor (Triparanol), desmosterol appears in the cerebrospinal fluid at a level 20 times higher than in normal patients (*299*). This phenomenon has been suggested as a possible way to diagnose brain tumors. Increased concentration of cho-

Table 10.5. Comparison of the fate of label from [2-^{14}C]MVA in normal and tumorous (Glioblastoma) human brains

Compound	% of Label in Neutral Lipids	
	Normal	Tumor
Squalene, prenols	32	49
Δ^8- and $\Delta^{8,24}$-Sterols	17	28
Cholestanol	2	0.05
Desmosterol	2	21
Cholesterol	47	2

Adapted from Galli et al. (299).

lesteryl esters, also a sort of reversion to an early developmental state, has been observed in various other diseases of the central nervous system, including subacute sclerosing panencephalitis, multiple sclerosis, sudano-philic leukodystrophy, gangliosidoses, Schilder's disease, and adrenocortical atrophy with diffuse sclerosis. In general, cholesteryl ester seems to increase as demyelination proceeds. The fatty acid pattern in the esters closely resembles that of brain phosphatidylcholine, and it has been suggested (300) that the cholesterol acts as a storage for the fatty acid produced in demyelination and in a reverse way as a fatty acid source during myelination. For a key to the literature see Ramsey and Davison (301).

The occurrence of desmosterol in unusually high concentrations in tumors and early developmental stages indicates a partial block, i.e., reduced enzyme concentration or activity, at the step involving the Δ^{24}-reductase. This enzyme can accept a variety of precursors, including lanosterol, and an accumulation of desmosterol could be paralleled by an accumulation of other Δ^{24}-sterols. For example, if there was reduced conversion of Δ^8- to Δ^7- to $\Delta^{5,7}$- to Δ^5-sterols, $\Delta^{8,24}$-sterols, $\Delta^{7,24}$-sterols, etc., could also accumulate, and indeed this happens in tumors (Table 10.5). If, however, only the Δ^{24}-reductase was impaired and the biosynthetic enzymes were indifferent to the presence and absence of the Δ^{24}-bond (which is the case), desmosterol would become essentially the only sterol present. This actually happens in L-cell mouse fibroblasts. These are transformed (tumor like) cells representing a line that can be grown in tissue culture and maintained and studied as one does microorganisms. No cholesterol is present. In its place is desmosterol with small amounts of a sterol believed to be 7-dehydrodesmosterol (302).

Tumors of the liver (hepatomas) are characterized by a different sort of enzymatic defect. In normal liver the HMG-CoA reductase is regulated by lipoproteins and the cholesterol present in the complex. Increased dietary cholesterol results then in a feedback inhibition of the reductase and a slower rate of cholesterol biosynthesis, which compensates for the dietary intake. In hepatomas this feedback is absent (*303*). The accumulation of 24-alkysterols in a variety of pathologic as well as normal situations has been reported. These included human mammary (*304, 305*) and brain tumors (*306*), human lipidoses (*307*), cow's milk (*308*), rat adrenals (*309*), rat liver (*310*), and rat hepatomas (*310*). When labeled sitosterol was injected intraperitoneally into rats bearing Morris hepatomas transplanted into the leg, label was subsequently found in the normal liver, the cancerous liver, as well as the remainder of the carcass, and the turnover of the sitosterol was greater than for cholesterol (*310*). Dietary absorption and a faster turnover rate of sitosterol compared to cholesterol has also been observed in man (*283*). Not enough work has yet been done to perceive the complete significance of these results, but tentatively it seems that, while healthy vertebrates strongly discriminate against gastrointestinal absorption of 24-alkylsterols and also selectively remove any that do enter the blood, species and probably individuals differ quantitatively in their discriminatory abilities. Furthermore, impaired discrimination seems to be associated with certain diseases. There is also, interestingly, good reason to believe that absorption of 24-alkylsterols is greater the more the sterol approximates the cholesterol structure. In rat adrenal glands the ratio of 24-methylcholesterol to 24-ethylcholesterol is greater than it is in the dietary sterol (*309*), and the data published for rat liver and hepatoma (*310*) as well as for cow's milk (*308*) suggest the same thing. This is reminiscent of selective absorption in insects (Section C.1.b). L-Cell mouse fibroblasts also incorporate cholesterol better than sitosterol (*311*), so the selection may not be only at the intestinal level in intact animals.

The relationship between cholesterol levels and disease is perhaps most dramatic in the case of arteriosclerosis. This was first observed in 1913 by Anitschkow (*312*), who was able to produce aortic lesions in the rabbit by feeding it cholesterol. The disease can also be induced in other animals, including primates. The rhesus monkey, for instance, when fed high concentrations of fat and cholesterol (which tend to be synergistic) has subsequently been shown to develop atherosclerosis (production of atheromas, i.e., lipid deposits, in the arterial wall) following a period of several months of hypercholesterolemia (elevated serum cholesterol, approximately greater than 250 mg/100 ml) (*313*). In the human population the incidence of cardiovascular disease and of atherogenesis in particular is statistically linked to blood lipids (Table 10.6). Cholesterol is present in the atheromas (atherosclerotic plaques); populations with a high average level of serum cholesterol have a higher reported mortality from coronary heart disease, and those with lower cholesterol levels have lower death rates as well as less atherosclerosis as determined postmortem (*278*). Data from the Framingham Study (*228*) (cf. Section C.2.b) indicate that the upper quartile of the population (of Framingham, Mass.) had moderate hypercholesterolemia

Table 10.6 Serum cholesterol and risk of coronary heart disease

	Risk of People with Levels of 265 mg % Compared to Those with Levels under 220 mg %	
Age	Men	Women
35–44	5.5	5.0
45–54	2.4	1.5
55–64	1.7	1.3
All ages	2.5	1.5

From the work of Kannel et al. (278) in the Framington Study of 5,128 people.

(250–350 mg/100 ml of serum). Depending on age and sex, these individuals are thought to have a risk of coronary heart disease two to five times higher than is found in the population with serum cholesterol values below the average of about 220 mg/100 ml. Detailed data on the incidence of the disease and its relationship to serum cholesterol have been published (314). In view of the facts just discussed, there has been much interest in finding ways to lower the serum cholesterol of people with hypercholesterolemia. One avenue would be to inhibit biosynthesis at some stage, and many compounds have been examined. Since total removal of endogenous cholesterol would obviously be expected to be fatal, in the simplest sense the inhibition should be quantitative and the inhibitor should have no other effects. No compound has completely satisfactorily approached this ideal at the clinical level. Among those, however, which appear to have some merit as a hypocholesterolemic drug is clofibrate, but its mechanism of action is not well understood (315–317). The other principle for lowering serum cholesterol depends on enhancing the rate of the cholesterol-to-bile acid metabolism, thereby removing cholesterol more quickly. This can be achieved with an anion-exchange resin, known as cholestyramine, which binds bile acids. The cholestyramine is taken orally. When it reaches the intestines, the bile acid is removed from the enterohepatic circulation and excreted. In man, bile acid is normally reabsorbed, circulating back to the liver and out again into the intestines 2–3 times per day (the enterohepatic circulation). By removing it from this cycle, cholestyramine increases the rate of bile acid excretion, enhances the conversion of cholesterol to bile acid, presumably through eliminating feedback, and consequently lowers the amount of cholesterol available for binding to lipoproteins in the blood. Because feeding cholestyramine (in gram-quantities per day) actually does lower serum cholesterol, apparently the bile acid depletion achieved is sufficient to override the ability of the HMG-CoA reductase to respond in a balancing increase in biosynthetic rate. For a key to the literature see Kim et al. (*317*), Nazir et al. (*318*), and Higgins et al. (*319*).

The obvious possibility that genetic factors play an important role in the regulation of cholesterol levels has begun to be examined in recent years, especially with experimental animals. In monkeys, cattle, and mice, estimates of the influence of heritable factors on the variability of plasma cholesterol levels are 56–99% and in chickens 26%. Furthermore, within a given species (examined in pigeons, monkeys, and man) it has been possible to show the existence of "hyperresponders" and "hyporesponders" to dietary cholesterol in terms of elevation of plasma cholesterol. The mechanism of the response has been elucidated in two selected lines (selected by inbreeding) of Show Racer pigeons. In one line the animals are hyporesponders and in the other hyperresponders. In the former, cholesterol absorption was lower (48 mg/day) than in the latter (58 mg/day), endogenous synthesis was the reverse, high (28 mg/day) in the hyporesponders and low (12 mg/day) in the hyperresponders, and excretion was greater in the hyporesponders. Thus, those animals that respond to dietary cholesterol by increasing their plasma cholesterol (by approximately 4-fold relative to the hyporesponders) had elevated abilities for absorption, depressed biosynthesis (presumably by feedback from the increased cholesterol load), and less capacity to excrete the sterol. This work with pigeons was done by Wagner and Clarkson (*320*), whose paper can be consulted as a key to the other literature.

As noted in Section C.2.c, cholesterol is present in blood both in the free and esterified forms (with fatty acids). Of the fatty acids present, linoleic acid is the most abundant in, at least, both man (50%) and the baboon (32%). Other fatty acids in decreasing relative abundance (in the baboon) are: oleic, palmitic, stearic, palmitoleic, arachidomic, and linoleic acids (*321*). In man, the highest percentage of total cholesterol in serum is carried by the LDL fraction, while in the baboon 55% is the HDL fraction (*321*). Esterification of the cholesterol occurs primarily in the blood through a transesterification from lecithin catalyzed by an enzyme (lecithin-cholesterol acyltransferase) known as LCAT, which is synthesized in the liver. For a detailed review see Norum and Gjone (*322*). In patients with certain hepatic disorders, the ester:free alcohol ratio is smaller than normal, and the reduction is believed to be due to impairment of hepatic LCAT synthesis (*323*). Familial LCAT deficiency also occurs in the human population (*322*). Such individuals suffer from corneal opacities, anemia, and in some cases renal failure and atherosclerosis (*322*). The propensity of arterial tissue (rather than blood) to esterify cholesterol similarly may be linked to atherosclerosis, since esters accumulate in atheromas and since in atherosclerotic arteries a higher proportion of fatty acid taken up by the artery proceeds to cholesterol esters (compared to that proceeding to phospholipid or triglyceride) than is so with the normal artery. For keys to the literature see Day and Proudlock (*324*) and Hashimoto and Dayton (*325*). Atherosclerotic lesions have been reported to contain small amounts of diesters (mostly oeate and palmitate) of 26-hydroxycholesterol, while normal arteries are believed to have only monoesters of this minor sterol (*326*). The relative ability of free and esterified cholesterol in an atheroma to equilibrate with plasma has also been studied (*327*).

In 1932, Kennaway and Cook (*328*) suggested that steroids might serve as precursors to polycyclic aromatic carcinogens, and in the following year methylcholanthrene was synthesized (*329, 330*) nonbiologically from a bile acid. Incorporation of C-18 into ring D enlarged this ring, and the fifth ring was made from the side chain (Scheme 10.8). Methylcholanthrene proved to be strongly carcinogenic (*329, 331*). An alternative polycyclic aromatic compound was subsequently synthesized by others (*332*) by a model of a biochemical route in which hormonal reactions were involved. A sterol was converted to pregnenolone, then the latter was rearranged to an "anthrasteroid" (rings A, B, and C linear), ring D was enlarged by the D-homosteroid rearrangement of a 17α-hydroxy derivative, and the compound was fully aromatized. Other, although linear, ways in which steroids could give polycyclic aromatic carcinogens have been considered. Unfortunately, as reasonable and attractive as the general hypothesis is, no support from such studies (*333*) as to the nature of constituents of urine and tissues of cancer patients has been found for the ideas at a biological level. For keys to the literature, see Nes and Ford (*332*), de Souza and Nes (*333*), Cook (*334*), Buu-Hoi (*335*), and Dannenberg (*336*). The polycyclic aromatic hydrocarbons in the environment and in archeologic deposits, however, may well come from steroids by nonbiological (or perhaps even microbial) processes related to those just discussed (Scheme 10.8).

D. LESS ADVANCED PHOTOSYNTHETIC SYSTEMS

1. Prokaryotic Organisms

Organisms that lack a nuclear membrane and other membraneous organelles (mitochondria, endoplasmic reticulum, etc.) are said to be prokaryotic. Among the photosynthetic systems, two types are prokaryotic, the photosynthetic bacteria and the blue-green algae. It was originally thought from negative attempts to show biosynthesis (*337*), as well as for other reasons (*338*), that the latter lacked sterols. The former have been believed also to lack sterols on the presumption that bacteria lack sterols (which is not true as a generalization; see Section B.1.c). Although the photosynthetic bacteria remain to be studied, blue-green algae have been well investigated in the last decade, and many species (all examined) have been shown to contain sterols. Reitz and Hamilton (*339*) and de Souza and Nes (*340*) were the first to demonstrate their presence in 1968. The latter authors (*340*) examined in great detail the filamentous blue-green alga *Phor-*

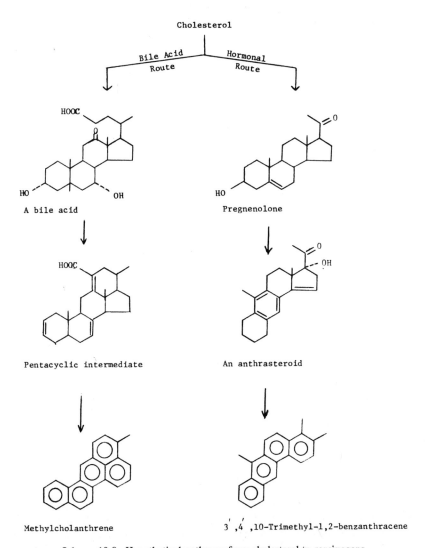

Scheme 10.8. Hypothetical pathways from cholesterol to carcinogens.

midium luridum, which was grown on a completely synthetic medium. Squalene, as well as seven sterols, was identified. The nature of the medium, the presence of squalene, and the unusual complexity of the sterol mixture proved the organism biosynthesized and did not just assimilate the sterols found (*340*). The sterol mixture was composed primarily (80%) of 24ξ-ethyllathosterol and its Δ²²-derivative in an abundance ratio of 3:2. The remaining 20% was constituted by cholesterol, 24ξ-ethylcholesterol and its Δ²²-derivative, as well as by 24ξ-ethyl-7-dehydrocholesterol and its

Δ^{22}-derivative. Of the Δ^5- and $\Delta^{5,7}$-sterols, the most abundant possessed a $\Delta^{5,7}$-system (15% of the total sterols). The sterols, therefore, consisted of a biosynthetic array of Δ^7-, $\Delta^{5,7}$-, and Δ^5-compounds in decreasing relative abundance. In all of them, except for small amounts of cholesterol, the 24ξ-ethyl group was present in the apparent absence of the 24-methyl group. The alkylation pathway must proceed in these algae only to a 24-methylenesterol, which is used exclusively for a second alkylation, and alkylation of the Δ^{24}-bond must be the predominant mode of metabolism compared to Δ^{24}-reduction.

Cholesterol and 24ξ-ethylcholesterol have also been isolated from *Anacystis nidulans* (*339*), *Fremyella diplosiphon* (*339*), three species of *Spirulina* (*341*), *Calothrix* sp. (*341*), *Nostoc commune* (*341*), and *Cyanidium caldarium* (*342*). In addition, the *Spirulina, Calothrix, Nostoc,* and *Cyanidium* species contain 24ξ-methylcholesterol. *Anacystis nidulans* and *Fremyella diplosiphon* contain, in addition to cholesterol and 24ξ-ethylcholesterol in each case, several unidentified peaks in the gas-liquid chromatogram, which appear from the published results (*339*) to include 24ξ-methylcholesterol. *Anabena cylindrica* seems to contain only cholesterol, 24ξ-methylcholesterol, and the latter's Δ^{22}-derivative (*343*). Δ^7-Sterols, notably 24ξ-methyl- and 24ξ-ethyllathosterol were also present in the *Spirulina, Calothrix,* and *Nostoc* species. *Cyanidium caldarium* as with *P. luridum,* contains some 24ξ-ethyl-7-dehydrocholesterol.

In summary, all blue-green algae examined contain cholesterol as a minor sterol, and, therefore, they must reduce the Δ^{24}-bond as a minor biosynthetic route. The major route is clearly Δ^{24}-alkylation in all cases. The algae are then divisible into genera according to the extent of alkylation (Table 10.7). Only the first C_1 transfer seems to occur in some (*Anabena*), in some the second C_1 transfer seems to occur to an extent that excludes 24-C_1 sterols as end products (*Phormidium*), and some comprise an intermediate type (*Spirulina, Calothrix, Nostoc,* and *Cyanidium*) in which the end products are composed of both 24-C_1 and 24-C_2 sterols. In all of the examined cases, Δ^5-sterols are present, and in most they are accompanied by Δ^7- and $\Delta^{5,7}$-sterols. If the latter two sterol types are taken to be intermediates, kinetic control of the pathway is not as highly developed as in other organisms in which Δ^5-sterols occur in the nearly complete absence of $\Delta^{5,7}$- and Δ^7-sterols. However, an alternative must be considered, namely, that the composition reflects fine-tuning of membranes to a particular environment of temperature, etc. In no case has the configuration at C-24 of blue-green algal sterols been determined, despite the use in the literature of configurationally meaningful names, e.g., sitosterol and chondrillasterol. The biosynthesis of sterols has been examined in two laboratories (*337, 339*) without success, but there can be little doubt (from the absence of sterols in the media and for other reasons) that biosynthesis does occur.

2. Eukaryotic Algae

The eukaryotic algae (which are those having nuclei and other subcellular organelles) are a diverse group of organisms, differing, among other things, in the extent of cellular differentiation, the structures of the photosynthetic pigments, and the presence or absence of locomotion. In addition, while most must always operate in a photosynthetic mode, some, e.g., the euglenoids, can live in the absence of light. Algae as a group do not possess an embryonic stage of ontogeny, nor do any have the extent of cellular differentiation encountered in the Embryophytes. They are generally classified according to the nature of their photosynthetic pigments, expressed roughly in their color, giving divisions (phyla) such as the red algae (Rhodophyta), brown algae (Phaeophyta), etc. Sterols were first recognized in algae by Willstätter and Page (344) in 1914 and examined in some detail by Heilbron and his associates (345, 346) during the 1930s. More recently, several groups of investigators have studied them with modern precision.

a. Red Algae (Rhodophyta) Thirteen species of red algae were originally collected by Heilbron et al. (345–347) off British shores, and based only on melting point data it was thought they contained sitosterol and one of its 24(28)-dehydroderivatives (fucosterol). In the late 1950s Tsuda et al. (348–350) examined 16 species in five orders collected in waters surrounding Japan. The Japanese investigators came to the remarkable conclusion for the time that, contrary to the previous reports on the Atlantic species, the Pacific species contained primarily cholesterol. This was the first unequivocal identification of cholesterol in the plant kingdom, and it established that this sterol is not exclusively, as had been thought, a product of animal metabolism. In 12 of the species, cholesterol was the only sterol identified, in three, cholesterol and 24-methylenecholesterol (ostreasterol), and in one, 24-dehydrocholesterol. In the following decade, Goodwin's group (351) in Wales reinvestigated the Atlantic species and came essentially to the same conclusion as had their Japanese colleagues. Of more than a dozen species in five orders, all had cholesterol either as the major or minor component. 24-Dehydrocholesterol (desmosterol) was discovered as the major sterol of two species and a minor sterol of several others. An Italian group (352) subsequently studying 17 species, presumably of Mediterranean origin, also found either cholesterol or its Δ^{22}- or Δ^{24}-derivatives and added to the list (from the order Nemalionales) the Δ^{23}-derivative (23-dehydrocholesterol), which they named liagosterol from its occurrence in the genus *Liagora*. It also occurs in *Scinaia* sp. Both *cis*- and *trans*-isomers were believed present. Still more intensive examination of 14 more species in Japan (353), Canada (354), and France (353, 356) revealed that red algae could be even more complex. Four species were found to contain cholestanol as the major sterol accompanied by lathosterol (353), several species contained 22-dehydrohalosterol (the C_{26}-analog of

Table 10.7. Classification of blue-green algae according to sterol composition[a]

Algae with 24-C$_1$ Sterols		Algae with 24-C$_2$ Sterols		Algae with 24-C$_1$ and 24-C$_2$ Sterols	
Species	Major Sterols[b]	Species	Major Sterols[b]	Species	Major Sterols[b]
Anabena cylindrica	$\Delta^{5,22}$-24-Methyl Δ^5-24-H Δ^5-24-Methyl	*Phormidium luridum*	$\Delta^{7,22}$-24-Ethyl Δ^7-24-Ethyl $\Delta^{5,7,22}$-24-Ethyl	*Cyanidium caladarium*	$\Delta^{5,7,22}$-24-Methyl Δ^5-24-Ethyl Δ^5-24-Methyl
				Spirulina platensis Mao I	Δ^5-24-Ethyl $\Delta^{5,24(28)}$-24-Ethyl[c] $\Delta^{5,22}$-24-Ethyl Δ^5-24-H $\Delta^{5,22}$-24-Methyl
				Spirulina platensis Mao II	Δ^5-24-Ethyl Δ^7-24-Ethyl Δ^7-24-Methyl
				Spirulina sp. (Mexico)	Δ^5-24-Ethyl Δ^5-24-H Δ^7-24-Ethyl $\Delta^{5,22}$-24-Ethyl Δ^7-24-Methyl
				Calothrix	$\Delta^{7,22}$-24-Ethyl $\Delta^{5,22}$-24-Methyl $\Delta^{5,24(28)}$-24-Ethyl[c]
				Nostoc commune	$\Delta^{7,22}$-24-Ethyl Δ^7-24-Methyl Δ^7-24-Ethyl

Fremyella diplosiphon	Unidentified sterol
	Δ^5-24-Ethyl
	Δ^5-24-H
	Sterol with g.l.c. of Δ^5-24-Methyl
Anacystis nidulans	Δ^5-24-Ethyl
	Unidentified sterol
	Δ^5-24-H
	Sterol with g.l.c. of Δ^5-24-Methyl

[a] All species contain cholesterol. The highest percentage found is approximately 25% in *Fremyella diplosiphon*. *Calothrix* and *Nostoc* species contain about 10%, the other species less. All species contained a complex mixture of sterols. Data have been taken from references cited in the text.
[b] The three most abundant sterols in descending order of amount are listed except in those cases where minor sterols need listing in order to justify the classification. In some cases more sterols than those listed have been identified (see text). The configuration at C-24 is unknown in all cases.
[c] Tentative identification.

22-dehydrocholesterol that lacks a CH_2 group in the side chain) and/or a related C_{26}-sterol as minor components (*353–355*), a variety of species contained 24-methylene-, 24-ethylidene, 24-methyl-, and 24-ethylsterols (*353–355*) in small amounts, and one species (*Rytiphlea tinctoria*) was found to contain principally 24ξ-methylcholesterol (*356*). *Rhodymenia palmata,* which contains cholesterol and desmosterol as 76% of the 4-desmethylsterol mixture, also contains small amounts of cycloartanol, indicating that cholesterol and desmosterol are derived by the cycloartenol rather than lanosterol route in this, and presumably other, red algae (*355*). Biosynthesis of cholesterol, desmosterol, 22-dehydrocholesterol, 24-methylenecholesterol, 24-ethylidenecholesterol, and 24ξ-methyl-22-dehydrocholesterol in *R. palmata* from acetate has been observed (*355*). The three sterols substituted at C-24 also were labeled from methionine containing ^{14}C in the methyl group. From neither labeled acetate nor methionine, however, did the C_{26}-sterol (which was present) incorporate label (*355*). Curiously, in 1961 *Porphridium cruentum,* when grown on a chemically defined medium, was reported (*357*) to lack sterols altogether. Since this is exceedingly rare in any organism, *P. cruentum* is worthy of further study.

In summary, in all but two (*R. tinctoria,* and *P. cruentum*) of the 50 or so species of red algae that have been studied in seven orders, the principal sterol bears an unalkylated side chain and is usually cholesterol itself (Table 10.8). In a few cases the major sterol is cholestanol, desmosterol, or 22-dehydrocholesterol. Small percentages of 23-dehydro-, 24-alkenyl-, and 24-alkylsterols have also been found, along with a C_{26}-sterol. Biosynthesis of all but the last-mentioned sterol has been demonstrated. Species containing nearly pure cholesterol include *Chondrus crispus* (in the family Gigartinaceae, order Gigartinales), living in tidal rock pools off the Cardiganshire coast of Britain, an unidentified species found floating off the beach at Miami, Florida, and the Japanese *Gelidium japonicum,* belonging to the order Gelidiales. A species containing mostly 22-dehydrocholesterol is *Hypnea japonica,* collected in Sagami Bay, Shizuoka Prefecture, Japan. From the latter collecting area was also obtained *Gelidium amansii,* family Gelidiaceae, order Gelidiales, which contained principally cholestanol and other Δ^0-sterols together with cholesterol, lathosterol, and 24-alkenyl- and 24-alkylsterols. Thus, the habitat alone cannot dictate the sterol composition. On the other hand, it may play a role, since *Rhodymenia palmata* from various sources has not been reported to have the same proportions of sterols in the mixture. The English workers (*351*) found it to be 99% desmosterol, while the desmosterol content found by the French workers (*355*) was only 56%, with 20% being cholesterol and the remainder being several other sterols, with and without a substituent at C-24, and traces of a C_{26}-sterol. A seasonal variation in the cholesterol-desmosterol ratio of both *R. palmata* (*358*) and *Halogaccian* sp. (*359*) has also been observed. These details warrant further investigation in order to under-

Table 10.8. Sterols of red algae (Nomenclature parent = cholestanol)

Order	Principal Sterol	Minor Sterols
Nemalionales (only two species)	Δ^5	$\Delta^{5,23}$(ca. 36%)
Gelidiales	Δ^5 or Δ^0	$\Delta^{5,22}$, Δ^5-24-C_2H_5, Δ^{22}, Δ^{22}-24-C_2H_5, Δ^7, Δ^0, Δ^0-24-CH_2, Δ^0-24-C_2H_5, C_{26}-$\Delta^{5,22}$, and C_{26}-Δ^{22}
Cryptonemiales	Δ^5 or Δ^0	$\Delta^{5,22}$, $\Delta^{5,22}$-24-CH_3, Δ^5-24-CH_2, Δ^5-24-C_2H_5, Δ^5-24-C_2H_4, Δ^{22}, Δ^7, Δ^{22}-24-CH_3, Δ^0-24-CH_2, Δ^0-24-C_2H_5, Δ^0-24-C_2H_4, and C_{26}-Δ^{22}
Gigartinales	Δ^5, $\Delta^{5,22}$, or $\Delta^{5,24}$	Δ^5, $\Delta^{5,22}$, $\Delta^{5,24}$, $\Delta^{5,22}$-24-CH_3, Δ^5-24-CH_2, Δ^5-24-C_2H_5, and Δ^5-24-C_2H_4
Ceramiales	Δ^5	$\Delta^{5,24}$
Rhodymeniales (only one species)	Δ^5 or $\Delta^{5,24}$	Δ^5, $\Delta^{5,22}$, Δ^5-24-CH_2, Δ^5-C_2H_4, $\Delta^{5,22}$-24-CH_3, Δ^0, and C_{26}-$\Delta^{5,22}$
Bangiales (only one species)	$\Delta^{5,24}$	Δ^5

Data derived from references 345–357.

stand the complicated ecology of the marine environment. Ikekawa and his associates (*353*) have pointed out that the stanol-containing algae live in the relatively deep sea and show a remarkable parallelism in sterol profiles with the deep sea jellyfish. Moreover, the species of algae in which stanols predominate come from two orders (Gelidiales and Cryptonemiales) in which other species contain essentially only Δ^5-sterols. While it would be a satisfying simplicity of sorts to find that the sterol patterns were only of a phylogenetic character, the present evidence compels us not to ignore possible environmental influences, which may, of course, be interrelated with the phylogenetic traits.

   b. Brown Algae (Phaeophyta)   A great many species of brown algae have been studied, beginning with the work in Heilbron's laboratory (*345, 346*). The algae vary from those that are essentially undifferentiated, microorganismic in character, e.g., *Sphacelaria* sp., to the great kelps of the Pacific Coast, which reach several hundred feet from a holdfast on the ocean floor to the surface of the water. All of these algae, in nearly 40 species of seven orders (Ectocarpales, Sphacelariales, Dictyotales, Chordariales, Dictyosiphonales, Laminariales, and Fucales), have so far been found to have a common Δ^5-sterol (fucosterol) in which C-24 bears a C_2 group and a $\Delta^{24(28)}$-bond. The stereochemistry is such that C-29 is on the same side (described as the *cis*-configuration) of the double bond in all examined cases. Fucosterol derives its name from its first isolation (*345*) from a common species on Atlantic shores, *Fucus vesiculosus*. This seaweed is recognizable in intertidal areas by its brown color, a holdfast to a rock, and flotation bladders that allow a foot or more of thallus to rise to the surface with the incoming tide. Fucosterol, which is accompanied by as much as 17% of 24-methylenecholesterol in some brown algae, does not occur in higher plants (Tracheophytes), but it is reported in marine invertebrates and red algae, which perhaps derive it from the Phaeophyta. The *trans*-isomer (isofucosterol) has never been found to accompany it in brown algae. Its Δ^7-isomer is conceivably an intermediate, but it also has not been found. Brown algae have, however, been reported in a few cases to contain small amounts (0.05–2.5%) of cholesterol (*359, 360*). It is unclear whether or not this represents contamination. The apparent occurrence of 24-hydroxy-24-vinylcholesterol (saringasterol) (*359, 361–363*) and 24-ketocholesterol (*359, 363, 364*) in some species very likely represents artifact formation by air oxidation of fucosterol (*363*). The early reports (*362*) of the existence of the C-20 epimer ("sargasterol") of fucosterol in *Sargassum ringgoldianum* and *Eisenis bicydis* (*349, 362*) have not been amenable to verification. Upon recent reexamination, Ikekawa et al. (*361*) found only fucosterol in one of these species. Theoretical reasons also exist for its not existing (see Chapter 2.) 7α-Hydroxyfucosterol and its dehydration product, *cis*-24-ethylidenecholesta-3,5-dien-7-one, which have been isolated in small amounts (*365*), are of uncertain origin. For earlier reviews from which details on species, etc., can be obtained, see Carter et al. (*346*), Miller (*366*), and Patterson (*367*), in addition to the more recent original papers quoted in the present writing. Biosynthesis of fucosterol in brown algae has been well documented as a part of fundamental mechanistic studies (see Chapter 9).

In summary, the Phaeophyta operate the biosynthetic pathway so as to produce the very unusual *cis*-24-ethylidenecholesterol (fucosterol). It is definitely accompanied on occasion by 24-methylenecholesterol and perhaps by cholesterol. Reductases for the $\Delta^{24(28)}$-bond must be absent, since no 24-methyl- or 24-ethylsterols have been observed to be present, except traces in one uncertain case (*359, 363*). Similarly, the absence of Δ^{22}-sterols, except a trace in one uncertain case (*359, 363*), indicates that a 22-dehydrogenase is probably not present, as it apparently is, for instance, in some red algae. There is also no evidence for environmental differences in the sterol composition of the kind suggested by recent work with the red algae. Of the red, green, and brown algae, the latter seems to be phylogenetically the most homogeneous in terms of the sterols present.

c. Yellow-brown Algae (Pyrrhyophyta) This division includes the dinoflagellates, which are responsible for "red tides." Only the latter have been investigated. The toxic *Gonyaulax tamarensis*, which has caused serious problems on North Atlantic coasts, has been recently found (*368*) to contain essentially only cholesterol in the 4-desmethyl fraction, but the 4α-monomethyl fraction contained an even larger amount (150%) of the previously unknown $4\alpha,23,24\xi$-trimethyl-22-dehydro-5α-cholestanol (dinosterol). This sterol is related to gorgosterol and its 23-desmethyl derivative found in the gorgonian marine invertebrates. On the assumption that the 24-methyl group of dinosterol is β-oriented, as it is in gorgosterol, gorgosterol is the Δ^5-derivative of dinosterol lacking a 4α-methyl group and possessing a cyclopropyl bridge between C-22 and C-23. A reasonable biosynthetic pathway (in which CH_3^+ is derived from 5-adenosylmethionine) is shown in Scheme 10.9. While the reasonable precursor Δ^{22}-24β-methylsterol (brassicasterol) in the Δ^5-series co-occurs in gorgonians with gorgosterol, a sterol with such a side chain has not (yet?) been found in the dinoflaggelate. Interestingly, however, there is mass spectroscopic reason to believe (*368*) that dinosterol occurs in zooxanthella, which are algal symbionts with gorgonians and may be the source of gorgosterol.

d. Golden-brown and Yellow-green Algae and Diatoms (Chrysophyta) This division is divided botanically into three classes. The studied (*369, 370*) flagellate species, belonging to the genus *Ochromonas*, which are also considered to be photosynthetic protozoa, are golden-brown algae of the class Chrysophyceae. The yellow-green algae are of the class Xanthophyceae. Species in three orders have been studied (*371*): *Botrydium granulatum* (Heterosiphonales), *Tribonema aeguale* (Heterotrichales), and *Monodus subterraneus* (Heterococcales). The diatoms belong to the class Bacil-

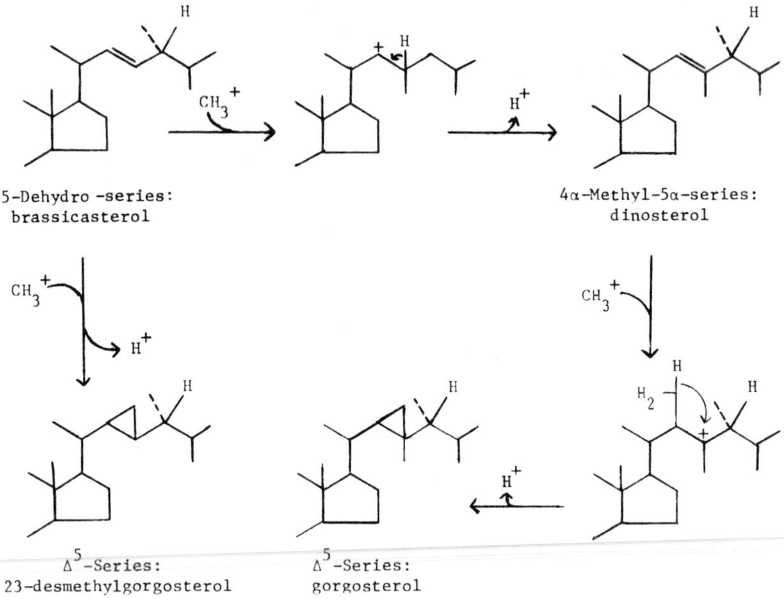

5-Dehydro -series:
brassicasterol

4α-Methyl-5α-series:
dinosterol

Δ⁵-Series:
23-desmethylgorgosterol

Δ⁵-Series:
gorgosterol

Scheme 10.9. Structures and possible biosynthetic relationships between dinoflaggelate and gorgonian sterols.

lariophyceae, and 12 species have been examined (*372–374*) in the genera *Nitzschia, Phaeodactylum, Navicula, Amphora, Biddulphia, Thallasiosira,* and *Fragilaria.* Except for some similarity in the photosynthetic pigments, these various algae are heterogeneous both by classic parameters and as seen in their sterol content. Although the dominant sterols in all cases possess a Δ^5-bond, the sterols of the three classes are quite different. All species (but one) contain principally 24-alkylsterols. Careful attention to C-24 has elucidated the configuration and shown it to be class-dependent. Cholesterol is present in some but not all species. Its relative amount varied enormously even within a single genus. Thus, it changes in the diatoms from 89% in *Nitzschia longissima,* through 11% in *N. ovalis,* to undetectable amounts in *N. alba.* In the Chrysophyceae it has not been found in the two phytoflaggelate (*Ochromonas*) species studied (*369, 370*), but it has been reported along with "sitosterol" in *Synura petersenii* (*375*). In the Xanthophyceae it is present and varies from 15 to 34% (*371*). The Xanthophyceae so far have the simplest and most uniform sterol composition, despite the variation just mentioned. The three investigated species (*371*) all contain only cholesterol and 24β-ethylcholesterol (clionasterol). Clionasterol, unfortunately, was identified as to configuration only by optical rotation, which is an uncertain parameter for contrasting it with sitosterol. The two *Ochromonas* species of Chrysophyceae are characterized

(369, 370) by having principally 22-$trans$-dehydroclionasterol (poriferasterol, distinguished readily from stigmasterol by melting point). In $O.$ $malhamensis$ it constitutes nearly 98% of the sterols present, while in $O.$ $danica$ it is accompanied by as much as 42% of other sterols, of which 24β-methylcholesterol (dihydrobrassicasterol), its 22-$trans$-dehydro-, and 7,22-$trans$-bisdehydroderivatives (brassicasterol and ergosterol) constitute half. The other half is composed of 7-dehydroporiferasterol and clionasterol in a 4:3 ratio. $O.$ $danica$ differs, therefore, from $O.$ $malhamensis$ in having substantial quantities of $\Delta^{5,7}$- (15%) and 24β-methylsterols (16%), as well as of sterols lacking the Δ^{22}-bond (15%). $Synura$ $petersenii$ (375) is quite different, as mentioned in a preceding sentence. Its "sitosterol" (which may well be clionasterol) in combination with cholesterol indicate that the alga (with Δ^5-24-H- and Δ^5-24ξ-ethylsterols) is more like the Xanthophyceae than the other two species of Chrysophyceae (which have $\Delta^{5,22}$-24β-ethylsterols and little or no Δ^5-24-H-sterol). The diatoms (Bacillariophyceae) are the most complex of the Chrysophyta, but this could be only a reflection of a greater number of species and genera having been examined. In half of the diatom species, a 24α-methylsterol is dominant (24α-methyl-22-$trans$-dehydrocholesterol, which we shall call diatomsterol). Diatomsterol (24-epibrassicasterol) is the main component in $Nitzschia$ $alba$ (90%), $N.$ $closterium$ (98%), $N.$ $ovalis$ (54%), $N.$ $frustulum$ (54%), $Navicula$ $pelleculosa$ (98%), and $Phaeodactylum$ $tricornatum$ (91%; a small form of $N.$ $closterium$). In another three species ($Biddulphia$ $aurita$, $Thallasiosira$ $pseudonana$, and $Fragilaria$ sp.), its 22-dihydroderivative,24α-methylcholesterol (campesterol), constitutes about 40%. One of these species ($B.$ $aurita$) also contains 21% of diatomsterol. Diatomsterol was identified as the α-epimer by Rubinstein and Goad (374) using PMR spectroscopy in the case of $Phaeodactylum$ $tricornatum$ (formerly known as $Nitzschia$ $closterium$ forma $minutissima$). However, some species, e.g., in the genus $Amphora$, can introduce a second C_1 group so as to make a 24-C_2-sterol dominant. Thus, in $Amphora$ $exiqua$, stigmasterol comprises 80% of the sterol mixture (373). The melting point of stigmasterol is about 15° higher than that of its epimer (poriferasterol), and it is on this basis that the configuration has been assigned (373). 24-Desalkylstigmasterol (22-dehydrocholesterol) constitutes most (17%) of the remaining sterol of $A.$ $exiqua$. This desalkylsterol also co-occurs with diatomsterol as a 33% component in $Nitzschia$ $ovalis$. The biosynthesis of the 24β-ethylsterols, clionasterol, and poriferasterol, in $Monodus$ and $Ochromonas$ genera, respectively, proceeds by the reduction of the 24-ethylidene group, since four H atoms from the methyl group of methionine are incorporated and since the 24-H atom is not lost (presumably having migrated to C-25) (375–377) and the references cited therein; see also Chapter 9). The pathway in $Monodus$ and $Ochromonas$ is known to proceed through cycloartenol (370, 371).

In summary, the dominant sterols of the Chrysophyta are a series comprised of cholesterol and 22-dehydrocholesterol together with their 24α- and 24β-alkyl (methyl and ethyl) derivatives. Of the 10 possibilities, only 24α-ethylcholesterol (in *S. petersenii*) has some question about it. The Chrysophyceae species (except perhaps for *S. petersenii*) are characterized by having 24β-ethylsterols, as may also the Xanthophyceae. The latter, however, seem both to lack the 22-dehydrogenase and to convert all of their 24-methylenesterol to the ethyl stage, while the former (except for *S. petersenii*, which resembles the Xanthophyceae) introduce a Δ^{22}-bond and reduce some of the 24-methylenesterol to the methyl stage. These two classes both generate their 24β-ethylsterol through the intermediacy of a 24-ethylidenesterol that is reduced directly. The class Bacillariophyceae is characterized by having in place of the 24β-alkylsterols, 24α-methyl- and 24α-ethylsterols. The respective Δ^{22}-derivatives, diatomsterol (24-epibrassicasterol) or stigmasterol, constitute more than 50% of the sterol mixture in two-thirds of the species examined in four of the seven genera, but they do not occur together in the same species. In the remaining three genera, campesterol is the major Δ^5-24α-alkylsterol. Cholesterol is present in most of the genera, becoming the dominant sterol in one diatom. Its 22-dehydroderivative, while not commonly an important constituent, is present at substantial levels (approximately 25%) in two diatoms. The relative amounts of the various sterols are highly varied from species to species, even within a single genus. Diatomsterol, for instance, which is dominant in many diatoms of the genera *Nitzschia, Navicula,* and *Phaeodactylum,* is completely absent not only in examined species of the genera *Thallasiosira, Amphora,* and *Fragilaria* but also in one species of *Nitzschia* as well. The Chrysophyta are related to the Rhodophyta, Phaeophyta, and Pyrrhyophyta in that the dominant 4-desmethylsterols of most species of these varied organisms possess a Δ^5-bond as well as by the fact that cholesterol has been found in amounts varying from traces to nearly 100% of the mixture in at least some species of all of the four divisions. Variations among the divisions are primarily in metabolism associated with the side chain, which is most pronounced and extensive in the Chrysophyta. Of these four divisions, only the Chrysophyta seem to have developed the operation of a reductase to the point where its action dominates the biosynthetic pathway, making 24-alkylsterols (by reduction of the alkyl group) the principal components of most of the species. In this respect (the presence of a reductase for the double bond derived from C_1 transfer) the Chrysophyta also resemble the Euglenophyta and Chlorophyta. The latter two divisions also contain primarily 24-alkylsterols, although they possess greater genetic variation in their metabolism of ring B. From a chemotaxonomic point of view, the individual sterols of the Chrysophyta could be used to distinguish the division from all others in the case of certain species, namely, those diatoms that contain diatomsterol which so far has not been found in any other plant whether algal or not. The other sterols of the Chrysophyta are quite common in one or another of the divisions. What really distinguishes the Chrysophyta is uniform completion of the Δ^5 pathway, coupled at the same time with highly variable metabolism of the side chain in terms of reduction versus alkylation of the $\Delta^{24(25)}$-bond, of the extent of alkylation, and of the configuration produced at C-24. In all of the other divisions, the kind and extent of side chain metabolism tends to be more uniform within the division or else there is not uniform completion of the Δ^5-pathway. Thus, the Rhodophyta usually do not alkylate C-24; the Phaeophyta usually carry out two C_1 transfers and do not reduce the consequent double bond; and the one Pyrrhyophyte examined only reduces the Δ^{24}-bond (except to give the specialized dinosterol). The one Euglenophyte examined operating in the green phase (for comparison with Chrysophyta) makes primarily Δ^7-sterols (roughly divided into equal amounts of 24-methyl and 24-ethyl components), and the Chlorophyta are highly variable both in the metabolism of the side chain and in ring B. The Chrysophyta are also the only algae known to possess both 24α- and 24β-ethylsterols. All other divisions appear at the present time to make only 24β-alkylsterols, if they have them at all.

   e. Euglenoids (Euglenaphyta) A number of algae are known that have little or no color (leucoforms) and hence lack photosynthetic ability. They have not been well studied biochemically except for one species among the Euglenaphyta (*Euglena gracilis*). This organism can operate either in a green, autotrophic, photosynthetic phase, or as a nonphotosynthetic, heterotrophic leucoform depending for its mode of existence in an interconvertible manner on the presence or absence of light. In the absence of light, not only are there no chloroplasts but, also, even protolasts are absent (*378, 379*), and the organism thus assumes certain characteristics of fungi. Interestingly, ergosterol, a common fungal sterol, was believed to be the principal sterol in both forms of *E. gracilis* (*380, 381*) as well as in *Astasis ocellata* and *Peranema trichophorum* (*369*). In a more recent and thorough study by Brandt et al. (*379*), however, ergosterol itself was not detected in *E. gracilis,* and $\Delta^{5,7}$-sterols (especially in the 24ξ-ethyl series) amounted to only a few percent of the mixture in either light or dark phases. Instead, Δ^5- and Δ^7-sterols with 24ξ-alkyl groups were found. In the green form, Δ^7-sterols accounted for 65% of the total (free, ester, and water-soluble) sterols and 98% of the free sterols, while in the leucoform only 5% of the total sterols and 47% of the free sterols were of the Δ^7-type. The remainder in all cases was composed of Δ^5-sterols, except for the 4% of $\Delta^{5,7}$-sterols already mentioned. In the green form, the free sterols were found to comprise 56% of the total sterols, but only 11% in the leucoform. The proportion of esters was the reverse: 1% in the green phase and 45% in the leucoform. About one-third of the sterols were water-soluble in both phases, and half or more of the water-soluble fraction was cholesterol, with 24ξ-ethylcholesterol as the other major component. In the green phase cholesterol was only 1% or less in the free condition and rose only 12% in the leucoform. In the green form the other free sterols were 24ξ-methyllathosterol (33%), 24ξ-methyl-22-*trans*-dehydrolathosterol (18%), 24ξ-ethyllathosterol (12%), and 24ξ-ethyl-22-*trans*-dehydrolathosterol (35%). In the leucoform the 24ξ-methyllathosterol and its 22-dehydro-derivative remained (30%), but their 24ξ-ethyl homologs nearly disappeared and were replaced by the Δ^5-analogs, 24ξ-ethylcholesterol, and 24ξ-ethyl-22-dehydrocholesterol. The ester and water-soluble sterols were always the Δ^5-sterols with 2–8% of $\Delta^{5,7}$-sterols. Brandt et al. (*379*) imply through the use of nomenclature (such as referring to chondrillasterol) that the configuration at C-24 was determined, but careful reading of the paper reveals that the β-configuration was only assumed. It would be most instructive to know what the configurations really are, since after Brandt et al. completed their work the existence of 24α-alkylsterols in algae was demonstrated in the case of diatoms. Biosynthesis of free, ester, and water-soluble forms of the sterols has been achieved in both green and white phases of *E. gracilis* from acetate (*379*), and in both phases squalene oxide leads to cycloartenol rather than to lanosterol (*382*).

In summary, based on the extensive examination of *E. gracilis* strain Z (*379, 382*), the Euglenaphyta biosynthesize sterols and do so through the cycloartenol route in both photosynthetic and nonphotosynthetic phases. 24ξ-Methyl- and ethylsterols with and without a Δ^{22}-bond are dominant in both phases, but 24-H-sterols (principally cholesterol) are present in small amounts. In the light phase, two-thirds of the sterols are of the Δ^7-type, the remainder being primarily Δ^5-sterols, but in the absence of light Δ^5-sterols become the major component and the percentage of 22-dehydrosterols decreases. There is also a shift in the proportion of free and bound sterols induced by light. In the green phase most of the sterols are free, but they are mostly bound in the leucoform. The reasons for these compositional shifts are obscure. There is also some conflict in the literature about the presence of ergosterol in euglenoids.

f. Green Algae (Chlorophyta) and the Charophyta   The green algae of all the algal divisions are believed to be closest to the higher plants and to occupy a central phylogenetic position (*383*). The precise relationships, of course, remain to be elucidated. Among the parameters that will have to be considered are the sterols and the biosynthetic pathways to them in these organisms. In recent years the details of this have been examined in some depth, especially by Patterson. For earlier reviews and a key to the literature see Nes (*384*), Patterson (*367*), and Miller (*366*).

A variety of orders (Chlorococcales, Ultrichales, Ulvales, Cladophorales, Oedogoniales, and Zygnematales) had been investigated in the laboratories of Bergmann (*385*), Heibron (*346, 347*), and others during the period 1935–1955. These investigators thought ergosterol, chondrillasterol, and perhaps zymosterol were present in the first-mentioned order, and sitosterol and perhaps fucosterol in the others, except that surprisingly none were found (*347*) in *Trentepohlia aurea* in the order Ultrichales (Chaetophorales). While ergosterol and chondrillasterol have been confirmed (*386, 387*) as the major sterols of some species, sitosterol and fucosterol probably do not occur in green algae. In every case for which good data are available, the green algal sterols are found to have 24β-alkylsterols rather than the α-epimers, despite recent assumptions to the contrary. Among the genera for which unequivocal melting point or PMR data are available are *Spirogyra* (Zygnematales), *Halimeda* and *Codium* (Siphonales), and *Chlorella* (Chlorococcales) (*388–391* and Nes and Patterson, unpublished observations). No difference in the configuration has been observed between 24-methyl- and ethylsterols, both having β-oriented alkyl groups. The phylogenetic, ecological, and functional significance of this configuration, however, warrants continued study of the epimeric question. Similarly, in those cases (*Nitella, Ulva, Enteromorpha, Chlorella,* and *Scenedesmus*) where 24-ethylidenesterols have been carefully examined, the configuration about the $\Delta^{24(28)}$-bond has been proven to be exclusively *trans* (*388, 392, 393*). In the Δ^5-series the compound is isofucosterol (also known as Δ^5-avenasterol) rather than fucosterol, and in the Δ^7-series it would be Δ^7-avenasterol (although not yet found in green algae) rather than its *cis*-isomer, which has no name, since it is not known to occur in either algae or higher plants.

The sterols of the green algae are the homologous series of 24-H-, 24β-methyl-, and 24β-ethylsterols with or without a Δ^{22}-bond in the Δ^7-, $\Delta^{5,7}$-, and Δ^7-series and/or on occasion the $\Delta^{25(27)}$-derivatives. This large array, however, does not generally occur together in the same species. In fact, the green algae are notable for having relatively well-defined species characteristics in their sterol compositions that are not necessarily dependent on presently used taxonomic classifications. Even two cell lines of the same "species" can be very different. A notable example is in the genus *Chlorella*. *C. ellipsoidea*, Gerneck, Indiana Culture Collection No. 246, is of a darker green color, foams less in culture, and grows faster than *C. ellipsoidea*, Gerneck, Indiana Culture Collection No. 247 (*394*). The sterol mixture of cells No. 246 is composed of ergosterol (35%), its $\Delta^{5,8(9),22}$-isomer (33%), 24β-methyllathosterol (17%, fungisterol), 24β-methyl-8(9)-dehydrocholesterol (10%), 5-dihydroergosterol (2%), two unidentified sterols (1%), and traces of 22-dihydroergosterol (*394*). Cells No. 247 contain 24β-ethyl-22-dehydrocholesterol (61%, poriferasterol), 24β-methylcholesterol (31%, dihydrobrassicasterol), 24β-ethylcholesterol (6%, clinasterol), cholesterol (1%), and 24β-methyl-22-dehydrocholesterol (1%, brassicasterol) (*395*). The two cell lines obviously differ in their ability to reduce the Δ^7-bond and introduce a second C_1 group. Cell line No. 246 can do neither. It also has a partial kinetic block in the introduction of the Δ^5-bond, a partial deficiency in the Δ^8- to Δ^7-conversion, and a very active $\Delta^{24(28)}$-reductase at the 24-C_1 stage. The result is a mixture primarily composed of 24β-methylsterols with two double bonds in ring B. Cell line No. 247, by contrast, has both an efficient Δ^7-reductase and second C_1-transferase and has well-developed kinetic control of the other steps in ring B, leading completely to Δ^5-sterols, most of which bear the 24β-ethyl group. These divergent cell lines perhaps should be reclassified into separate species, but the species problem evident here is reflected also at the genus level, again especially well demonstrated in the genus *Chlorella*. There are species in this genus that have only Δ^7-sterols, a larger number with only $\Delta^{5,7}$-sterols, and a still larger group with only Δ^5-sterols. To compound the taxonomic and phylogenetic problem, there are species in different genera with essentially the same sterol mixture, as in the *Cladophora* and *Pithophora* genera, and genera in two different orders, e.g., in the Chlorosphaerales and Chlorococcales, in which the sterol composition is only quantitatively different.

Chlorella fusca (*388*), C. vulgaris (*387, 396*), C. emersonii (*367*), C. glucotropha (*367*), C. miniata (*367*), Scenedesmus obliquus (*387, 397*), and Oocystis polymorpha (*398*), all (with the exception of the report of 0.4% cholesterol in O. polymorpha) contain only Δ^7-sterols. Most (approximately 80%) of the mixture is composed of 24β-ethyllathosterol and its 22-*trans*-dehydroderivative (chondrillasterol). The remainder consists of the corresponding 24β-methylsterols (fungisterol and 5-dihydroergosterol, respectively). The Δ^{22}-sterol at the 24-C_2 level (chondrillasterol) is present in greatest amount (approximately two-thirds) and at the 24-C_1 level the least, to the extent of having not been found at all in some cases. The report (*399*) of spinasterol in *Hydrodictyon reticulatum* (Chlorococcales) presumably means the sterol was chondrillasterol and adds an eighth species to the list of those with Δ^7-sterols. Six species of *Chlorella* viz., *simplex* (*386*), *ellipsoidea* (*394*), *nocturna* (*386*), *sorokiniana* (*386*), *vannilii* (*386*), and *candida* (*386*) have $\Delta^{5,7}$-sterols composed in most cases primarily of ergosterol (70%) and its 22-dihydroderivative (12%, 24β-methyl-7-dehydrocholesterol). In one case (*C. ellipsoidea—246*) ergosterol is only 35%, and the remainder is composed of sterols described in the preceding paragraph. A seventh species (*C. pyrenoidosa*) is reported in the older literature (*385*) to contain ergosterol. *Chlamydomonas rheinhardi* in the order Volvocales also has only $\Delta^{5,7}$-sterols but includes the 24-C_2 level of alkylation (ergosterol and 7-dehydroporiferasterol, amounting to 44% and 56%, respectively).

The algae known to contain Δ^5-sterols are more numerous. They also have greater variety in the side chain. The order Ulvales is so far the simplest, with no 24-methyl- or 24-ethylsterols. Two species (*Enteromorpha intestinales* and *Ulva lactura*) contain only isofucosterol, and in one (*E. linza*) it is the major sterol (*360, 393*). However, in *U. pertussa* Kjellman (Anaaosa), isofucosterol is only a 15% component, its 24-C_1 analog (ostreasterol) a 3% component, and cholesterol the major (74%) sterol, with 8% unidentified (*360*). The next most uniform are the two studied species of Siphonales. Both contain 94% of a Δ^5-24β-ethylsterol; in *Halimeda incrassata* 24β-

ethylcholesterol (clinoasterol) itself occurs as the major component, along with 4% of 24β-methylcholesterol (dihydrobrassicasterol) and 2% of cholesterol (*388*), while in *Codium fragile* the major sterol is 25(27)-dehydroclionasterol (clerosterol named for its first isolation from a Tracheophyte of the *Clerodendrum* genus) and the minor sterol (6%) is 24β-methyl-25(27)-dehydrocholesterol (codisterol) (*389*). The one examined (*388*) species of Chlorosphaerales (*Cocomyxa elongata*) is similar to *H. incrassata* in that 24β-ethyl- and 24β-methylsterols are present, but in *C. elongata* the ethyl component is divided into clionasterol (33%) and its 22-dehydroderivative (19%, poriferasterol), and the dihydrobrassicasterol is increased in amount to 48%, with no cholesterol detected. The species of Chlorococcales (*Chlorella ellipsoidea*—247, *C. saccharophilia*, and *C. pringsheimii*) that have Δ^5-sterols (*388, 395, 396*) are almost the same in their composition as the Chlorosphaerales. In all three *Chlorella* species, poriferasterol, clionasterol, and dihydrobrassicasterol occur, as they do in the Chlorosphaerales, but in the Chlorococcales species poriferasterol is the major component (approximately two-thirds), dihydrobrassicasterol is next in amount (one-quarter), and clionasterol is least (a few percent). From *C. ellipsoidea*—247 1% each of cholesterol and brassicasterol have also been isolated. In one species of Zygenematales belonging to the genus *Spyrogyra*, cholesterol and its 24β-methyl and ethyl homologs along with their Δ^{22}-derivaties are also all present in amounts, respectively, of 11%, 12%, 39%, 6%, and 32% (*388*). It differs from *C. ellipsoidea*—247 only in the relative amounts of the sterols present, and even in that not drastically. The two investigated (*388*) species of Cladophorales (*Cladophora flexnosa* and *Pithophora* sp.) have the largest array of sterols. Not only are cholesterol and its two homologs present together with the latter's Δ^{22}-derivatives, but 24-methylenecholesterol (ostreasterol) and isofucosterol occur. The two $\Delta^{24(28)}$-sterols are in fact dominant, comprising 54–66% of the mixtures, with cholsterol (22–28%), clionasterol (6–10%), poriferasterol (2%), brassicasterol (1–2%), and dihydrobrassicasterol (0–2%) following in lesser amounts. A Japanese marine alga (*Chaetomorpha crassa*) is also reported (*360*) to contain 13% of ostreasterol, and cholesterol (31%) and its 24ξ-methyl- (10%) and ethyl (40%) homologs, along with 24ξ-methyl-22-dehydrocholesterol.

Two species (*Nitella flexilis* and *Chara vulgaris*) belonging to the order Charales have been investigated (*392*). Both are identical to each other in composition and contain 36% of isofucosterol and 58% of clionasterol. This order is frequently assigned to the Chlorophyta, but some phycologists (*383*) place it in a separate division, the Charophyta.

Biosynthesis of sterols occurs in all examined cases. Especially important conclusions have derived from the use of the inhibitors AY-9944 (*400–401*) (which inhibits the Δ^8-to Δ^7-isomerase and the Δ^7-reductase) and the more broadly based triparanol (*402, 403*) (which inhibits the Δ^8- to Δ^7-isomerase, the Δ^7-reductase, the second C_1-transferase, and the mixed-function oxidase that oxidizes the 14α-methyl group before its removal). The more significant facts are as follows. From inhibited cultures, cycloartenol, cyclolaudenol, 24-methylenecycloartanol, and pollinastanol, but not lanosterol, are isolable. Both cycloartenol and lanosterol are efficiently used when presented to *Chlorella* species (*404*), and both give the naturally occurring 4-desmethyl mixture in uninhibited cultures. In the same genus 24β-methylcholesta-8,14-dien-3β-ol (identifiable in inhibited cultures) and $14\alpha,24\beta$-dimethylcholesta-8-en-3β-ol yield (*395*) 24β-methylcholesterol, but not its 22-dehydroderivative, despite the fact that both of the latter two sterols naturally occur in the species used (*C. ellipsoidea*—247). In *Trebouxia*, 24-methylenesterols fail to yield 24-methylsterols, and 24-ethylidenesterols do not lead to 24-ethylsterols (*405*). Similar results were found with several species of *Chlorella* (*406–408*), but not with all. *Chlorella ellipsoidea*— 247 will reduce fucosterol to 24ξ-ethylcholesterol, which does not proceed to the naturally occurring 24β-ethyl-22-dehydrocholesterol, and 24-methylenecholesterol undergoes a second C_1 transfer but little or no $\Delta^{24(28)}$-reduction (*404, 409*). 24β-Methylsterols do not yield 24β-ethylsterols and 24β-dihydrolanosterol gives cholesterol but not C_{28}- or C_{29}-sterols in *C. ellipsoidea*—247 (*410*). 24β-Methyl and 24β-ethylsterols of *Trebouxia* species arise through the intermediacy of $\Delta^{25(27)}$-sterols that are reduced at the 25(27)-bond (*411, 412*). All five of the H atoms in the 24-ethyl group of poriferasterol in *Chlorella* are derived from the methyl group of methionine (*406*). This precludes the intermediacy of a 24-ethylidenesterol.

The biosynthetic information, coupled with knowledge of the structures that occur, can be interpreted in the following way. The $\Delta^{24(25)}$-bond can be either alkylated or reduced but not introduced. Reduction occurs to the greatest extent in the Cladophorales and Zygnematales, where cholesterol amounts to 11–28% of the mixture, and in *Chaetomorpha crassa*, where it is reported as a 70% component. Except for *C. crassa*, which is unique, all other species primarily alkylate the $\Delta^{24(25)}$-bond. This can happen immediately after cyclization to cycloartenol to give 24-methylenecycloartanol. Alkylation also occurs, at least in *Codium fragile*, *Trebouxia* sp., and *Chlorella sorokiniana*, to give $\Delta^{25(27)}$-24β-methylsterols. Since cyclolaudenol is isolable from triparanol-treated cultures of *C. sorokiniana*, the $\Delta^{25(27)}$-route of alkylation also can happen immediately after cyclization. A third route, 24β-C_1 transfer with concomitant introduction of a Δ^{22}-bond, probably occurs to give Δ^{22}-24β-methylsterols, such as brassicasterol, in, at least, *Chlorella ellipsoidea*—247, since brassicasterol does not arise from its 22-dihydroderivative. The pathway following cyclization and the first C_1 transfer proceeds through $\Delta^{8,14}$-, to Δ^8-sterols, which sequentially give $\Delta^{5,8}$-, $\Delta^{5,7}$-, and Δ^5-sterol. At some stage the $\Delta^{24(28)}$-bond of the 24-methylenesterol undergoes a second C_1 transfer. The same three mechanisms described for the first C_1 transfer are possible and probably will occur. The sterols bearing a 24-*trans*-ethylidene group in Cladophorales, Ulvales, and Charales must arise directly with concomitant $\Delta^{24(28)}$-introduction. In one species (*Trebouxia* sp.) of Chlorococcales and one (*Codium fragile*) of the two studied species of Siphonales, the second C_1 transfer occurs with introduction of a $\Delta^{25(27)}$-bond. The Δ^{22}-route of alkylation is probably the process by which the Δ^{22}-24β-ethyl structure of poriferasterol arises in *Chorella*, as it is for the Δ^{22}-24β-methyl structure of brassicasterol. Indeed, because there is no evidence for the existence of a Δ^{22}-dehydrogenase and because there is actually evidence against it at both 24-C_1 and 24-C_2 levels, all of the Δ^{22}-sterols in Chlorophyta probably arise by this route. The absence of Δ^{22}-sterols in a given alga is then interpretable not as the selected absence of a dehydrogenase in the given species compared to one with Δ^{22}-sterols, but rather as difference in the alkylation route. Further examples would be Siphonales, in which the $\Delta^{25(27)}$-route is known to operate and no Δ^{22}-sterols occur, and Ulvales and Charales, where the $\Delta^{24(28)}$-route clearly occurs from the presence of 24-ethylidenecholesterol (isofucosterol), but again no Δ^{22}-sterols are present, even though in Charales 24β-ethylcholesterol (clionasterol) occurs together with the isofucosterol. The clionasterol may be derived from the isofucosterol (or related $\Delta^{24(28)}$-sterol) by reduction, but further assessment will have to await studies with methionine. An alternative would be that it arises by the $\Delta^{25(27)}$-route. At the moment, though, the presence of the $\Delta^{24(28)}$-reductase in *Chlorella* speaks for a $\Delta^{24(28)}$-origin of clionasterol, at least in this organism.

A simplifying assumption can be made that obviously, however, requires further experimental examination. Let us assume that all 24β-ethylsterols lacking a Δ^{22}-bond arise through alkylation with $\Delta^{24(28)}$-introduction ("$\Delta^{24(28)}$-alkylation") except in the order Siphonales (where "$\Delta^{25(27)}$-alkylation" occurs), that all 24β-methylsterols lacking a Δ^{22}-bond arise through alkylation with $\Delta^{25(27)}$-introduction ("$\Delta^{25(27)}$-alkylation"), and that all Δ^{22}-sterols arise by alkylation with Δ^{22}-introduction ("Δ^{22}-alkylation"). We can now understand most of the known data. Ulvales and Charales must possess primarily or only the "$\Delta^{24(28)}$-alkylation," which is kinetically completed to the 24-C_2 stage, and Ulvales must lack, and Charales have partially, a $\Delta^{24(28)}$-reductase. Similarly, Siphonales must have only the "$\Delta^{25(27)}$-alkylation," and *Halimeda* would have, and *Codium* would not have, a $\Delta^{25(27)}$-reductase. The various Chlorococcales species would have, depending on the species, all of the mechanisms, as they do for all the choices for metabolism of ring B. The similarity of the sterol content of the Chlorosphaerales and Zygnematales of the Δ^5-containing Chlorococcales suggests their mechanisms of alkylation to be similar. This would include a "Δ^{22}-alkylation" at the 24-C_1 and 24-C_2 levels, a "$\Delta^{24(28)}$-alkylation" for 24β-ethylsterols, and a "$\Delta^{25(27)}$-alkylation" for 24β-methylsterols. Among the $\Delta^{5,7}$-sterol-containing species, *Chlamydomonas* would have only the "Δ^{22}-alkylation" at the 24-C_2 level, and both "Δ^{22}-alkylation" and "$\Delta^{24(28)}$-alkylation" at the 24-C_1 level. This species has only Δ^{22}-sterols, but its 24-ethylsterols must arise from a

24-methylenesterol. On the other hand, *Chlorella ellipsoidea*—246 contains only 24β-methylsterols with and without a Δ^{22}-bond. It must follow both "Δ^{22}- and $\Delta^{25(27)}$-alkylation," as do other *Chlorella* species. The Δ^7-sterol-containing algae would also have both "Δ^{22}- and $\Delta^{25(27)}$-alkylation," with the former predominating at the 24-C_2 level, and with the latter predominating at the 24-C_1 level. Again, "$\Delta^{24(28)}$-alkylation" must also occur at the 24-C_1 level to allow a second C_1 transfer. Since all but two species of Chlorophyta and Charophyta have principally 24-C_2-sterols, "$\Delta^{24(28)}$-alkylation" at the 24-C_1 level is the major route of metabolism of the Δ^{24}-bond.

In summary, the sterols of some six orders of Chlorophyta and one order of Charophyta arise through cycloartenol and comprise a set of 24-H-, 24-methylene-, 24-*trans*-ethylidene-, 24β-methyl-, and 24β-ethyl-, Δ^{22}-24β-methyl-, and Δ^{22}-24β-ethylsterols in the Δ^7-, $\Delta^{5,7}$-, and Δ^5-series. There is a strong species dependence on which of these sterols are present in consequential amounts, especially with regard to unsaturation in ring B. It seems that the algae are Δ^7-, $\Delta^{5,7}$- or Δ^5-producers, without mixing the series in a given species. This indicates the existence of substantial differences in the genes for the Δ^5-dehydrogenase and Δ^7-reductase. Both appear to be absent or unexpressed, yielding Δ^7-sterols in five species of the genera *Chlorella* and in one known species each in *Scenedesmus, Oocystis,* and *Hydrodictyon* of the order Chlorococcales, while both are present in seventeen of the other 29 or so examined species giving only Δ^5-sterols. In seven *Chlorella* and one *Chlamydomonas* species, all in the orders Chlorococcales and Volvocales, the Δ^7-reductase is deficient, yielding $\Delta^{5,7}$-sterols. The order Chlorococcales has, so far, the largest number of species that seem either to have lost or never had enzymes to complete the Δ^5-pathway. Another peculiarity at the order level is in Ulvales. The four examined species all possess only $\Delta^{24(28)}$-sterols of the 24-C_1, or 24-C_2 types and appear, as in the case of brown algae, to lack a $\Delta^{24(28)}$-reductase. They differ from the brown algae, however, in the stereochemical manner by which they introduce the second C_1 group. In the green algae the configuration about the $\Delta^{24(28)}$-bond is *trans*, in contrast to *cis* in the brown algae. Also, unlike other algae, there are unquestionably two, and perhaps three, mechanisms of introduction of alkyl groups at C-24 operative in Chlorophyta. They differ by the position ($\Delta^{24(28)}$, $\Delta^{25(27)}$, and Δ^{22}) of the double bond that results. The Charophyta seem to be similar to the Chlorophyta in that they contain 24-*trans*-ethylidene- and 24β-ethylsterols. Differences in side chain metabolism can be associated with taxonomic classifications and explained at mechanistic and enzymatic levels but only to a limited and tentative extent. Substantial uncertainties exist that will require more experimental work to resolve.

3. Lichens

Two different organisms (an alga and a fungus) living together symbiotically give what is known as a lichen. The algal component is called a phycobiont and the fungus a mycobiont. In some cases it has been possible to separate the two, culture them individually, and then recombine them to reestablish the lichen (*413, 414*). This would lead one to expect a lichen to possess both algal and fungal steroids, and such is the case. Commonly lichens are composed of a green alga (Chlorophyta) and an Ascomycete. The latter usually contains 24β-methylsterols dominated by ergosterol. The former have a much more complex mixture that is species-dependent, but 24β-ethylsterols frequently are present. The earlier literature reports the presence of "ergosterol" in rough agreement with expectation. A more precise recent study (*415, 416a*) of the common foliose lichen *Xanthoria parietina*, composed of the algae *Trebouxia decolorans* and a fungus with the same name as the lichen,found it to contain primarily poriferasterol, ergosterol, and the latter's $\Delta^{5,8,22}$-isomer (lichesterol). Separate culture of the phycobiont yielded poriferasterol with smaller amounts of clionasterol, brassicasterol, 24β-methylcholesterol, and cholesterol itself. The mycobiont, on separate culture, proved to contain the ergosterol and lichesterol found in the lichen together with smaller amounts of $\Delta^{7,22}$-, $\Delta^{7,22,24(28)}$-, and $\Delta^{7,24(28)}$-24β-methylsterols (5-dihydroergosterol, 22-dehydroavenasterol, and avenasterol, respectively). In another recent study (*416b*) the lichens *Lobaria pulmonaria*, *Lobaria scrobiculata*, and *Usnea longissima* yielded principally ergosterol, episterol, fecosterol, and lichesterol, with minor amounts of C_{27}-, C_{28}-, and C_{29}-sterols with one and two double bonds.

E. MORE ADVANCED PHOTOSYNTHETIC ORGANISMS

1. Bryophyta

The Bryophyta are constituted by the classes Anthocerotae (hornworts), Hepaticae (liverworts), and Musci (mosses) with one, three, and five genera, respectively. Some are aquatic, although none is marine. In general, they are more adapted to terrestrial life than are the algae. Bryophytes, some of which have structures superficially resembling roots, stems, and leaves, lack real vascular structures and tend to be an intermediate form between the algae and truly vascular plants. They differ from the latter (Tracheophyta) not only in the development of vascularization but also in the relationship between the gametophytic and sporaphytic generations. With the exception of the hornworts, where partial independence of the sporophyte occurs, the gametophyte is the observable green plant, and the essentially colorless sporophyte lives more or less parasitically with it. In sexual reproduction the sperm requires water to swim to the egg. Bryophytes are poorly studied in relation to their steroids. Part of the reason is difficulty in obtaining large amounts of pure samples. Owing to the lack of vascularization and reproductive habit, the organisms are small, forming dense growths in shady, cool places to hold moisture, and the resultant vegetation is usually strongly mixed with bacteria, algae, fungi, and invertebrate animals (worms, insects, snails, etc.). Only *Sphagnum* and other mosses appear to have been examined (*417–419*). The reported sterols are 24ξ-methyl- and 24ξ-ethylcholesterol. Unidentified sterols occur as esters in sporophytes of the liverwort *Lophocolea heterophylla* (*420*). In view of the biologically intermediate status of the Bryophyta, more extensive study (configuration, alkylation mechanisms, etc.) would certainly be of value.

2. Tracheophyta

The division (or phylum) Tracheophyta includes highly diverse plants that are grouped together by the presence in varying degrees of sophistication of a vascular system that allows them to transport water, nutrients, and metabolic products throughout the organism. This in turn permits the existence of a large organism with a great deal of cellular differentiation. In the very old subphylum Psilopsida, represented today by only two genera, there are no true roots, and in the subphylum Lycopsida, also ancient, with only four extant genera, true roots are present but not always well developed. In all the other groups of Tracheophytes, sophisticated vascularization of the underground parts occurs, giving a real root. This is important, because the observable morphological characteristics of a root allow efficient assimilation and transport of water and dissolved substances. In the Tracheophytes, especially those with roots, we see a number of other developments, among which are specialization of photosynthetic tissue to give a leaf and an evolution in various reproductive aspects. The sporophyte is the dominant "generation," and in all but a few cases, e.g., the beautiful Indian pipes seen in moist forests, it is photosynthetic. Considerable variation exists among and within the subphyla in the way the gametes are formed and protected as well as in the manner of union and subsequent development of the zygote. In the seed plants, the embryonic sporophyte is encapsulated for protection and provided with food before it is released into the environment. The structures in the parent that are responsible for this and related phenomena and the degree to which protection is provided serve taxonomically to distinguish the gymnosperms ("naked seeds") and angiosperms. The latter produce a flower, and the seed develops within an ovary that is derived from a leaf-like structure known as a carpel. In the gymnosperm, the carpel has not metamorphosed into an ovary, and the seed develops on its surface in a more exposed position.

Despite a great deal of interest in Tracheophyte sterols over many years and despite both the variety of the plants and the ease with which they can be collected, our knowledge of the relationship between sterol structure and occurrence has only recently become sophisticated. All the plants studied have sterols that are unsaturated in ring B, and in some cases, e.g., *Calendula officinalis* (*421*) and *Zea mays* (*524*), stanols are present as trace components. From many, e.g., seeds from *Pisum sativum* (peas) (*422*) as well as from carrots and tomatoes (*423*), *Aster scaber* (*424*), eggplant (*Solanum melongeana*), and avocado (*Persea gratissima*) (*425*), squalene has also been obtained. Its isolation from peas constituted its discovery in photosynthetic organisms and, together with its biosynthesis (*422, 423*) and with the conversion of mevalonate to sitosterol (*426*), opened the field of Tracheophytes to the same kind of biosynthetic investigation as had previously been done in animals and in yeast.

As early as 1906, Windaus and Hauth (*427*) isolated stigmasterol from the Calabar bean. This sterol, named for the genus of plant (*Physostigma venenosum*) from which it was obtained, was the first tracheophyte sterol known. Consequently, it has attracted much attention. In addition, it possesses a Δ^{22}-bond that allows degradation of the side chain. The insolubility of its tetrabromide and existence of simple ways to regenerate the dienic sterol made it easy to be isolated in a pure condition. It therefore had a prominent place in early structural work of plant sterols and their correlation with animal sterols. However, despite assumptions to the contrary, it is only rarely the major sterol, as in banana peel (*428*) and ivy (*429*), and usually is either absent or found only in a small amount. For instance, in an analysis of vegetable oils from 19 nuts and seeds (walnut, pecan, cashew, pistacchio, pine, almond, Sal fat, Japan wax, Tohaku oil, Chaulmoogra oil, Perilla oil, Tung oil, Akamegashiwa oil, hemp seed, mustard, Illipe butter, poppy seed, Capsicum, and Fugara) containing Δ^5-sterols, Jeong et al. (*430*) found only one (Tung oil) in which stigmasterol exceeded 24-methylcholesterol in amount. Stigmasterol was found to constitute, on the average, only 7%, varying from traces to 18% of the mixture. Sitosterol, the major sterol, varied from 45% to 91% (average 67%), and 24-methylcholesterol from 4% to 28% (average 14%). Cholesterol varied from traces to 9%. Examination of many more seeds containing Δ^5-sterols in several laboratories (*430–436*) reveals the same sort of values. The average value for stigmasterol was only 8%, with a range from none or traces to 26%. The major component (sitosterol) had an average value of 64%, ranging from 38% to 93%; 24-methylcholesterol, ranging from 2% to 30%, had an average of 16%; and cholesterol varied from trace amounts to 3%, except in several cases in the Cruciferae, e.g., *Cheiranthus cheri,* where it was 12–15%. Stigmasterol is absent in most of the Cruciferae, and cholesterol and its 24-methyl and ethyl homologs are always present. In many but not all Cruciferae species, especially of the genus *Brassica*, brassicasterol is present. Knights and Berrie (*432*) have made an extensive study of this family. In still other studies involving various plants and plant parts (Tables 10.9 and 10.10), much the same results have been found. On the other hand, in plants primarily containing Δ^7-sterols, the Δ^{22}-compounds are frequently in large amount, and spinasterol, in contrast to its Δ^5-analog, is quite often a major sterol (Table 10.11).

Sitosterol (24α-ethylcholesterol) was first isolated in 1926 from wheat germ oil by Anderson et al. (*464*) and named accordingly (Greek "sito"

Table 10.9. Some plants of category I-A[a]

Family	Genus and Species	Part	Dominant Sterols[b]	Ref.
Lycopsidaceae	*Lycopodium complanatum*[c]	Fronds and stems	Sitosterol (40) Ergosterol (21) Stigmasterol (17) Epiergosterol (11) Dihydrobrassicasterol (9) Campesterol (2)	437 438
Polypodiaceae	*Dryopteris noveboracensis* (*Thelypteris*) (*New York fern*)	Fronds	Sitosterol (69) Campesterol (8) Dihydrobrassicasterol (5) Cholesterol (8) Dihydrospinasterol (5) Lathosterol (4) 24ξ-Methyllathosterol (ca. 1)	437
Polypodiaceae	*Polystichum acrostichoides* (Christmas fern)	Fronds	Sitosterol (72) Campesterol (9) Dihydrobrassicasterol (4) Cholesterol (8) 24α-Ethyllathosterol (?) (7)	437
Polypodiaceae	*Dennstaedtia punctilobula* (hay-scented fern)	Fronds	Sitosterol Campesterol Dihydrobrassicasterol	437
Osmundaceae	*Osmunda cinnamomea* (cinnamon fern)	Fronds	Sitosterol Campesterol Dihydrobrassicasterol	437
Ginkgoaceae	*Ginkgo biloba*	Leaves (male)	Sitosterol Campesterol Dihydrobrassicasterol	437 439

			Cholesterol Other (traces)	
Pinaceae	*Pinus pinea* (stone pine)	Embryo same as endosperm	Sitosterol Campesterol Dihydrobrassicasterol	437
Magnoliaceae	*Liriodendron tulipifera* (tulip tree)	Leaves	Sitosterol (ca. 90) Stigmasterol Campesterol Dihydrobrassicasterol	440
Podophyllaceae (Berberidaceae)	*Podophyllum peltatum* (May apple)	Leaves	Sitosterol (80) Stigmasterol (11) Other (9)	440
Ericaceae	*Kalmia latifolia* (laurel)	Leaves	Sitosterol	437
Leguminosae	*Pisum sativum* (pea)	Embryo	Sitosterol Stigmasterol Campesterol Dihydrobrassicasterol	440
Leguminosae	*Glycine max* (soybean)	Embryo	Sitosterol (53) Stigmasterol (19) Campesterol (14) Dihydrobrassicasterol (ca. 6) Isofucosterol (3) Dihydrospinasterol (3) Avenasterol (1) Cholesterol (<0.5)	431, 440
Musaceae	*Musa sapientum* (banana)	Peel	Stigmasterol (92) 24ξ-Ethylcholesterol (6) 24ξ-Methylcholesterol (2)	428

Continued

Table 10.9. *Continued.*

Family	Genus and Species	Part	Dominant Sterols[b]	Ref.
Cruciferae	*Brassica oleracea* (cabbage)	Leaf	Sitosterol (69) Campesterol (20) Dihydrobrassicasterol (10) Cholesterol (1)	440
Surianaceae	*Suriana maritima*	Whole	Sitosterol	441
Euphorbiaceae	*Euphorbia polygonifolia*	Aerial parts	Sitosterol	442
Compositae	*Calendula officinalis*	Flowers	Sitosterol 24ξ-Methylcholesterol (<5%) Dihydrospinasterol 24ξ-Methyllathosterol	421
Gramineae	*Hordeum vulgare* (barley)		Sitosterol 24ξ-Methylcholesterol	443
Solanaceae	*Nicotiana tabacum* (tobacco)		Stigmasterol Others	444
Solanaceae	*Dioscorea xanthocarpum*		Sitosterol Others	445

| Solanaceae | Dioscorea tokoro | Stigmasterol Others | 444 |

| Solanaceae | Withania somnifera | Isofucosterol (37)
 24ξ-Methylcholesterol (26)
 Sitosterol (19) (α-orientation presumed from ethylidenesterol's presence)
 Stigmasterol (9) (α-orientation presumed from presence of ethylidenesterol as well as from Δ^{22})
 24-Methyldesmosterol (7)
 24-Ethyldesmosterol (?) (1) | 446 |

[a] Category I refers to plants with 24α-alkylsterols in greater amount than 24β-alkylsterols. In all cases studied of plants of this category, a 24-α-ethylsterol is the major single component and is not contaminated with its 24-epimer. Category A refers to plants with sterols bearing primarily or exclusively the Δ^5-bond. The plants included are those for which the sterols have been examined configurationally by NMR (*Lycopodium*, the four ferns following it, *Ginkgo*, *Pinus*, *Liriodendron*, *Podophyllum*, *Kalmia*, *Pisum*, and *Glycine*), by m.p. stigmasterol or of sitosteryl acetate (*Suriana*, *Euphorbia*, *Dioscorea xanthocarpum*, and *rice*) or are known to lose the 24-H atom of cycloartenol (*Hordeum*, *Pinus*, *Calendula*, *Nicotiana*, and *Dioscorea*), or have 24-ethylsterols accompanied by *trans*-24-ethylidenesterols (*Withania*). Sitosterol when identified only by the m.p. of its acetate probably also contains the 24-methylcholesterols, since the m.p. is nearly always about 5° too high, indicative of such contamination.

[b] These are the 4,4,14-trisdesmethylsterols which appear in sufficient quantity to be identified. They are listed in descending order of amount. Where exact or approximate figures are reported, the percentage of the sterol in the mixture is given in parentheses.

[c] *Lycopodium complanatum* sterols are primarily of the 24α-alkyl type, and for this reason the plant is included in the list. However, it is very unusual in the high quantity of $\Delta^{5,7}$-sterols, the high amount of 24-methylsterols, and the dominance of the 24β-configuration in the latter. It really constitutes an intermediate category between I and II and between A and C.

Table 10.10. Some plants very probably of category I-A[a]

Family	Genus and Species	Part	Dominant Sterols	Ref.
Bromeliaceae	*Tillandsia usneoides* (Spanish moss)	Whole	Sitosterol Stigmasterol 24ξ-Methylcholesterol Cholesterol	448,449
Gramineae	*Saccharum officinarum* (sugar cane)	Leaves	Sitosterol (38) Stigmasterol (37) 24ξ-Methylcholesterol (25)	450,451
Gramineae	*Prosopis spicigera*	Leaves	Sitosterol (60) Stigmasterol (24) 24ξ-Methylcholesterol (12) Cholesterol (4)	452
Gramineae	*Sorghum vulgare*	Seeds	Sitosterol 24ξ-Methylcholesterol Stigmasterol Cholesterol Isofucosterol Avenasterol Methylenecholesterol Methylenelathosterol	436
Compositae	*Helianthus annus* (sunflower)	Seeds	Sitosterol (59) Dihydrospinasterol (11) Stigmasterol (10) 24ξ-Methylcholesterol (9) Peposterol (?) (4) Isofucosterol (4) Cholesterol (1) 24ξ-Methyllathosterol (1)	453

Family	Species	Part	Sterols (%)	Ref.
Compositae	*Eupatorium perfoliatum*	Leaves and twigs	Avenasterol (1) $\Delta^{7,9(11),24(28)}$-Stigmastatrienol (<1) Sitosterol (60) Stigmasterol (40)	454
Compositae	*Digitalis lanata*	Whole	Sitosterol (75) Stigmasterol (25)	455
Solanaceae	*Nicotiana suaveolens*	Root	Stigmasterol (39) 24ξ-Methylcholesterol (30) Sitosterol (29) Cholesterol (2)	456
		Parts above ground	Sitosterol (46) Stigmasterol (26) 24ξ-Methylcholesterol (21) Cholesterol (7)	
Solanaceae	*Nicotiana langsdorffii*	Root	Stigmasterol (55) 24ξ-Methylcholesterol (32) Sitosterol (11) Cholesterol (2)	456
		Parts above ground	Sitosterol (44) Stigmasterol (28) Cholesterol (18) 24ξ-Methylcholesterol (10)	
Palmaceae	*Cocos nucifera* (coconut)	Seed oil (fruit similar)	Sitosterol (58) Isofucosterol (14) Stigmasterol (13) 24-Methylcholesterol (8) Dihydrospinasterol (6) Cholesterol (1)	431

Continued

Table 10.10. *Continued.*

Family	Genus and Species	Part	Dominant Sterols	Ref.
Palmaceae	Palm	Oil	Sitosterol (70) Stigmasterol (11) 24ξ-Methylcholesterol (9) Isofucosterol (6) Cholesterol (3) Dihydrospinasterol (1)	431
Leguminosae	*Arachis hypogaea* (peanut)	Seed oil	Sitosterol (64) 24ξ-Methylcholesterol (15) Stigmasterol (9) Isofucosterol (8) Dihydrospinasterol (3) Avenasterol (1) Cholesterol (<0.5)	431
Gramineae	*Zea mays* (corn)	Seed oil	Sitosterol (66) 24ξ-Methylcholesterol (23) Stigmasterol (6) Isofucosterol (4) Dihydrospinasterol (1) Avenasterol (<0.5) Cholesterol (<0.5)	431
Gramineae	(Rice)		Sitosterol (49) 24ξ-Methylcholesterol (28) Stigmasterol (15) Isofucosterol (5) Avenasterol (2) Dihydrospinasterol (1) Cholesterol (<0.5)	431

Family	Species	Plant part	Sterols (%)	Ref.
Gramineae	*Triticum vulgare* (wheat)	Seed oil	Sitosterol (67) 24ξ-Methylcholesterol (22) Isofucosterol (6) Dihydrospinasterol (3) Avenasterol (2) Stigmasterol (<0.5) Cholesterol (<0.5)	431
Oleaceae	*Olea europaea* (olive)	Fruit oil	Sitosterol (91) Dihydrospinasterol (4) 24ξ-Methylcholesterol (2) Isofucosterol (2) Avenasterol (<0.5)	431
Malvaceae	*Gossypium hirsutum* (cotton)	Seed oil	Sitosterol (93) 24ξ-Methylcholesterol (4) Isofucosterol (2) Stigmasterol (1) Avenasterol (<0.5) Dihydrospinasterol (<0.5) Cholesterol (<0.5)	431
Cruciferae	*Brassica rapa* (rapeseed)	Seed oil	Sitosterol (58) Campesterol (25) Brassicasterol (10) Dihydrospinasterol (5) Isofucosterol (2)	431
Cruciferae	41 species in 21 genera	Seeds	Sitosterol 24-Methylcholesterol Cholesterol Others, depending on species	432a

Continued

Table 10.10. *Continued.*

Family	Genus and Species	Part	Dominant Sterols	Ref.
Rubiaceae	*Coffea* sp. (coffee)	Seeds	Sitosterol (54) Stigmasterol (20) 24ξ-Methylcholesterol (19) Isofucosterol (6) Dihydrospinasterol (1) Cholesterol (<0.5)	431
Compositae	*Lactuca sativa* (lettuce)	Seeds	Sitosterol (52) 24ξ-Methylcholesterol (14) Stigmasterol (12) Avenasterol (6) Isofucosterol (4)	432b
Linaceae	*Linum usitatissimum* (linseed)	Seeds	Sitosterol (46) 24ξ-Methylcholesterol (29) Isofucosterol (15) Stigmasterol (8) Cholesterol (2)	432c
Solanaceae	*Solanum dulcamara*	Leaves	Cholesterol (34) Sitosterol (29) Stigmasterol (24) 24ξ-Methylcholesterol (6) Brassicasterol (3) Isofucosterol (3) Methylenecholesterol (1)	457

Leguminosae	*Phaseolus vulgaris* (beans)	Sitosterol (57)
		Stigmasterol (34)
		24ξ-Methylcholesterol (6)
		Isofucosterol (2)

[a] Category I-A refers to plants with primarily 24α-alkylsterols bearing a Δ^5-bond. Listed in this table are cases where the sterol composition is or approximates the homologous series of 24-H, 24-methyl, 24-ethyl but for which configurational data is uncertain. From Table 9 the homologous series will be seen to be typical of category I-A. Plants of category B (24β-alkyl) have so far been found to have only 24-ethylsterols. Stigmasterol completely replaces the two lowest homologs in category I-A plants. Consequently, the presence of a 24-ethylcholesterol and its Δ^{22}-derivative alone probably also indicates the 24α configuration, and plants of this sort are included.

Table 10.11. Some plants of category I-B[a]

Family	Genus and Species	Part	Dominant Sterols (%)	Ref.
Cucurbitaceae	*Cucurbita pepo*	Leaves (same as Pericarp of fruit)	Spinasterol (42) Dihydrospinasterol (36) Avenasterol (16) Peposterol (?) (5) 24ξ-Methyllathosterol (1) Lathosterol (0.2)	437
Chenopodiaceae	*Spinacea oleracea*	Leaves	Spinasterol (40) Dihydrospinasterol (40) Avenasterol (8) Methylenelathosterol (8) Other (2)	475,506
Compositae	*Aster scaber*	Roots	Spinasterol	424
Cucurbitaceae	*Cucumis melo*	Fruit	Spinasterol (major)	458–460
Cucurbitaceae	*Citrullus vulgaris*	Fruit	Spinasterol (major)	458–460
Theaceae	*Camellia japonica*	Oil	Spinasterol (45) Dihydrospinasterol (45) Avenasterol (6) Methylenelathosterol Other (1)	506
Theaceae	*Camellia sasangua*	Oil	Dihydrospinasterol (60) Spinasterol (28) Avenasterol (6) Methylenelathosterol (1) Other (5)	506

Theaceae	*Thea sinensis*	Oil	Spinasterol (59) Dihydrospinasterol (33) Methylenelathosterol (4) Avenasterol (2)	506
Sapotaceae	*Butyrospermum parkii*	Seeds	Spinasterol (43) Dihydrospinasterol (37) Avenasterol (11) Methylenelathosterol (6) Other (3)	506
Gramineae	Alfalfa	Oil	Spinasterol (46) Dihydrospinasterol (40) Methylenelathosterol (7) Avenasterol (5) Other (2)	506

[a] In category I-B are plants with principally or exclusively sterols with 24α-alkyl groups and a Δ^7-bond. Included in the list are only those cases for which NMR or other unequivocal configurational data exist.

implying grain). The older prefix "β" was meant to imply not configuration but a difference from "α-" and "γ-sitosterol." Since neither of the latter two "sterols" are true entities (465–468), it has become common practice to drop the "β" from the name. Although the sterol from wheat germ oil has not been the subject of unequivocal configurational analysis, nuclear magnetic resonance spectroscopy of sitosterol from a dozen other plants has demonstrated that it has the 20β-methyl and 24α-ethyl configurations and is not contaminated by its epimers (437, 440). The absolute configuration of stigmasterol at C-24 was demonstrated by Tsuda et al. (469), through degradation and correlation of the side chain fragment with a substance, the configuration of which was known from x-ray data. Because, upon reduction of the Δ^{22}-bond, stigmasterol is converted to a sterol with the same NMR spectrum as natural sitosterol (440), stigmasterol and sitosterol must have the same (α) configuration, in view of the fact that the 24-epimer (clionasterol) of sitosterol has a different spectrum (440). Through the use of NMR coupled with other modern analytical techniques, a number of vascular plants, ranging from the Lycopsida through the Filicopsida to the less and more advanced Pteropsida, have now been fully and unequivocally characterized. Some previous assumptions have been validated and others revised.

The dominant sterols of all Tracheophytes studied lack C-30 through C-32 and possess a ring B with either a Δ^5- or a Δ^7-bond. In some cases, the Δ^5-sterols are accompanied by smaller amounts of Δ^7-sterols, but the reverse seems to be rare if existent at all. In a few cases, $\Delta^{5,7}$-sterols are present. They have been detected in trace amounts by ultraviolet spectroscopy (470), but only in two cases, Lycopodium complanatum (437, 438), and the Rangpur lime (471), do they accumulate sufficiently to allow isolation. In the former case, ergosterol is present together with what is thought on the basis of NMR data to be its 24-epimer. In the latter case, ergosterol and/or its epimer are present. In contrast to algae and fungi, no Tracheophytes are known that contain principally $\Delta^{5,7}$-sterols. All Tracheophytes are also characterized by having principally 24-alkylsterols as end products. Furthermore, the dominant sterols of Tracheophytes usually contain either principally or exclusively a side chain that is saturated or, less commonly, one containing Δ^{22}- or $\Delta^{25(27)}$-bonds, or both. This means as a first approximation that the dominant sterols of the investigated cases fall, except and refined in what follows, primarily into the homologous series: cholesterol, 24-methycholesterol, and 24-ethylcholesterol and/or, but less commonly, the analogous series with a Δ^7-bond (lathosterol, etc.). Stigmasterol and its Δ^7-analog (spinasterol) are also frequent companions of cholesterol and lathosterol. The analogous Δ^{22}-derivatives of the 24-methyl homologs are rare. As will be seen, other sterols also occur, and in some cases are the dominant ones. Tables 10.12 to 10.14 summarize the names and structures of the important sterols.

Table 10.12. 24-C$_1$- and 24-C$_2$-Cholesterols with and without a Δ^{22}-bond

Structure and Name	Substitution	Structure and Name
Δ^5-series		$\Delta^{5,22\text{-}trans}$-Series
Campesterol	R = H, R' = CH$_3$	Epibrassicasterol[a]
Dihydrobrassicasterol	R = CH$_3$, R' = H	Brassicasterol
Sitosterol	R = H, R' = C$_2$H$_5$	Stigmasterol
Clionasterol[b]	R = C$_2$H$_5$, R' = H	Poriferasterol[a]
Ostreasterol (methylenecholesterol)	R and R' = CH$_2$	
Isofucosterol	R and R' = trans-CHCH$_3$[c]	Unknown[a]
Fucosterol[a]	R and R' = cis-CHCH$_3$[c]	Unknown[a]

[a] Unknown in Tracheophytes.
[b] Observed in Tracheophytes in only one uncertain case.
[c] The terms cis and trans refer to the relationship of the methyl group (C-29) to C-23.

Table 10.13. 24-C_1- and 24-C_2-Lathosterols with and without a Δ^{22}-bond

Structure and Name	Substitution	Structure and Name
Δ^7-Series		$\Delta^{7,22}$-*trans*-Series
Epifungisterol (unknown but probably occurs)	R = H, R' = CH_3	Unknown
Fungisterol	R = CH_3, R' = H	Dehydrofungisterol
Schottenol (Dihydrospinasterol)	R = H, R' = C_2H_5	Spinasterol
Epischottenol (Dihydrochondrillasterol)	R = C_2H_5, R' = H	Chondrillasterol
Methylenelathosterol	R and R' = CH_2	
Avenasterol	R and R' = *trans*-$CHCH_3{}^a$	Unknown
Unknown	R and R' = *cis*-$CHCH_3{}^a$	Unknown

[a]The terms *cis* and *trans* refer to the relationship of the methyl group (C-29) to C-23.

Table 10.14. $\Delta^{25(27)}$-Sterols

Structure and Name	Nuclear Series	Structure and Name
Codisterol[a]	Cholesterol	Clerosterol or 25(27)-Dehydroclionasterol (Δ^{22}-*trans*-derivative = 22-dehydroclerosterol = 25(27)-dehydroporifasterol)
25(27)-Dehydrofungisterol[a]	Lathosterol	25(27)-Dehydrodihydrochondrillasterol (Δ^{22}-*trans*-derivative = 25(27)-dehydrochondrillasterol)
Cyclolaudenol	Cycloartenol	Unknown

[a] Not yet detected in Tracheophytes but possible on biosynthetic grounds as is its Δ^{22}-derivative.

Cholesterol itself was first isolated from a Tracheophyte in 1963 by Johnson, Bennett, and Heftman (*472*), who obtained it from *Solanum tuberosum* and *Dioscorea spiculiflora*. In the intervening years it has been found to be fairly common. Both it and its Δ^7-analog, lathosterol, have nearly always been found to be present in smaller amount than their 24-alkylderivatives. *Solanum dulcamara* leaves are an example of a case in which cholesterol is the major single component (34%) (*457*). The remaining sterols contain six 24-alkenylated and 24-alkylated sterols comprised principally of sitosterol (29%). More commonly, cholesterol is either not observable or constitutes only at most a few percent of the mixture. Lathosterol, like cholesterol, was first isolated from animals. The recognition that it also occurs in plants is very recent. It was observed in several mixtures by gas-liquid chromatography in the period 1965–1975. In at least one case (the New York fern) reported in 1977 (*437*), it was separated chromatographically from the other sterols and unequivocally identified in the pure state by, among other things, nuclear magnetic resonance and mass spectroscopy.

The 24-methyl-Δ^5-sterols usually occur in Tracheophytes with both the 24α- and 24β-configurations (*437, 440*). 24α-Methylcholesterol was first isolated by Fernholz and MacPhillamy (*473*) from seeds that belong to the genus *Brassica* and species *campestris*. It was named campesterol for the species, the genus having already been so honored, as will be seen subsequently, but it was the genus and the plant part taken that, unknowingly to the early authors, were really important. Seeds of the *Brassica* genus are now known (*474*) to be unusual, in that they contain only the 24α-methyl epimer. This facilitated its proof of structure, as did the fact that, when it occurs together with its 24β-methyl epimer, campesterol is the dominant sterol of the pair (*437, 440*). The 24β-methyl epimer (dihydrobrassicasterol) was first identified in soybeans and other Tracheophytes in 1976 by Nes, Krevitz, and Behzadan (*440*) using nuclear magnetic resonance spectroscopy. While it occurs in configurationally pure form in algae, which constituted the first known natural occurrence, it so far always is found in Tracheophytes mixed with campesterol (except in *Brassica* seeds). 24ξ-Methyllathosterol has recently been identified by gas-liquid chromatography and mass spectroscopy in several vascular plants, e.g., the New York fern (*437*). For reasons not clear, its amount is always very small even when all the sterols contain the Δ^7-bond, and too little has been obtained to investigate the configuration. By analogy to the Δ^5-case, it probably occurs as an epimeric mixture (epifungisterol and fungisterol).

24α-Ethyllathosterol (schottenol, dihydrospinasterol) was apparently first isolated in a pure form and configurationally examined with nuclear magnetic resonance spectroscopy by Amarego, Goad, and Goodwin (*475*) in 1973 using spinach leaves (*Spinacea oleracea*).

Twenty years earlier, Idler, Kandutsch, and Baumann (*476*) isolated it or its 24-epimer as a 3% component of the sterols from wheat. Since the wheat sterols probably are of the 24α-ethyl variety, the isolation of Idler et al. (476) constitutes the discovery of 24α-ethyllathosterol in vascular plants. It was named schottenol by Djerassi and his associates when they found it in *Lophocereus schottii* (477). Its 24β-epimer (dihydrochondrillasterol, epischottenol) has not been observed so far, although it is found in algae.

The Δ²²-derivatives of the 24-alkylsterols of vascular plants were first discovered some 60 years ago in the case of 22-*trans*-dehydrositosterol (stigmasterol), as described earlier in this section. Three years later in 1909, Windaus and Welsh (478) isolated the analogous 24β-methylsterol from seeds of *Brassica rapa* and named it brassicasterol (22-*trans*-dehydro-24β-methylcholesterol) in honor of the genus. The 24α-epimer (diatomsterol) of brassicasterol has so far been found only in algae (diatoms), and the 24β-epimer (poriferasterol) of stigmasterol is known to occur only in algae and marine invertebrates. However, the Δ²⁵⁽²⁷⁾-derivative of poriferasterol [known as 22-*trans*-,25(27)-bisdehydroclionasterol, 25(27)-dehydroporiferasterol, 22-*trans*-dehydroclerosterol, or 22-*trans*,25(27)-bisdehydro-24β-ethylcholesterol] and the analogous derivative of clionasterol [25(27)-dehydroclionasterol, 25(27)-dehydro-24β-ethylcholesterol, or clerosterol] have recently been discovered in Tracheophytes (Table 10.15). 25(27)-Dehydroporiferasterol was first found (in *Clerodendrum campbellii*) and configurationally elucidated in Goodwin's laboratory (461, 462) in 1970. Its 22-dihydro derivative (clerosterol) was configurationally elucidated by Nes et al. (437) in a sample from *Kalanchoe daigremontiana*, where it occurs together with its Δ²²-derivative (437). It was first isolated in 1966 from *Clerodendrum infortunatum* by Manzoor-I-Khuda (463). 24β-Ethylsterols were also discovered in the same period by Sucrow and his associates (458–460) in the seeds of the family Cucurbitaceae. The latter sterols are the Δ⁷-analogs of clerosterol and 22-*trans*-dehydroclerosterol. They are, respectively, 25(27)-dehydro-24β-ethyllathosterol [25(27)-dehydrodihydrochondrillasterol] and 22-*trans*-25(27)-bisdehydro-24β-ethyllathosterol [25(27)-dehydrochondrillasterol]. The Δ⁷-analog of stigmasterol is spinasterol. It was isolated by Hart and Heyl (479) from spinach (*Spinacea oleracea*) and named accordingly in 1932. Its structure was elucidated by Barton and Cox (480), and by Fieser, Fieser, and Chakravarti (481), and more recently confirmation has been afforded by nuclear magnetic resonance spectroscopy (437, 475). Its 24β-epimer (chondrillasterol) has not been observed in vascular plants.

The sterols described in the preceding paragraphs are the ones comprising what appear to be the common dominant sterols of Tracheophytes; however, a number of others are known. They presumably are intermediates, since in most cases they occur in small amounts. Thus, 24(28)-*trans*-dehydrositosterol [*trans*-24-ethylidenecholesterol, isofucosterol] was isolated as an 8% component of *Pinus pinea* seeds in 1969 (482). A decade earlier

Table 10.15. Some plants of category II[a]

Family	Genus and Species	Part	Dominant Sterols (%)	Ref.
			Category B	
Cucurbitaceae	*Cucurbita pepo*	Seeds	25(27)-Dehydrodihydrochondrillasterol (54)	458–460
			25(27)-Dehydrochondrillasterol (23)	
			Spinasterol (23)	
Cucurbitaceae	*Cucumis sativus*	Seeds	25(27)-Dehydrochondrillasterol (8)	458–460
			25(27)-Dehydrodihydrochondrillasterol (10)	
			Spinasterol (10)	
Cucurbitaceae	*Cucumis melo*	Seeds	25(27)-Dehydrochondrillasterol (61)	458–460
			25(27)-Dehydrodihydrochondrillasterol (26)	
			Spinasterol (13)	
Cucurbitaceae	*Citrullus vulgaris*	Seeds	25(27)-Dehydrochondrillasterol (58)	458–460
			25(27)-Dehydrodihydrochondrillasterol (27)	
			Spinasterol (15)	
			Category A	
Crassulaceae	*Kalanchoe daigremontiana*	Mature plant	25(27)-Dehydroclionasterol (50) (Clerosterol)	437
			25(27)-Dehydroporiferasterol (50) (22-*trans*-Dehydroclerosterol)	
Verbenaceae	*Clerodendrum infortunatum*		25(27)-Dehydroclionasterol (Clerosterol)	463
Verbenaceae	*Clerodendrum campbellii*		25(27)-Dehydroporiferasterol (22-*trans*-Dehydroclerosterol)	461,462

[a] Plants of category II contain principally or exclusively sterols with the 24β-alkyl configuration. *Clerodendrum* and *Kalanchoe* are in category II-A and have Δ⁵-sterols, while Cucurbitaceae seeds having principally Δ⁷-sterols are in category II-B.

it was found to be the second most abundant sterol in seeds of *Avena sativa* (*483, 484*) and later called "Δ^5-avenasterol." Its Δ^7 isomer is "Δ^7-avenasterol." We shall use the term "avenasterol" to refer only to the Δ^7-compound (*trans*-24-ethylidenelathosterol). In *Vernonia anthelmintica* seeds, avenasterol constitutes as much 35% of the sterol mixture (*485-487*). This species is also remarkable for containing principally (approximately 65%) the $\Delta^{8,14}$-diene corresponding to avenasterol (*485-487*). The compound, which has the structure (*486*) of 24-*trans*-ethylidenecholesta-8,14-dien-3β-ol, has been called vernosterol (*485*). Traces of Δ^5- and Δ^7-24ξ-ethylsterols are also present. The derivatives of isofucosterol and avenasterol with Δ^{22}- and/or $\Delta^{25(27)}$-bonds are unknown as plant products. The $\Delta^{24(25)}$-analogs, however, while not fully characterized, have been reported. 24(25)-Dehydrositosterol (24-ethyldesmosterol) is believed to occur as a very minor sterol in *Withania somnifera* (*446*), and its Δ^7-analog (peposterol) is a trace component in *Helianthus annus* seeds (*453a*), *Cucurbita pepo* leaves (*437*), and elsewhere (*453b*). The 24-methyl analog [24-methyldesmosterol, 24(25)-dehydro-24-methylcholesterol] has been isolated from *Withania somnifera* and well characterized (*446*). *Seseli indicum* contains a sterol in which the common Δ^5- or Δ^7-bond is replaced by a $\Delta^{9(11)}$-bond. It [24α-ethylcholesta-9(11),22-*trans*-dien-3β-ol] has been named indosterol by its discoverers, Gupta and Gupta (*488*), and is the $\Delta^{9(11)}$-analog of spinasterol (Scheme 10.10). Indosterol may be the dominant sterol of the plant. Unfortunately, it is not clear in the publication (*488*) whether other sterols are present, but, since it is reported to be isolable in a pure condition just by chromatography on alumina or silica gel lacking silver nitrate, there is the strong suggestion that it is indeed the dominant sterol. Methylene-cholesterol (ostreasterol), first discovered in crustacea, was found to be the dominant sterol of many pollens by Barbier et al. (*489*) in 1960. In the next decade it was discovered as a minor component in several other plant tissues, although it is not commonly accumulated sufficiently to be observed. Pollen is clearly highly specialized in its ability to make or accept (through transport) mainly this $\Delta^{24(28)}$-sterol. For a further discussion, see below.

Several sterols with an extra hydroxyl group are known. They include macdougallin (14α-methylcholest-8-en-3β-,6α-diol) from the cactus *Peniocereus macdougalli* (*490*), its 14-desmethyl derivative (peniocerol) (Scheme 10.10) from *P. fosterianus* (*491*), and 22α-hydroxycholesterol from a Norwegian lily, *Narthecium ossifragum* (*492, 493*). Hydroxy-ketosterols include viperidinone (9α,14α-dihydroxy-6-ketolathosterol) from *Wilcoxia viperina* (*494*) and carpesterol (22β-hydroxy-6-keto-24α-ethyl-4α-methyllathosterol), which occurs (*495*) as the 3-benzoate in *Solanum xanthocarpum* along with sitosterol. Carpesterol and viperidinone are related structurally to the insect moulting hormones. From sugar cane (*Saccharum officinarum*), in addition to the common Δ^5-sterols, small amounts of 7α-hydroxysitosterol (ikshusterol), its 7β-epimer (epiikshusterol), and 5α,6β-dihydroxysitostanol

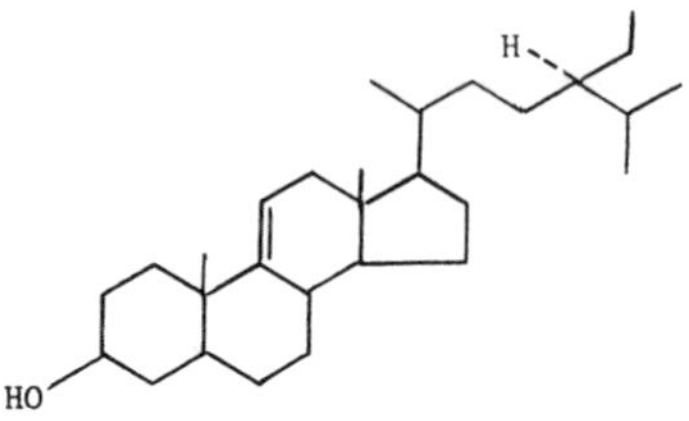

Indosterol 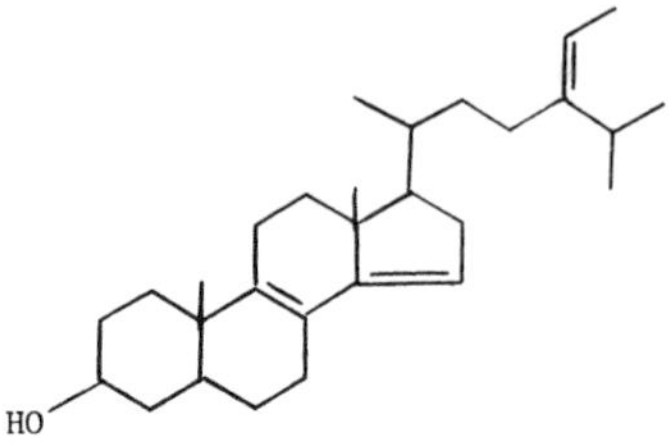   Vernosterol

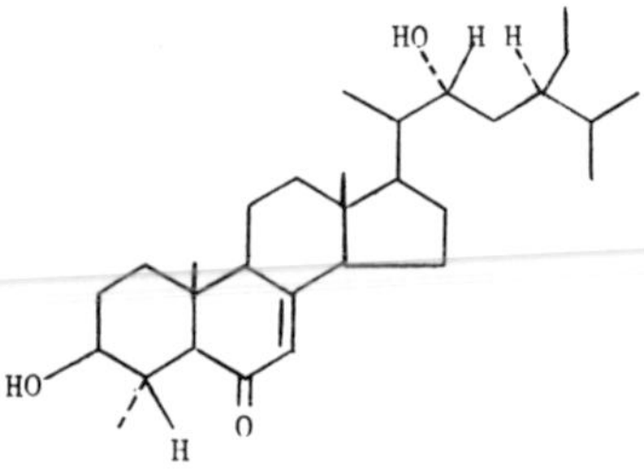

Carpesterol   Peniocerol
(Occurs as 3-Benzoate)

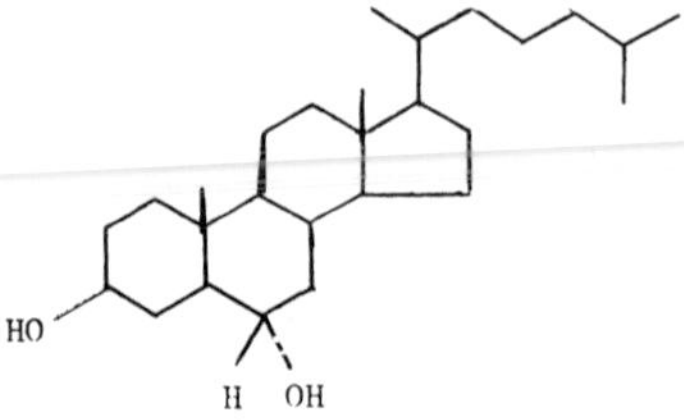

Scheme 10.10. Some uncommon steroids of Tracheophytes (configurations at the ring junctures and at C-17 and C-20 are as in 5α-cholestane).

have been isolated (451). The occurrence of both epimers at C-7 suggests that these compounds are artifacts derived by nonbiological oxidation of sitosterol. Spanish moss (*Tillandsia usneoides*) has similarly yielded (448, 449) diols (cycloart-23-ene-3β,25-diol, as well as its 25-methoxy analog and cycloart-25-ene-3β,24ξ-diol) that conceivably could result from air oxidation (of cycloartenol), as could 24,25-epoxycycloartanol, which has been isolated from this source. Spanish moss has an unusually large surface area for a higher plant. However, cycloart-23-ene-3β,25β-diol has been isolated from other plants. For a review of these and many other oxygenated 9(19)-cyclosterols, see Boar and Romer (496).

Several quantitatively minor sterols retaining one or more of the methyl groups at C-4 and C-14, which, however, are believed to be of importance biosynthetically, were obtained in pure form in the decade between 1955 and 1965 (Scheme 10.11). Lophenol (4α-methyllathosterol) was first isolated in 1958 from the cactus *Lophocereus schottii* (497). Its *trans*-24-ethylidene derivative (citrostadienol, 24-trans-ethylidenelophenol) was discovered in grapefruit peel in the same period (498). 24-Methylenelophenol (grami-

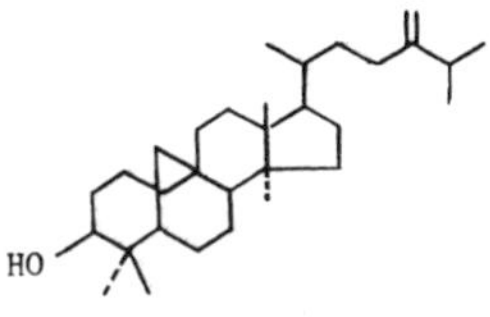

Methylenecycloartanol 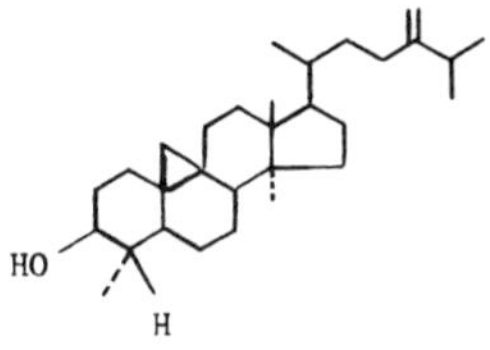   Cycloeucalenol 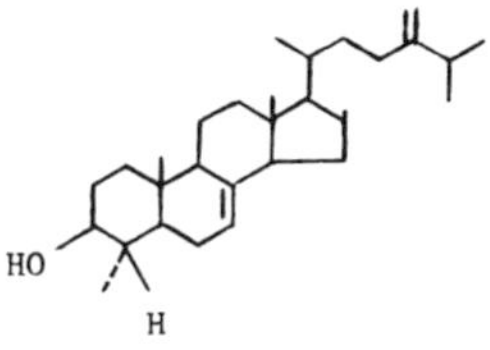   Gramisterol

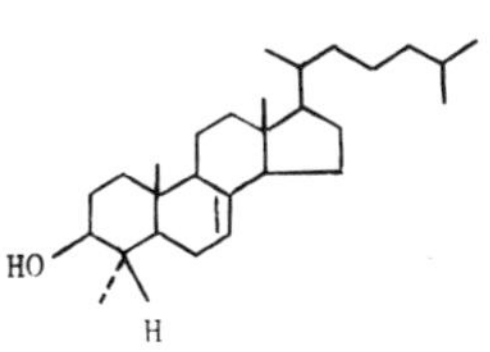

Lophenol 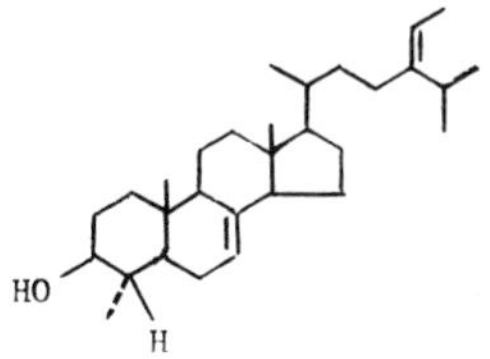   Citrostadienol 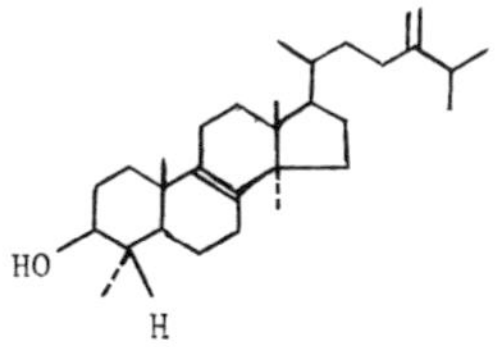   Obtusifoliol

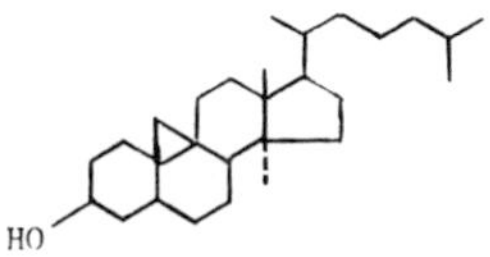

Pollinastanol 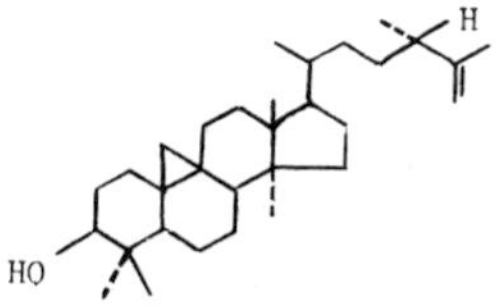   Cyclolaudenol 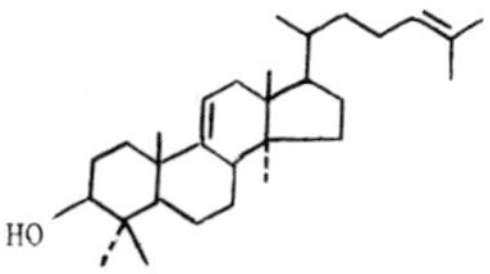   Parkeol

Scheme 10.11. Some intermediates retaining one or more methyl groups at C-4 and C-14 (except for C-9 in the 9,19-cyclo-series, configurations at ring junctures, C-17 and C-20 are as in 5α-cholestane).

sterol) was first reported in sugar cane (Graminaceae) leaves (genus *Saccharum*) in 1965, and its 14α-methyl-homolog, in which a Δ^8-bond is present in place of the Δ^7-bond (obtusifoliol), was found in *Euphorbia obtusifolia* (*499*) a few years earlier. 24-Methylenecycloartanol was discovered in 1957 in rice (*500,501*) and its 4-desmethyl derivative (cycloeucalenol, 24-methylene-4α,14α-dimethyl-9,19-cyclo-5α-cholestanol) in wood from *Eucalyptus microcorys* (*502, 503*) and *Swietenia mahagoni* (*504*) in the late 1950s. 24-Methylenelanosterol is unknown in vascular plants. The $\Delta^{9(11)}$-analog [parkeol, lanost-9(11),24-dien-3β-ol] of lanosterol was found in "shea butter" from the kernels of *Butyrospermum parkii* in the family *Sapotaceae* in 1956 (*505*, see also *506*) and more recently its 24-methylene derivative [24-methylenelanost-9(11)-en-3β-ol] was obtained from the same source

(*507*). Also recently, 25(27)-dehydro-24ξ-ethyllophenol was isolated from *Clerodendrum campbellii* (*461*). The ethyl groups at C-24 are probably β-oriented. Much earlier, 25(27)-dehydro-24β-methylcycloartanol (cyclolaudenol) was discovered. The interesting compound pollinastanol (4,4-desmethylcycloartanol, 14α-methyl-9,19-cyclo-5α-cholestan-3β-ol), which may be on the pathway to lathosterol and cholesterol in Tracheophytes, was first isolated from Compositae pollen (*508*). The structure has been confirmed by x-ray crystallography (*509*). Its 4α-hydroxy-24-methylene derivative (surianol) represents 0.01% of *Suriana maritima*, a pantropical shrub. (*441*). This amount is 50% of the sitosterol content. For a review of the occurrence of these and many other 9(19)-cyclosterols, see Boar and Romer (*496*), and for their quantitative values in various plants see Itoh et al. (*510, 511*). For a discussion of cycloartenol and lanosterol see Chapter 9. Some structures are shown in Scheme 10.11.

There are several hundred families in the Tracheophyta, culminating in no less than 175,000 species of angiosperms. While nothing like this large number of plants has been studied, enough have been systematically and precisely examined to begin to see some of the rules governing occurrence. Species in a given family and especially a given genus have proved to be very closely related to one another in their dominant sterols. In all cases of which the authors are aware, the principal sterol bears a 24-C_2 group. In all cases, it is an ethyl group, except in the genus *Vernonia*, where it is a 24-*trans*-ethylidene group (*485–487*). When the principal sterol is present in less than 50% of the mixture, more than 50% of the mixture is still comprised by 24-C_2-sterols. This generalization includes representatives of the Lycopodia, Filicopsida, as well as lower and higher Gymnospermae and lower and higher Angiospermae in the Pteropsida. Several dozen families (and a great many more species) have been investigated, which becomes a significant percentage of the extant botanical groupings. There can, therefore, be little doubt that vascular plants have a very strong biosynthetic and presumably functional preference for a sequence of two C_1 transfers, one to C-24 and one then to C-28. Moreover, except so far in *Vernonia*, where isomerization to $\Delta^{24(25)}$-sterols is inhibited, the majority of families have at the mature stage a pathway (presumably through isomerization of 24-*trans*-ethylidenesterols and reduction of the resulting $\Delta^{24(25)}$-sterol) leading to 24α-ethylsterols. Most families also have Δ^5-sterols, which means that 24α-ethylcholesterol (sitosterol) is the most common of the principal sterols encountered. In Table 10.9 is a list of the plants for which sitosterol has been shown clearly to be the major sterol both in a quantitative and a configurational sense. This listing and what is subsequently discussed have been achieved in several ways, all of which depend both on isolation of the components in a pure state and on some form of quantitation of the relative amounts of the components. The most certain method for structural elucidation has included the combined use of mass and nuclear magnetic resonance spectroscopy on the separated components. However, the discrimination between stigmasterol and its 24-epimer can be made through the melting points of their pure free alcohols and of sitosterol and its 24-epimer through the melting points of their pure acetates. Since there seems to be a difference in the pathway to 24α- and 24β-alkylsterols (24-H loss in the former, and retention in the latter), labeling evidence can also be used to discriminate between the epimeric alternatives. Less secure but probably valid as a configurational assessment is the ratio of the components. It will be seen from Table 10.9 that, when sitosterol is dominant, its 24-methyl homolog, and frequently its 24-H homolog, as well as its Δ^{22}-derivative, are usually present. On the other hand, when the major sterols are in the Δ^7- or 24β-ethyl series, the 24-methylsterols are negligible or not present at all. Furthermore, in the 24β-ethyl series the $\Delta^{25(27)}$-bond is not reduced in the well examined recent cases. These facts mean that the presence of the homologous series (with significant amounts of 24-methylsterol) and/or the presence of a Δ^{22}-sterol lacking a $\Delta^{25(27)}$-bond can tentatively be used to imply the presence of sterols primarily of the 24α-alkyl series, including only the 24α-epimer at the 24-ethyl level. The presence of the homologous series implies further that the sterols have a Δ^5-bond. Available data therefore permit us to assemble a further list (Table 10.10) of plants that very probably possess the same sterols as those in Table 10.9. Further examples can be found in the literature, with varying degrees of certainty. The majority of vascular plant families for which unequivocal information is available (Table 10.9) or for which reasonable estimates can be made, e.g., Table 10.10, have sterols containing primarily or exclusively a Δ^5-bond, sterols with a 24-ethyl group that is exclusively α-oriented, and 24-methylsterols primarily of the α configuration. Plants in which the 24α-alkylsterols are dominant have been classified by Nes et al. (437) as being in category I and those with primarily Δ^5-sterols as category A. Most examined plants are therefore of category I-A.

Plants of category II-A (437) contain principally or exclusively Δ^5-24β-alkylsterols. They are so far limited to mature tissue (leaves) of plants in the genus *Clerodendrum* (investigated species being *campbellii* and *infortunatum*) in the family Verbenaceae and in the genus *Kalanchoe* (species *diagremontiana*) in the family Crassulaceae. The latter contains both 25(27)-dehydroclionasterol (clerosterol) and its Δ^{22}-derivative [25(27)-dehydroporiferasterol]. *C. campbellii* contains only the Δ^{22}-derivative, and *C. infortunatum* contains apparently only clerosterol (configuration at C-24 inferred from the work with *C. campbellii*). The sterols of both *C. campbellii* and *K. daigremontiana* unequivocally (NMR and other data) contain the 24β-ethyl structure. "Clerosterol" has also been reported (512) in the leaves of a species of the Compositae (*Enhydra fluctuans*) along with "stigmasterol" and "stigmasta-5,22,25-trien-3β-ol," but without adequate data for any of the three. The "stigmasterol" lacks any data, as does the trienol, and the "clerosterol" was characterized by melting point, rotation, and infrared spectra. A methylene absorption at 890 cm^{-1} could have been from a 24- rather than a 25-methylene group. "Clerosterol," along with "24-methylenecholesterol" and "stigmasterol," have also been reported in the embryo axes and cotyledons of *Calendula officinalis* (*513*). At the time of this writing, the crucial structural paper was in press and not available to the authors. Since in *Clerodendrum campbellii* (*461, 462*) and *Kalanchoe daigremontiana* (*437*) only $\Delta^{25(27)}$-24β-ethylsterols are found, the species of *Calendula* and *Enhydra* warrant further investigation. Is the "stigmasterol" poriferasterol? Is the clerosterol its 24α-epimer? What are the relative quantities? The problem is further complicated by ontogeny, because clerosterol does not seem to be present in mature tissues (*421*). Ontogenetic changes of other sorts are already known, as is described in what follows.

Plants with principally or exclusively Δ^7-sterols have been designated as category B. All investigated genera and species of the Cucurbitaceae are in this category (*437*). While mature tissue (leaves and pericarp of the fruit) of the pumpkin (*Cucurita pepo*) contains only Δ^7-24-ethylsterols with the α-orientation (spinasterol and its 22-dihydro derivative) (*437*), pumpkin seeds (as well as seeds in other genera of the family), which are principally composed of an embryo, contain mainly (*514*) Δ^7-24β-ethylsterols [25(27)-dehydrochondrillasterol and its 22-dihydro derivative] with structures analogous to clerosterol and its Δ^{22}-derivative (*458–460*). These embryos in the family Cucurbitaceae are therefore of category II-B, while the mature plants are of category I-B, as shown in Table 10.16.

Plants or tissues with dominant sterols lacking an asymmetric C-24 but with a 24-C$_2$ group (*trans*-24-ethylidene) we shall call category III$_a$ and those with a 24-C$_1$ group (24-methylene), category III$_b$. *Vernonia anthelmintica* seeds are of category III$_a$, since they contain principally isofucosterol and its $\Delta^{8,14}$-derivative. One wonders whether the leaves would be of category I-B or perhaps of I-A? There is clearly a biosynthetic block in the seeds in the conversion of the 24-ethylidene sterol to a 24-ethylsterol. Since the 24-ethylidene sterols in the examined cases of vascular plants are precursors via $\Delta^{24(25)}$-intermediates to 24α-ethylsterols (and not to the 24β-epimers, which are thought to arise through $\Delta^{25(27)}$- intermediates resulting directly from C$_1$-transfer), completion of the pathway in the mature tissue should lead to one or both of the Δ^7-pair of 24α-ethylsterols, dihydrospinasterol/spinasterol, or one or both of the corresponding Δ^5-sterols, sitosterol/stigmasterol. This and other ontogenetic phenomena are summarized in Table 10.16.

While 24-methylcholesterol usually exists as the epimeric pair, campesterol-dihydrobrassicasterol in a 2:1 mixture, respectively, an extensive investigation (*432, 515*) of the family Cruciferae has revealed that brassi-

Table 10.16. Ontogenetic and related phenomena

Plant	Developmental Stage	Sterol Feature	Probable Enzymatic Explanation
Cucurbita (Cucurbitaceae)	Embryonic	Category II	Change from
Cucurbita (Cucurbitaceae)	Mature	Category I	$\Delta^{25(27)}$ to $\Delta^{24(28)}$ pathway
Brassica (Cruciferae)	Embryonic	Δ^{22}-24β-Methyl but no 24β-methyl	
Brassica (Cruciferae)	Mature	24β-Methyl but little or no Δ^{22}-derivative	Development of Δ^{22}-reductase or loss of Δ^{22}-dehydrogenase
Vernonia (Compositae)	Embryonic	Category III$_a$	Lack of $\Delta^{24(28)}$-isomerase
Vernonia (Compositae)	Embryonic	$\Delta^{8,14}$ in large amount; Δ^7 also present	Partial lack of 14-reductase and complete lack of 5-dehydrogenase
Vernonia (Compositae)	Mature	If change occurs, expect 24α-ethyl and perhapsΔ^5, but not studied	Development of $\Delta^{24(28)}$-isomerase and $\Delta^{24(25)}$-reductase and, if plant is genetically of category A, development of Δ^5-dehydrogenase and Δ^7-reductase

casterol, which is found in many of the seeds, disappears during germination and seedling development of *Brassica* species (Table 10.17). Moreover, seeds of *Brassica rapa* contain only campesterol as the 24-methyl component (*474*), but the mature leaf of *Brassica oleracea* has the usual epimeric mixture of campesterol and dihydrobrassicasterol (*440*). Moreover, brassicasterol is only a rare component of tissues of plants other than certain Cruciferae species, e.g., in the genus *Brassica*. These facts suggests that the dihydrobrassicasterol is being converted to brassicasterol by dehydrogenation at C-22,23 in the early phases of ontogeny but not in the later ones, on the assumption that dihydrobrassicasterol arises through the $\Delta^{25(27)}$-pathway of alkylation with cyclolaudenol probably being the first alkylated intermediate. The presence of the $\Delta^{25(27)}$-bond may induce homoallylic dehydrogenation to give the $\Delta^{22,25,(27)}$-dienic structure. This structure is well documented in the ethyl homolog both in the Δ^7-series (Cucurbitaceae) and Δ^5-series (*Clerodendrum* and *Kalanchoe*). The enzyme that is responsible for the homoallylic dehydrogenation may also be primitive, while dehydrogenation of the saturated side chain may be more advanced. This would explain why the Δ^{22}-24β-methyl, but not the Δ^{22}-24α-methyl structure, is found in early ontogenesis. Loss of the more primitive character with development would then also explain the disappearance of brassicasterol and appearance of dihydrobrassicasterol. Other explanations, of course, also come to mind, but, regardless of the reason, which can be examined at evolutionary, functional, and mechanistic levels, there can be no doubt of the fact of ontogenetic changes in the genus *Brassica*, whose mature tissues are similar in their sterol content to most other plants, implying unusual character only in the seeds.

Because most vascular plants are of category I-A, with sitosterol the most frequently encountered and in greatest amount, because algae and fungi are most commonly of category II, because Cucurbitaceae plants undergo an ontogenetic change from category II to category I, and because Δ^7-sterols must necessarily precede Δ^5-sterols, it has been suggested (*437*) that the most highly evolved sterols have the Δ^5-24α-alkyl structure with sitosterol at the apex. The early appearance of Δ^5-24α-alkylsterols in diatoms and of sitosterol itself in *Lycopodium* indicates that the evolution of the sterol pathway can occur to its highest level while other biological characteristics remain well below their peak. Conversely, the presence of vascular plants of categories II (*Kalanchoe, Clerodendrum,* etc.) and B (Cucurbitaceae, Theaceae, etc.) means that various other characteristics can evolve faster than the sterol pathway. Based on these ideas, some more detailed analyses of plant phylogenesis have been made (*437*), and additional efforts in this direction should be fruitful.

From work on the geranium (*Pelargonium hortorum*), Nicholas and his associates (*516*) have concluded that sterols (and their esters) are biosynthesized by all plant parts, and that the leaves are the primary source, from which they are also transported to other tissues (*517*).

Table 10.17. Changes in sterol composition during development in the Cruciferae

Plant	Age (days)	24-H	24-CH$_3$	24-C$_2$H$_5$	Δ^{22}-24-CH$_3$	Δ^{22}-24-C$_2$H$_5$	24-CHCH$_3$
				% of Mixture (Cholesterol and Its Derivatives)			
Brassica rapa (rapeseed)	0	3	22	62	13	Trace	Trace
	8	4	26	50	17	2	2
	14	5	19	64	6	2	4
Brassica oleracea (cabbage)	0	Trace	26	61	13	—	—
	5	2	32	55	9	3	—
	19	8	26	55	5	4	2
Raphanus sativus (French breakfast)	0	2	24	62	9	—	3
	5	4	25	60	9	2	Trace
	19	6	23	61	6	5	Trace
Cheiranthus cheri (blood-red)	0	15	20	52	—	—	4
	19	17	23	53	—	—	4
	33	5	23	70	—	—	2

From Ingram et al. (*515*).

Pollen seems to be the only case in which a given tissue may have a sterol composition dramatically different from that of the whole plant. Extensive surveys (16 families) have been made by Barbier and his associates (*518* and references cited) and by others (*519*) that indicate the frequent occurrence of large amounts of $\Delta^{24(28)}$-sterols. Thus, cornseed oil is 66% sitosterol, 23% 24-methylcholesterol, <1% cholesterol, 6% stigmasterol, and 5% other, but corn pollen is 9% sitosterol, 13% 24-methylcholesterol, 5% cholesterol, 9% stigmasterol (or isofucosterol), and 65% methylenecholesterol. Methylenecholesterol or isofucosterol is found as the sterol in the largest amount in the mixtures from about half of the two dozen investigated species (Table 10.18). In the other half, most have principally sitosterol and one stigmasterol, in keeping with most plants as a whole, but two have mostly cholesterol. There seems to be no clear correlation with genus or family as to the pollen sterols, nor does the habitat or the method of collection (by bees or by people) influence the content.

Sterols frequently and perhaps always occur both as the free alcohols, as esters, and at least sometimes as glycosides. Steryl esters of fatty acids were first prepared by Tanret at the turn of the century (*520, 521*). They were recognized in plants by Oxford and Raistrick in 1933 (*522*), and during the next three decades several investigators did further work on their occurrence. For keys to the literature see Kuksis and Beveridge (*523*), who examined the preparation and properties of the esters, and Kemp and Mercer (*524*). The latter authors (*524*) in 1968 were the first to make a detailed analysis of the esters in a given plant. They found that shoots, roots, scutella, and endosperms of 10-day-old corn (*Zea mays*) seedlings all contained esters of 4,4,14-trimethyl-, 4α-methyl-, and 4,4,14-trisdesmethylsterols. Increasing amounts were found with decreasing nuclear methylation, the trisdesmethyl steryl esters accounting for 90% of the total. All of the common sterols were found in the ester fraction, including cholesterol, 24-methylcholesterol, 24-methyl- and 24-ethylcholestanol (in endosperm only), stigmasterol, obtusifoliol, methylenelophenol, cycloeucalenol, ethylidenelophenol, cycloartenol, and methylenecycloartanol, as well as the pentacycles, α- and β-amyrin. The fatty acids obtained from the esters after hydrolysis varied in chain length from C-12 to greater than C-22 with both even and odd numbers present, except for C-13, which was absent. Odd numbers tended to be in smaller amount than even numbers. From C_{14} to C_{18}, both saturated and monounsaturated acids occurred. The di- and triunsaturated C-18 acids also were present, but only saturated above C-18. In greatest abundance were $C_{16:0}$, $C_{16:1}$, $C_{18:1}$, and $C_{18:2}$, with considerable variation, depending on the plant part. Thus, shoots were especially rich in $C_{16:0}$, while scutellum was very rich in $C_{18:2}$. The main monounsaturated fatty acids of shoot were palmitoleic ($C_{16:1}$) and oleic ($C_{18:1}$), appearing in esters principally of cholesterol, sitosterol, and stigmasterol. In root, scutellum, and endosperm, the main monounsaturated fatty acid was oleate ($C_{18:1}$), appearing principally in esters of sitosterol and its epimeric 24-

methyl homologs. The scutellum and endosperm together contained 80% of the steryl ester in the seedling, which was mainly sitosteryl linoleate ($C_{18:2}$). Cholesteryl ester fraction of the mixture was greatest in the shoot. For greater detail, the original paper, which has a wealth of information, should be consulted. In a subsequent study by Nordby and Nagy (525), of three or four varieties each in four species of *Citrus* (orange, grapefruit, lemon, and lime), the major acid in the juice sac lipid was linoleic, varying from 10% to 56% of the total acid in esters. Other important ones were $C_{16:0}$, $C_{16:1}$, $C_{18:1}$, and $C_{18:2}$. The exact relative amounts were species dependent. Fatty acids of longer chains were also present. In all citrus varieties, C_{24} was the most prominent of these longer chain acids, and they were found primarily in sterols retaining nuclear methyl groups. Work in the laboratory of Nicholas (516) showed that 4,4,14-trimethylsteryl esters underwent only slight conversion to 4-desmethylsterols, while the free alcohols of the trimethylsterols showed pronounced turnover, presumed to be to the desmethylsterols. This suggests that esters do not function as intermediates, but rather in some other capacity, probably as a reserve for fatty acids or sterols or both.

Kemp and Mercer (526) have studied the sterol and steryl ester compostion of subcellular organelles of corn (*Zea mays*) shoots. Only 1% of the steroid isolated from organelles was esterified, and the nuclear fraction had the most ester, and the microsomal fraction the least. The microsomal and mitochondrial fractions contained the bulk of the sterols, and they lacked methyl groups at C-4 and C-14. Esters of linoleic acid were more abundant in microsomal and mitochondrial fractions than in the nucleus and chloroplast. In all four organelles, stigmasterol and the homologous series of cholesterol and its 24-methyl and 24-ethyl derivatives were present in the ester fraction as well as the free alcohol fraction (Table 10.19), but two notable phenomena were observed. The proportion of cholesterol in the ester fraction of all four organelles was much higher than that in the free alcohols. In the nucleus, it constituted 90% of the steryl esters, 53% in the chloroplast, and about a third of the other two organelles. Second, the nucleus was unusually rich in free cholesterol, which comprised 22% of the mixture, compared to 1-2% in the other three organelles. Cholesterol and its esters thus seem to play a special nuclear role, and its esters may play some role distinct from that of other sterols in other organelles as well. Brandt and Benveniste (527), using bean leaves (*Phaseolus vulgaris*), also have observed a high percentage of cholesterol (and isofucosterol) in the ester fraction of various subcellular organelles. They noted further a relatively low level of stigmasterol. The same sterols found in the leaf as a whole were found in the subcellular organelles, but their relative amounts varied. The most dramatic difference was in chloroplasts and mitochondria, where cholesterol was a quarter of the sterols, compared to 1% of the leaf as a whole.

Steryl glycosides and their acylated (on the sugar) derivatives have

Table 10.18. Sterols of pollen

Plant	Sterol (Nomenclature Base: Cholesterol)						
	24-H	24-CH$_3$	24-C$_2$H$_5$	Δ^{22}-24-C$_2$H$_5$	24-CH$_2$	24-CHCH$_3$	Ref.
Elaeis guineensis (Oil palm)							
Free sterol	2	25	14	—	—	56	528
Esterified sterol	11	11	37	6	—	35	527
Trifolium pratense (Red clover)	3	6	3	6	82	6	527
Carneigiea gigantee (Saguaro cactus)	Trace	6	Trace	Trace	94	Trace	527
Brassica nigra (Mustard)	9	15	7	32	37	32	527
Sisymbrium irio (London-rocket)	15	12	18	12	37	12	527
Secale cereale (Rye)	7	17	13	15	49	15	527
Phleum pratense (Timothy)	3	13	13	10	62	10	527
Zea mays (Corn)	5	13	9	9	65	9	527
Baccharis viminea (Mule fat)	Trace	11	74	11	4	11	527
Juniperus utahensis	16	17	50	11	7	11	527
Polygonum sp. (Heartsease)	21	8	29	17	21	17	527

Hydrophyllum capitatum (Waterleaf)	4	16	39	26	15	26	527
Pinus sylvestris (Scotch pine)	7	14	54	16	9	16	527
Pino mugo			65				527
Alnus glutinosa (European alder)	2.5	11	64	17	6	17	527
Populus nigra (Lombardy popular)	15	15	61	6	3	6	527
Populus fremontii (Cottonwood)	59	7	15	5	6	5	527
Hypochaeris radicata (Cat's ear)	90						527
Malus sylvestris (Apple)					60		527
Salix sp. (Willow)					50		527
Calluna vulgaris (Heather)				80			527
Taraxacum officinale (Dandelion)			38				527
Aesculus hippocastanum (Sweet chestnut)			74				527
Corylus avellana (Hazel)			75				527
Helianthus annus (Sunflower)			42				527

Table 10.19. Subcellular distribution of sterols and their esters in *Zea mays*

| | Percent Composition of Mixture of Cholesterol and Derivatives[a] | | | | | | | |
| | Free Alcohol | | | | Ester | | | |
Organelle	24-H	24-CH$_3$	24-C$_2$H$_5$	Δ^{22}-24-C$_2$H$_5$	24-H	24-CH$_3$	24-C$_2$H$_5$	Δ^{22}-24-C$_2$H$_5$
Nuclei	22	9	51	18	90	1	8	1
Chloroplasts	2	13	59	26	53	10	36	3
Mitochondria	1	12	61	26	35	11	48	9
Microsomes	1	12	60	27	32	9	52	8

[a]From Kemp and Mercer (526).

been isolated from a number of Tracheophytes as well as from other organisms. They are thought to be of very wide occurrence. Their existence has been known for more than half a century, but only recently has interest in them been substantial. While glycosides of the sterols retaining nuclear methyl groups have not been isolated, cholesterol and its 24-methyl and 24-ethyl derivatives, as well as stigmasterol, spinasterol, and other 4-desmethylsterols, are known in glycosidic form (528-543). Usually the sugar is glucose (Scheme 10.12), but the mannosides (541), galactosides

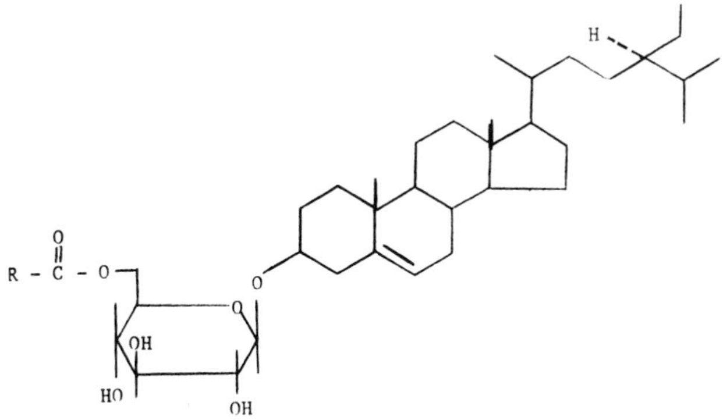

Scheme 10.12. Structure of sitosteryl-β-D-(6-O-fattyacyl)-glucopyranoside.

(539), and gentiobiosides (543) are also known. The glucosides frequently also are acylated at the primary alcoholic group of C-6 of the sugar. The glycosides usually occur as mixtures that more or less reflect the structures of the dominant sterols. Thus, if sitosterol is the major sterol, sitosteryl glycoside is the major glycoside occurring together with glycosides of the minor sterols, or if spinasterol is the major sterol, its glycoside is found. An example is with whole tissues of corn (540), soybean (542), and sorghum (436), as shown in Table 10.20, which should be compared with Tables 10.9 and 10.10 on the total sterols. However, strong enrichment of cholesteryl glycoside occurs in the pellet from centrifugation at 25,000 × g of Pisum sativum (534). The fatty acid composition of the acyl moiety is much like that of steryl esters. Palmitic, stearic, oleic, linoleic, and linolenic are usually the main constituents. Examples of analytical values are shown in Table 10.21. Biosynthesis occurs in subcellular particles. The sugar substrate is its uridine diphosphate, and UDP-glucose glucosyltransferase catalyzing coupling to the sterol is (in Pisum sativum seedlings) concentrated in axis tissue, where its highest activity is found in the fraction sedimenting between 13,000 and 25,000 × g (534). The enzyme has been solubilized with Triton X-100 from cotton seeds and fibers, purified, and its properties studied in detail (544). It was highly specific for UDP-glucose,

Table 10.20. Sterol composition of fatty acyl glycosides

Plant	24-H	24-CH$_3$	24-C$_2$H$_5$	Δ^{22}-24-C$_2$H$_5$
		% of Mixture (Nomenclature Base: Cholesterol)		
Zea mays	—	26	69	5
Glycine max	—	20	51	29
Sorghum vulgare	7	23	60	11

From Aneja and Harries (*540*), Kiribuchi et al. (*539*) and Palmer and Bowden (*436*).

Table 10.21. Fatty acid composition of the acyl portion of steryl glucosides

Plant	16:0	16:1	18:0	18:1	18:2	18:3
	% Composition by Chain Length and Double Bonds					
Corn	71	—	4	12	12	1
Soybean	38	1	8	12	39	3
Potato tuber	51	2	9	1	24	5

Adapted from Aneja and Harries (*540*).

showing only slight activity (18% or less) with ADP-glucose, GDP-glucose, CDP-glucose, TDP-glucose, or the UDP derivatives of galactose and mannose. However, it was relatively unspecific toward cholesterol, sitosterol, and stigmasterol, all being glycosylated at rates varying less than a factor of two. A quantitative comparison of free sterols, their esters, and their glycosides in *Sorghum vulgare* reveals 86% of the sterols are present as free alcohols, 13% as esters, and 1% as glycosides (*436*).

Gibberellic acid has been found to increase the specific and total activities of MVA kinase in embryonic axes of germinating *Corylus avellana* seeds (*545*). This is accompanied by increased biosynthesis of sterols and their esters in the axes but not in the cotyledons (*546*). Young growing tissues of *Phaseolus aureus* (Mung bean) contained more sterols than older tissues, and with age there was an increasing proportion of stigmasterol (*547*). In the Mung bean, naphthalene acetic acid (NAA) stimulated sterol biosynthesis in both wounded surfaces and intact tissues (*548*). Increased sterol content induced by NAA occurred primarily in the zone of growth associated with elongation (*549*).

In the early phases (24 hr) of germination of either gymnosperms (*550*) or angiosperms (*551*) the rate of formation of squalene is much faster than the rate of the hydrocarbon's metabolism. With subsequent development (several days) of the embryo, metabolic enzymes become active. These phenomena are reflected in the fate of label from [2-^{14}C]MVA. During the first day of germination most of the label appears in squalene and very little in cyclized products, but later the reverse is true. It has been pointed out (550, 551) that, because the formation of squalene is anaerobic and its metabolism to sterols, etc., is aerobic, the developmental change, which is independent of whether or not β-amyrin or sterols constitute the cyclized product, may constitute an evolutionary recapitulation of phylogeny.

In summary, Tracheophytes are unique among living things in having in most cases the homologous 24α-ethyl- and 24α-methylcholesterols often accompanied by cholesterol itself. The amounts of these three sterols are such that they parallel the size of the substituent at C-24 ($C_2 > C_1 > H$). The 24α-ethyl component often is split into the sterols with (stigmasterol) and without (sitosterol) a trans-Δ^{22}-bond. While the 24α-methyl component (campesterol) is not split in this way, the 24β-methyl component (dihydrobrassicasterol) is, on rare occasions (some Cruciferae species). Intermediate Δ^7-, $\Delta^{24(28)}$-, and, more rarely, $\Delta^{5,7}$-, and $\Delta^{8,14}$-sterols can be present in significant amounts, and in some cases one or more become dominant, as in the Cucurbitaceae and Theaceae, when Δ^7-sterols replace Δ^5-sterols. Less frequently, mature plants with only 24β-ethylsterols (usually retaining a $\Delta^{25(27)}$-bond) are found, and in one family (Cucurbitaceae) the seeds have 24β-ethylsterols and develop into plants with 24α-ethylsterols. These and other facts suggest an evolutionary development toward Δ^5-24α-ethylsterols that is crowned by sitosterol. Sterols occur in vascular plants both as the free alcohols and as esters composed usually from the fatty acids. The sterols found in the ester fraction are the same as in the free alcohol fraction, but the ester fraction has more cholesterol in it. Sterols also occur as glycosides, commonly of glucose, but also of other sugars. The glycosides (usually as fatty acid esters at C-6 of the sugar) reflect the structures of the dominant sterols. No glycosides are known in which methyl groups occur at C-4 or C-14. Sterols have been found in subcellular organelles, and some work has been done on other subjects, such as translocation. Except for pollen, where $\Delta^{24(28)}$-sterols are frequently dominant (explaining their occurrence in bees), there is no striking tissue specialization. The composition of the sterol mixture, for instance, in roots, leaves, fruits, and seeds has little variance in a given plant except for certain cases. If there is a functional difference in the various sterols, it presumably is manifested at the subcellular level, where more work would be fruitful. A large variety of sterols retaining one or more of the methyl groups at C-4 and C-14 occur in small amounts, and many of them have additional oxygen atoms. Some, lacking extra oxygenation, such as methylenecycloartanol, cyclolaudenol, and obtusifoliol, play a role as intermediates between cycloartenol and the dominant sterols. The function of others is obscure, although the ones with the Δ^7-6-keto moieties found in the ecdysones may play a role in defense against insects.

LITERATURE CITED

1. P. R. Rao and J. W. Beard, Natl. Cancer Inst. Monogr. 17:673 (1964).
2. L. H. Frommhagen, C. A. Knight, and N. K. Freeman, Virology 8:176 (1959).
3. H. B. White, Jr., S. S. Powell, L. G. Gafford, and C. C. Randall, J. Biol. Chem. 243:4517 (1968).
4. R. M. Franklin, in E. Berger and J. L. Melnick (eds.), Progress in Medical Virology. Vol. 4. Hafner, New York, 1962. p. 1.
5.′ P. L. Smith, The Biology of Mycoplasmas. Academic Press, New York, 1971.
6. D. G. H. Edward and E. A. Freundt, J. Gen. Microbiol. 62:1-2 (1970).
7. H. von Behring, Hoppe-Seyler's Z. Physiol. Chem. 192:112 (1930).
8. A. Hammerschlag, Monatsh. Chem. 10:9 (1889).
9. H. Dam, Biochem. J. 28:820 (1934).
10. (a) A. Snog-Kjaer, I. Prange, and H. Dam, Experientia 11:316 (1955); (b) A. Snog-Kjaer, I. Prange, and H. Dam, J. Gen. Microbiol. 14:256 (1956); (c) R. S. Rosenfeld and L. Hellman, J. Lipid Res. 12:192 (1971).
11. (a) G. Parmentier and H. Eyssen, Biochim. Biophys. Acta 348:279 (1974); (b) I. Bjorkhem and J. A. Gustafsson, Eur. J. Biochem. 21:428 (1971).
12. K. Schubert, G. Rose, R. Tümmler, and N. Ikekawa, Hoppe-Seyler's Z. Physiol. Chem. 339:293 (1964).
13. K. Schubert, G. Rose, and C. Hörhold, Biochim. Biophys. Acta 137:168 (1967).
14. K. Schubert, G. Rose, H. Wachtel, C. Hörhold, and N. Ikekawa, Eur. J. Biochem. 5:246 (1968).
15. R. H. Siefferd and R. J. Anderson, Hoppe-Seyler's Z. Physiol. Chem. 239:270 (1936).
16. S. Dauchy, F. Kayser, and J. Villoutreix, Compt. Rend. Soc. Biol. 150:1974 (1956).
17. S. Dauchy, and F. Kayser, Bull. Soc. Chim. Biol. 40:1533 (1958).
18. C. W. Bird, J. M. Lynch, F. J. Pirt, W. W. Reid, C. J. W. Brooks, and B. S. Middleditch, Nature 230:473 (1971).
19. A. Van Dorsselaer, A. Ensminger, C. Spyckerelle, M. Dastillung, O. Sieskind, P. Arpino, P. Albrecht, G. Ourisson, P. W. Brooks, S. J. Gaskell, B. J. Kimble, R. P. Philip, J. R. Maxwell, and G. Eglington, Tetrahedron Lett. 1349 (1974).
20. C. Anding, M. Rohmer, and G. Ourisson, J. Am. Chem. Soc. 98:1274 (1976).
21. A. Fiertel and H. P. Klein, J. Bacteriol. 78:738 (1959).
22. (a) T. G. Tornabene, M. Kates, E. Gelpi, and J. Oro, J. Lipid Res. 10:294 (1969); (b) J. K. G. Kramer, S. C. Kushwaha, and M. Kates, Biochim. Biophys. Acta 270:103 (1972).
23. G. Suzue, K. Tsukada, C. Nakai, and S. Tanaka, Arch. Biochem. Biophys. 123:644 (1968).
24. J. Han and M. Calvin, Proc. Natl. Acad. Sci. U.S.A. 64:436 (1969).
25. R. L. Conner and W. J. Van Wagtendonk, J. Gen. Microbiol. 12:31 (1955).
26. A. T. Soldo and W. J. Van Wagtendonk, J. Protozool. 14:596 (1967).
27. R. L. Conner, J. R. Landrey, E. S. Kaneshiro, and W. J. Van Wagtendonk, Biochim. Biophys. Acta 239:312 (1971).
28. G. G. Holz, J. A. Erwin, and B. Wagner, J. Protozool. 8:297 (1961).
29. G. G. Holz, B. Wagner, J. Erwin, J. J. Britt, and K. Bloch, Comp. Biochem. Physiol. 2:202 (1961).

30. G. G. Holz, J. Erwin, B. Wagner, and N. Rosenbaum, J. Protozool. 9:359 (1962).
31. R. L. Conner, F. B. Mallory, J. R. Landrey, and C. W.L. Iyengar, J. Biol. Chem. 244:2325 (1969).
32. F. B. Mallory and R. L. Conner, Lipids 6:149 (1971).
33. W. R. Nes, P. A. G. Malya, F. B. Mallory, K. A. Ferguson, J. R. Landrey, and R. L. Conner, J. Biol. Chem. 246:561 (1971).
34. W. R. Nes, A. Alcaide, J. R. Landrey, F. B. Mallory, and R. L. Conner, Lipids 10:140 (1975).
35. W. R. Nes, K. Krevitz, S. Behzadan, G. W. Patterson, J. R. Landrey, and R. L. Conner, Biochem. Biophys. Res. Commun. 66:1462 (1975).
36. A. S. Beedle, P. J. Pettler, H. H. Rees, and T. W. Goodwin, FEBS Lett. 55:88 (1975).
37. F. B. Mallory, J. T. Gordon, and R. L. Conner, J. Am. Chem. Soc. 85:1362 (1963).
38. Y. Tsuda, A. Morimoto, T. Sano, Y. Inubushi, F. B. Mallory, and J. T. Gordon, Tetrahedron Lett. 1427 (1965).
39. J. T. Gordon and T. H. Doyne, Acta Cryst. 21(Suppl.):A-113 (1966).
40. F. B. Mallory, R. L. Conner, J. R. Landrey, J. M. Zander, J. B. Greig, and E. Caspi, J. Am. Chem. Soc. 90:3563 (1968).
41. E. Caspi, J. M. Zander, J. B. Greig, F. B. Mallory, R. L. Conner, and J. R. Landrey, J. Am. Chem. Soc. 90:3563 (1968).
42. E. Caspi, J. B. Greig, and J. M. Zander, Biochem. J. 109:931 (1968).
43. R. L. Conner and F. Ungar, Exp. Cell Res. 36:134 (1964).
44. M. S. Shorb, B. E. Dunlap, and W. O. Pollard, Proc. Soc. Exp. Biol. Med. 118:1140 (1965).
45. R. L. Conner, J. R. Landrey, C. H. Burns, and F. B. Mallory, J. Protozool. 15:600 (1968).
46. W. R. Nes, Lipids 9:596 (1974).
47. (a) H. Dixon, C. D. Ginger, and J. Williamson, Comp. Biochem. Physiol. 41B:1 (1972); (b) T. von Brand, P. McMahon, E. J. Tobie, M. J. Thompson, and E. Mosettig, Exp. Parasitol. 8:171 (1959); (c) S. Halevy, L. Avivi, and H. Katan, J. Protozool. 13:480 (1966).
48. (a) E. Heftmann, B. E. Wright, and G. Liddel, Arch. Biochem. Biophys. 91:266 (1960); (b) E. Lederer, Quart. Rev. Chem. 453 (1969).
49. J. D. Weete, Phytochemistry 12:1843 (1973).
50. J. D. Weete, Fungal Lipid Biochemistry. Plenum, New York, 1974.
51. J. W. Hendrix, Mycologia 58:307 (1966).
52. C. G. Elliott, M. R. Hendrie, B. A. Knights, and W. Parker, Nature 203:427 (1964).
53. R. H. Haskins, A. P. Tulloch, and R. G. Micetoch, Can. J. Microbiol. 10: 187 (1964).
54. J. W. Hendrix, Science 144:1028 (1964).
55. J. A. Leal, J. Friend, and P. Holliday, Nature 203:545 (1964).
56. W. N. Harnish, L. A. Berg, and V. G. Lilly, Phytopathology 54:895 (1964).
57. J. W. Hendrix, Phytopathology 55:790 (1965).
58. C. G. Elliott, M. R. Hendrie, and B. A. Knights, J. Gen. Microbiol. 42:425 (1966).
59. C. G. Elliott, J. Gen. Microbiol. 51:137 (1968).
60. E. Schlosser and D. Gottlieb, Arch. Microbiol. 61:246 (1968).
61. B. A. Knights, Phytochemistry 9:70 (1970).
62. J. H. Adler, M. Young, and W. R. Nes, Lipids, in press.
63. R. B. Holtz and L. C. Schisler, Lipids 7:251 (1972).

64. (a) L. I. Strigina, Y. N. Elkin, and G. B. Elyakou, Phytochemistry 10:2361 (1971); (b) G. R. Pettit and J. C. Knight, J. Org. Chem. 27:2696 (1962).
65. (a) J. D. Weete and J. L. Laseter, Lipids 9:575 (1974); (b) J. Alais, A. Lablache-Combier, L. Lacoste, and G. Vidal, Phytochemistry 15:49 (1976).
66. Y. S. Chen and R. H. Haskins, Can. J. Chem. 41:1647 (1963).
67. M. J. Vacheron and G. Michel, Phytochemistry 7:1645 (1968).
68. F. Blank, F. E. Shorland, and G. Just, J. Invest. Dermatol. 39:91 (1962).
69. G. A. Bean, G. W. Patterson, and J. J. Motta, Comp. Biochem. Physiol. 43B:935 (1973).
70. N. J. McCorkindale, S. A. Hutchinson, B. A. Pursey, W. J. Scott, and R. Wheeler, Phytochemistry 8:861 (1969).
71. L. L. Jackson and D. S. Frear, Phytochemistry 7:654 (1968).
72. R. T. van Aller, H. Chikamatsu, N. J. de Souza, J. P. John, and W. R. Nes, Biochem. Biophys. Res. Commun. 31:842 (1968).
73. K. Hunter and A. H. Rose, Biochim. Biophys. Acta 260:639 (1972).
74. O. N. Brewik, J. L. Owades, and R. F. Light, J. Org. Chem. 19:1734 (1954).
75. K. Petzoldt, M. Kühne, E. Blanke, K. Kieslich, and E. Kasper, Justus Liebigs Ann. Chem. 709:203 (1967).
76. W. R. Nes, J. H. Adler, and B. Sekula, unpublished observations.
77. (a) G. Goulston, E. I. Mercer, and L. J. Goad, Phytochemistry 14:457 (1975); (b) E. I. Mercer and D. J. R. Carrier, Phytochemistry 15:283 (1976).
78. H. K. Lin, R. J. Langenbach, and H. W. Knoche, Phytochemistry 11:2319 (1972).
79. G. Ourisson, P. Crabbe, and O. Rodig, Tetracyclic Triterpenes. Holden-Day, San Francisco, 1964. pp. 147-150.
80. C. G. Anderson and W. W. Epstein, Phytochemistry 10:2713 (1971).
81. M. J. Kulshreshtha, D. K. Kulshreshtha, and R. P. Rastogi, Phytochemistry 11:2369 (1972).
82. N. Entwistle and A. D. Pratt, Tetrahedron 25:1449 (1969).
83. A. W. Barksdale, T. C. McMorris, R. Seshadri, T. Arunachalam, J. A. Edwards, J. Sundeen, and D. M. Green, J. Gen. Microbiol. 82:297 (1974).
84. A. W. Barksdale, Science 166:831 (1969).
85. M. Henze, Hoppe-Seyler's Z. Physiol. Chem. 41:109 (1904).
86. C. Dorée, Biochem. J. 4:72 (1909).
87. W. Bergmann, J. Marine Res. 8:137 (1949).
88. W. Bergmann, in M. Florkin and H. S. Mason (eds.), Comparative Biochemistry. Academic Press, New York, 1962. pp. 103-162.
89. W. Bergmann, D. H. Gould, and E. M. Low, J. Org. Chem. 10:570 (1945).
90. F. R. Valentine and W. Bergmann, J. Org. Chem. 6:452 (1941).
91. W. R. Nes, K. Krevitz, and S. Behzadan, Lipids 11:118 (1976).
92. T. R. Erdman and R. H. Thomson, Tetrahedron 28:5163 (1972).
93. E. Fattorusso, S. Magno, C. Santacroce, and D. Sica, Gazz. Chim. Ital. 104:409 (1974).
94. (a) L. Minale and G. Sodano, J. Chem. Soc. Perkin I:1888 (1974); (b) L. Minale and G. Sodano, J. Chem. Soc. Perkin I:2380 (1974); (c) Y. M. Sheikh and C. Djerassi, Tetrahedron 30:4095 (1974); (d) P. DeLuca, M. DeRosa, L. Minale, and G. Sodano, J. Chem. Soc. Perkin I:2132 (1972).
95. (a) M. DeRosa, L. Minale, and G. Sodano, Comp. Biochem. Physiol. 45B: 883 (1973); (b) M. J. Walton and J. F. Pennock, Biochem. J. 127:471 (1972).
96. (a) W. Bergmann, R. J. Feeney, and A. N. Swift, J. Org. Chem. 16:1337

(1951); (*b*) W. Bergmann and J. P. Dusza, Liebig's Ann. Chem. 603:36 (1957).

97. Y. Toyama and T. Takagi, Mem. Fac. Eng. Nagoya Univ. 7:156 (1955).
98. W. Bergmann, M. J. McLean, and D. Lester, J. Org. Chem. 8:271 (1943).
99. L. S. Ciereszko, M. A. Johnson, R. W. Schmidt, and C. B. Koons, Comp. Biochem. Physiol. 24:899 (1968).
100. N. C. Ling, R. Hale, and C. Djerassi, J. Am. Chem. Soc. 92:5281 (1970).
101. (*a*) F. J. Schmitz and T. Pattabhiraman, J. Am. Chem. Soc. 92:6073 (1970); (*b*) E. L. Enwall, D. Van der Helm, I. N. Hsu, T. Pattabhiraman, F. J. Schmitz, R. L. Spraggins, and A. J. Weinheimer, J. Chem. Soc. Chem. Commun. 215 (1972).
102. J. H. Block, Steroids 23:421 (1974).
103. F. Haurowitz and H. Waelsch, Liebig's Ann. Chem. 161:300 (1926).
104. R. E. Middlebrook and C. E. Lane, Comp. Biochem. Physiol. 24:507 (1964).
105. H. E. Van Aarem, H. Vonk, and D. I. Zandee, Arch. Int. Physiol. Biochim. 72:606 (1964).
106. S. Yasuda, Comb. Biochem. Physiol. 48B:225 (1974).
107. K. C. Gupta and P. J. Scheuer, Steroids 13:343 (1969).
108. J. P. Engelbrecht, B. Tursch, and C. Djerassi, Steroids 20:121 (1972).
109. P. A. Voogt, J. M. Van De Ruit, and J. W. A. Van Rheenen, Comp. Biochem. Physiol. 48B:47 (1974).
110. (*a*) J. P. Ferezou, M. Devys, and M. Barbier, Experientia 28:407 (1972); (*b*) J. P. Ferezou, M. Devys, and M. Barbier, Experientia 28:153 (1972).
111. T. van Brand, Z. Vergleich Physiol. 8:613 (1928).
112. E. S. Faust and T. W. Tallquist, Arch. Exp. Pathol. Pharmakol., Naunym-Schmiedeberg's 57:367 (1907).
113. L. F. Salisbury and R. J. Anderson, J. Biol. Chem. 129:505 (1939).
114. S. Cmelick and Z. Bartl, Hoppe-Seyler's Z. Physiol. Chem. 305:170 (1956).
115. G. J. Frayha, Comp. Biochem. Physiol. 39B:167 (1971).
116. G. J. Frayha, Comp. Biochem. Physiol. 49B:93 (1974).
117. G. J. Frayha, Comp. Biochem. Physiol. 27:875 (1968).
118. G. A. Digenis, R. E. Thorson, and A. Konyalian, J. Pharm. Sci. 59:676 (1970).
119. G. J. Frayha and D. Fairbairn, Comp. Biochem. Physiol. 28:1115 (1969).
120. G. J. Frayha and D. Fairbairn, J. Parasit. 54:1144 (1968).
121. T. M. Smith, T. J. Brooks, and V. G. Lockard, Lipids 5:854 (1970).
122. D. Fairbairn and R. N. Jones, Can. J. Chem. 34:182 (1956).
123. R. J. Cole and L. R. Krusberg, Comp. Biochem. Physiol. 21:109 (1967).
124. W. F. Hieb and M. Rothstein, Science 160:778 (1968).
125. M. Rothstein, Comp. Biochem. Physiol. 21:109 (1967).
126. J. D. Willett and W. L. Downey, Biochem. J. 138:233 (1974).
127. J. D. Willett and W. L. Downey, Comp. Biochem. Physiol. 45B:139 (1973).
128. R. I. Bolla, P. P. Weinstein, and C. Law, Comp. Biochem. Physiol. 43B:487 (1972).
129. S. R. Dutky, W. E. Robbins, and J. V. Thompson, Nematologica 13:140 (1967).
130. R. J. Cole and S. R. Dutky, J. Nematol. 1:72 (1969).
131. W. F. Hieb, E. L. R. Stokstad, and M. Rothstein, Science 168:143 (1970).
132. (*a*) J. A. Wooton and L. D. Wright, Comp. Biochem. Physiol. 5:253 (1962); (*b*) P. A. Voogt, J. W. A. Van Rheenen, and D. I. Zandee, Comp. Biochem. Physiol. 50B:511 (1975).

133. F. Bock and F. Wetler, Hoppe-Seyler's Z. Physiol. 256:33 (1938).
134. Y. Naya and M. Kotake, Bull. Chem. Soc. Japan 40:880 (1967).
135. M. Kobayashi and H. Mitsuhashi, Steroids 24:399 (1974).
136. A. J. Clark and K. Bloch, J. Biol. Chem. 234:2578 (1959).
137. H. Lipke and G. Fraenkel, Annual Review of Entomology, 1. Annual Reviews, Inc., Palo Alto, Calif., 1956. p. 17.
138. R. B. Clayton, J. Biol. Chem. 235:3421 (1960).
139. R. B. Clayton, A. M. Edwards, and K. Bloch, Nature 195:1125 (1962).
140. J. N. Kaplanis, W. E. Robbins, H. E. Vroman, and B. M. Bryce, Steroids 2:547 (1963).
141. D. I. Zandee, Nature 195:815 (1962).
142. D. I. Zandee, Archs. Int. Physiol. Biochim. 74:435 (1966).
143. D. I. Zandee, Comp. Biochem. Physiol. 20:811 (1967).
144. S. I. Teshima and A. Kanazawa, Comp. Biochem. Physiol. 38B:597 (1971).
145. A. Van Den Ord, Comp. Biochem. Physiol. 13:461 (1964).
146. J. Lewkowitsch, Z. Unfersuch. Nahr. U. Genussm 13:552 (1907).
147. M. Tsujimoto, J. Coll. Eng. Tokyo Imp. Univ. 4:63 (1908).
148. T. Menozzi and A. Moreschi, Atti. Acad. Nazl. Lincei, Rend. Classe, Sci. Fis. Mat. Nat. 19:126 (1910).
149. W. Bergmann, J. Biol. Chem. 107:527 (1934).
150. H. Wieland and A. Kotzschmar, Liebig's Ann. Chem. 530:152 (1937).
151. J. L. Noland, Arch. Biochem. Biophys. 52:323 (1954).
152. E. D. Bergmann and Z. H. Levinson, Nature 182:723 (1958).
153. A. J. Clark and K. Bloch, J. Biol. Chem. 234:2589 (1959).
154. W. E. Robbins, R. C. Dutky, R. E. Monroe, and J. N. Kaplanis, Ann. Entomol. Soc. Amer. 55:102 (1962).
155. F. J. Ritter and W. H. J. M. Wientjens, TNO Nieuws 22:381 (1967).
156. N. Ikekawa, M. Suzuki, M. Kobayashi, and K. Tsuda, Chem. Pharm. Bull. 14:834 (1966).
157. M. J. Thompson, J. N. Kaplanis, W. E. Robbins, and J. A. Svoboda, in R. Paoletti and D. Kritchevsky (eds.), Advances in Lipid Research. Vol. II. Academic Press, New York, 1973. pp. 219-265.
158. J. A. Svoboda and W. E. Robbins, Science 156:1637 (1967).
159. M. J. Thompson, S. J. Louloudes, W. E. Robbins, J. A. Waters, J. A. Steele, and E. Mosettig, Biochem. Biophys. Res. Commun. 9:113 (1962).
160. M. Barbier and D. Bogdanovsky, Comp. Acad. Sci. Paris 252:3497 (1961).
161. J. Pain, M. Barbier, D. Bogdanovsky, and E. Lederer, Comp. Biochem. Physiol. 6:233 (1962).
162. W. H. Brown and E. E. Felauer, Nature 190:88 (1961).
163. P. T. Russell and W. R. Nes, J. Miss. Acad. Sci. 11:49 (1965).
164. M. Barbier, M. F. Hügel, and E. Lederer, Bull. Soc. Chim. Biol. 42:91 (1960).
165. M. Barbier, Ann. Abeille 9:243 (1966).
166. K. Ubik and J. Vrkoc, Insect. Biochem. 4:281 (1974).
167. H. J. Veith, M. Barbier, J. Pain, and B. Roger, Comp. Biochem. Physiol. 47B:459 (1974).
168. K. G. Goodnight, and H. W. Kircher, Lipids 6:166 (1971).
169. W. B. Heed and H. W. Kircher, Science 149:758 (1965).
170. H. M. Chu, D. M. Norris, and L. T. Kok, J. Insect Physiol. 16:1379 (1970).
171. C. Djerassi, G. W. Krakower, A. J. Lemin, L. H. Liu, J. S. Mills, and R. Villetti, J. Am. Chem. Soc. 80:6284 (1958).
172. D. R. Idler, P. M. Wiseman, and L. M. Safe, Steroids 16:451 (1970).
173. D. R. Idler, L. M. Safe, and E. F. MacDonald, Steroids 18:545 (1971).

174. G. W. Patterson, M. W. Khalil, and D. R. Idler, J. Chromat. 115:153 (1975).
175. D. R. Idler, M. W. Khalil, J. D. Gilbert, and C. J. W. Brooks, Steroids 27:155 (1976).
176. J. Viala, M. Devys, and M. Barbier, Bull. Soc. Chim. Fr. 3626 (1972).
177. M. Kobayashi and H. Mitsuhashi, Steroids 26:605 (1975).
178. S. I. Teshima, A. Kanazawa, and T. Ando, Comp. Biochem. Physiol. 47B: 507 (1974).
179. P. A. Voogt, Comp. Biochem. Physiol. 31:37 (1969).
180. P. A. Voogt, Ph.D. Dissertation, University of Utrecht, Holland, 1970.
181. P. A. Voogt, Comp. Biochem. Physiol. 39B:139 (1971).
182. P. A. Voogt and D. J. Van Der Horst, Arch. Int. Physiol. Biochim. 80:293 (1972).
183. P. A. Voogt, Comp. Biochem. Physiol. 50B:505 (1975).
184. P. A. Voogt, Comp. Biochem. Physiol. 50B:499 (1975).
185. S. I. Teshima and A. Kanazawa, Comp. Biochem. Physiol. 44B:881 (1973).
186. S. I. Teshima and A. Kanazawa, Comp. Biochem. Physiol. 47B:555 (1974).
187. U. H. M. Fagerlund and D. R. Idler, Can. J. Biochem. Physiol. 39:1347 (1961).
188. U. H. M. Fagerlund and D. R. Idler, Can. J. Biochem. Physiol. 39:505 (1961).
189. W. Bergmann and H. A. Stansbury, J. Org. Chem. 9:281 (1944).
190. A. Kossell and S. Edlbacher, Hoppe-Seyler's Z. Physiol. Chem. 94:264 (1915).
191. M. Kobayashi and H. Mitsuhashi, Tetrahedron 30:2147 (1974).
192. M. Kobayashi, R. Tsuru, K. Todo, and H. Mitsuhashi, Tetrahedron 29:1193 (1973).
193. M. Kobayashi, R. Tsuru, K. Todo, and H. Mitsuhashi, Tetrahedron Lett. 2935 (1972).
194. A. G. Smith, I. Rubinstein, and L. J. Goad, Biochem. J. 135:443 (1973).
195. L. J. Goad, I. Rubinstein, and A. G. Smith, Proc. Royal Soc. (London), Ser. B 180:223 (1972).
196. Y. M. Sheikh, M. Kaisin, and C. Djerassi, Steroids 22:835 (1973).
197. A. G. Smith and L. J. Goad, Biochem. J. 142:421 (1974).
198. (a) A. G. Smith and L. J. Goad, Biochem. J. 146:25 (1975); (b) A. G. Smith and L. J. Goad, Biochem. J. 123:671 (1971).
199. S. I. Teshima and A. Kanazawa, Comp. Biochem. Physiol. 52B:437 (1975).
200. P. A. Voogt, Int. J. Biochem. 4:42 (1973).
201. P. A. Voogt and J. Over, Comp. Biochem. Physiol. 45B:71 (1973).
202. A. G. Smith and L. J. Goad, Biochem. J. 146:35 (1975).
203. A. G. Smith, G. Goodfellow, and L. J. Goad, Biochem. J. 128:1371 (1972).
204. R. F. Nigrelli and S. Jakowska, Ann. N.Y. Acad. Sci. 90:884 (1960).
205. A. B. Turner, D. S. H. Smith, and A. M. Mackie, Nature 233:209 (1971).
206. T. Yasumoto, T. Watanabe, and Y. Hashimoto, Bull. Jap. Soc. Sci. Fisheries 30:357 (1964).
207. S. Ikegami, Y. Kamiya, and S. Tamura, Tetrahedron Lett. 3725 (1972).
208. S. Ikegami, Y. Kamiya, and S. Tamura, Agr. Biol. Chem. 36:1087 (1972).
209. H. I. Bolker, Nature 213:904 (1967).
210. G. A. Blondin, J. L. Scott, J. K. Hummer, B. D. Kulkarni, and W. R. Nes, Comp. Biochem. Physiol. 17:391 (1966).
211. S. C. Saxena and D. I. Zandee, Arch. Int. Physiol. Biochim. 77:673 (1969).
212. W. R. Nes, J. W. Cannon, N. S. Thampi, and P. A. G. Malya, J. Biol. Chem. 248:484 (1973).

213. (a) T. Takagi, T. Maeda, and Y. Toyama, Mem. Fac. Eng. Nagoya Univ. 8: 169 (1956); (b) A. Alcaide, J. Viala, F. Pinte, M. Itoh, T. Nomura, and M. Barbier, Compt. Rend. Acad. Sci. Paris 273, Ser C, 1386 (1971).
214. E. G. Gross and V. Deulofeu, J. Chem. Soc. Chem. Commun. 711 (1967).
215. M. J. Thompson, W. E. Robbins, and G. L. Baker, Steroids 2:505 (1963).
216. A. Windaus and O. Stange, Hoppe-Seyler's Z. Physiol. Chem. 244:218 (1936).
217. R. Schoenheimer, Hoppe-Seyler's Z. Physiol. Chem. 192:86 (1930).
218. (a) L. F. Fieser, J. Am. Chem. Soc. 73:5007 (1951); (b) L. F. Fieser, J. Am. Chem. Soc. 75:4395 (1953).
219. S. Shefer, S. Hauser, and E. H. Mosbach, J. Biol. Chem. 241:946 (1966).
220. S. Shefer, S. Hauser, and E. H. Mosbach, J. Lipid Res. 7:763 (1966).
221. I. Björkhem and K. E. Karlmar, Biochim. Biophys. Acta 337:129 (1974).
222. D. R. Idler and C. A. Baumann, J. Biol. Chem. 195:623 (1952).
223. W. M. Stokes, W. A. Fish, and F. C. Hickey, J. Biol. Chem. 220:415 (1956).
224. W. M. Stokes, W. A. Fish, and F. C. Hickey, J. Biol. Chem. 232:347 (1958).
225. E. Schulze, Ber. der Deutsch. Chem. Gessel. 5:1075 (1872).
226. J. C. Drummond and L. C. Baker, J. Soc. Chem. Ind. 48:232T (1929).
227. H. Windaus and R. Tschesche, Hoppe-Seyler's Z. Physiol. Chem. 190:51 (1930).
228. L. Ruzicka, E. Rey, and A. C. Muhr, Helv. Chim. Acta 27:472 (1944).
229. T. A. Miettinen, Ann. Clin. Res. 3:264 (1971).
230. J. E. van Lier and L. L. Smith, Biochemistry 6:3269 (1967).
231. C. J. W. Brooks, W. A. Harland, and G. Steel, Biochim. Biophys. Acta 125:620 (1966).
232. J. E. van Lier and L. L. Smith, Lipids 6:85 (1971).
233. A. Ercoli and P. de Ruggieri, J. Am. Chem. Soc. 75:3284 (1953).
234. W. Kline and W. M. Stokes, J. Chem. Soc. 1979 (1954).
235. N. Koizumi, M. Morisaki, N. Ikekawa, A. Suzuki, and T. Takeshita, Tetrahedron Lett. 2203 (1975).
236. Y. Y. Lin and L. L. Smith, Biochim. Biophys. Acta 348:189 (1974).
237. (a) G. Galli, E. Grossi-Paoletti, and J. F. Weiss, Science 162:1495 (1968); (b) J. F. Weiss, G. Galli, and E. Grossi-Paoletti, J. Neurochem. 15:563 (1968).
238. J. E. Van Lier and L. L. Smith, Texas Rept. Biol. Med. 27:168 (1969).
239. A. N. Davison and M. Wajda, J. Neurochem. 9:427 (1962).
240. J. McC. Howell, A. N. Davison, and J. Oxberry, Res. Vet. Sci. 5:376 (1964).
241. A. N. Davison, J. Dobbing, R. S. Morgan, and G. Wright, Lancet 1:658 (1959).
242. G. Brante, Acta Physiol. Scand., 18 (Suppl.):63 (1949).
243. R. T. Ramsey, R. T. Aexel, and H. J. Nicholas, J. Biol. Chem. 246:6393 (1971).
244. B. E. Gustafsson, J. A. Gustafsson, and J. Sjövall, Acta Chem. Scand. 20: 1827 (1966).
245. R. S. Rosenfeld and L. Hellman, J. Lipid Res. 12:192 (1971).
246. H. Eyssen and G. Parmentier, Am. J. Clin. Nutrition 27:1329 (1974).
247. G. Parmentier and H. Eyssen, Biochim. Biophys. Acta 348:279 (1974).
248. N. McIntyre, K. Kirsch, and K. J. Isselbacher, J. Lipid Res. 12:336 (1971).
249. B. A. Vela and H. F. Acevedo, J. Clin. Endocrinol. Med. 29:1251 (1969).
250. H. F. Acevedo and E. A. Campbell, Steroids 16:569 (1970).
251. E. Lederer and P. Kitchen, Bull. Soc. Chim. Biol. Paris 27:419 (1945).
252. N. Nicolaides, Science 186:19 (1974).
253. T. Nikkari, P. H. Schreibman, and E. H. Ahrens, J. Lipid Res. 15:563 (1974).

254. A. K. Bhattacharyya, W. E. Connor, and A. R. Spector, J. Clin. Invest. 51: 2060 (1972).
255. N. Nicolaides and S. Rothman, J. Invest. Derm. 24:125 (1955).
256. (a) D. R. Romsos, G. L. Allee, and G. A. Leveille, Proc. Soc. Exp. Biol. Med. 137:570 (1971); (b) J. Avigan, D. Steinberg, and M. Berman, J. Lipid Res. 3:216 (1962).
257. J. M. Dietschy and J. D. Wilson, N. Engl. J. Med. 282:1241 (1970).
258. D. Kritchevsky, Cholesterol. John Wiley, New York, 1958.
259. R. P. Cook, Cholesterol. Academic Press, New York, 1958. pp. 145-180.
260. A. N. Davison and M. Wajda, Nature (London) 183:1606 (1959).
261. M. Smith and L. Eng, J. Am. Oil Chem. Soc. 42:1013 (1965).
262. M. Cuzner, A. N. Davison, and A. Gregson, Ann. N.Y. Acad. Sci. 122:86 (1965).
263. M. Cuzner, A. N. Davison, and A. Gregson, Biochem. J. 101:618 (1966).
264. A. A. Kahn and J. P. Folch-Pi, J. Neurochem. 14:1099 (1967).
265. A. N. Davison, Adv. Lipid Res. 3:171 (1965).
266. J. J. Kabara, Prog. Brain Res. 40:363 (1973).
267. R. Paoletti, E. Grossi-Paoletti, and R. Fumagalli, in A. Lajtha (ed.), Handbook of Neurochemistry. Plenum Press, New York, 1969. pp. 195-221.
268. C. Serougne and F. Chevallier, Exp. Neurol. 44:1 (1974).
269. A. Keys, O. Mickelsen, E. V. O. Miller, E. R. Hayes, and R. L. Todd, J. Clin. Invest. 29:1347 (1950).
270. A. Keys, J. Gerontol. 7:201 (1952).
271. I. H. Page, E. Kirk, W. H. Lewis, W. R. Thompson, and D. D. Van Slyke, J. Biol. Chem. 111:613 (1935).
272. N. W. Barker, Ann. Int. Med. 132:685 (1939).
273. M. C. Roberts, Br. Vet. J. 130:xvi (1974).
274. D. Kritchevsky, Trans. N.Y. Acad. Sci. 32:821 (1970).
275. K. K. Carroll and R. M. G. Hamilton, Lipids 8:635 (1973).
276. G. V. Mann, G. Pearson, T. Gordon, and T. R. Dawber, Am. J. Clin. Nutrition 11:200 (1962).
277. A. Kagan, T. R. Dawber, W. B. Kannel, and N. Revotskie, Fed. Proc. 21, No. 4, Part II, Suppl. 11:52 (1962).
278. W. B. Kannel, W. P. Castelli, T. Gordon, and P. N. McNamara, Ann. Int. Med. 74:1 (1971).
279. E. Quintao, S. M. Grundy, and E. H. Ahrens, J. Lipid Res. 12:233 (1971).
280. A. Keys, O. Mickelsen, E. V. O. Miller, and C. B. Chapman, Science 112: 79 (1950).
281. C. Sylven and B. Bergstrom, J. Lipid Res. 10:169 (1969).
282. R. G. Gould, R. J. Jones, G. V. LeRoy, R. W. Wissler, and C. Bruce Taylor, Metabolism, 18:652 (1969).
283. G. Salen, E. H. Ahrens, and S. M. Grundy, J. Clin. Invest. 49:952 (1970).
284. C. G. Beames, H. H. Bailey, C. O. Rock, and L. M. Schanbacher, Comp. Biochem. Physiol. 47A:881 (1974).
285. M. C. Ritter and M. E. Dempsey, Biochem. Biophys. Res. Commun. 38: 921 (1970).
286. M. C. Ritter and M. E. Dempsey, J. Biol. Chem. 246:1536 (1971).
287. M. C. Ritter and M. E. Dempsey, Proc. Natl. Acad. Sci. U.S.A. 70:265 (1973).
288. T. J. Scallen, M. W. Schuster, and A. K. Dhar, J. Biol. Chem. 246:224 (1971).
289. M. E. Dempsey, Ann. Rev. Biochem. 43:983 (1974).
290. T. J. Scallen, M. V. Scrikantaiah, B. Seetharam, E. Hansbury, and K. Gavey, Fed. Proc. 33:1733 (1974).

291. M. A. Macheboeuf, Bull. Soc. Chim. Biol. Fr. 11:485 (1929).
292. V. P. Skipski, *in* G. J. Nelson (ed.), Blood Lipids and Lipoproteins: Quantitation, Composition, and Metabolism. Wiley-Interscience, New York, 1972. pp. 471–583.
293. R. G. Dennick, K. J. Worthington, D. R. Abramovich, and P. D. G. Dean, J. Neurochem. 22:1019 (1974).
294. (*a*) R. B. Ramsey and A. N. Davison, J. Lipid Res. 15:249 (1974); (*b*) P. Samuel, A. Schussheim, S. Liebermann, and E. Don, Pediatrics 54:222 (1974); (*c*) J. A. Story and D. Kritchevsky, Experientia 30:243 (1974).
295. R. D. Adler, A. L. Metzger, and S. M. Grundy, Gastroenterology 66:1212 (1974).
296. G. Salen, Ann. Intern. Med. 75:843 (1970).
297. G. Salen and S. M. Grundy, J. Clin. Invest. 52:2822 (1973).
298. G. Salen and A. Polito, J. Clin. Invest. 51:134 (1940).
299. (*a*) G. Galli, M. Galli-Kienle, F. Cattabeni, A. Fiecchi, E. Grossi-Paoletti, and R. Paoletti, *in* G. Weber (ed.), Advances in Enzyme Regulation. Vol. 8. Pergamon, New York, 1970. pp. 311–321; (*b*) R. Fumagalli, E. Grossi-Paoletti, and R. Paoletti, Ann. New York Acad. Sci. 472 (1969).
300. E. Grossi-Paoletti, C. R. Sirtori, J. F. Weiss, and R. Paoletti, Adv. Exp. Biol. Med. 4:457 (1968).
301. R. B. Ramsey and A. N. Davison, J. Lipid Res. 15:249 (1974).
302. G. H. Rothblatt, C. H. Burns, R. L. Conner, and J. R. Landrey, Science 169:880 (1970).
303. M. S. Brown, J. L. Goldstein, and M. D. Siperstein, Fed. Proc. 32:2168 (1983).
304. E. A. Day, G. T. Malcorn, and M. F. Beeler, Metab. Clin. Exp. 18:646 (1969).
305. G. S. Gordon, M. E. Fitzpatric, and W. P. Lubich, Trans. Assoc. Am. Physicians 80:183 (1967).
306. R. Paoletti, G. Galli, E. Grossi-Paoletti, A. Fiecchi, and A. Scala, Lipids 6:134 (1971).
307. M. K. Rao, E. G. Perkins, W. E. Connor, and A. K. Bhattacharyya, Lipids 10:566 (1975).
308. V. P. Flanagan and A. Ferretti, Lipids 9:471 (1974).
309. M. Prost, B. F. Maume, and P. Padieu, Biochim. Biophys. Acta 360:230 (1974).
310. W. R. Nes, N. S. Thampi, and J. T. Lin, Cancer Res. 32:1264 (1972).
311. G. H. Rothblatt and C. H. Burns, J. Lipid Res. 12:653 (1971).
312. N. Anitschkow, Bietr. Path. Anat. 56:379 (1913).
313. G. E. Cox, C. B. Taylor, L. G. Cox, and M. A. Counts, A.M.A. Arch. Pathol. 66:32 (1958).
314. The Framingham Study. An Epidemiological Investigation of Cardiovascular Disease. Sections 10-23. Washington, D.C., U.S. Government Printing Office, Washington, D.C., 1969.
315. S. M. Grundy, E. H. Ahrens, G. Salen, P. H. Schreibman, and P. J. Nestel, J. Lipid Res. 13:531 (1972).
316. H. S. Sodhi, B. J. Kudchodkar, L. Horlick, and C. H. Wedner, Metabolism 20:348 (1971).
317. D. N. Kim, K. T. Lee, J. M. Reiner, and W. A. Thomas, J. Lipid Res. 15:326 (1974).
318. D. J. Nazir, L. Horlick, B. J. Kudchodkar, and H. S. Sodhi, Circulation 46:95 (1972).
319. M. J. P. Higgins, D. Brady, and H. Rudney, Arch. Biochem. Biophys. 163:271 (1974).

320. W. D. Wagner and T. B Clarkson, Proc. Soc. Exp. Biol. Med. 145:1050 (1974).
321. J. P. Kotze, J. S. Neuhoff, G. P. Engelbrecht, G. J. Van Der Merwe, J. P. DuPlessis, and L. P. Horn, Atherosclerosis 19:469 (1974).
322. K. P. Norum and E. Gjone, Scand. J. Clin. Lab. Invest. 33:191 (1974).
323. J. B. Simon, D. L. Kepkay, and R. Poon, Gastroenterology 66:539 (1974).
324. A. J. Day and J. W. Proudlock, Atherosclerosis 19:253 (1974).
325. S. Hashimoto and S. Dayton, Proc. Soc. Exp. Biol. Med. 145:89 (1974).
326. J. D. Gilbert, C. J. W. Brooks, and W. A. Harland, Biochim. Biophys. Acta 270:149 (1972).
327. S. N. Jagannathan, W. E. Connor, W. H. Baker, and A. K. Bhattacharyya, J. Clin. Invest. 54:366 (1974).
328. E. Kennaway and J. W. Cook, Chem. Ind. (London) 521 (1932).
329. J. W. Cook and G. A. D. Haslewood, J. Chem. Soc. 428 (1934).
330. H. Wieland and E. Dane, Hoppe-Seyler's Z. Physiol. Chem. 219:240 (1933).
331. J. W. Cook and G. A. D. Haslewood, Chem. Ind. (London) 758 (1933).
332. W. R. Nes and D. L. Ford, J. Am. Chem. Soc. 85:2137 (1963).
333. N. J. de Souza and W. R. Nes, Cancer Res. 27:1969 (1967).
334. J. W. Cook, J. Chem. Soc. 1210 (1950).
335. N. P. Buu-Hoi, Cancer Res. 24:1511 (1964).
336. H. Dannenberg, Z. Krebsforsch. 62:217 (1957).
337. E. Y. Levin and K. Bloch, Nature 202:4927 (1964).
338. P. W. Carter, I. M. Heilbron, and B. Lythgoe, Proc. Roy. Soc. (London), Ser. B 128:82 (1939).
339. R. G. Reitz and J. G. Hamilton, Comp. Biochem. Physiol. 25:401 (1968).
340. N. J. de Souza and W. R. Nes, Science 162:363 (1968).
341. C. Paoletti, B. Pushparaj, G. Florenzano, P. Capella, and G. Lercker, Lipids 11:266 (1976).
342. J. Seebach and R. Ikan, Plant Physiol. 49:457 (1972).
343. S. Teshima and A. Kanazawa, Nippon Suisan Gakkaishi 38:1197 (1972).
344. R. Willstätter and H. J. Page, Liebig's Ann. Chem. 404:237 (1914).
345. I. M. Heilbron, R. F. Phipers, and H. R. Wright, J. Chem. Soc. 1572 (1934).
346. P. W. Carter, I. M. Heilbron, and B. Lythgoe, Proc. Roy. Soc. (London), Ser. B 128:82 (1939).
347. I. M. Heilbron, J. Chem. Soc. 79 (1942).
348. K. Tsuda, S. Akagi, and Y. Kishida, Science 126:927 (1957).
349. K. Tsuda, S. Akagi, and Y. Kishida, R. Hayatsu, and K. Sakai, Chem. Pharm. Bull. (Tokyo) 6:724 (1958).
350. K. Tsuda, K. Sakai, K. Tanabe, and Y. Kishida, J. Am. Chem. Soc. 82: 1442 (1960).
351. G. F. Gibbons, L. J. Goad, and T. W. Goodwin, Phytochemistry 6:677 (1967).
352. E. Fattorusso, S. Magno, C. Santacroce, D. Sica, G. Impellizzeri, S. Mangiafico, G. Oriente, M. Piattelli, and S. Sciuto, Phytochemistry 14:1579 (1975).
353. I. Chardon-Loriaux, M. Morisaki, and N. Ikekawa, Phytochemistry 15:723 (1976).
354. D. R. Idler and P. Wiseman, Comp. Biochem. Physiol. 38A:581 (1971).
355. J. P. Ferezou, M. Devys, J. P. Allais, and M. Barbier, Phytochemistry 593 (1974).
356. A. Alcaide, M. Barbier, P. Potier, A. M. Magueur, and J. Teste, Phytochemistry 8:2301 (1969).
357. S. Aaronson and H. Baker, J. Protozol. 8:274 (1961).

358. D. R. Idler and P. Wiseman, Comp. Biochem. Physiol. 35:679 (1970).
359. L. M. Safe, C. J. Wong, and R. F. Chandler, J. Pharm. Sci. 63:464 (1974).
360. N. Ikekawa, N. Morisaki, K. Tsuda, and T. Yoshida, Steroids 12:41 (1968).
361. N. Ikekawa, K. Tsuda, and N. Morisaki, Chem. Ind. 1179 (1966).
362. K. Tsuda, R. Hayatsu, Y. Kishida, and S. Akagi, J. Am. Chem. Soc. 80:921 (1958).
363. B. A. Knights, Phytochemistry 9:903 (1970).
364. A. M. Motzfeldt, Acta Chem. Scand. 24:1846 (1970).
365. N. Ikekawa, N. Morisaki, and K. Hirayama, Phytochemistry 11:2317 (1972).
366. J. D. A. Miller, in R. A. Levin (ed.), Physiology and Biochemistry of Algae. Academic Press, New York, 1962. p. 364.
367. G. W. Patterson, Lipids 6:120 (1971).
368. Y. Shimizu, A. Maktoab, and A. Kobayashi, J. Am. Chem. Soc. 98:1059 (1976).
369. B. L. Williams, T. W. Goodwin, and J. F. Ryley, J. Protozool. 13:227 (1966).
370. M. C. Gershengorn, A. R. H. Smith, G. Goulston, L. J. Goad, and T. W. Goodwin, Biochemistry 7:1698 (1968).
371. E. I. Mercer, R. A. London, I. S. A. Kent, and A. J. Taylor, Phytochemistry 13:845 (1974).
372. T. G. Tornabene, M. Kates, and B. E. Volcani, Lipids 9, 279 (1974).
373. D. M. Orcutt and G. W. Patterson, Comp. Biochem. Physiol. 50B:579 (1975).
374. I. Rubinstein and L. J. Goad, Phytochemistry 13:485 (1974).
375. R. P. Collins and K. Kalnins, Comp. Biochem. Physiol. 30:779 (1969).
376. E. I. Mercer and W. B. Harris, Phytochemistry 14:439 (1975).
377. A. R. H. Smith, L. J. Goad, and T. W. Goodwin, Phytochemistry 11:2775 (1972).
378. M. Lefort, Comp. Rend. Acad. Sci. (Paris) 258:4318 (1964).
379. R. D. Brandt, R. J. Pryce, C. Anding, and G. Ourisson, Eur. J. Biochem. 17:344 (1970).
380. A. I. Stern, J. A. Schiff, and H. P. Klein, J. Protozol. 7:52 (1960).
381. L. Avivi, O. Iaron, and S. Halevy, Comp. Biochem. Physiol. 21:321 (1967).
382. C. Anding, R. D. Brandt, and G. Ourisson, Eur. J. Biochem. 24:259 (1971).
383. R. M. Klein and A. Cronquist, Quart. Rev. Biol. 42:106 (1967).
384. W. R. Nes, Adv. Lipid Res., in press.
385. M. Klotsky and W. Bergmann, J. Am. Chem. Soc. 74:1601 (1952).
386. G. W. Patterson, Comp. Biochem. Physiol. 31:391 (1969).
387. G. W. Patterson, Plant Physiol. 42:1457 (1967).
388. G. W. Patterson, Comp. Biochem. Physiol. 47B:453 (1974).
389. I. Rubinstein and L. J. Goad, Phytochemistry 13:481 (1974).
390. M. J. Thompson, S. R. Dutky, G. W. Patterson, and E. L. Gooden, Phytochemistry 11:1781 (1972).
391. W. R. Nes, K. Krevitz, J. Joseph, W. D. Nes, B. Harris, and G. Gibbons, Lipids, in press.
392. G. W. Patterson, Phytochemistry 11:3481 (1972).
393. G. F. Gibbons, L. J. Goad, and T. W. Goodwin, Phytochemistry 7:983 (1968).
394. G. W. Patterson, M. J. Thompson, and S. R. Dutky, Phytochemistry 13:191 (1974).
395. L. B. Tsai, G. W. Patterson, C. F. Cohen, and P. D. Klein, Lipids 9:1014 (1974).

396. G. W. Patterson and R. W. Kraus, Plant Cell Physiol. 6:211 (1965).
397. I. Iwata, H. Nakata, M. Mizuschima, and Y. Sakurai, Agr. Biol. Chem. 25:319 (1961).
398. D. M. Orcutt and B. Richardson, Steroids 16:429 (1970).
399. S. Hunek, Phytochemistry 8:1313 (1969).
400. L. G. Dickson, G. W. Patterson, C. F. Cohen, and S. R. Dutky, Phytochemistry 11:3473 (1972).
401. L. G. Dickson and G. W. Patterson, Lipids 7:635 (1972).
402. J. T. Chan and G. W. Patterson, Plant Physiol. 52:246 (1973).
403. J. T. Chan, G. W. Patterson, S. R. Dutky, and C. F. Cohen, Plant Physiol. 53:244 (1974).
404. L. B. Tsai and G. W. Patterson, Phytochemistry 15:1131 (1976).
405. L. J. Goad, F. F. Knapp, J. R. Lenton, and T. W. Goodwin, Biochem. J. 129:219 (1972).
406. J. H. Adler and G. W. Patterson, Plant Physiol. 53:S-13 (1974).
407. Y. Tomita, A. Uomori, and H. Minato, Phytochemistry 9:555 (1970).
408. Y. Tomita, A. Uomori, and E. Sakurai, Phytochemistry 10:573 (1971).
409. G. W. Patterson and E. G. Karlander, Plant Physiol. 42:1651 (1967).
410. L. B. Tsai, J. H. Adler, and G. W. Patterson, Phytochemistry 14:2599 (1975).
411. Z. A. Wojchiechowski, L. J. Goad, and T. W. Goodwin, Biochem. J. 136: 405 (1973).
412. L. J. Goad, F. F. Knapp, J. R. Lenton, and T. W. Goodwin, Biochem J. 129:12 (1972).
413. V. Ahmadjian, Ann. Rev. Microbiol. 19:1 (1965).
414. V. Ahmadjian, Symbiosis 1:35 (1966).
415. J. R. Lenton, L. J. Goad, and T. W. Goodwin, Phytochemistry 12:1135 (1973).
416. (a) J. R. Lenton, L. J. Goad, and T. W. Goodwin, Phytochemistry 12:2249 (1973); (b) S. Safe, L. M. Safe, and W. S. G. Maass, Phytochemistry 14: 1821 (1975).
417. D. A. J. Ives and A. N. O'Neill, Can. J. Chem. 36:434 (1958).
418. A. Marsili and I. Morelli, Phytochemistry 7:1705 (1968).
419. A. Marsili and I. Morelli, Phytochemistry 9:651 (1970).
420. R. J. Thomas, Phytochemistry 14:623 (1975).
421. J. Sliwoski and Z. Kasprzyk, Phytochemistry 13:1451 (1974).
422. E. Capstack, Jr., D. J. Baisted, W. W. Newschwander, G.A. Blondin, N. L. Rosin, and W. R. Nes, Biochemistry 1:1178 (1962).
423. D. A. Beeler, D. G. Anderson, and J. W. Porter, Arch. Biochem. Biophys. 102:26 (1963).
424. M. Tada, T. Takahashi, and H. Koyama, Phytochemistry 13:670 (1974).
425. R. W. Lewis, Phytochemistry 11:417 (1972).
426. (a) D. J. Baisted, E. Capstack, Jr., and W. R. Nes, Biochemistry 1:537 (1962); (b) D. J. Baisted and W. R. Nes, J. Biol. Chem. 238:1947 (1963); (c) H. J. Nicholas, J. Biol. Chem. 237:1481 (1962).
427. A. Windaus and A. Hauth, Chem. Ber. 39:4378 (1906).
428. F. F. Knapp and H. J. Nicholas, Phytochemistry 8:207 (1969).
429. J. R. Hillman, B. A. Knights, R. McKail, Lipids 10:542 (1975).
430. T. M. Jeong, T. Itoh, T. Tamura and T. Matsumoto, Lipids 9:921 (1974).
431. T. Itoh, T. Tamura, and T. Matsumoto, J. Am. Oil. Chem. Soc. 50:122 (1973).
432. (a) B. A. Knights and A. M. M. Berrie, Phytochemistry 10:131 (1971); (b) B. A. Knights and B. S. Middleditch, Phytochemistry 11:1177 (1972); (c) B. A. Knights and B. S. Middleditch, Phytochemistry 11:1183 (1972).
433. B. S. Middleditch and B. A. Knights, Phytochemistry 11:1183 (1972).

434. B. A. Knights, Phytochemistry 11:1177 (1972).
435. R. T. van Aller, H. Chikamatsu, N. J. de Souza, and W. R. Nes, J. Biol. Chem. 6645 (1969).
436. M. A. Palmer and B. N. Bowden, Phytochemistry 14:1813 (1975).
437. W. R. Nes, K. Krevitz, J. Joseph, W. D. Nes, B. Harris, G. F. Gibbons, and G. W. Patterson, Lipids, in press (1977).
438. W. R. Nes, K. Krevitz, S. Behzadan, G. W. Patterson, J. R. Landrey, and R. L. Conner, Biochem. Biophys. Res. Commun. 66:1462 (1975).
439. H. W. Kircher, Phytochemistry 9:1879 (1970).
440. W. R. Nes, K. Krevitz, and S. Behzadan, Lipids 11:118 (1976).
441. R. E. Mitchell and T. A. Giessman, Phytochemistry 10:1559 (1971).
442. A. N. Starratt, Phytochemistry 8:795 (1969).
443. J. R. Lenton, L. J. Goad, and T. N. Goodwin, unpublished observations quoted in L. J. Goad, J. R. Lenton, F. F. Knapp, and T. W. Goodwin, Lipids 9:582 (1974).
444. Y. Tomita and A. Uomori, Chem. Commun. 1416 (1970).
445. M. R. Heble, S. Narayanaswami, and M. S. Chadha, Science 145:1145 (1968).
446. W. J. S. Lockley, D. P. Roberts, H. H. Rees, and T. W. Goodwin, Tetrahedron Lett. 43:3773 (1974).
447. A. M. Metwally, A. M. Habib, and S. M. Khafagy, Planta Medica 25:68 (1974).
448. A. M. Atallah and H. J. Nicholas, Phytochemistry 10:3139 (1971).
449. C. Djerassi and R. McCrindle, J. Chem. Soc. 4034 (1962).
450. G. Osske and K. Schreiber, Tetrahedron 21:1559 (1965).
451. S. S. Deshmane and S. Dev, Tetrahedron 27:1109 (1971).
452. K. Jewers, M. J. Nagler, K. A. Zirvi, and F. Amir, Phytochemistry 15:238 (1976).
453. (a) E. E. Homberg and H. P. K. Schiller, Phytochemistry 12:1767 (1973); (b) E. E. Homberg, Phytochemistry 15:1361 (1976).
454. X. A. Dominquez, J. A. Quintanilla, and M. P. Rojas, Phytochemistry 13: 673 (1974).
455. R. D. Bennett and E. Heftmann, Steroids 14:403 (1969).
456. A. L. S. Cheng, M. J. Kasperbauer, and L. G. Rice, Phytochemistry 10: 1481 (1971).
457. V. G. Willuhn and J. Kostens, Planta Medica 25:115 (1974).
458. W. Sucrow and A. Reimerdes, Z. Naturforsch. 23b:42 (1968).
459. W. Sucrow and B. Girgensohn, Chem. Ber. 103:750 (1970).
460. W. Sucrow, B. Schubert, W. Richter, Chem. Ber. 104:3689 (1974).
461. L. M. Bolger, H. H. Rees, E. L. Ghisalberti, L. J. Goad, and T. W. Goodwin, Tetrahedron Lett., 3043 (1970).
462. L. M. Bolger, H. H. Rees, E. L. Ghisalberti, L. J. Goad, and T. W. Goodwin, Biochem. J. 118:197 (1970).
463. M. Manzoor-I-Khuda, Tetrahedron 22:2377 (1966).
464. R. J. Anderson, R. L. Shriner, and G. O. Burr, J. Am. Chem. Soc. 48:2987 (1926).
465. M. J. Thompson, W. E. Robbins, and G. L. Baker, Steroids 2:505 (1963).
466. R. B. Bates, A. D. Brewer, B. A. Knights, and J. W. Rowe, Tetrahedron Lett. 6163 (1968).
467. H. Linde, N. Ergenc, and K. Meyer, Helv. Chim. Acta 49:1246 (1966).
468. I. Nishioka, N. Ikekawa, A. Yagi, T. Kawasaki, and T. Tsukamoto, Chem. Pharm. Bull. (Tokyo) 13:379 (1965).
469. K. Tsuda, Y. Kishida, and R. Hayatsu, J. Am. Chem. Soc. 82:3396 (1960).
470. C. E. Bills, in W. N. Sebrell, Jr., and R. S. Harris (eds.), The Vitamins. Vol. 2. Academic Press, New York, 1954. p. 149.

471. H. Yokoyama and M. J. White, Phytochemistry 7:493 (1968).
472. D. F. Johnson, R. D. Bennett, and E. Heftmann, Science 140:198 (1963).
473. E. Fernholz and H. B. MacPhillamy, J. Am. Chem. Soc. 63:1155 (1941).
474. L. J. Mulheirn, Tetrahedron Lett. 3175 (1973).
475. W. L. F. Amarego, L. J. Goad, and T. W. Goodwin, Phytochemistry 12: 2181 (1973).
476. D. R. Idler, A. A. Kandutsch, and C. A. Baumann, J. Am. Chem. Soc. 75: 4325 (1953).
477. C. Djerassi, G. W. Krakower, A. J. Lemin, L. H. Zin, and J. S. Mills, J. Am. Chem. Soc. 80:6284 (1958).
478. A. Windaus and A. Welsh, Chem. Ber. 42:612 (1909).
479. M. C. Hart and F. W. Heyl, J. Biol. Chem. 95:311 (1932).
480. D. H. R. Barton and J. D. Cox, J. Chem. Soc. 1354 (1948).
481. L. F. Fieser, M. Fieser, and R. N. Chakravarti, J. Am. Chem. Soc. 71:2226 (1949).
482. R. T. van Aller, H. Chikamatsu, N. J. de Souza, J. P. John, and W. R. Nes, J. Biol. Chem. 244:6645 (1969).
483. D. R. Idler, S. W. Nicksic, D. R. Johnson, V. W. Meloche, H. A. Schuette, and C. A. Baumann, J. Am. Chem. Soc. 75:1712 (1953).
484. B. A. Knights, Phytochemistry 4:857 (1965).
485. J. A. Fioriti, M. G. Kolor, and R. P. McNaught, Tetrahedron Lett., 2971 (1970).
486. D. J. Frost and J. P. Ward, Rec. Trav. Chim. 89:1054 (1970).
487. D. J. Frost and J. P. Ward, Rec. Trav. Chim. 89:186 (1970).
488. G. S. Gupta and N. L. Gupta, Tetrahedron Lett. 1221 (1974).
489. M. Barbier, M. F. Hygel, and E. Lederer, Bull. Soc. Chim. Biol. 42:91 (1960).
490. J. C. Knight, D. I. Wilkinson, and C. Djerassi, J. Am. Chem. Soc. 88:790 (1966).
491. C. Djerassi, R. D. H. Murray, and R. Villotti, J. Chem. Soc. 1160 (1965).
492. A. Stabursvik, Acta Chem. Scand. 7:1220 (1953).
493. K. Tsuda and R. Hayatsu, J. Am. Chem. Soc. 81:5987 (1959).
494. C. Djerassi, J. C. Knight, and H. Brockmann, Jr., Chem. Ber. 97:3118 (1964).
495. J. A. Beisler and Y. Sato, J. Org. Chem. 36:3946 (1971).
496. R. B. Boar and C. R. Rober, Phytochemistry 14:1143 (1975).
497. C. Djerassi, G. W. Krakower, A. J. Lemin, L. H. Liu, J. S. Mills, and R. Villotti, J. Am. Chem. Soc. 80:6284 (1958).
498. Y. Mazur, A. Weizmann, and F. Sondheimer, J. Am. Chem. Soc. 80:6293 (1958).
499. A. G. Gonzalez and L. Breton, Anales Real Soc. Espan. Fis. Quim. (Madrid), Ser. B 55:93 (1959).
500. G. Ohta and M. Shimizu, Chem. Pharm. Bull. (Tokyo) 5:40 (1957).
501. G. Ohta, Chem. Pharm. Bull. (Tokyo) 8:9 (1960).
502. J. S. G. Cox, F. E. King, and T. J. King, J. Chem. Soc. 1384 (1956).
503. J. S. G. Cox, F. E. King, and T. J. King, J. Chem. Soc. 514 (1959).
504. L. Amoros-Marin, W. I. Torres, and C. F. Asenyo, J. Org. Chem. 24:411 (1959).
505. W. Lawrie, F.S. Spring, and H. S. Watson, Chem. Ind. 1458 (1956).
506. T. Itoh, T. Tamura, and T. Matsumoto, Lipids 9:173 (1974).
507. T. Itoh, T. Tamura, and T. Matsumoto, Lipids 10:454 (1975).
508. M. F. Hugel, M. Barbier, and E. Lederer, Bull. Soc. Chim. Fr. 2012 (1964).
509. A. Ducruix, C. P. Billy, M. Devys, M. Barbier, and E. Lederer, Chem. Commun. 929 (1973).

510. T. M. Jeong, T. Itoh, T. Tamura, and T. Matsumoto, Lipids 10:634 (1975).
511. T. Itoh, T. Tamura, and T. Matsumoto, J. Am. Oil Chem. Soc. 50:300 (1973).
512. N. R. Krishnaswamy and S. Prasanna, Phytochemistry 14:1663 (1975).
513. G. Adler and Z. Kasprzyk, Phytochemistry 14:723 (1975).
514. W. Sucrow, M. Slopianka, and H. W. Kircher, Phytochemistry, 15:1533 (1976).
515. D. S. Ingram, B. A. Knights, I. J. McEvoy, and P. McKay, Phytochemistry 7:1241 (1968).
516. A. M. Atallah, R. T. Axel, R. B. Ramsey, and H. J. Nicholas, Phytochemistry 14:1529 (1975).
517. A. M. Atallah, R. T. Axel, R. B. Ramsey, S. Threlkeld, and H. J. Nicholas, Phytochemistry 14:1927 (1975).
518. L. N. Standifer, M. Devys, and M. Barbier, Phytochemistry 7:1361 (1968).
519. F. I. Opute, Phytochemistry 14:1023 (1975).
520. C. Tanret, Compt. Rend. Acad. Sci. (Paris) 147:75 (1889).
521. C. Tanret, Ann. Chim. Phys. 15:313 (1908).
522. A. E. Oxford, and H. Raistrick, Biochem. J. 27:1176 (1933).
523. A. Kuksis and J. M. R. Beveridge, J. Org. Chem. 25:1209 (1960).
524. R. J. Kemp and G. I. Mercer, Biochem. J. 110:111 (1968).
525. H. E. Nordby and S. Nagy, Phytochemistry 13:443 (1974).
526. R. J. Kemp and E. I. Mercer, Biochem. J. 110:119 (1968).
527. R. D. Brandt and P. Benveniste, Biochim. Biophys. Acta 282:85 (1972).
528. M. LePage, J. Lipid Res. 5:587 (1964).
529. M. E. McKillican, J. Am. Oil Chem. Soc. 41:554 (1964).
530. W. Eichenberger and E. C. Grob, FEBS Lett. 11:177 (1970).
531. T. Kiribuchi, C. S. Chen, and S. Funahashi, Agr. Biol. Chem. Japan 29: 265 (1965).
532. P. B. Bush and C. Grunwald, Plant Physiol. 50:69 (1972).
533. J. Meance and M. R. Daperon, Compt. Rend. Acad. Sci. (Paris) 277:849 (1973).
534. T. Y. Fang and D. J. Baisted, Phytochemistry 15:273 (1976).
535. S. A. I. Rizvi, J. Lal, and P. C. Gupta, Phytochemistry 10:670 (1971).
536. G. Willuhn and J. Kostens, Phytochemistry 14:2055 (1975).
537. E. Ali, V. S. Giri, and S. C. Pakrashi, Phytochemistry 14:1133 (1975).
538. D. V. Myhre, Can. J. Chem. 46:3021 (1968).
539. T. Kiribuchi, N. Yasumatsu, and S. Funahashi, Agr. Biol. Chem. Japan 31:1244 (1967).
540. R. Aneja and P. C. Harries, Chem. Phys. Lipids 12:351 (1974).
541. W. Eichenberger and W. Menke, Z. Naturforsch. 216:859 (1966).
542. M. Kiribuchi, T. Mizunaga, and S. Funahashi, Agr. Biol. Chem. Japan 30: 770 (1966).
543. (a) V. Hariharan and S. Rangaswami, Phytochemistry 10:621 (1971); (b) I. Khana, R. Seshadri, and T. R. Seshadri, Phytochemistry 13:199 (1974).
544. W. T. Forsee, R. A. Laine, and A. D. Elbein, Arch. Biochem. Biophys. 161:248 (1974).
545. P. R. Shewry, N. J. Pinfield, and A. K. Stobart, Phytochemistry 13:341 (1974).
546. P. R. Shewry and A. K. Stobart, Phytochemistry 13:347 (1974).
547. J. M. C. Geus, Phytochemistry 12:103 (1973).
548. J. M. C. Geus, Phytochemistry 14:975 (1975).
549. J. M. C. Geus and J. C. Vendrig, Phytochemistry 13:919 (1974).

550. M. L. McKean and W. R. Nes, Lipids, 12:382 (1977).
551. W. R. Nes, D. J. Baisted, E. Capstack, Jr., W. W. Newschwander, and P. T. Russell, *in* T. W. Goodwin (ed.), Biochem. of the Chloroplast. Vol. 2. Academic Press, New York, 1967. pp. 273-282.

Chapter
11

Function
of
Steroids

A. **General Comments** 535
B. **Membranes** 536
    1. *History and Concepts* 536
    2. *Isolation of Sterols and Related Molecules from Membranes* 538
    3. *Structure-Function Correlations in vivo* 539
    4. *Structure-Activity Correlations in Model Systems* 554
C. **Hormones** 557
    1. *Progesterone* 557
    2. *Adrenocortical Steroids* 568
    3. *Androgens* 575
    4. *Estrogens* 578
    5. *Metabolism of Mammalian Hormones* 584
    6. *Nonmammalian Hormones and Their Metabolism* 587
    7. *Metabolism by Microorganisms* 587
    8. *Hormone Effects on Target Cell Nuclei* 588
    9. *Ecdysones* 588
D. **Bile Acids and Bile Salts** 590
    1. *Occurrence* 590
    2. *Biosynthesis* 594
    3. *Sequencing of Bile Acid Biosynthesis* 600
    4. *Physiology* 602
E. **Vitamin D** 604
    1. *Discovery of Vitamin D* 604
    2. *Mechanism of Vitamin D Formation* 606
    3. *Physiology* 610
Literature Cited 616

A. GENERAL COMMENTS

Steroids play four main roles: as architectural components of membranes, as hormones, as gastrointestinal emulsifying agents (bile alcohols and acids), and as precursors to the vitamins D. In all but the first case, which involves the monohydroxy sterols themselves and perhaps their esters and glycosides, the active agent has at least two oxygenated carbon atoms, and in most hormonal and bile cases the steroidal molecule has been cleaved in the side chain, while cleavage in the nucleus occurs to give the vitamins D. The hormones, bile alcohols and acids, and the vitamins D are all metabolites of the sterols. Sterols therefore play a dual role, viz., as membraneous components and as precursors to hormones, etc. In addition, there are many steroidal molecules in plants, e.g., the alkaloids and sapogenins, for which no clear function is yet known. With a few exceptions, the function of the other polycyclic isopentenoids also remains a mystery. However, the wide occurrence of the amyrins, lupeol, etc., strongly suggests they have a part in the biological process.

B. MEMBRANES

1. History and Concepts

The discovery that sterols act as membraneous components has been the result not of one stroke of genius but of a slow accumulation of information during the last half century. Serious consideration of the structure of the membraneous cytoplasmic envelopes began in 1925 with the work of Gorter and Grendel (1), who examined the lipid content of the functionally prokaryotic erythrocyte and showed that there was a sufficient amount present to cover the surface of the cell and act as a limiting membrane. A decade later, Danielli and Davson (2) suggested a rough model for membrane structure involving what has come to be known as a "lipid leaflet." The first clear indication that sterols are involved came from work on nervous tissue during the 1930s and 1940s. It was found to be very rich in cholesterol. With the later advent of the ability to isolate a membrane, cholesterol was shown to reside in the myelin sheath. The dimensions of this membrane were determined (3) in 1962 and Vandenheuvel (4, 5) was able to construct a molecular model of interdigitated cholesterol and phospholipid which had the observed dimensions. Just before this, Robertson (6) proposed the so-called "unit membrane" hypothesis, which involved a lipid leaflet in a sandwich between protein. The idea of a "unit membrane" implies that all membranes have this sort of architecture, which more precisely entails two layers of phospholipid oriented so that the polar phosphate ends of the molecule are extended outward and the alkyl chains inward. Van der Walls attraction is presumed in the model to hold the two layers ("lipid bilayer") together, while polar forces would bind the protein to the phosphate ends. The involvement of sterol has tacitly been assumed but rarely given much attention until very recently. An exact analysis of the amount of cholesterol in the erythrocyte membrane became available in

1964 (7); this demonstrated that the myelin sheath was not unique in possessing sterol. In the succeeding decade, many other membranes were found to contain sterol. These included mitochondria (8), microsomes (8, 9), and the cytoplasmic membrane of yeast (10) and the prokaryotic choleplasmas (11). In addition, the prokaryotic blue-green algae, at least as the whole cell, were found to possess sterols (Chapter 10). In fact, the only membranes examined that are not thought to contain sterol were the inner (but not outer) membrane of yeast mitochondria (12), the envelope of bacteria (see Ref. 13 for a key to the literature), and the membranes of the eukaryotic, protozoan Tetrahymena pyriformis. In the latter case, however, the sterol's role is played by the closely related tetrahymanol, and it can be replaced by sterol (14). Since bacteria do contain sterols, at least in some cases (Chapter 10), the reported absence of membraneous sterols in these organisms bears reexamination. Simple color tests for cholesterol will not qualify as adequate methodology, and a search for, among others, stanols, sterols methylated in the nucleus, and for other polycyclics such as tetrahymanol should be made. It should also be mentioned at this point that all of the lipid (sterol, etc.) in mycoplasmas is thought to be in the membrane and that all subcellular particles isolated from vascular plants contain sterol (see Chapter 10).

The facts just described can leave no doubt that sterols play a role as membraneous components. However, this does not prove whether or not it is a minor or a major role and to what extent it is general. The first evidence that it is the primary function came from an investigation of the nutrient requirements of insects. They were all found to require sterol. A particularly good assay technique was found to be the amount of material necessary to permit larval growth and development of larvae into pupae (pupation). Experimentally taking advantage of this, in 1959 Clark and Bloch (15) were able to examine whether or not the added sterol underwent metabolism in the course of inducing pupation. What they discovered was that most of the sterol is not metabolized. In particular, they found that, while cholesterol alone would support pupation, cholestanol alone will not. On the other hand, with subminal amounts of cholesterol, cholestanol did induce pupation in what they called a "sparing effect." Then, when larvae of the hide beetle (Dermestes vulpinus) were reared on a minimal 1:4-mixture of cholesterol and cholestanol, respectively, and the sterols were reisolated 34 days later from the healthy animals, the cholestanol was recovered unchanged. This striking effect led Clark and Bloch (15) to conclude that the sterol must have played a nonmetabolic role, since it was necessary but underwent no chemical change.

Insects are by no means the only organism that have been shown to have a sterol requirement. A few years before the work of Clark and Bloch (15), Andreasen and Stier (16) demonstrated that yeast under anaerobic conditions will grow only if sterol (and an unsaturated fatty acid) is present in the medium, and Conner, van Wagtendonk, and Miller (*17*) and Vishniac and Watson (*18*) found that the protozoa *Paramecium aurelia* and *Labyrinthula vitellina* had sterol requirements under any condition. More recently, sterol has been reisolated from *P. aurelia* (*19*) as well as from anaerobically grown yeast (*20*). In the latter case, if the added sterol was the organism's natural ergosterol, no metabolism was observed, even when the initial concentration in the medium was close to the minimal requirement. It appears, therefore, that quite generally in biological systems sterols act primarily in an architectural way rather than through metabolism. Further evidence for this conclusion, which was suggested in 1974 by Nes (*21*), comes from the following facts. The cholesterol of the human body has a rather slow turnover rate, which is still slower in brain tissue (see Chapter 10). During germination of peas, when the organism is highly active metabolically, growing, and producing new tissue (roots, stem, etc.), incorporation of label into sterol is bearly detectable from [2-^{14}C]MVA, and no measurable increase in the total amount of sterol is observed (*22*). In germinating pine seeds, while substantial amounts of label proceed to sterol, the total amount of newly biosynthesized sterol is not consequential compared to the sterol already present, and MVA proceeds in any event primarily to other substances, e.g., geranylgeranyl pyrophosphate (*23*). Finally, a common role for sterols in all organisms can be inferred (*21*) from the commonality of the structures (Δ^5-, $\Delta^{5,7}$-, or Δ^7-4,4,14-trisdesmethylsterols with or without a 24-alkyl group) that are found in the otherwise enormously different kinds of organisms in the evolutionary hierarchy (Chapter 10). When one looks carefully at the trememdous diversity (Chapters 7, 9, and 10) of compounds that can be derived from squalene, the nearly ubiquitous occurrence of end products with closely similar structures (the dominant sterols) can only be reasonably interpreted as implying a common function (*21*). That this function is a membraneous one follows not only from the data already cited but from the information discussed in what follows.

2. Isolation of Sterols and Related Molecules from Membranes

The difficulty in isolating pure membranes, even with modern centrifugal techniques, is still great, and the number of defined cases is limited. More information is available on particulate matter as a whole. However, all pure membranes studied from eukaryotic cells as well as from the prokaryotic choleplasmas have been found to have sterols (Table 11.1). Similarly, all subcellular particles have been found to possess sterols. Although esters and glycosides do occur, the sterol is always primarily (approximately 90%) in the free form. See, for instance, the discussion on Tracheophytes in Chapter 10 for a more detailed analysis of this. This leads to the compelling conclusion that sterols act in a membraneous way principally as the free 3β-hydroxy compound. A corollary, which is less secure, is that the

Table 11.1. Composition of some membranes

Membrane	Sterol	% Sterol in Lipid Leaflet	Ref.
Myelin	Cholesterol	25	24
Erythrocyte	Cholesterol	25	7
Endoplasmic reticulum (animal)	Cholesterol	6–8	8,9
Mitochondria (animal)	Cholesterol	2–5	8
Yeast protoplast	24(28)-Dehydro-ergosterol[a]	13	10
Neurospora crassa outer mitochondrial membrane	Ergosterol	16	12
Choleplasma	Cholesterol[b]	2	11

[a]24(28)-Dehydroergosterol is the dominant sterol of this yeast strain.
[b]Cholesterol was derived from the medium.

free sterol content of a cell (or of a whole differentiated tissue or organism) is a measure of the membraneous sterol. The one pentacycle, incidentally, that is known to be present in membranes (tetrahymanol) also occurs in the free form. Furthermore, during the process of myelination there is a drop in the percentage of sterol present as ester, in agreement with the general thesis. This is not to say that esters and glycosides may not play a membraneous role, too. In fact, there are increasing reasons for believing that they do. An intriguing hypothesis, put forward by Smith (25, 26), proposes that the steryl glucoside found in mycoplasmas acts as a carrier of glucose through the cytoplasmic envelope. He cites as evidence the fact that cholesteryl acetate is also present, and he suggests that this is derived from the glucose that is oxidized while still attached to the sterol. This idea warrants further examination in fungi and higher plants, where glycosides have been well documented, and more thorough study of glycosides in mammalian tissue would be interesting.

3. Structure-Function Correlations in vivo

a. Systems Studied   In most cases, the sterol already present in a membrane cannot be experimentally removed and still leave an intact membrane in which one sterol can be replaced with another for study of the relationship between structure and activity. There are, however, some "tricks" that can lead to the same result. Partial (55%) depletion of the cholesterol in erythrocytes has been achieved by an exchange process with an added phospholipid (lecithin) that will complex with it, but the method has not been exploited for structure-activity correlations. A biosynthetic block in the sterol pathway can be achieved either naturally—notably in insects, certain protozoa, the choleplasmas, and certain fungi—or artificially. The artificial block is achievable by genetic alteration with nitrous acid, nystatin, etc., producing mutants, or it can be induced temporarily and at will by placing an organism capable of deriving energy through glycolysis in an anaerobic environment. The mechanism of nitrous acid mutation is presumably through direct nucleic acid changes that are not reversible. The mechanism of the "mutation" induced by nystatin is more complicated. It is really an adaptation. With successively increasing concentrations of nystatin, which damages the membrane by complexing with the sterol (27, 28 and references cited therein), the yeast responds to give nystatin-resistant cells by successively removing steps in the ergosterol pathway. However, the alteration is not permanent, and the cells will revert to ones producing ergosterol in the absence of nystatin. It follows that the sterol intermediates to ergosterol complex less readily, but this has not been studied yet, except qualitatively, in that cholesterol lacking the $\Delta^{5,7,22}$-24β-methyl groups will form a complex (28). On the other hand, the inhibitory mechanism of anaerobiosis is well understood. The pathway from MVA stops at squalene, which accumulates (29, 30). This permits the replacement of ergosterol with other sterols for quantitative examination. Andreasen and Stier (16) were the first to do such studies, which have been expanded by others. An approach to the anaerobic situation has also been achieved by growing yeast in a medium rich in glucose, which induces a fermentive metabolism. Qualitative information has been derived from yeast by genetic alteration, which eliminates only late steps in the pathway so as to produce cells with sterols lacking various features, e.g., the 24β-methyl group. That they still live implies that the group eliminated is not obligatory. Unfortunately, one cannot show by this method, as one can with, say, anaerobic yeast or with insects, what features are inconsistent with activity, since no viable cells would be isolable. One also cannot study as easily the effect of synthetic sterols. Careful comparison of growth curves of the mutants with normal cells and studies of other parameters could be carried out, but they usually have not been performed. A summary of the methods is given in Table 11.2.

    b. Results The results (Tables 11.3–11.5) of studies carried out so far lead to the important conclusion that all membranes have certain structural requirements in common. They are clearly associated with the three-dimensional character of the molecule, in contrast to the ability of the molecule to undergo metabolism. A particularly clear example comes from the capacity of cholestanol to support the growth of as varied organisms as an insect (15) and anaerobic yeast (20, 47). A stanol, of all possibilites, is the least highly functionalized and would require oxidation just to place it in a chemical position to undergo metabolism. This is not to say that stanols are intrinsically the best architectural components, because the introduction of double bonds can have a powerful effect on the three-dimensional condition of the molecule. This is particularly true of double bonds in the side chain, which necessarily place substituents on either side of the π-system in a *cis-* or *trans*-relationship. Thus, (Z)-17(20)-dehydro-cholesterol has C-22 and the remainder of the side chain to the left (*cis*-oriented with respect to C-13). It fails to support the growth of anaerobically grown yeast, while its (E)-isomer, with the bulk of the side chain to the right, does support growth (*50*). A second effect of a double bond could be to act as a binding site to polar parts of either protein or phospholipid. There is no direct experimental evidence for this, however, attractive as the idea is, especially in terms of double bonds in the nucleus. Perusal of Chapter 10 will reveal that nearly all biological systems contain dominant sterols with a double bond in ring B. In most cases it is at C-5, less commonly at C-7, and occasionally (certain algae, protozoa, and fungi) the $\Delta^{5,7}$-diene system is dominant. On very rare occasions, a major sterol has Δ^8-, $\Delta^{5,8}$-, or in one case $\Delta^{8,14}$-unsaturation, but it will be seen ring B is involved even in these cases. Of the possibilities, the Δ^5-sterols with only the one double bond in ring B are by far the most common both in animals and plants. Whether the double bond represents a fine-tuning of the stereochemistry or a binding site is unclear. Its stereochemical effect is not large. The A/B-ring junction has approximately the space requirements of a stanol in the 5α-series (A/B-*trans*). The double bond does, however, have the effect of removing the axial 6β-H atom and of placing C-6 and C-7 in slightly different positions. Similarly, the Δ^7-bond alters the precise positions of C-6 and C-7 and removes an axial H atom, but the latter is on the α rather than the β face in the corresponding saturated case. In the $\Delta^{5,7}$-diene, both axial H atoms disappear. A third possible reason for the strong tendency toward Δ^5-sterols is their homoallylic effect on the C—O bond at C-3. Donation of electrons through an inductive effect, analogously to the well studied 3,5-cyclosteroid rearrangement, should strengthen the H—O bond and therefore weaken somewhat and fine-tune any H bonding of the sterol to phospholipid or protein.

The hydroxyl group at C-3 is the one polar functionality that is an absolute necessity. Cholestane, which stereochemically mimics the sterols, fails to have any activity in a variety of systems (yeast, mycoplasmas, etc.). Knowing that the sterol interdigitates with the phospholipid in the lipid leaflet, one might conclude that the OH group functions as the H donor in an H bond with the oxygen atoms of the phosphate moiety of the phospholipid, but the true situation is probably more complicated than this for two reasons. In model membranes, the phosphate group is hydrated (*51, 52*), which should prevent close approach of the steroidal OH group. Secondly, cholesteryl methyl ether will support growth of anaerobic yeast, albeit not as well as will cholesterol, indicating that the oxygen is acting as an H acceptor since no H atom is present on the oxygen and no hydrolysis occurs (*20*). Tentatively, it would seem that the OH group immerses itself in the

Table 11.2. Systems for studying membraneous structure-activity correlations in vivo by sterol replacement

Organism	Methodology	Principal	Ref.
Erythrocytes	Incubation with lecithin then with sterol	Original cholesterol partially removed	31,32
Insects	Rear larvae on sterol; measure pupation, etc.	Natural biosynthetic block induces sterol requirement	15
Certain protozoa	Culture on sterol; measure growth, etc.	Natural biosynthetic block induces sterol requirement (*Paramecium*) or permits replacement (*Tetrahymena*) of pentacycle	17
Certain fungi	Culture on sterol; measure sexual function	*Phytophthora* and *Pythium* require exogenous sterols for reproduction presumably through biosynthetic block	33–37
Choleplasmas	Culture on sterol; measure growth, etc.	Natural biosynthetic block induces sterol requirement in carotenol-less mycoplasmas	26
Yeast	Select live cells after treatment with nystatin; determine sterol structure	Nystatin-resistant cells have sterol block	38–40
Yeast	Culture on thiamine; determine sterol structure	Thiamine induces low respiratory level reducing rate of oxidative steps in sterol biosynthesis after squalene	41
Yeast	Select live cells after 99% death induced by HONO; culture on sterols and determine growth, etc.	HONO-resistant cells have biosynthetic block prior to lanosterol	42
Yeast	Culture anaerobically in presence of sterols; measure growth, etc.	Block induced in epoxidation and C-30-32 removal; squalene accumulates	16

Table 11.3. Sterol requirements of mycoplasmas[a]

Sterol	Mycoplasma arthritidis[b]	T-Mycoplasmas[c]
Squalene	0	—
Geraniol	0	—
Solanesol	0	—
Cholesterol	+	+
Cholesteryl esters (propionate to laurate)	+	0
Cholesteryl esters (myristate to linoleate)	0	—
3-Epicholesterol	0	—
5α-Cholestan-3β-ol	+	+
5α-Cholestan-3α-ol	0	0
5β-Cholestan-3β-ol	0	0
5β-Cholestan-3α-ol	0	0
7-Dehydrocholesterol	—	+
Ergosterol	+	+
Sitosterol		+
Stigmasterol	+	+
Cholestan-3-one		0
5α-Cholestane	0	—
Progesterone	0	—
Testosterone	0	—

[a] A plus sign indicates growth response. A zero indicates no growth response and in some cases (5β-sterols and 3-epicholesterol with T-strain) inhibition of cholesterol. A dash means no report.
[b] Smith (26), pp. 137–138.
[c] Rottem et al. (43).

polar milieu acting perhaps partially in the capacities of both H donor and H acceptor. The relative importance of the two effects could well depend on the membrane in question.

Only minor alterations in the stereochemistry of the nucleus are permitted by membranes. This follows first of all from the nearly universal occurrence of sterols, which either have or closely approximate the all-trans-anti-arrangement of the ring junctions. In addition, sterols with an A/B-cis-junction fail to have membraneous activity as measured by growth-support. Similarly, the quantitative dominance of sterols lacking the methyl groups at C-4 and C-14 both in whole cells as well as in isolated membranes indicates that the axial protrusions of the 4β- and 14α-methyl groups on either side of the molecule are deleterious, from which one can conclude the thickness of the molecule in the front-to-back direction has limits in terms of membraneous function. Furthermore, the removal of the equatorial 4α-methyl group indicates limitations of the thickness in the top-to-bottom direction. The three-dimensional requirements related to C-4 may have to do with the H-bonding ability of the 3β-hydroxyl group. It is well known from chromatographic data that the ability of this group to H bond to alumina or silica gel depends on the substitution at C-4, with

Table 11.4. Sterols of some yeasts adapted, mutated, or otherwise changed

Mutant Strain	Principal Sterols	Comments	Ref.
Porphyrin deficient	14α-Methylfecosterol Lanosterol Obtusifoliol	Requires ergosterol for growth	44,45
Nys-3	24β-Methylcholesta-8,22-dien-3β-ol (major)		40
Nys-30	24β-Methylcholesta-7,22-dien-3β-ol (80%)		27
Nys-200	24-Methylenecholesta-7,22-dien-3β-ol (80%)		27
Nys-300	24-Methylenecholest-8-en-3β-ol (90%) (fecosterol)		27
pol-1	$\Delta^{5,24}$-, $\Delta^{5,7,24}$- and $\Delta^{5,7,22,24}$-Cholestapolyenols		46
pol-2	Δ^{8}-, $\Delta^{8,22}$-, and $\Delta^{5,8,22}$-24β-Methylcholestapolyenols		46
pol-3	$\Delta^{7,22}$-, $\Delta^{8,22}$-, $\Delta^{7,22,24(28)}$- and $\Delta^{8,22,24(28)}$-24β-Methyl-cholestapolyenols		46
Olerg 2-1 from HONO	4,4-Dimethylsterols (major) 4α-Methylsterols (minor) 4,4-Desmethylsterols (<1%)	Requires ergosterol, stigmasterol, or sitosterol. Cholesterol less efficient	42
Thiamine altered	Ergosterol replaced by another sterol		41

Table 11.5. Sterol requirements of anaerobic yeast[a]

Sterol	Study 1[b]	Study 2[c]	Study 3[d]
24β-Methylcholesta-5,7,22-*trans*-trien-3β-ol (Ergosterol)	100	+	+
24β-Metylcholesta-5,22-*trans*-dien-3β-ol (Brassicasterol)	100	+	—
24β-Methylcholesta-5-en-3β-ol	77	—	+
Cholest-7-en-3β-ol (Lathosterol)	38	—	—
Cholest-5-en-3β-ol (Cholesterol)	24	+	+
Cholest-5,7-dien-3β-ol	23	—	+
Cholest-5,24-dien-3β-ol	—	+	—
5α-Cholestan-3β-ol	24	+	—
Cholesta-4,6-dien-3β-ol	17	—	—
Cholest-4-en-3β-ol	12	—	—
Cholesteryl Methyl Ether	8	—	—
5α-Cholestan-3α-ol	8	+	—
5β-Cholestan-3β-ol	—	0	—
Cholest-5-en-3α-ol	5	—	—
Cholest-5-en-3-one	2	—	—
Cholest-4-en-3-one	—	0	—
5α-Cholestane	0	0	—
24α-Ethylcholest-5-en-3β-ol (Sitosterol)	—	+	+
24α-Ethylcholesta-5,22-*trans*-dien-3β-ol (Stigmasterol)	—	—	+
24α-Methylcholest-5-en-3β-ol (Campesterol)	—	—	+
Lanosterol	—	+	—
Lupeol	—	0	—
Androst-5-en-3β,17β-diol	—	0	—

[a] A plus sign indicates growth, a zero no growth, and a dash not studied. In study 1 the numbers indicate the cell count relative to ergosterol after 3 days. They reflect primarily (but not exclusively) rates of growth. Thus, while cholesteryl methyl ether gives only 8% as many cells as ergosterol at 3 days, after one week the population approaches the cholesterol case. The numbers in the table are derived from yeast recently (<1 month) subjected to anaerobic conditions. With cultures well adapted (6–12 months) to the lack of oxygen, cholesterol has a value of 100.
[b] Nes et al. (*20, 49*).
[c] Proudlock et al. (*47*).
[d] Hossack and Rose (*48*).

increasing substitution decreasing the H bonding. Direct studies of the ability of sterols with nuclear methyl groups to function in a membraneous capacity have not received much attention in a quantitative sense. It would be surprising if the presence of methyl groups at C-4 and/or C-14 induced an absolute loss of activity in all systems, and indeed it does not. The one clear case is with *Tetrahymena pyriformis*, in which the pentacyclic tetrahymanol is the organism's natural pentacycle and is localized in the limiting membrane (*14, 53*). Some bacteria (Chapter 10) also have high proportions of sterols with nuclear methyl groups. In yeast, however, mutants producing only nuclear-methylated sterols require 4-desmethylsterol for growth (Table 11.4). This conflicts with the report that lanosterol will support the growth of yeast under anaerobic conditions (*47*). A possible explanation for the discrepancy is that the anaerobic conditions used were not sufficiently strict. It is extremely difficult to prevent enough oxygen from entering the system to allow some endogenous biosynthesis. In a recent paper (*48*), for instance, reporting the effects of exogenous sterols on "anaerobically" grown yeast, 29% of the sterol found in membranes was derived from endogenous biosynthesis when the medium contained cholesterol. On the other hand, careful studies (*20*) on the effect of drastically limited oxygen show that yeast produces a higher ratio of lanosterol to ergosterol than when oxygen is abundant. Slow growth under these semianaerobic conditions suggests that lanosterol may function to some degree as a membraneous component, perhaps sparing rather than replacing ergosterol. There is, in any event, little question that ergosterol will support growth quantitatively in a far superior fashion. In the absence of oxygen, no growth occurs; with limited oxygen and an accumulation of lanosterol, only a few million cells/per milliliter are obtained; while in the presence of ergosterol but no oxygen, 100 million cells/per milliliter result in the same time period (*20*). A preference for 4,4,14-trisdesmethylsterols is also shown by *Tetrahymena pyriformis*. When sterols, e.g., cholesterol, campesterol, ergosterol, sitosterol, stigmasterol, and others are added to the medium, growth occurs as it does in their absence (*54–59*), but biosynthesis of the natural pentacycle (tetrahymanol) is inhibited (*59, 60*) and the sterol is found in its place in the membranes (*14, 61*). Thus, the weight of evidence leads to the compelling conclusion that the dimensions of the molecule are critical. Both the growth studies and natural occurrence indicate the best architectural fit is achieved by the 4,4,14-trisdesmethylsterols bearing stereochemistry with or approximating the all-*trans-anti*-arrangement. As this is departed from, there is presumably a loss in membraneous functionality, a part of which may be compensated for by adjustments in the phospholipid. In *T. pyriformis*, for instance, sterol-grown cells exhibit a shortening of the fatty acyl chain length, lowering in the degree of unsaturation, and a discrimination between $\Delta^{6,11}$- and $\Delta^{9,12}$-$C_{18:2}$-acids (*61*).

The importance of the all-*trans-anti*-arrangement in the nucleus undoubtedly derives from its flatness. Alternate carbon atoms lie approximately in a plane, with the two planes containing the two series of alternate carbon atoms lying parallel to one another. The nucleus is therefore like a table-top, flat but with thickness. Axial or equatorial groups project from this "table-top" at various positions. One can analyze approximately what this latter detail is from conformational and configurational considerations.

A more exacting analysis has been made by physical measurements of several kinds, among which is x-ray diffraction. The work on the latter method, pioneered in the 1930s by Bernal (*62*) and carried further by his associate Crowfoot (*63, 64*), has been extended recently by Duax (*65–67*) and others. The atomic coordinates of cholesteryl chloride were first reported by Carlisle and Crowfoot in 1945 (*63*). Structures of more than 234 steroids have now been examined. For a key to the literature and detailed presentations see Duax and Norton (*66*), Duax et al. (*65, 67*), and Romers et al. (*68*). The bond distances in Δ^5-sterols are all close to 1.53 Å (1.51–1.56), except for the C-5,6 distance, which is 1.32 Å. The bond angles for the tetrahedral carbon atoms are slightly more than the theoretical 109°, as is shown in Scheme 11.1. The annular carbon atoms of the nucleus are all

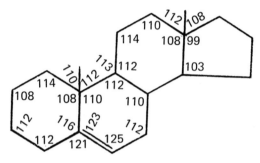

Scheme 11.1. Bond angles in Δ^5-steroids. Data are from Duax et al. (*66*) and averages for 15 compounds. Angles are rounded to nearest degree.

unequivocally in the chair form and lie with 1 Å of a plane (zero plane), passing through the molecule as shown for the saturated 5α-androstane derivatives in Scheme 11.2. The angular methyl groups protrude about 1.5 Å above this plane at roughly 90°. The equatorial 3β-hydroxyl group lies somewhat less than 1 Å below the zero plane and the C—O bond projects away from the nucleus in a plane tilted slightly toward the zero plane passing through the molecule. The axial 3α-hydroxyl group projects down from the zero plane, extending somewhat more than 2 Å from it. In 3-keto steroids the oxygen also projects down and 1.5–2.0 Å from the zero plane. The 17β-substituent projects slightly above the zero plane. In the 5β-series (Scheme 11.3), a very different situation arises in which all of ring A projects down at nearly 90°. The side chain projects at a small angle above the zero plane in the direction shown by the 17β-hydroxy substituent of the diols shown in Schemes 11.2 and 11.3. The preferred skew conformation about the 17(20)-bond of sterols bearing a 20α-H atom places C-22 to the right ("right-handed" side chain) in the usual view of the molecule with the nuclear β face toward the observer and C-3 to the left (*69, 70*). When C-22 lies to the left ("left-handed" side chain), the molecule has no membrane-

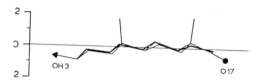

3β-Hydroxy-5α-androstan-17-one

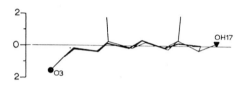

17β-Hydroxy-5α-androstan-3-one

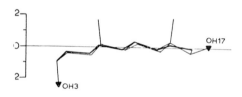

5α-Androstan-3α,17β-diol

Scheme 11.2. Structures of all *trans-anti*-steroids as deduced from x-ray data (66). The molecule is viewed on its edge. The scale on the left is in angstroms.

ous activity. This has been demonstrated (50) by comparative studies of sterols with normal and iso-configurations at C-20. Sterols with a 20β-H have a preferred skew conformation in which the side chain is left-handed, and they fail to support the growth of anaerobic yeast, while their isomers with a 20α-H and a right-handed conformation do support growth (Table 11.6). That the effect is conformational [at the 17(20)-bond] rather than configurational (at C-20) was demonstrated by obtaining parallel results with left- and right-handed $\Delta^{17(20)}$-sterols that lack asymmetry at C-20. The latter [E-configuration at the 17(20)-bond, also called *trans*] did, and the former (Z- or *cis*-configuration) did not support growth. Similarly, only the sterols with right-handed side chains were metabolized by *T. pyriformis* to give their $\Delta^{5,7,22}$-derivatives (50). The most active molecules, therefore, are elongated parallelograms of approximately 4 Å thickness with the terminus

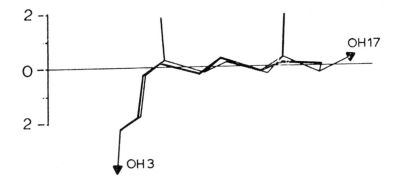

5β-Androstan-3α,17β-diol

Scheme 11.3. Structure of a *cis-anti-trans-anti-trans*-steroid as deduced from x-ray data (*66*). The molecule is viewed on its edge. The scale on the left is in angstroms.

Table 11.6. Membrane dependence on side chain stereochemistry[a]

Structure (R = Remainder of cholesterol side chain)			
Growth Supporting		Inactive	

[a] From Nes et al. (*50*).

of the side chain at one end and the polar hydroxyl group at the other, as is shown in Scheme 11.4. The overall thickness is determined by the angular methyl groups on one side and on the other by the plane containing the axial H atoms on alternate carbon atoms, which include C-3. In Schemes 11.2 and 11.3 the thickness can be visualized from the top of the angular methyl groups (which would include the H atoms, altogether approximately 2Å from the zero line) to the bottom of the axial H atoms on the lower plane of carbon atoms. Although these H atoms are not shown, the C—H bond distance is 1.5 Å, which, when added to the displacement of a few

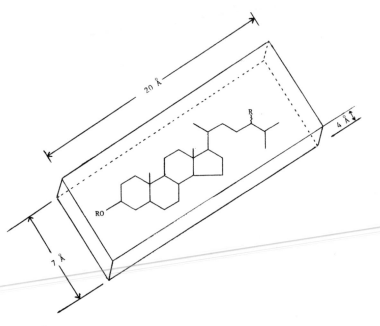

Scheme 11.4. Elongated, flat character of membraneous steroids.

tenths of an Å of the bottom carbon plane, gives about 2 Å from the zero plane.

If one rotates tetrahymanol around an axis halving the molecule in the central ring, the stereochemistry of the molecule (except for the OH group, the converse on either side of the line) deduced in part by x-ray diffraction (71) is such that ring A, in terms of orientation on the biosynthetic cyclase (electrophilic attack of H^+ on the double bond), becomes ring E (Scheme 11.5) when compared to a steroid. Conversely, biosynthetic ring E bearing the hydroxyl group (derived by nucleophilic attack) becomes ring A when compared to a steroid; i.e., in a functional sense it is possible to designate ring A as that one containing the hydroxyl group. It will be

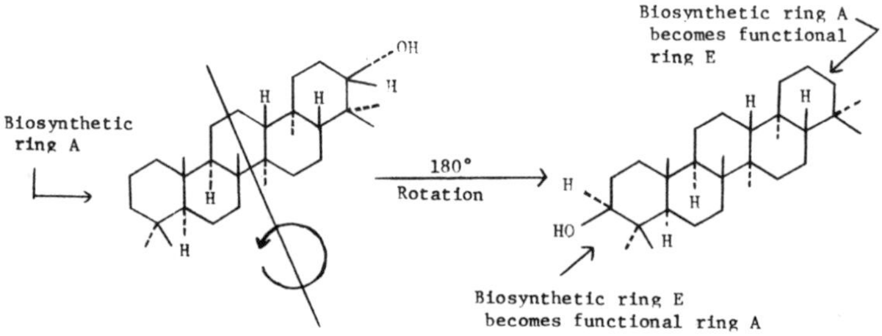

Scheme 11.5. Structure of tetrahymanol illustrating its relationship to sterols.

seen from Scheme 11.5 that tetrahymanol then mimics the shape of a sterol. More precisely, it is exactly the same as lanosterol except for 1) an 8β-methyl group in place of an 8β-H atom, a 13β-H atom in place of a 13β-CH$_3$ group, enlargement of ring D, transfer of C-21 to C-17, and cyclization of the 17β side chain. The primary effect of these changes is to thicken slightly the molecule in places when compared to the sterols. Since otherwise it retains the flat character and approximate length of sterols, it is not surprising that it can act as a membraneous component in a specialized system. It is interesting to note in this regard that tetrahymanol is biosynthesized by a variety of species of the genus *Tetrahymena* (72) (as well as in plants), but only the species *T. pyriformis* grows well in the absence of lipid supplements (73).

The necessity of sterols (or substances that mimic them) for membranes of eukaryotic organisms is apparently violated to some extent by the fungus *Phytophthora cactorum*, the mycelium of which contains no sterols (37). However, sterols, e.g., cholesterol and cholestanol, stimulate vegetative growth (74) and they are necessary for oospore formation (37, 75). The number of oospores produced thus becomes a means of quantifying the effectiveness of various structures, as does the time required to produce them. Cholesterol, ergosterol, and stigmasterol all induce oospore production in abundant quantity in 5–6 days, while Δ^4- and Δ^5-cholestenone, $\Delta^{4,6}$-cholestadienone, 5β-cholestanone, cholestane, 20-keto-, 17-keto-, and 17β-hydroxy steroids, squalene, and sodium acetate produce no more than do unsupplemented cultures (37). A precise comparison of sterol structures yielded the following relative activities: sitosterol = isofucosterol = fucosterol = stigmasterol > cholesterol = 7-dehydrocholesterol > ergosterol > cholestanol (75). It is clear that a substituent at C-24 and a Δ^5-bond (preferably but not necessarily in the absence of a Δ^7-bond) enhance the activity and that a Δ^{22}-bond is essentially neutral. As in other systems (Tables 11.3 and 11.5), the hydroxyl group at C-3 and an A/B-*trans*-junction were necessary (37).

It has been thought (47, 48) that anaerobic yeast displays little specificity for sterol structure. This has probably been brought about by difficulties in excluding oxygen. Under rigorous conditions (no sterol yielding no growth), cholesterol is only about one-quarter as effective as ergosterol in promoting growth and the cholesterol-supplemented cells display pathology (pseudomycelia and early death) (49). Much the same though not identical behavior is induced by 5α-cholestan-3β-ol (cholestanol), and removal of the hydroxyl group to give 5α-cholestane abolishes all activity (Table 11.5). Yeast's natural sterol (ergosterol) is characterized by a $\Delta^{5,7}$-diene system and a Δ^{22}-24β-methyl side chain. The importance of these is in the reverse order; i.e., the most important is the 24β-methyl group, followed by its conjunction with the Δ^{22}-unsaturation, followed by the $\Delta^{5,7}$-diene system. The deleterious effects of cholesterol are reversed if the side chain is restored by using brassicasterol, the Δ^{22}-24β-methyl derivative of cholesterol (20). The presence of the $\Delta^{5,7}$-system under natural conditions seems, therefore, to be more a result of a phylogenetic block in biosynthesis than of a feedback derived from greater functionality of the homoannular diene system. Conversely, the presence of the alkylated (and unsaturated) side chain is clearly not simple happenstance, since it confers a higher degree of functionality on the molecule. The relative orders given are derived from yeast cultures soon after they are placed in an anaerobic environment. With time (6 months), the structural specificity lessens, for reasons that are not clear. Older anaerobic cultures still show better growth with ergosterol than with cholesterol, but the difference is much less than with new cultures (20). This adaptation may have to do with increasing repression of the mitochondria through successive generations. During early phases, while not functioning in respiration, the mitochondria may still perform biosynthetic roles that are compensated for in later stages. If the mitochondrial membrane has a greater specificity for the alkylated side chain than does, say, the cytoplasmic membrane, the differential results with the new and old cultures would be explicable. In concert with this explanation is the fact that in aerobic cultures the C_1-transferase is known to be localized in (or on) the mitochondria (76), even though there can be no question that ergosterol is not only in the mitochondrial (12) but also in the cycloplasmic (10, 77) membrane. Moreover, with another fungus (Aspergillus fenelliae) surviving "mutants" are resistant to successive treatment with polyene antibiotics (high levels of amphotericin B and low levels of nystatin). Cells resistant to the former lacked ergosterol and those resistant to the latter have some ergosterol and a new sterol. Lack of ergosterol was associated with reduced growth rate, poor asexual reproduction, and loss of sexual reproduction.

Detailed differences between various membranes in their requirements for structural features of sterols is displayed in systems other than fungal ones. While it is commonly believed that all animals or animal-like organisms require cholesterol (usually therefore referred to as the "zoosterol"), this is not so. A more correct generalization is that all examined vertebrates both biosynthesize cholesterol and utilize it as their dominant sterol in membranes. This is paralleled, at least in L-cell mouse fibroblasts (79), by the following order of cellular incorporation from the medium: cholesterol > cholestanol > sitosterol. However, the fly Drosophila pachea as well as the protozoan Paramecium aurelia are characterized by an inability either to biosynthesize or to utilize cholesterol (19, 80, 81). In the former case, development of larvae requires a Δ^7- or $\Delta^{5,7}$-sterol with a 24-H (lathosterol or 7-dehydrocholesterol) or 24α-ethyl group (schottenol or 7-dehydrositosterol). The intermediate Δ^7-24β-methyl structure (24β-methyllathosterol or ergosterol) is inactive. Paramecium aurelia similarly will not grow on cholesterol or ergosterol (Table 11.7) but will on Δ^5-24-ethylsterols. In both

Table 11.7. Sterol requirements of animals and protozoa incapable of utilizing cholesterol[a]

Organism	Active Sterols	Metabolite	Inactive Sterols
Paramecium aurelia	Stigmasterol Clionasterol Sitosterol Poriferasterol 7-Dehydrostigmasterol	7-Dehydrostigmasterol $\Delta^{5,7}$ $\Delta^{5,7}$ $\Delta^{5,7}$	Cholesterol Erosterol 7-Dehydrocholesterol 22-Dehydrocholesterol 7,22-Bisdehydrocholesterol
Drosophila pachea	Lathosterol 7-Dehydrocholesterol 7-Dehydrositosterol (but animals infertile)	7-Dehydrocholesterol	Cholesterol Sitosterol Stigmasterol 24β-Methyllathosterol Ergosterol

[a] From Conner et al. (*19*), Heed and Kircher (*80*), and Goodnight and Kircher (*81*).

P. aurelia and *D. pachea* the active sterols with a double bond in ring B are converted to $\Delta^{5,7}$-sterols. The protozoan introduces a Δ^{7}-bond into Δ^{5}-sterols and the insect does the converse. A requirement for $\Delta^{5,7}$-sterols is also shown by the beetle *Xylaborus ferrugineus* (*82*).

4. Structure-Activity Correlations in Model Systems

If one mixes a phospholipid with a sterol in chloroform and removes the solvent, a complex (a so-called "liposome") is produced that can then be suspended in an appropriate aqueous (or other) medium and its properties examined. Liposomes can also be obtained by direct mixing in aqueous media. Phospholipids from a variety of sources and complexed with several steroids have been studied in a manner such as this. Among the properties investigated is the degree of order in the liposome, which can be estimated by electron-spin resonance (ESR) of nitroxides attached to one of the components (so-called "spin labeling"). The angle between the nitroxide and the lipid lamellae influences the hyperfine splittings in the spectra (*83*). The ESR technique gives results (*84*) that parallel those obtained from growth and related in vivo studies. 5α-Cholestan-3β-ol yields highly ordered systems with brain phospholipids or erythrocyte ghosts partially depleted of cholesterol, while 5α-cholestanone causes only a low degree of ordering, and 5α-cholestane produces none indicating the oxygen function at C-3 is important. Similarly, 5β-cholestan-3β-ol and lanosterol have only slight effectiveness, and squalene has none. The technique is less effective, however, than the studies in vivo in discriminating fine detail of the side chain, since sitosterol and ergosterol were about as effective as cholesterol, and since even in the absence of a side chain and an inverted configuration at C-5 (5β-cholestan-3β-ol) ordering was observed. Its 3-epimer was without ordering activity, as were 20-keto- and 17-hydroxy-steroids (*84*). Methoxy, carbonyl oxygen, or chloro substituents at C-3 drastically reduce the ordering (*85*).

The ability of cholesterol to condense, i.e., to restrict, the volume of phospholipid layers was observed as early as 1925 by Leathes (*86*). A wide variety of spectroscopic and other techniques has verified that this results from restriction of the alkyl chains in the phospholipid by some sort of interdigitation of the sterol. See Darke et al. (*87*) and Phillips and Finer (*88*) for a key to the literature.

The idea of a condensing effect also implies a strong temperature dependence of the ability of the fatty acyl chains to orient themselves. At some critical point, T_c, analogous to a melting point, a phase transition will occur. Below it, high order ("crystallization") is achieved, while above it (the "liquid crystalline" or "fluid state") much more motion (conformational equilibria) occurs. T_c can be determined by measuring some rate parameter against temperature. A graph of the reciprocal of the absolute temperature (usually plotted on the x axis) against the log of the parameter (growth, rate, etc.) will give two intersecting straight lines with different slopes (an Arrehnius plot). The temperature of the discontinuity (break) is T_c. The addition of cholesterol to many liposome and membrane preparations has been found to lower T_c. Cholesterol decreases chain mobility and reduces mean molecular area when phospholipids are in the liquid-crystalline state and increases chain mobility in the gel state. See de Kruyff et al. for a key to the literature (89). The concept of "fluidity" is returned to in a subsequent paragraph. When dispersed in water, lecithin and cholesterol can form an equimolar complex, and NMR data indicate the lecithin phosphate group and the sterol hydroxyl group are juxtaposed (87). Moreover, when less than equimolar amounts are present, NMR indicates there is a clustering of the sterol molecules coincident with a clustering of lecithin molecules (88). Differential scanning calorimetry (89) shows that clustering is nonrandom. Cholesterol interacts preferentially with the phosphatidyl choline species with the lowest transition temperature. With spin-labeled sterol in liposomes, the spin label is orientated nearly perpendicularly to the lamellar plane of the phospholipid (90). Force-area measurements (91) of liposomes indicate that sterols lie perpendicularly to the air-water interface. Minimal area per molecule is achieved only with 3β-hydroxysterols in the A/B-*trans*-series or with those approximating it (Δ^5-, $\Delta^{5,7}$, etc.). With mycoplasmas the presence of cholesterol reduces permeability to glycerol and erythritol, and this has been related to the sterol's condensing effect (92). With egg lecithin liposomes, similar permeability effects were found (93), and sterols with a 24-H atom were more effective than those with a 24α- or 24β-alkyl substituent. Sterols with inverted (3α or 5β) stereochemistry or lacking a side chain were ineffective. Cholesterol reduces the energy content of phase transitions of lecithin as measured by differential scanning calorimetry for either liposomes prepared from mycoplasma lipids or with the intact membranes themselves (92). 3-Epicholesterol, 5α-androstan-3β-ol, and cholesta-4,6-dien-3-one failed to show such an effect, in agreement with the importance of an equatorial hydroxyl group and the presence of an alkyl side chain.

By the use of the spin-labeling technique (94) with egg lecithin liposomes, the effect of the length of the side chain has been found to be crucial. When the side chain is shorter by more than three carbon atoms, ordering of the fatty acyl chains falls off rapidly. When the side chain is alkylated in the homologous series cholesterol, 24α-methyl- and 24α-ethyl-cholesterol, there is a slight preference for incorporation of the unalkylated sterol into egg lecithin liposomes (95). When the sterol of the lecithin-sterol liposome was allowed to exchange with the cholesterol of erythrocytes, the erythrocytes again favored the cholesterol (95).

In another study (96) Arrehnius plots of yeast mitochondrial ATPase activity showed that, with increasing ergosterol content of the organelle (in the range of 7–105 mg/g of mitochondrial protein), the temperature of the discontinuity decreases as much as 17°, proving that the effect of the sterol on membrane architecture is also manifest on the activity of membrane-bound enzymes. Similarly, when ergosterol is replaced by 24β-methylcholesta-8,22-dien-3β-ol, a decrease in the phase-transition temperature of the mitochondrial membrane occurs when the activity of the C_1-transferase is used as the rate parameter (97). With membranes of *Mycoplasma mycoides* grown on ample cholesterol, no break in the Arrehnius plots of the ATPase activity is detectable, but when the organism is adapted to low cholesterol concentrations (yielding membranes with 3% of the lipid rather than 25% being cholesterol) breaks occur that depend on the structure of the fatty acyl chains in the phospholipid (98, 99). The native cells are also capable of growing at lower temperatures. This and other facts are interpreted (98, 99) to mean that the sterol maintains the other lipids in a "fluid state." In mycoplasma cells the presence of sterol can be demonstrated to have a variety of other effects, e.g., on permeability and osmotic fragility (98, 99) as well as on interaction with polyene antibiotics (100), which are also believed to be associated with the "fluidity."

The concept of "fluidity" has been most well investigated with liposomal models. Among these are combinations of cholesterol with dipalmitoyl or egg lecithin. A variety of techniques (NMR, ESR, x-ray diffraction, permeability, scanning calorimetry, Raman spectroscopy, etc.) have allowed exploration of the physical properties of these systems. See Lippert and Peticolas (101) for a key to the literature. What has been found, as introduced previously in terms of Arrhenius plots, is that there is a transition point (at temperature T_c) at which the fatty acyl chains of the phospholipid proceed from a highly ordered, semicrystalline condition (below T_c) to a less ordered state (above T_c). The former is often called the "gel" phase and the latter the "liquid-crystalline" phase. Two sorts of effects of cholesterol were observed in the late 1960s. Below T_c the fatty acyl chains become more mobile than otherwise would be the case, while above it the reverse happens, i.e., they become more restricted than in the absence of sterol. The comparison, it should be noted, is being made of the mobility of the chains at a given temperature in the presence and absence of sterol; then the comparison is made again at another temperature that is on the other side of T_c. Ladbrooke, Williams, and Chapman (102) have interpreted the results to mean that sterol disrupts the crystalline lattice (below T_c) by interdigitation between the fatty acyl chains, thereby reducing the crystallinity (increasing the "fluidity") of the gel phase. On the other hand, above T_c, where increased conformational motion of the fatty acyl chains would normally lead to the liquid-crystalline phase, the presence of sterol packed between the layers of chains decreases their capacity for conformational freedom (sometimes called "flexing"), making this phase more rigid than it would otherwise be. The net result of the sterol's presence is to reduce the difference between the two phases insofar as freedom of motion of the fatty acyl chains is concerned. For instance, abrupt changes at 1,100 cm^{-1} in the Raman spectrum of dipalmitoyl lecithin occur when T_c is passed, but in the presence of sterol the changes in the spectrum while present are subdued (broadened), corresponding to a diffuse change in the conformation of the fatty acyl chains (*101*). Furthermore, the energy absorbed in passing through T_c from below it to above it (obtained by calorimetry) is less in the presence of sterol. This reduction in the difference between the two phases leads to opposite effects of the sterol above and below T_c. Not only does sterol induce fluidity below T_c and rigidity above it, but permeability to glycerol or glycol is enhanced below it and decreased above it (*103*). The presence of sterol also probably influences the interaction of proteins (*104*) and has been shown to affect the action of ionophores on Rb$^+$ movement through bilayers (*105*). X-ray analysis of aqueous liposomes has yielded the dimensions of the system and shown that the maximum allowable amount of sterol is 30%, corresponding to about a 1:1-molar ratio of sterol and lecithin (*106*).

The ability of sterols to interact with phospholipids (and proteins) is undoubtedly a result of their unusual mix of hydrophobic (*107*) and steric characteristics. For most membranes this mix appears to be best achieved with free sterols, but, as discussed in Chapter 10, subcellular particles of plants are well known to have some of their sterols present as esters. The presence of esters in animal organelles is also known. In particular, cholesteryl 14-methylhexadecanoate has been isolated (*108*) from rat ribosomes and evidence presented to indicate that is is essential for the activity of the peptide elongation factors, transferases I and II.

C. HORMONES

1. Progesterone

a. Isolation and Biosynthesis in Animals   Progesterone was first isolated in 1934 simultaneously by four groups of investigators (*109–113*) from the corpora lutea of sow ovaries. It required the glands of 50,000 animals to yield 20 mg. Subsequently, it was identified in various other endocrine tissues. Progesterone is a crucial intermediate in the biosynthesis of hormones of the adrenal cortex, ovaries, and testes; it also plays a hormonal role itself.

Although as early as 1945, Bloch (*113*) presented evidence for the conversion of injected cholesterol in a pregnant woman to urinary pregnanediol, which was found a few years earlier (*114*) to be a progesterone metabolite, the real breakthrough in the study of hormone biosynthesis came from the development of techniques with the isolated adrenal gland. In the late 1940s, Hechter (*115*) developed a perfusion system whereby he could add precursors to the perfusate and examine products in the effluent. Various reasonable pathways had already become obvious to him as well as to others. For a detailed review of the history see Hechter (*116*). Pregnenolone, the 20-ketone corresponding to cholesterol already known to be present in endocrine tissue (*117*), was an obvious intermediate to progesterone, which itself was envisioned as a further intermediate to the corticords, androgens, and estrogens. In the early 1950s, Hechter and his associates (*118*) perfused [^{14}C]cholesterol and obtained labeled cortisol and corticosterone. Shortly thereafter it was found that adrenal homogenates would yield the same results (*119, 120*). Then, in the mid-1950s, Gurin and his associates (*121, 122*) demonstrated that cholesterol proceeded first to pregnenolone and suggested that 20α-hydroxycholesterol was an intermediate. At the same time the conversion of pregnenolone to progesterone was demonstrated by Samuels (*123, 124*) and by the Hechter group (*119*) (Scheme 11.6). The reaction involves oxidative cleavage of the side chain at the 20(22)-bond. The fragment comprised by C-22 to C-27 was identified as isocaproic acid (2-methylpentanoic acid) (*122*). The rupture of the 20(22)-bond occurs in several steps that involve a sequence problem.

20α,22β-Dihydroxycholesterol as well as the 20α- and 22β-monohydroxycholesterols have been isolated (or identified by tracer techniques) from adrenal glands (*125–133*). Both 20α-hydroxycholesterol, known as (20*S*)-20-hydroxycholesterol in the *R*,*S*-notation, and 22β-hydroxycholesterol, known as (22*R*)-22-hydroxycholesterol, have been converted to pregnenolone (*125, 128, 129, 134*) and both have been converted to 20α,22β-dihydroxycholesterol, known as (20*R*,22*R*)-20,22-dihydroxycholesterol, a nomenclature inversion occurring in the *R*,*S*-notation at C-20 compared to 20α-hydroxycholesterol (*128, 129, 134*). Moreover, the dihydroxysterol has been converted to pregnenolone (*129*). These various investigations therefore indicate that cholesterol is first monohydroxylated either at C-20 or C-22, followed by introduction of a second hydroxyl group at the position not previously attacked. The dihydroxycholesterol is then cleaved to give pregnenolone. However, both monohydroxysterols have not been simultaneously identified. Thus, in a recent study, Burstein, Middleditch, and Gut (*128*) incubated cholesterol with an acetone-dried powder preparation of adrenocortical mitochondria. They obtained 22β-hydroxycholesterol and 20α,22β-dihydroxycholesterol but no 20α-hydroxycholesterol. On the other hand, Roberts, Bandy, and Lieberman (*125*) and Shimizu, Hayano, Gut, and Dorfman (*129*) have converted 20α-hydroxycholesterol to pregnenolone (and to dihydroxycholesterol) with adrenal preparations. The reasons for these discrepancies are not clear. A possible explanation lies in metabolism at C-3. The 3-sulfate of 20α-hydroxycholesterol is converted to pregnenolone in high yield (*125*), suggesting along with other evidence that the unesterified sterol may not be a true intermediate.

The mechanism of the cleavage of the hydroxylated intermediate(s) unquestionably involves mixed-function oxidases (*131*). The oxygen atoms

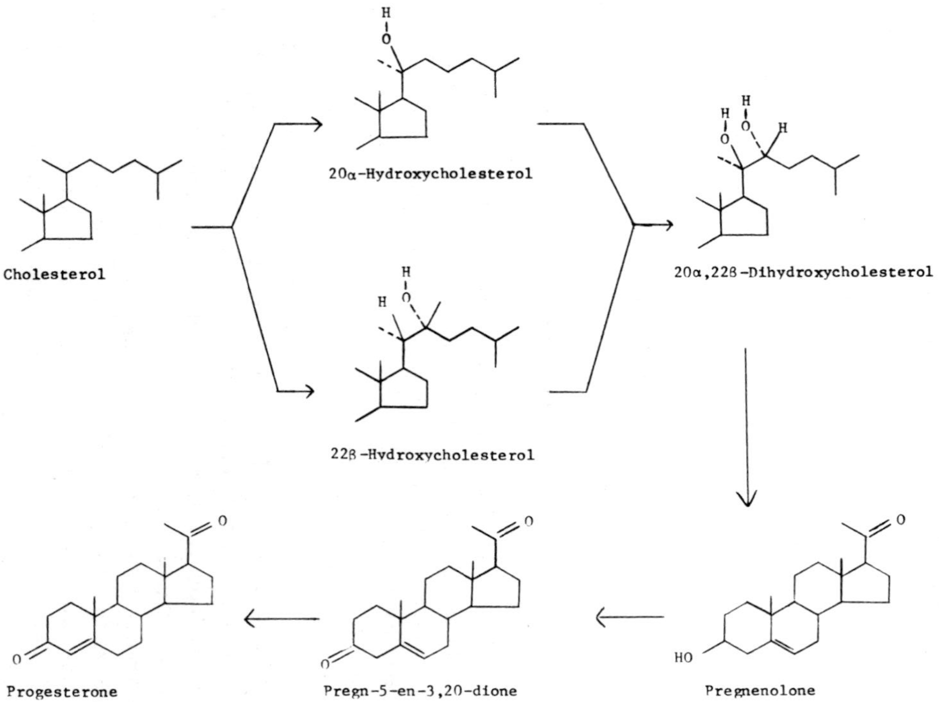

Scheme 11.6. Pathway from cholesterol to progesterone.

at C-20 and C-22 of the 22β-hydroxy- and 20α,22β-dihydroxycholesterols are derived from molecular oxygen (128) and the cleavage is aerobic and dependent on reduced pyridine nucleotide (131). Since neither (E)- nor (Z)-20 (22)-dehydrocholesterol proceeds to pregnenolone and since (20R,22R)-20,22-epoxycholesterol also does not yield pregnenolone (135), a suggested (136–138) pathway through a monohydroxycholesterol that undergoes dehydration, epoxidation, and hydrolytic opening of the epoxy ring to give the dihydroxycholesterol seems to be excluded (135). This is corroborated by retention of [18]O in the dihydroxysterol when 20α-hydroxycholesterol labeled at C-20 with [18]O is the substrate (135), as well as by the origin of the oxygen at C-20 and C-22 in [18]O$_2$ (128). However, (20R,22S)-20,22-epoxycholesterol does proceed to pregnenolone in a yield about one-sixth as great as cholesterol does (135). Does this mean the epoxide is on the pathway after, rather than before, the dihydroxycholesterol? Little is actually known about the process beyond this point. For reasons not understood in detail, 20α-hydroxycholesterol, pregnenolone, and various other steroids inhibit the cleavage of cholesterol (139–141). The involvement of metallo complexes in the cleavage has been suggested (142). Cleavage can occur when C-22 is incorporated into a benzene ring (142). A 20α-ethyl group also does not prevent cleavage. Evidence that the physiological sequence of events for the formation of steroid hormones occurs through the usual process of conversion of acetate to sterol has been obtained through the degradation of radioactive cortisol derived from labeled acetate (143). The expected labeling pattern was observed.

The further metabolism of pregnenolone to progesterone proceeds by microsomal pyridine nucleotide-dependent oxidation of the hydroxyl group at C-3 to a keto group giving pregn-5-en-3,20-dione (Δ^5-pregnenedione), which is isomerized to the Δ^4-derivative (progesterone) (124, 144–146). The isomerization reaction, which is a separate step, has been well studied mechanistically using an induced bacterial enzyme. While acid catalysis results in a "push-pull" process with incorporation of an H atom at C-6 from the medium (147), with the isomerase an internal 1,3-migration occurs from C-6 to C-4 (148).

As already mentioned, steroidal sulfates may be involved in hormone biosynthesis. It is worth noting that, following the isolation of cholesteryl sulfate from bovine adrenals (149), it has been found in many other mammalian tissues and fluids. Cholesteryl sulfate has also been identified in eggs of the sea urchin (*Anthoeidaris crassispina*) (150), and this and other steryl sulfates are present in starfish (*Asterias rubens*) (151, 152).

b. Isolation, Biosynthesis, and Metabolism in Plants Pregnenolone has been isolated from a number of plants, including *Xysmalobium undulatum* (153). Its biosynthesis from cholesterol has been documented in *Digitalis purpurea* (154) and *Haplopappus heterophyllus* (155a), and its conversion to progesterone in *Digitalis lanata* (*156, 157*), *Holarrhena floribunda* (*155b*), and plant tissue cultures (*158*). Progesterone has been isolated from *Holarrhena floribunda* (*159a*) and apples (*159b*). Interest in the presence and metabolism of these steroids in plants stems in part from studies of the biosynthesis of cardenolides that bear a five-membered lactone ring at C-17. In 1964, Tschesche and Lilienweiss (*160*) found that cardenolides were formed from pregnenolone in *Digitalis lanata*. A few years later, Heftmann and his associates (*157*) obtained progesterone as well as a number of other steroids from pregnenolone in this plant, and Caspi and Lewis (*156*) demonstrated that progesterone would proceed to the cardenolides. Progesterone may be reduced to 5β-pregnenedione, hydroxylated at C-14, and condensed with an appropriate C_2 or related unit to give such cardenolides as digitoxigenin. Substantiating evidence is that the diketone is formed from pregnenolone in *D. lanata* (*157*), but a sequence problem exists relative, for instance, to the 14-hydroxylation (*161, 162*). Support for the general pathway through a steroidal 20-ketone comes from an analysis of the fate of C atoms from mevalonic acid. [2-^{14}C]Mevalonic acid yields labeled digitoxigenin, but no ^{14}C appears in the side chain (*162–165*). This proves the removal of the original C-22 and its reintroduction. Examination of the structure reveals that C-23 is at the carboxyl stage, suggesting that C-22 and C-23 are derived from C-2 and C-1, respectively, of acetyl CoA (or malonyl CoA). In agreement, [1-^{14}C]acetate labels digitoxigenin at C-23 (*165*), while [3'-^{14}C]MVA labels it at C-21 (*165*) and [3-^{14}C]MVA at C-20 (*166*). The physiological intermediacy of a 3-ketone was also demonstrated by the loss of the 3α-H atom of pregnenolone in proceeding to digitoxigenin (*167*). The sequence shown in Scheme 11.7 represents one of several possible pathways, and a number of steps have been ignored, e.g., hydroxylation at C-21. 21-Hydroxylation of progesterone itself would give desoxycorticosterone. While this has actually been demonstrated in *D. lanata* (*168*), hydroxylation probably does not take place at this stage physiologically for several reasons (*168, 169*). 14β-Hydroxylation is believed to be a better candidate for the first step after pregnenolone. 7α-tritio-20α-Hydroxycholesterol leads to labeled digitoxigenin and other cardenolides in *D. lanata* but to unlabeled progesterone (*155*), in agreement with the early introduction of the 14β-hydroxyl group.

In *Strophanthus* species, cardenolides, exist with 5β-hydroxyl groups, e.g., periplogenin, which is 5β-hydroxydigitoxigenin, and with C-19 oxidized to the aldehyde stage, e.g., periplogenin, which is 5β-hydroxydigitoxigenin, and with C-19 oxidized to the aldehyde stage, e.g., strophanthidin, which is the C-19 aldehyde of periplogenin (Scheme 11.8). Progesterone also leads to these compounds and to 5β-hydroxy intermediates in *S. kombé* (*170*). Pregnenolone is probably also the prescursor of the six-membered lactone ring constituting the side chain of the bufadienolides (*171*) and of

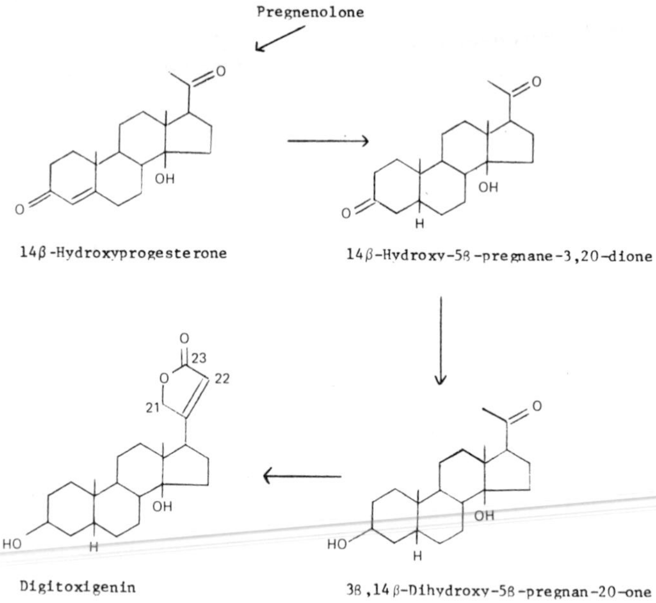

Scheme 11.7. A possible pathway for the conversion of progesterone to a cardenolide.

various C_{21}-alkaloids, e.g., halophyllamine, which is pregnenolone with NH_2 replacing the 3β-OH group. This and related subjects has been reviewed in greater detail by Singh et al. (172).

Many of the lactones just discussed occur naturally as glycosides at C-3, sometimes with unusual sugars, e.g., cymarose. Thus, the k-strophanthoside is the trioside, glucosyl-glucosyl-cymarosyl-strophanthidin, cymarose being a 3-methoxy-2-desoxy-hexose. These glycosides have powerful effects on the cardiovascular system of animals. Known collectively as "cardiac glycosides," they have been used as arrow poisons. The poisons of toads (bufotoxins such as bufotalin) are not glycosides. They occur as the free steroid and as suberylarginine esters, both of which are pharmacologically active.

c. Function of Progesterone   As discussed in the previous sections, pregnenolone and progesterone have an important role to play as precursors to other steroids. This will be extended in subsequent sections dealing with the origin of the other hormones. However, while pregnenolone is known only to play such a role, progesterone is a hormone in its own right. It is beyond the scope of this book to discuss the physiology in depth, but it can be summarized as follows. In response to a brief elevation in the blood concentration of luteinizing hormone (LH), which is a polypeptide from the pituitary gland, ovulation occurs, i.e., the mature (Graafian) follicle on the surface of an ovary ruptures, and the egg (ovum) inside it

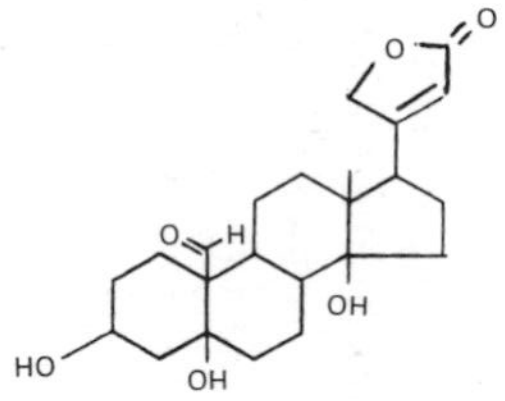

Strophanthidin

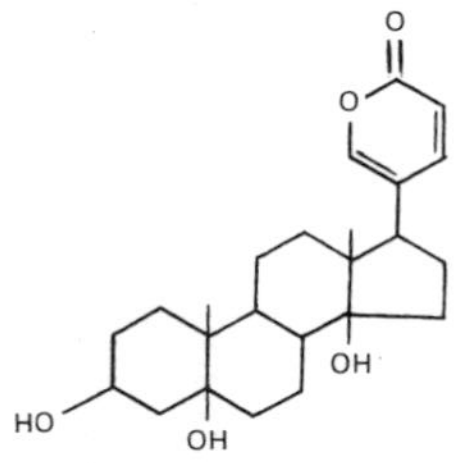

Helebrigenin

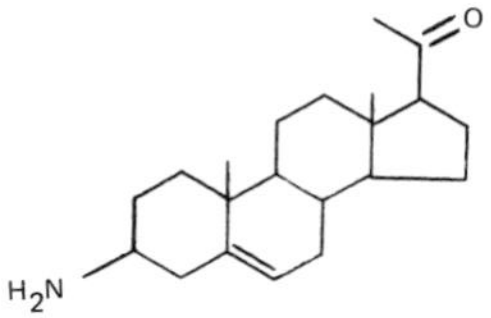

Halophyllamine

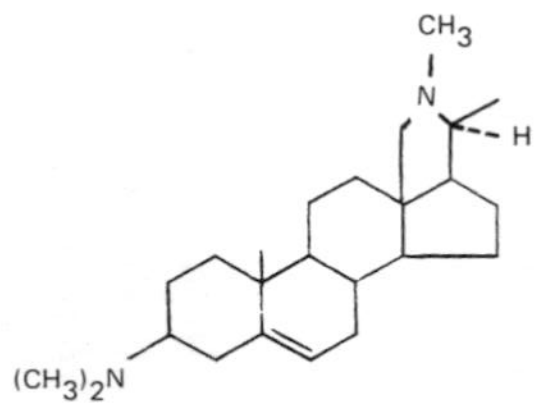

Conessine

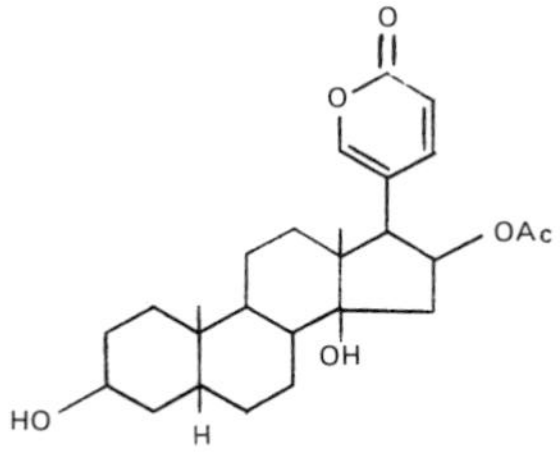

Bufotalin

Scheme 11.8. Some steroids bearing the C atoms of pregnenolone.

is transferred in a still rather mysterious process to one of the Fallopian tubes. The ruptured follicle then reconstitutes itself in a remarkable and very poorly understood metamorphosis to give a new endocrine gland, known from its yellowish color (from β-carotene) as a corpus luteum. Evidence exists that the carotenoid is biosynthesized in the gland but for what purpose is obscure. The corpus luteum then functions to biosynthesize progesterone, which is secreted into the blood. This is known as the luteal phase of estrus or menstrual cycles. During the period before ovulation (follicular phase), estrogen is produced; among other things, it functions to sustain the uterus. The estrogen-stimulated uterus is then acted on by the progesterone to induce differentiation of the cells in the inner lining (endometrium). This differentiation is necessary for implanation of the somewhat developed (blastocyst) zygote (fertilized ovum), which has descended through and from the Fallopian tube if fertilization has occured. It is from this process of initiating preparation for gestation that progesterone derives its name.

A number of other physiological effects of progesterone are known that may be species dependent. Among them, and of great importance, is its action as an inhibitor of FSH and LH secretion, manifested through the hypothalmic-pituitary axis. When the blood level of progesterone is high, these pituitary hormones are not secreted, and follicles (which bear ova) do not mature, ovulation does not occur, no cycle ensues, and, if pregnancy has occurred, gestation is allowed to proceed. In the event that an ovum is not implanted, the progesterone level drops, inducing removal of the endometrium, which in man and other higher primates is excreted through the vaginal opening (bleeding). In animals lacking a menstrual cycle, it is resorbed. If implantation has occurred, membranes form around the developing embryo, one of which is known as the chorion. This produces a polypeptide very similar in structure to LH, which is known as chorionic gonatotrophin (CG). The CG, taking the place of the LH, which has disappeared, maintains and stimulates the corpus luteum (which otherwise would retrogress, forming a corpus albicans) and not only prevents the progesterone level from decreasing but may actually elevate it, thereby maintaining the proliferated endometrium and implantation and, through hypothalamic-pituitary feedback, preventing a new cycle. During the later stages of pregnancy, the placenta secretes progesterone. The progesterone levels in the blood of both men and women have been the subject of much study. For a detailed review of this and other hormones in blood, see Gray and Bacharach (173). In men, in ovariectomized or anovulatory women, or during the follicular phase of the menstrual cycle, the progesterone concentration is low (approximately 0.5 μg/100 ml of peripheral blood) and the adrenal cortex may be the source, while in pregnancy it attains a level of approximately 5 μg/100 ml in the first trimester (0–13 weeks), which rises to approximately 20 μg/100 ml in the third trimester. In the luteal phase of the menstrual cycle, progesterone rises to approximately 2 μg/ml in peripheral blood.

Progesterone is rapidly metabolized by reduction and other reactions to a variety of other steroids. These include pregnanediol (5β-pregnane-3α,20α-diol) (Scheme 11.9), 17-ketosteroids, and steroids hydroxylated in the nucleus. These metabolites are "conjugated," i.e., they are converted to sulfate esters or to glycosides of glucuronic acid, which is the C-6 carboxylic acid corresponding to D-glucose, and then are excreted in the urine. The detail of the metabolism is species dependent. In man, about 20% of the progesterone is accounted for as pregnanediol glucuronide. It is also present in the pigtail monkey, the baboon, and the chimpanzee. However, in the rhesus monkey, almost none is found as this end product. In both the rhesus monkey and the baboon, androsterone (3α-hydroxy-5α-androstan-17-one) has been identified as a progesterone metabolite along with more polar steroids. There are reasons for believing that the hormone is primarily oxidized to smaller molecules that become a part of other metabolic processes. Depending on the species, the intermediates are reduced, conjugated, and excreted. For a key to the literature on metabolism see Reddy et al. (174). The presence of pregnanediol glucuronide in human urine is the basis of assays for progesterone in blood, for the determination of secretion rates, and for the determination of pregnancy.

Since progesterone inhibits ovulation via the hypothalmic-pituitary axis (175, 176), it and several synthetic progestogens (steroids with progestational activity) act as contraceptives. Oral doses of 300 mg of progesterone were found effective by Pincus and his associates (177–179). Much greater oral efficacy was found with certain 19-norsteroids, notably norethynodrel, [17α-ethinyl-5(10)-estren-17-ol-3-one] and its Δ^4-isomer (17α-ethinyl-19-nortestosterone) (Scheme 11.10). A large-scale study of these compounds by Pincus began in Puerto Rico in 1955, and later was extended by the original investigators as well as by others. The effective "pill" was found to require only 10 mg of a 19-norsteroidal progestogen, which was mixed with 0.1 mg of a synthetic estrogen (the 3-methyl ether of 17α-ethinylestradiol). For reasons not clear, cessation of administered estrogen produces bleeding (sloughing of the endometrium), known as "withdrawal bleeding." Thus, when the "pill" is taken with periodic lapses, ovulation is prevented but periodic bleeding still occurs. This maintains the outward appearance of a normal cycle and keeps the endometrium cycling and healthy. More recently, in the use of "sequential pills," the estrogen is administered for about half of the menstrual cycle and progestogen the other half, in an attempt to mimic the physiological sequence. The "pill" is 99.9% effective, but has some side effects in certain individuals. When the dose is reduced to 0.1–0.5 mg/day of progestogen alone ("micro dose pills"), effectiveness at the slightly lowered 95–97% level is maintained, but the mechanism of action is believed to lie, among others, in alterations in the cervical mucus

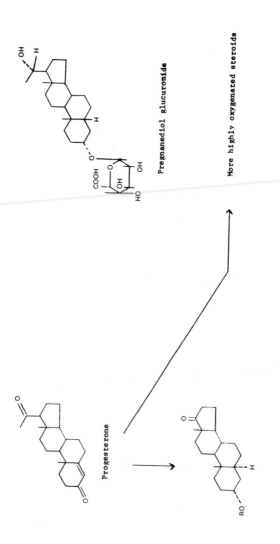

Scheme 11.9. Mammalian metabolism of progesterone in blood.

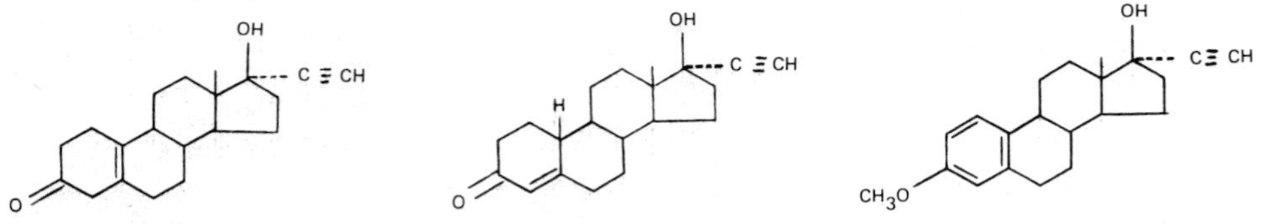

Norethynodrel 17α-Ethinyl-19-nortestosterone 17α-Ethinylestradiol methyl ether

Scheme 11.10. Some ingredients of the contraceptive pill.

rather than in ovulation suppression. A pill containing a long-acting estrogen and a short-acting progestogen that can be given once a month is under investigation.

2. Adrenocortical Steroids

a. Isolation and Function   As early as 1930, Swingle, Pfiffner, Hartman, Brownell, and others demonstrated that extracts of the adrenal gland would maintain the life of animals from which the glands had been removed. In the absence of such therapy it was known that all species would die within a week or two following adrenalectomy. During the next and succeeding decades more than three dozen steroids were isolated in pure form in several laboratories by Kendall, Mason, Reichstein, Wintersteiner, Pfiffner, Simpson, Tait, and their co-workers. 21-Hydroxyprogesterone (desoxycorticosterone, DOC), synthesized in 1937 (*180*) and a year later isolated (*181*), was the first adrenocortical steroid ("adrenocorticoid") to show substantial activity (*182*). In controlling electrolyte and water balance in adrenalectomized animals, it mimicked to some extent the normal function of the gland. However, it did not restore the animals to their prior state. Cortisol ($11\beta,17\alpha,21$-trihydroxyprogesterone) and its 11-keto analog, cortisone, were isolated in 1937 (*183*) and 1936 (*184–187*), respectively. The yield of hormone was only about 1 mg/kg of gland. Despite a small supply, as early as 1940–1941, cortisone was found to have a strong effect on carbohydrate metabolism, having anti-insulin character and producing glycosuria in large doses (*188–191*). On the other hand, it did not have the effect on sodium retention or on survival that DOC possessed (*192, 193*). This proved that the physiological behavior of the adrenal cortex could be divided into at least two phenomena, control of electrolytes on the one hand and of carbohydrates on the other, with each activity residing principally in different hormones. In the late 1940s, sufficient material was obtained by partial synthesis from bile acids, and cortisone, followed later by cortisol, was shown to ameliorate the symptoms of patients with Addison's disease (hypofunction of the adrenal cortex). These two hormones also were dramatically effective in relieving the symptoms of rheumatoid arthritis (*194, 195*). The latter observation was prompted in the mind of Hench (*194, 195*) by the fact that spontaneous remissions occurred during pregnancy, surgical procedures, and other stressful situations. Selye earlier had demonstrated the involvement of the adrenal cortex in regulating the response to stress. A steroid, corticosterone ($11\beta,21$-dihydroxyprogesterone) closely related to cortisol (actually 17-desoxycortisol) was also isolated in 1937 (*183, 196*). It too failed to have life-maintenance properties, and was largely ignored in the flurry of activity over the behavior of cortisone in rheumatoid arthritis, which is a prevalent disease. It did, however, possess weak glucocorticord behavior. Finally, in the mid-1950s the 18-oxygenated hormones, 18-hydroxycorticosterone (*197*) and its 18-aldehyde, aldosterone

(*198-202*), were isolated. It was in these latter steroids that the principal mineralocortical behavior of the gland was shown to reside. Aldosterone, in particular, displayed an ability to relieve Addisonian symptoms and to prevent death in adrenalectomized animals. It was 30-100 times as active as DOC. Subsequently, with the development of analytical techniques, the concentration of hormones in blood could be measured. This allowed definition of what hormones are actually secreted. For a detailed discussion of the history and chemistry see Nes (*203*). The physiology and biochemistry have been reviewed in depth in the books edited by Eisenstein (*204*) and Gray and Bacharach (*173*).

Although several dozen steroids are present in the gland, including progesterone, androgens, and estrogens, as well as a variety of 20-hydroxy- and 3-hydroxy-C_{21}-compounds, only some of these leave the gland in consequential amounts. Exactly which and in what amounts is a subject of some controversy. The problem is complicated by their being present both in the free and "conjugated" form as well as being bound at least in some cases to carrier proteins. Furthermore, there is a variation with biological and environmental parameters. The best estimates, however, are that the principal activity of the adrenal secretion in man resides in cortisol, corticosterone, and aldosterone. In peripheral plasma they are thought to have concentrations in the unconjugated form of roughly 10 μg/100 ml, 1 μg/100 ml, 10 μg/100 ml, respectively. While all of these amounts are small, it is worth noting that the value for aldosterone is three orders of magnitude less than that of cortisol. This is reflected in the concentrations in the adrenal gland (Table 11.8) and explains why nearly 20 years elapsed between the isolations of cortisol and aldosterone. Aldosterone is replaced by 18-hydroxycorticosterone in the rat. In addition to the C_{21} steroids, the adrenals secrete the C_{19} steroid, dehydroepiandrosterone, and its sulfate. This compound is actually the major steroid (Table 11.8) derived from the adrenals and the principal 17-keto steroid of blood, regardless of origin, and is excreted in human urine in relatively large amounts (2-10 mg/day). Despite this, almost nothing is known about the physiological reason for its presence. In view of the fact that it is an ester of a Δ^5-steroid and a

Table 11.8. Adrenal steroid concentrations[a]

	Sheep Adrenal (μg/gland)	Human Peripheral Plasma (μg/100 ml)
Cortisol	26	10
Corticosterone	5	1
Aldosterone	0.22	0.01
Dehydroepiandrosterone Sulfate	—	100

[a]Adapted from P. F. Dixon, M. Booth, and J. Butler, J. P. Coughlan, and J. R. Blair-West, and W. R. Eberlein, J. Winter, and R. L. Rosenfeld, in Gray and Bacharach (*173*).

strong acid, the possibility of its undergoing the 3,5-cyclosteroid rearrangement has been investigated, but no evidence was obtained for this reaction occurring in vivo (205). It circulates bound, primarily to albumin (206). Similarly, most of the cortisol is protein-bound in plasma, to albumin, and especially to an α-globulin known as corticosteroid-binding globulin (CBG) (207), also known as transcortin (208). The binding to albumin has been studied as a function of concentration (209). Other steroids, such as progesterone, are also bound to CBG (210).

Glucocorticoid activity is closely associated with the presence of an 11β-hydroxyl group. A 17α-hydroxyl group enhances but is not necessary for such activity. Cortisone, which is reductively metabolized to cortisol, may have no activity in its own right. Cortisol is the most active of the natural glucocorticoids. So-called "glucocorticoid" behavior is complicated and only very poorly understood. It has many components, many of which are not directly related to carbohydrate metabolism. Long, Katzin, and Fry (211) in 1940 were the first to call attention to the complicated effects produced by adrenalectomy which could be alleviated by adrenal extracts. In the years since then, with the use of pure hormones, the original findings have been verified and extended. Glucocorticoids induce deposition of glycogen in the liver and to a smaller extent in the muscle. No effect on kidney glycogen results. The hormones also lead to increased blood glucose. In the liver, increased glucose production actually occurs, as does an increase in ketone bodies. Perhaps most striking is an increase in RNA and protein synthesis in the liver, giving the so-called anabolic effect of the glucocorticoids. This effect seems to be unique to hepatic tissue, since corticoid treatment generally results in protein depletion from most body tissues and an increase in urinary excretion of nitrogen as urea (catabolic effect). The hepatic phenomena, which occur in 2-4 hr, are currently thought to be the primary hormonal effects, and those in other tissues, which occur 12-24 hr later, are thought to result from the hepatic changes. For a detailed discussion see Ashmore and Morgan in the book edited by Eisenstein (204). Activity of a number of hepatic enzymes having to do with glucose, amino acids, and urea is increased. These include glycogen synthetase, sugar phosphatases, aldolase, transaminases, and arginase. The overall effect of glucocorticoids tentatively appears to be the conversion of body protein to amino acids, which in the liver are converted to urea and glucose.

In addition to the above-mentioned metabolic effects, the glucocorticoids dramatically suppress the inflammatory reaction, which is a major reason why they are useful clinically in the treatment of rheumatoid arthritis, eye diseases associated with inflammation, etc. This may be associated with potentiation of the vasoconstrictive action of norepinephrine. Glucocorticoids also decrease resistance to infection, which may be related to effects on leukocytes and to the ability of the hormones to inhibit antibody production. The symptoms of infection, such as inflammation, are also reduced.

The importance of the 11β-hydroxyl group is unquestionably related to its electronic rather than its steric qualities. This has been demonstrated by strong potentiation of the ability to induce glycogen deposition when a halogen is placed either on C-9 or C-12, and the effect increases as the halogen becomes smaller (I, Br, Cl, F). For instance, 9α-fluorocortisol is 11 times as active as cortisone, the chloro analog 4 times as active, and the bromo and iodo analogs 0.3 and 0.1 times as active, respectively (212). 9α-Fluorocortisone and 9α-chlorocortisone are 9 and 4 times as active, respectively, as cortisone (212). While reduction of the Δ^4-bond destroys activity and cannot be restored by the halogen, lost activity by removal of the 21- and 17α-hydroxyl groups is restored. Thus, both 9α- and 12α-fluoro-11β-hydroxyprogesterone are 80-90% as active as cortisone in liver glycogenesis (213). The influence of the halo group in the hepatic glycogen assay is paralleled by an increase in anti-inflammatory activity, 9α-flurocortisol, for instance, being 7 times as active as cortisol in anti-inflammatory behavior. Increasing the π-electrons conjugated with the 3-keto group also increases glucocorticoid activity. The 1,2-dehydro derivatives of cortisone and cortisol (prednisone and prednisolone, respectively) are about 3.5 times as active as the parent hormones. Methyl substituents on the β face inhibit activity, indicating that interaction of the hormone with the receptor site occurs on the front side. For a detailed discussion of structure-activity relationships see the review by Nes (203).

Mineralocortical behavior is induced by the presence of a 21-hydroxy group on a 3-keto-Δ-^{4}-steroid and is greatly enhanced by an oxygen atom on C-18 at the hydroxyl or especially at the aldehydo stages. 21-Hydroxy-progesterone (DOC) as well as cortisone, etc., exhibit some activity of this sort. It is measured by an increase in retention of sodium ion and excretion of potassium ion. Aldosterone is the most active of the natural hormones. The presence of the 11β-hydroxyl group in aldosterone also induces some glucocorticoid behavior. Aldosterone is believed to act directly on the distal convoluted tubule of the kidney, causing reabsorption of Na^+ but increasing the passage of H^+, K^+, NH_4^+, and Mg^{++}. As a result of changing the ion balance, water balance is also affected. During water diuresis, aldosterone increases clearance of water. From studies by Edelman et al. (214), it is thought that aldosterone stimulates RNA synthesis, in turn inducing formation of a protein involved in sodium transport. The effect of the hormone on the kidney (and bladder) in influencing Na^+ transport is believed to be its primary action, from which a variety of other effects ensue. For a detailed discussion see Mulrow in the book edited by Eisenstein (204). The most serious effect of adrenalectomy has to do with alteration of the electrolyte balance, which is also seen in various adrenal insufficiencies, e.g., Addison's disease.

b. Biosynthesis and Control   The adrenocortical steroids (corticords) are derived from pregnenolone (Scheme 11.11). Three transformations are involved: oxidation of the 3β-hydroxyl group and isomerization of the Δ^5-bond establishing the Δ^4-3-keto system, hydroxylations at C-21, C-11β, C-17α, and C-18 as the case may be, and, for aldosterone, oxidation of C-18 to the aldehydo stage. A severe sequence problem exists here that has not been fully resolved and that is species dependent. Cortisol was first obtained from cholesterol in the studies described in the foregoing discussion of the biosynthesis of progesterone. There can be no doubt that progesterone can be an intermediate leading sequentially through 17α-, 21-, and 11β-hydroxylations to cortisol. This is believed to be the major sequence in man and perhaps most vertebrates. The rat and mouse seem to differ from man in the relative activity of the 17α-hydroxylase. If it is fully active, cortisol becomes dominant, while if it has low activity, corticosterone becomes dominant. In man, the first of these alternatives arises, and in rats and mice, the second. In addition, the changes in ring A can be postponed from the first to a later step, i.e., pregnenolone is 17α-hydroxylated and then dihydroxylated to yield cortisol. Currently, this is thought to be a minor but not inconsequential route depending on the species. Glucocorticoid production occurs primarily in the two innermost zones (zona reticularis and zona fasciculata) of the cortex.

18-Oxygenation occurs primarily in the zona glomerulosa, where a sequence problem also exists. The primary pathway is currently thought to be via 21-, 11β-, and 18-hydroxylation of progesterone in the order given, followed by oxidation, presumably by pyridine nucleotide, of the 18-hydroxyl group. There are some reasons for believing that the 18-hydroxysteroid, when acting as an intermediate, remains protein bound, perhaps involving a sulfur bond. For a detailed discussion of corticoid sequences see the review by Samuels in the book edited by Eisenstein (*204*).

Cleavage of 17α-hydroxypregnenolone at the 17(20)-bond leads to dehydroepiandrosterone (DHEA). The 17-keto group to some extent is then reduced to the 17β-alcohol giving androstenediol. Both DHEA and the diol have been found in adrenal venous blood, and both can be converted to the corresponding Δ^4-3-ketones, androstenedione and testosterone, respectively. These are androgens and are responsible for androgenic phenomena emanating from the adrenal cortex. If the relative activities of the biosynthetic enzymes in the gland shift strongly in favor of the route through DHEA to the Δ^4-3-ketones, serious abnormalities in sexual phenomena result. Metabolism of the 11β-hydroxycorticords can also take this route, leading to 11-oxygenated C_{19} steroids, e.g., 11-hydroxytestosterone, which retain androgenicity. Masculinizing adrenal carcinomas have enzymatic patterns of this sort.

Control (Scheme 11.12) of the secretion of glucocorticords resides in adrenocorticotrophic hormone (ACTH), which is a polypeptide of some 39

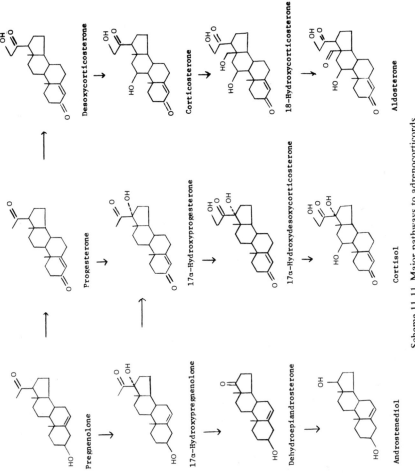

Scheme 11.11 Major pathways to adrenocorticords.

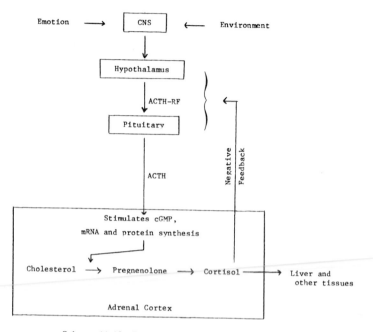

Scheme 11.12. Regulation of glucocorticoid secretion.

amino acid units formed in the pituitary gland. ACTH stimulates the growth and maintains the integrity of the adrenal gland itself and also increases the adrenocorticoid secretion. The secretion of ACTH is in turn regulated by a polypeptide "releasing factor" (ACTH-RF) secreted by the hypothalamus, located at the base of the brain, and which appears to be partially under the control of the brain proper. Thus, primary control of the corticoid secretion lies in the so-called hypothalamic-pituitary axis (which refers to the interrelationship between two glands) and in the central nervous system (CNS). Emotional and environmental factors that are known to induce changes in the adrenal secretion [Selye's (215) general adaptation syndrome; see also DeWied et al. (216)] are presumably mediated through the CNS via the hypothalamic-pituitary axis. Periodicity (diurnal, etc.) in the adrenal secretion also is apparently mediated at or above the hypothalamic level. However, there is in addition an internal regulation in the endocrine system that is probably independent of the CNS. Cortisol exerts a negative feedback on the hypothalamic-pituitary axis, reducing the secretion of ACTH. As the blood level of ACTH rises, so does the level of cortisol, but the increased concentration of the cortisol induces its own regulation by inhibiting ACTH. The mechanism by which ACTH stimulates corticoid secretion has been extensively studied. In his perfusion studies (cf. Section C.1), Hechter found that the conversion of cholesterol to progesterone was increased in the presence of ACTH but that the pituitary hormone did not influence subsequent steps. Ensuing examination in several laboratories with tissue slices, tissue cultures, etc., has confirmed that the polypeptide stimulates the cleavage at the 17(20)-bond but only in an indirect way. Cyclic nucleotides ("the second messenger") are involved in some still incompletely understood manner. At physiological concentrations of ACTH, cGMP (but not cAMP) is elevated in isolated adrenal cells (217) and cGMP stimulates the hydroxylation of cholesterol at C-20 (218) without having any effect on the conversion of 20α-hydroxycholesterol or pregnenolone to corticoids (218). The suggestion has been made by Sharma (218), on the basis of these and other facts, that cGMP is responsible for the formation or processing of a mRNA, which then is translated by means of a cGMP- or cAMP-dependent phosphorylation factor. Mostafapour and Tchen (219) also regard the ultimate effect of ACTH as being an increase in the concentration of an essential protein produced by a stimulation of a long-lived mRNA. The rate-controlling step in the cleavage of cholesterol is thought (217, 218) to be 20α-hydroxylation, since, among other things 20α-hydroxycholesterol is converted to corticoids (220) in the system used to study the cyclic nucleotides as discussed above, but it should be remembered that the sequence of hydroxylations is not known with certainty. Control of mineralocorticoid secretion has not been as well studied as has glucocorticoid regulation. While aldosterone secretion is generally presumed to be mediated by ACTH, for which some support is available, there are additional factors involved. Indeed, the primary regulatory agent is believed to be the renin-angiotensin system. Plasma electrolyte concentrations also are influential. See Davis in the book edited by Eisenstein (204) for a thorough discussion of this subject. The biochemical mechanisms involved are still unknown.

3. Androgens

a. *Isolation and Function* The androgens (Greek andros, man) are a group of C_{19} steroids that induce certain aspects of maleness (secondary sex characteristics). It was observed thousands of years ago that castration of boys would prevent the development of the genitalia, the normal physique (musculature, etc.), voice, hair, aggressiveness, and the ability to inseminate, all of which are characteristic of a man. Castration of mature men also had profound effects, although generally much less severe. In the intervening centuries, similar phenomena were found in other animals, and Berthold was able to show in 1849 that transplanted testes would reverse effects of castration (atrophy of the cock's comb). This led to the supposition, proved true through the use of extracts, that the testes produce a hormone that elicits male characteristics. Dorfman and Shipley (221) should be consulted for a detailed discussion of the history of the subject. In 1928 androgenic activity was observed in urine. Butenandt (222) then succeeded in isolating a pure entity from this source that had potent androgenicity. This compound (androsterone) proved to be the 17-ketone derived from 3-epicholestanol, and it became evident that androgenicity is associated with the absence of a side chain. A few years later, David et al. (223) isolated a closely related steroid bearing a 17β-hydroxyl group and a 3-keto-Δ^4-system from bull testes. They named it testosterone. Two decades later, Dorfman and his associates (224) isolated the corresponding ketone (androstenedione) from human testes, and a variety of other steroids have since been isolated, some of which are clearly intermediates. Recently it has been possible to examine the constituents of the spermatic venous blood. Surprisingly, not only are testosterone and androstenedione present but so are 17α-hydroxyprogesterone, dehydroepiandrosterone (the 17-ketone corresponding to cholesterol), and the sulfates of testosterone and pregnenolone, depending on the species. For a key to the literature, see Steinberger and Steinberger (225). The Leydig cells are thought to be the main source of testicular androgens, but, while there is no question that they have biosynthetic capacity, there is reason to believe the seminiferous tubules and Sertoli cells may also be sources of hormone (225). The sequence of biosynthetic events in testicular tissue is strongly dependent on maturation, although not in a way that is easy to interpret. During early life testosterone is formed in the rat, but at about 20 days of age androsterone and 5α-androstanediol take its place, in turn disappearing after about 40 days, at which time testosterone reasserts itself (225–227).

The physiology of maleness is understood on the one hand in very gross parameters and on the other in some very precise details. Unfortunately, little progress has been made in interrelating the two. Based primarily on the effects of castration, androgens are believed, among other things, to support development of the penis, scrotum, seminal vesicles, prostate, vas deferens, epididymis, Cowper's gland, and prepetial gland, to allow normal sexual behavior and deepening of the voice, and to induce formation of pubic and axillary hair. Studies of hypogonadism have added strength to some of these conclusions. Thus, in cases where the penis has not grown, administration of testosterone rectifies the situation. In women, exogenous or endogenous (adrenocortical tumors, etc.) androgens also induce some of these changes, e.g., growth of facial hair and enlargement of the clitoris. Administration of testosterone also maintains spermatogenesis in the hypophysectomized rat, and Leydig cell secretions are capable of initiating spermatogenesis in prepuberal human testes. The role of androgens has been discussed in depth elsewhere (221, 225, 226).

b. Biosynthesis and Control   In the 1950s and 1960s, after the clear demonstration that cholesterol leads to hormones in the adrenal cortex, various workers showed that testes will form testosterone and other androgens de nove from acetate through cholesterol via pregnenolone, progesterone, and their 17α-hydroxy derivatives, followed by cleavage at the

17(20)-bond, as is shown in Scheme 11.13. Evidence for several sequences, e.g., 17α-hydroxylation before or after 3-keto-Δ⁴-formation, exists as it does in the adrenal cortex, but no testicular preference has been elucidated.

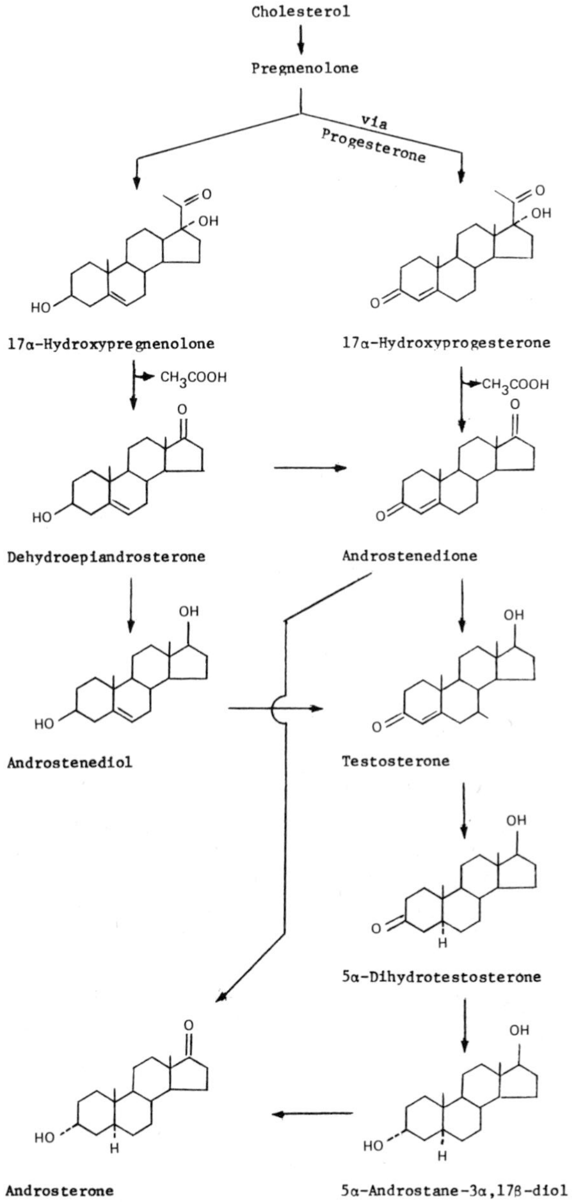

Scheme 11.13. Biosynthesis of androgens.

Unlike the adrenal cortex, where 11β-, 17α-, 18-, and 21-hydroxylations all occur, the testicular route proceeds exclusively through 17α-hydroxylation. Since the adrenal cortex also shares with testes the ability to form androgens by eliminating acetate through 17(20)-cleavage, the testes have the simpler metabolic pattern. They also seem to have an enhanced capacity for reduction of the 17-keto group.

In the 1920s and 1930s, it was unequivocally demonstrated by several investigators that spermatogenesis is under the control of the pituitary gland (hypophysis). With the discovery of the mechanism of action of ACTH, it was obvious to believe that a hypophysial gonadotrophin played exactly the same role in testes, but this has not yet been conclusively demonstrated. The pituitary gland is thought to secrete a polypeptide (interstitial cell stimulating hormone, ICSH) that is the same as or similar to the better studied female counterpart (luteinizing hormone, LH) and/or another polypeptide (chorionic gonadotrophin, CG), with activity in the female similar to that of LH (see Section C.1). Chorionic gonadotrophin and/or ICSH have been reported to stimulate testicular secretion of testosterone, to enhance incorporation of acetate into the hormone, and to promote the conversion of cholesterol to testosterone. From these findings and analogy, it is thought that a pituitary factor (ICSH, LH, etc.) possesses ACTH-like behavior in the testes. The literature has been reviewed recently in detail (225). For various details of function, biosynthesis, and control, also see the book by Paschkis et al. (228) and the one edited by McKerns (229).

c. *Structure-Activity Correlations* Nonendocrine tissue is importantly involved both in the inactivation and activation of the androgens. Testosterone is about 10 times as active as androstenedione (in the capon's comb assay) and therefore the reduction-oxidation that controls their relative amounts is of great physiological importance. Since the oxido-reductases are found in other tissues, the full regulation of androgenic physiology is a very complicated matter requiring much more study before a full understanding will be had. Close similarities in the activities of testosterone and 5α-dihydrotestosterone, together with the demonstration that nonendocrine tissues will reduce the Δ⁴-bond, have led to the hypothesis that it is actually only the saturated 3-ketone that may be androgenic (230–237). This finds support in the androgenicity of other saturated steroids, which are unlikely to be converted to the corresponding Δ⁴-3-ketones. Structure-activity correlations (203), some of which are shown in Table 11.9, reveal that the simultaneous presence of a 17β-hydroxy group and an oxygen atom at C-3 in a steroid with a *trans*-A/B-fusion (or one approximating it in the Δ⁵-steroids) are required for activity as measured by the promotion of a capon's comb growth.

4. Estrogens

a. *Isolation and Function* The term "estrogen" is derived from the idea that a chemical induces "estrus," the phenomenon associated with

Table 11.9. Relative activities of steroids in the capon's comb assay[a]

Steroid	Activity Relative to Testosterone
Testosterone	100
17α-Methyl-5α-dihydrotestosterone	100
5α-Androstan-17β-ol-3-one	70
5α-Androstane-3α,17β-diol	60
17α-Methyltestosterone	50
17α-Methyl-5α-androstane-3α,17β-diol	50
17α-Ethyltestosterone	20
Androsterone	15
5-Dehydroandrosterone	15
Androstenedione	11
5α-Androstane-3,17-dione	11
Dehydroepiandrosterone	7
5α-Androstane-3α,17α-diol	5
17-Epitestosterone	3
5α-Androstan-3β,17β-diol	2
3β-Chloro-5-androstan-17-one	0
5β-Androstan-3α-ol-17-one	0

[a] Adapted from Nes (*203*) and references cited therein.

the female's biological ability for and behavioral acceptance of successful mating with a male. Rats and guinea pigs, for instance, show rapid and complete loss of mating interest folowing ovariectomy. Based on the female's response to mounting by the male, the loss is nearly completely restored in the rat by injections of an ovarian steroid (estradiol) (*238*), proving the existence of hormonal regulation. Castration also has other profound effects. If it occurs before sexual maturity in women, the genital tissues, mammary glands, and pubic and axillary hair fail to develop, but, unlike the lower animals, libido is not much affected. Similarly, libido is not cyclic in normal, mature women, in contrast to many infraprimates, where cyclicity is thorough, e.g., in seasonal breeders. Women, and the higher primates also, undergo a period of bleeding ("menses" from the Greek word "men" through the Latin "mensis" for month) at the end of the cycle from sloughing of the uterine endometrium. The term "menstrual cycle" is therefore used for women and the higher primates, and it implies a special case of an "estrus cycle" in which behavioral cyclicity and resorption of the uterine lining are absent. Despite such categorization, there is little really fundamental knowledge of the physiology of estrogens, the administration of which will not reverse the effects of castration in the more or less complete manner which the adrenal steroids will do in the case of adrenalectomy. Estrogens can, however, be shown to have at least a supporting role for a variety of sex-related (vagina, mammary glands, uterus, etc.) as well as unrelated (skin, etc.) tissues. With the availability of pure hormones and methods for analysis, investigators have concentrated on a definition of biosynthesis, metabolism, normal and abnormal blood concentrations, and estrogen-induced changes in protein biosynthesis and lipid metabolism. Estrogens are thought to be produced by the ovarian follicles, but this is probably not the only source.

Allen and Doisy developed a bioassay for estrogenicity that depends on the ability of the test material to induce estrus in the rat or mouse. This allowed a way to screen biological sources for estrogenicity, and, together with the observation of Aschheim and Zondek in 1927 that urine of pregnant women is estrogenic, allowed Doisy (*239a*) and Butenandt (*239b*) simultaneously in 1930 to isolate estrone (Scheme 11.14). This proved to be a C_{18} steroid with *trans*-B/C- and C/D ring junctures, as in cholesterol, but differing from the latter in that the side chain was replaced by a 17-keto group and ring A was aromatized. The same year Marrian (*240*) reported the isolation of the corresponding $16\alpha,17\beta$-dihydroxy derivative (estriol) from pregnancy urine. Then a few years later Doisy and his co-workers (*241*) isolated the 17β-hydroxy compound (estradiol) from sow's ovaries, and Wintersteiner and his colleagues (*242*) obtained the same diol from pregnant mare's urine. Horse urine (and feminizing adrenocortical tumors) also contains estrogens in which both rings A and B are aromatic, e.g., equilenin. Horses are interesting for still another reason. Bioassay of stallion urine gives a higher titer of estrogenicity than that of a pregnant mare and a thousand times higher than that of a nonpregnant woman! Could this be diet? Reports of estrogens in plants are abundant. The well documented cases, however, are of nonsteroidal materials, notably isoflavones, e.g., genistein and its 7-methyl ether (prunetin) and 4'-methyl ether (biochanin-A). The claim that estrone occurs botanically, e.g., in palm seeds and willow catkins, has not been verified, although the development of floral structures that, of course, are highly sexual strongly suggests hormonal implication. Strangely, no attempts seem to have been made to investigate whether steroidal hormones are present in flowers, despite the fact that many aspects of Angiosperm reproduction are similar to what happens in vertebrate animals. These include the presence of an ovary, and a tube through which the sperm (pollen) travels to the ovum, and the bearing of the new life in a "uterus," the fruit, which is a metamorphosed ovary. As discussed in an earlier section, there can be no doubt that plants can make progesterone; why not estrogens? Flower coloring is clearly related to libido, since it encourages pollination through an insect vector, and the morphology of the flower undoubtedly requires special chemicals. The physiology and biochemistry of sex in higher plants is a remarkably neglected science.

   b. Structure-Activity Correlations   There can be no doubt that estrogenicity is integrally associated with aromaticity, as is reviewed in detail elsewhere (*203*). Very simple phenols, e.g., 4-cyclohexylphenol, and aro-

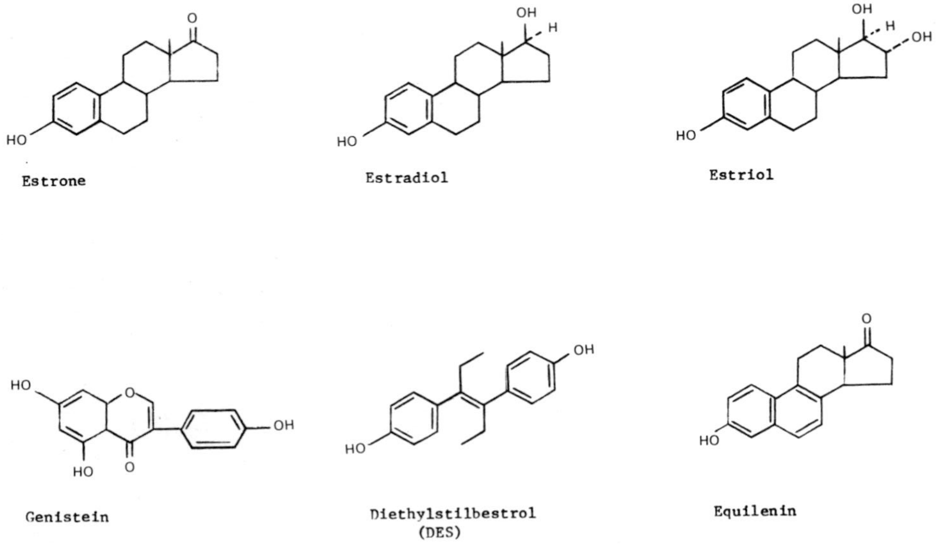

Scheme 11.14 Estrogenic compounds.

matic hydrocarbons, e.g., *trans*-stilbene, are estrogenic. Those nonaromatic compounds, e.g., androstenedione, which display this type of activity are theoretically or experimentally capable of aromatization in vivo. The importance of aromaticity would seem at least in part to be due to its effect on an hydroxyl group, i.e., to make it more acidic (phenolic). The active compounds are primarily phenolic, but those that are not can readily be presumed to be hydroxylated after administration. It is well known that hydroxylative metabolism of endogenous (phenylalanine, etc.) and exogenous (polycyclic carcinogens) aromatic compounds occurs in animals. The first requirement, then, seems to be phenolic character. This is followed by three-dimensional characteristics. The closer the molecule approximates estradiol in structure, the greater is the probability that the estrogenicity will increase. This is dramatically illustrated by diethylstilbestrol (Scheme 11.14), which closely mimics estradiol in structure without itself being a steroid. It has very powerful estrogenic behavior and has been used widely clinically (until recently), since it is much easier to synthesize commercially than the mammalian estrogens. Its *cis*-isomer, which places "ring D" down close to ring A, no longer resembles estradiol, and the activity falls as one would expect on stereochemical grounds. The presence of additional hydroxyl groups on the steroid molecule tends to reduce estrogenicity in the usual assays, but, especially in the case of estriol, this generalization needs further examination. There are reasons for believing that it plays a special role, particularly in human pregnancy. Since some 65 different assays have been used in assaying estrogenicity, but rarely more than one or two for a given series of compounds, a fully quantitative comparison of structure-activity relationships, especially as they relate to physiology, remains to be accomplished.

  c. Biosynthesis   That the ovary is a biosynthetic source of estrogen was demonstrated in 1953 by Werthessen, Schwenk, and Baker (*243*), who perfused sow ovaries with [^{14}C]acetate and obtained labeled estrone and estradiol, and 2 years later testosterone yielded estrone in vivo in horses (*244*). Subsequently, canine and human ovaries were shown to produce estrogens, and [^{14}C]acetate led in vivo to both urinary estrone and equilenin in the horse. In 1961, ovaries were also shown to produce androstenedione and 17β-hydroxy intermediates, and progesterone and testosterone led to estrogens. It became evident from these studies, which are reviewed by O'Donnell and Preedy in the book edited by Gray and Bacharach (*173*), that estrogens are derived by an extension of the androgen pathway in which the 3-keto-Δ^4-system in ring A undergoes additional α,β-desaturation (at C-1,2) and C-19 is lost, with resultant establishment of the benzenoid system by enolization. It was also clear that androstenedione would lead to estrone, and testosterone to estradiol, by such a process. This left the question of sequence preferences, e.g., androstendione to estrone to estradiol versus androstenedione to testosterone to estradiol to estrone, the question of oxidation-reduction at C-17 in peripheral tissues, and the mechanism of the dehydrogenation and C-19-elimination to be resolved. Considerable progress has been made in the latter case.

In 1959, Ryan (245) found that the microsomal fraction of human placental tissue readily aromatizes steroids, and this system has been used extensively for mechanistic and related studies. Estrogen biosynthesis in ovaries seems to be under some sort of gonadotrophic control, which makes this tissue a difficult experimental tool. The exact nature of the control is not known. Short-term treatment with LH or FSH produces no stimulation of estrogen biosynthesis in the rat's ovary, but long-term treatment with pregnant mare's serum gonadotrophin does (246). With placental tissue, Dorfman and his associates (247) showed that 19-hydroxy- and 19-oxoandrostenedione are excellent substrates for the aromatization reaction yielding estrone and, respectively, formaldehyde and formic acid. This indicates the involvement of a hydroxylase, which allows functionalization of the angular methyl group. It was immediately appreciated (248) that a concerted enolization would then eliminate C-19 and after ketonization would produce a 19-nor-Δ^4-3-ketone (Scheme 11.15). Dehydrogenation of

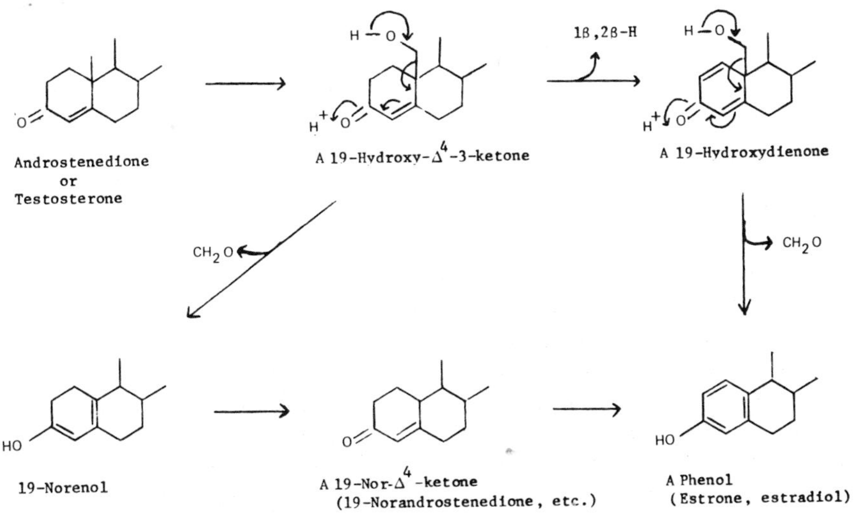

Scheme 11.15 Mechanism of estrogen biosynthesis.

the latter ketone at C-1,2 would lead to the final phenolic structure. In agreement, 19-norandrostenedione readily aromatizes and both it and its C_{19} analog, androstenedione, require NADPH and oxygen to do so (249). 19-Norsteroids will not only aromatize in both placental and ovarian preparations (250–251), but they have been isolated from mare's follicular fluid (252). The two H atoms lost from C-1,2 both have the β configuration, as is shown in extensive studies by Brodie et al. (*248, 249, 253, 254*). The sequence of events is not entirely certain but is thought to proceed essentially in the order just discussed, i.e., hydroxylation of C-19 with or (more likely) without oxidation to the aldehydo stage, followed by elimination of C-19, desaturation, and enolization to the phenol. An alternative sequence involving desaturation of the 19-hydroxysteroid followed by eliminative aromatization is simpler and may (also) occur. For detailed considerations and a key to the literature see Ganguly, Cheo, and Brodie (*255*). 1β-Hydroxylation and aromatization seem to be mediated by the same enzyme, and 17-keto substrates are preferred to 17β-hydroxy ones. Inhibitors of the process have been well studied (*256*). Steroids with close similarities to the expected intermediates will decrease the rate of reaction. Aromatization also occurs in bacteria (*Bacillus sphaericus*), but by a different mechanism. The stereospecificity of the dehydrogenation is different, and the $NADPH/O_2$ requirement is absent (*257*). Estriol is believed to arise by 16α-hydroxylation prior to aromatization (*258*).

The estrogen concentration in the blood of women rises a few days after the beginning of the menstrual cycle, reaching a high near ovulation, and during the luteal phase it again reaches a minimum. The amounts involved at the peak are about 0.05 μg/100 ml decreasing to approximately 0.01 μg/100 ml at the base. Estrone is the major constituent, with estradiol and estriol accounting for the remainder. Estrogens have higher levels in the latter part of pregnancy, where estriol becomes dominant (approximately 10 μg/100 ml), followed by estrone (approximately 5 μg/100 ml) and estradiol (approximately 2μg/100 ml). The value in men is approximately that of the minimum value of women. Direct testicular excretion of estrone and estradiol has been demonstrated (*259*). For a more thorough discussion of blood values see O'Donnell and Preedy in the book edited by Gray and Bacharach (*173*).

5. Metabolism of Mammalian Hormones

The increase in the blood levels of hormones is the result of increased biosynthesis. Little or no hormone or precursors later than cholesterol are stored in the glands of origin. The steroidal mass in the blood therefore results from secretion by the endocrine glands, if we include such temporary tissues as the placenta and corpus luteum in this category, along with the permanent glands (adrenal cortex, testes, and ovaries). The distribution of the mass, however, in terms of individual compounds is in part determined by metabolism in target and other tissues, notably the liver. Target tissues convert the secreted form into derivatives. One of the more interesting examples of this has to do with andogenicity. Hair, the growth of which is stimulated by androgens, is imbedded in the hair follicle, which in turn is imbedded in the skin, and skin is known to reduce testosterone to its 5α-dihydro derivative. The breadth of the subject is illustrated by human gingiva, which will convert estrone to estradiol as well as metabolize progesterone, androsenedione, and cortisol (*260* and references cited). Conversion of testosterone to estrogens also is thought to occur in peripheral tissues (*259* and references cited), which strongly suggests along with testicular secretion of the latter (*259*) that the female hormones play a functional role in the male. Conversely, adrenocortical C_{19}-steroids in the female may be metabolized in peripheral tissues to more or less active androgenic materials. Of intriguing interest is the case of adrenal dehydro-epiandrosterone sulfate. Munson et al. (*261*) discovered it in human urine in 1944, and in 1961 Lieberman and his associates (*262*) showed that it was both interconverted with its free alcohol and through the latter converted to androsterone and etiocholanolone. Since androsterone is an active androgen, study of this and other such metabolism should greatly increase our understanding of endocrine phenomena in secondary sexual characteristics.

The fall in the hormonal concentration following cessation of biosynthesis and secretion is the result of hepatic (and perhaps other) metabolism of several kinds that result in derivatives recognized by the kidneys for urinary excretion. In consequence, the mass of the blood steroid decreases. The activity of the blood steroid also decreases independent of excretion as a result of the metabolism, because most of the products lack hormonal behavior. The most well described of such metabolites are products of reduction. In the C_{21} series, all hormones are inactivated by reduction of the 3-keto-Δ^4-system, and such compounds appear in the urine. Important human examples are pregnanediol from progesterone (Scheme 11.9), tetrahydrocortisol ($3\alpha,11\beta,17\alpha,21$-tetrahydroxy-$5\beta$-pregnan-20-one) (*263*) from cortisol, and the analogous steroid from aldosterone (*264*). Stereoisomers at C-3, C-5, and C-20 also are excreted. Similar liver reductions of testosterone (*265*) and androstenedione occur, yielding, e.g., etiocholanolone, its 17β-hydroxy analog, 5β-androstane-$3\alpha,17\beta$-diol, and the epimers, 5α-androstane-$3\alpha,17\beta$-diol and 5α-androstane-$3\beta,17\beta$-diol (Scheme 11.16). Reduction of the Δ^4-bond occurs before reduction of the 3-keto group (*266*). Hydroxylations at various positions also occur, e.g., at C-1, C-2, C-6, and C-16 (*267* and references cited). Most of the urinary metabolites occur as "conjugates," i.e., glycosides (primarily glucuronic acid), sulfates, etc. For a detailed discussion of the conjugates, see Hadd and Blickenstaff (*268*). Species differences occur. Notable is the conversion of estradiol to it 17α-epimer by rabbits (*269, 270*), which also forms the diglucoside (3-glucuronoside-17α-N-acetylglucosaminide) of the latter but not the former (*270*). Rat adrenals seem to lack the ability to oxidize the 18-hydroxy group or to 17α-hydroxylate, producing corticosterone and 18-hydroxycorticosterone in place of cortisol and aldosterone.

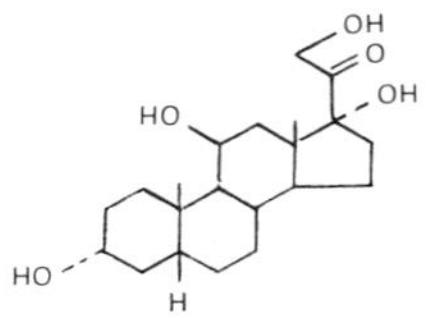

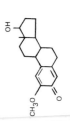

5α-Androstane-3β,17β-diol

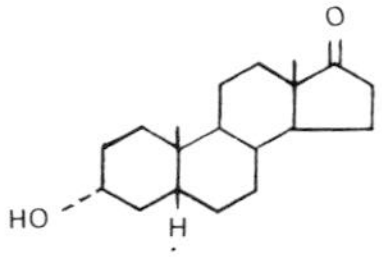

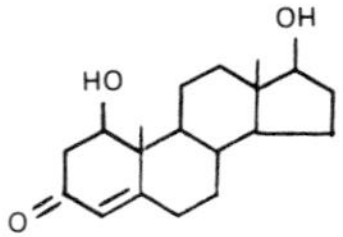

1β-Hydroxytestosterone

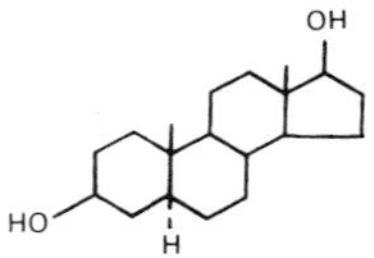

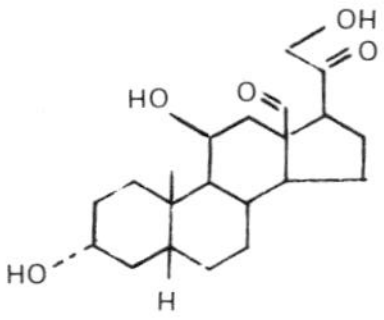

2-Methoxyestrone

Etiocholanolone

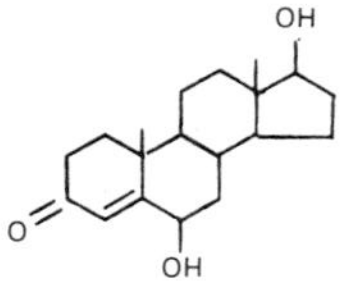

6β-Hydroxytestosterone

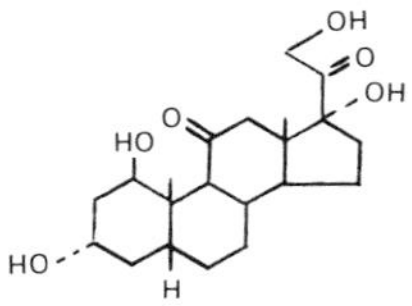

1β-Hydroxytetrahydrocortisone

Tetrahydrocortisol

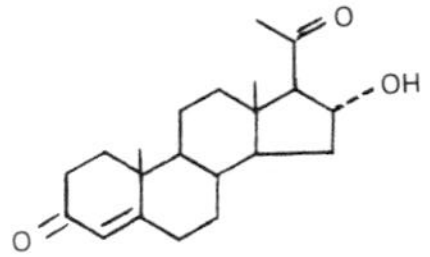

16α-Hydroxyprogesterone

Tetrahydroaldosterone

Scheme 11.16. Some hormone metabolites.

6. Nonmammalian Hormones and Their Metabolism

In animals below mammals, there is a certain but only a limited amount or morphological homology in the endocrine system compared to that in the higher vertebrates. The anatomical relationships that exist suggest that the hormones would be the same as those in mammals. The extent to which they are different, especially in the case of adrenal tissue, which morphologically diverges substantially in lower vertebrates, complicates the problem experimentally as well as theoretically. Some progress has been made, however, in examining the problem, and many similarities between higher and lower forms have been found. In the duck, the bullfrog, and many but not all reptiles, the corticoids lack a 17α-hydroxyl group. A common reptilian pattern consists of corticosterone, its 18-hydroxy derivative, and aldosterone, which arise in the usual way from cholesterol. For a key to the literature see Mehdi and Sandor (271). Reptiles also can produce 11β-hydroxyl-androstenedione and testosterone, and the latter two are interconvertible (271). In 1959, Phillips and Mulrow (272) reported the head kidney of the killifish (*Fundulus heteroclitus*) was capable of corticoid biosynthesis. This has been extensively substantiated in a variety of teleosts in the intervening years. For instance, Arai et al. (273), who should be consulted for a key to the literature, making a study of the rainbow trout (*Salmo gairdneri*) showed that head kidneys containing interrenal tissue are capable of biosynthesizing cortisol, corticosterone, 18-hydroxycorticosterone, testosterone, and 11β-hydroxytestosterone, while the body kidney and corpuscles of Stannius produced only reduced steroids in the 5α and 5β series, e.g., 5α- and 5β-pregnane-3,20-dione. Although the corpuscles of Stannius, in agreement with the latter biochemical work, are thought on ultrastructural grounds not to be an analog of the adrenals in the goldfish and the eel, some reports exist on hormone production by this tissue. Testosterone, which is androgenic in teleosts, has been obtained from testicular tissue of the rainbow trout, but testicular tissue of this species also produces 11β-hydroxy- and 11-ketotestosterone. See Arai et al. (273) for a key to the literature. In some fish 11-oxygenated C_{19} hormones are the principal 17-ketosteroids of peripheral blood. Elasmobranchs are interesting in that 1α-hydroxycorticosterone is produced by their interrenal tissue (274).

7. Metabolism by Microorganisms

Microorganisms (fungi and bacteria) have a substantial ability to metabolize hormones and related steroids. Hydroxylations at essentially all positions have been observed. An important industrial example is the conversion of progesterone to 11α-hydroxyprogesterone by soil molds (275a,b). Isomerization of the Δ^5-3-ketones to Δ^4-3-ketones occurs in the bacterium *Pseudomonas testosteroni* (276), and 3-ketosteroids are desaturated at C-1,2 and/or C-4,5 by a variety of microorganisms (*Nocardia, Corynebacterium,*

Pseudomonas, Streptomyces, etc.), and when 19-norsteroids are substrates, ring A is aromatized to give estrogens (*277, 278* and references cited). Dienone-phenol rearrangements also occur with opening of ring B (9,10-secosteroids) and aromatization of ring A (*279, 280* and references cited) with *Pseudomonas, Arthrobacter,* and *Mycobacterium* sp.

8. Hormone Effects on Target Cell Nuclei

A great deal of recent work indicates that hormones mediate biochemical processes by influencing protein biosynthesis. Especially extensive work has been done with estrogens and progesterone. The current view, extensively discussed by O'Malley and Means (*281*), is that following uptake of the hormone, it is bound to a cytoplasmic receptor-protein, which transports it to the nucleus. There the complex is bound to a specific site on the genome (chromatin DNA and acidic protein) that activates the transcriptional apparatus resulting in new mRNAs (and other RNA molecules). The latter, on transport to the cytoplasm, induce ribosomal synthesis of proteins (enzymes, etc.), which in turn lead to the ultimate response associated functionally with the hormone.

9. Ecdysones

Arthropod molting, the process by which the exoskeleton changes, is under hormonal control. In 1954, Butenandt and Karlson (*282a*) isolated an active substance from pupae of *Bombyx mori* which they named ecdysone, and they later proved by degradation and x-ray studies that it was a steroid.

Its full structure including stereochemistry has been elucidated. While it was originally thought to be biosynthesized in the prothoracic gland, acting on a stimulus by "brain hormone," the actual physiology is much more complicated. In the first place, six active steroids have now been isolated from insects, etc., giving a family of hormones instead of a single ecdysone, and the abdomen can, at least in some cases, be a biosynthetic site. Second, in additon to inducing a molt, a variety of actions of ecdysones have been demonstrated (Table 11.10). Third, in the course of searching for possible anticancer agents in plants, Nakanishi et al. (*283a*) in 1966 made the startling discovery that leaves of *Podocarpus nakii* contain ecdysones. In the succeeding decade, the phenomenon of ecdysones in plants was found indeed to be common. About a hundred botanical families, ranging through all of the Tracheophyta, have been shown to have active substances. Specifically, activity resides in the Lycopsida, Filicopsida, and the Gymnospermae, as well as in both monocots and dicots in the Angiospermae. The concentration of ecdysone in plants, which can be as much as 1%, is actually several orders of magnitude higher than in animals, in which the hormone is usually present at levels of 10^{-5} to 10^{-9}%, and it is known that plants containing ecdysones are fed upon by insects, e.g.,

Table 11.10. Ecdysone action in insects[a]

Order	Response	Dose (μg)
Neuroptera	Larval pupation	0.5
Ioptera	Larval molting	0.03
Hemiptera	Larval molting	0.75
Hymenoptera	Larval development	6.7
Lepidoptera	Larval pupation	0.5
Lepidoptera	Pupal development	10.0
Diptera	Larval development formation	0.01
Diptera	Larval puff induction	

[a] From P. Karlson in the book edited by Burdette (*282b*).

Morus and *Podocarpus* species, used as food by moths of the genera *Bombyx* and *Milionia*. As in the case of sex and adrenocortical hormones, the ecdysones are thought to have an influence on nucleic acids, although the field is not as well examined as the mammalian case. For a detailed discussion of the physiology and biochemistry see Burdette (*282b*) and other reviews (*283b,c*). Biosynthesis has been achieved in plants (*283d*) and in insects (*282b*). A sequence problem exists for which some information is available. Forty different ecdysones have been isolated from plants and they include all but one (20,26-dihydroxy-α-ecdysone) of the six that have been found in animals.

The fundamental hormonal structure is that of a Δ^7-6-ketone, and all steroids with this feature are sometimes referred to generically as "ecdysones," although the details of structure versus activity have yet to be examined fully. The great majority of such compounds isolated are also $2\beta,3\beta,14\alpha,20\alpha,22\beta$-pentols in the A/B-*cis*-series. This basic structure (Scheme 11.17) is represented by ponasterone A found in 10 plant genera, including *Osmunda, Podocarpus,* and *Taxus*. β-Ecdysone (also known as crustecdysone, ecdysterone, isoinokosterone, polypodine A, and commisterone) is 25-hydroxyponasteron A. β-Ecdysone has been isolated from insects and crustacea as well as from more plants than any other ecdysone. α-Ecdysone is the latter's 20-desoxy derivative and was the original isolate from the *Bombyx mori*. It also occurs in plants. The many other compounds are variants, depending on such factors as the presence and absence of a C_1 or a C_2 group at C-24, the presence of additional hydroxyl groups, the presence of double bonds, and stereochemical differences. Some examples are pterosterone (24ξ-hydroxyponasterone A), amarasterone B (29-hydroxy-24α-ethylponasterone A), and the lactones derived from 26(or 27)-hydroxy derivatives that have been oxidized to the carboxyl stage, as is shown in Scheme 11.17.

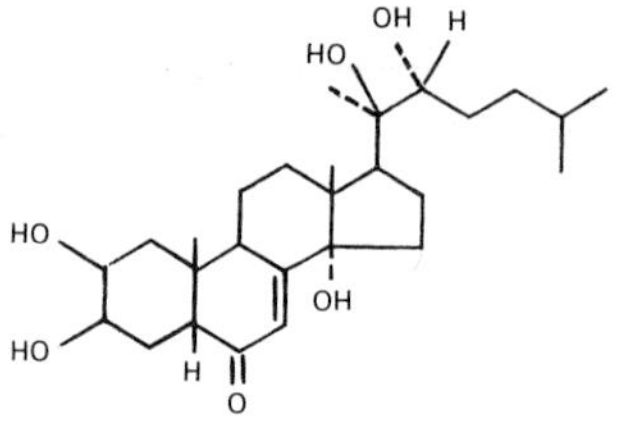

Ponasterone A

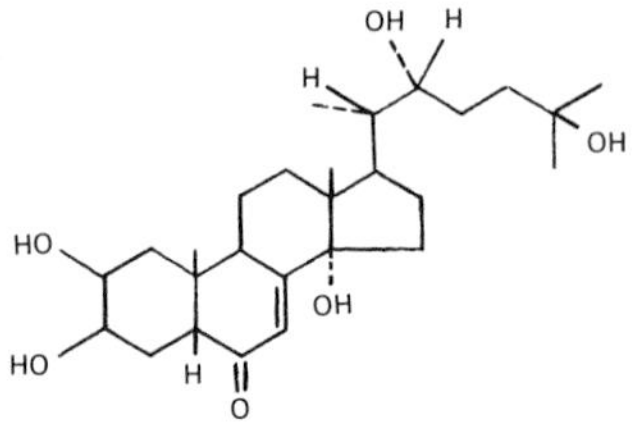

α -Ecdysone

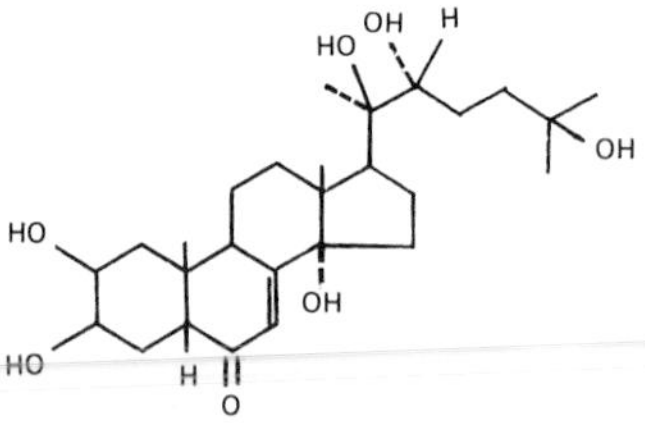

ß -Ecdysone

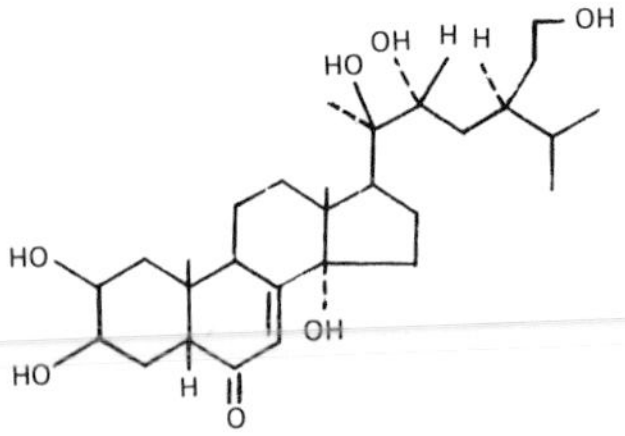

Amarasterone B

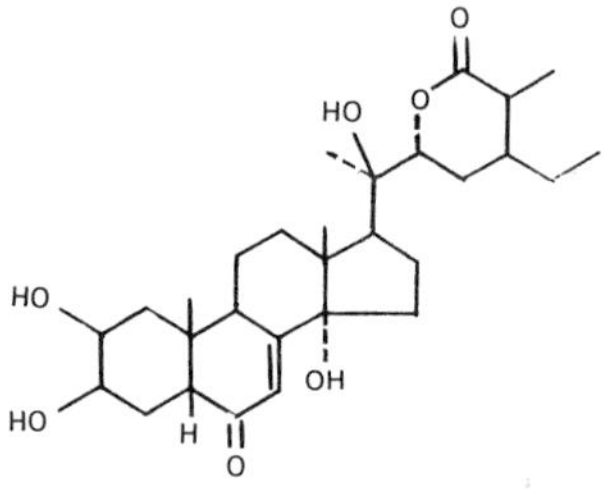

Capitasterone

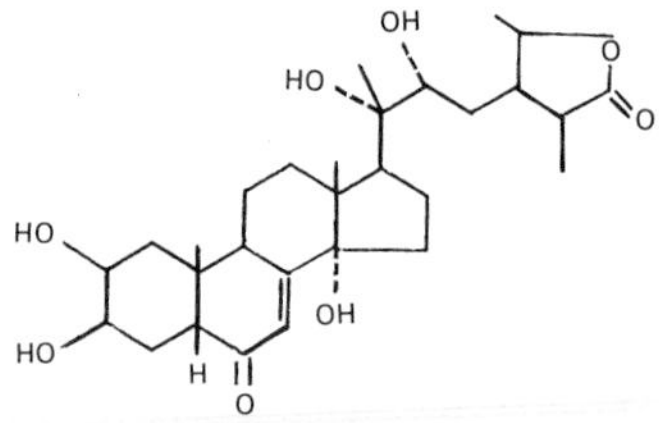

Cyasterone

Scheme 11.17. Some ecdysones.

D. BILE ACIDS AND BILE SALTS

1. Occurrence

Bile salts are polyfunctionalized products of cholesterol metabolism excreted in the bile of mammals and many other vertebrates. In mammals, the 3β-hydroxyl group is epimerized to the 3α position and the configuration at C-5 is inverted from the configuration in cholestanol (A/B *trans* to A/B *cis*). Hydroxyl groups having the α orientation also are common at C-7 and C-12. All three hydroxyl groups, when present, are on the same side of the steroid nucleus. Because of this agreement, bile salts have both a polar and a nonpolar face. Mammalian bile salts are also distinguished by a C-24 carboxylic group on the side chain and the absence of the terminal isopropyl group of cholesterol. The carboxyl group is conjugated to glycine or taurine, which also contributes to the polarity of the molecule in addition to the hydroxyl groups. When the carboxyl group is free, these compounds are termed "bile acids." Bile salts are the conjugates of the acids. The common bile acids of man and many mammals are shown in Scheme 11.18, and the taurene and glycine conjugates of cholic acid are depicted in Scheme 11.19 as an example of the bile salts.

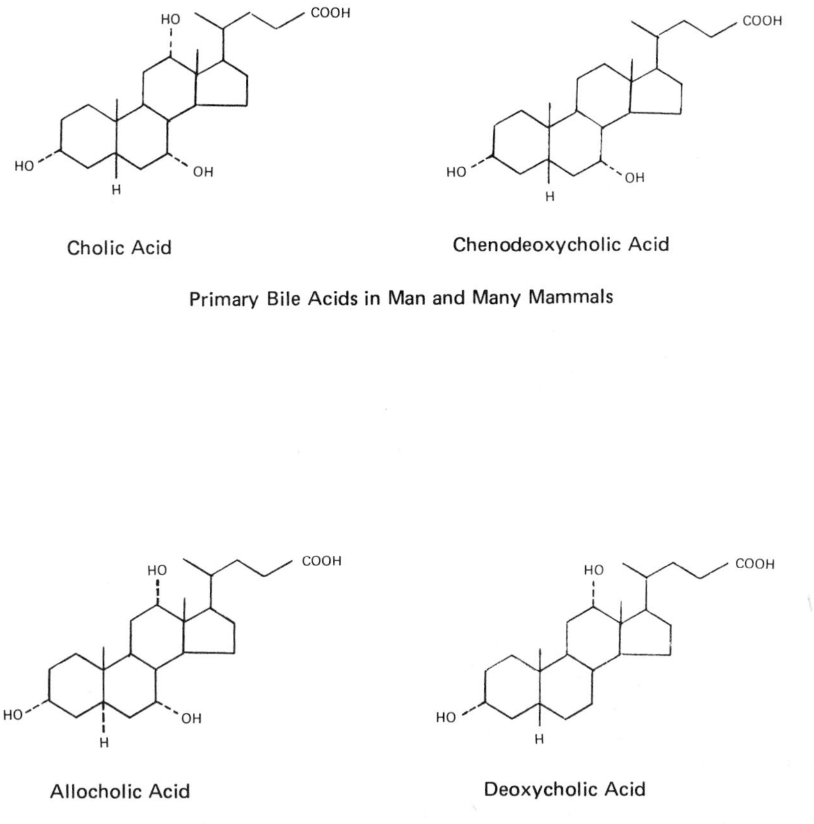

Cholic Acid

Chenodeoxycholic Acid

Primary Bile Acids in Man and Many Mammals

Allocholic Acid

Deoxycholic Acid

Scheme 11.18. Common mammalian bile acids.

Certain bile salts predominate among mammalian groups. Dihydroxy bile acids and sometimes hydroxy-keto acids usually conjugated to glycine are more common in herbivores. In carnivores, on the other hand, taurine conjugates of the trihydroxy bile acids predominate. Omnivores appear to have a mixture of all of the above kinds of bile salts. The herbivorous ruminants appear to be an exception in that their bile salts are similar to those of man. Certain bile acids are unique to a few families and suborders, e.g.,

$NH_2CH_2CH_2SO_3H$

Taurine

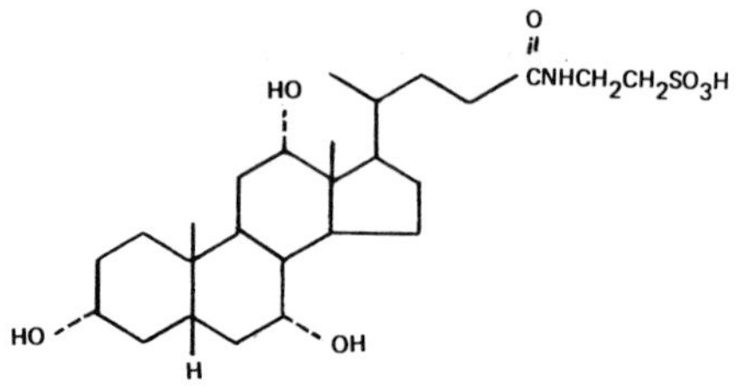

HO

$\overset{O}{\overset{\|}{C}}NHCH_2CH_2SO_3H$

HO

HO

H

OH

Taurocholic Acid

NH_2CH_2COOH

Glycine

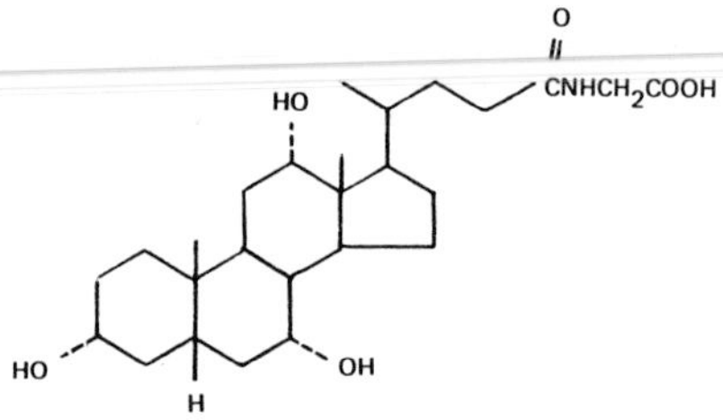

HO

$\overset{O}{\overset{\|}{C}}NHCH_2COOH$

HO

HO

H

OH

Glycocholic Acid

Scheme 11.19. Taurine and glycine conjugates of cholic acid.

α- and β-muricholic acid ($3\alpha,6\beta,7\alpha$- and $3\alpha,6\beta,7\beta$-trihydroxycholanic acid) in the Murinae, phocaecholic acid ($3\alpha,7\alpha,23\xi$-trihydroxycholanic acid) in the Pinnipedia, and hyocholic acid ($3\alpha,6\alpha,7\alpha$-trihydroxycholanic acid) in the Suidae (*284*).

Steroids in the bile of lower vertebrates more closely resemble cholesterol than the bile salts of mammals (Scheme 11.20). A bile alcohol ester (myxinol disulfate) is found in the hagfish, a representative of the most primitive vertebrate group, Cyclostomata. Myxinol disulfate has 27 carbon atoms and a 3β-hydroxyl group as in cholesterol, but C-7, C-16, and C-26 have been oxidized and the C-3 and C-26 hydroxyl group are esterified to sulfate. The nucleus of chimaerol sulfate isolated from a member of the Chondrichthyes resembles the bile salts of mammals; however, the compound retains 27 carbon atoms, and bears a C-26 hydroxyl group esterified to sulfate. Bile salts such as taurocholic acid are found in many bony fishes, but steroids in the bile of the coelacanth and the amphibians are interme-

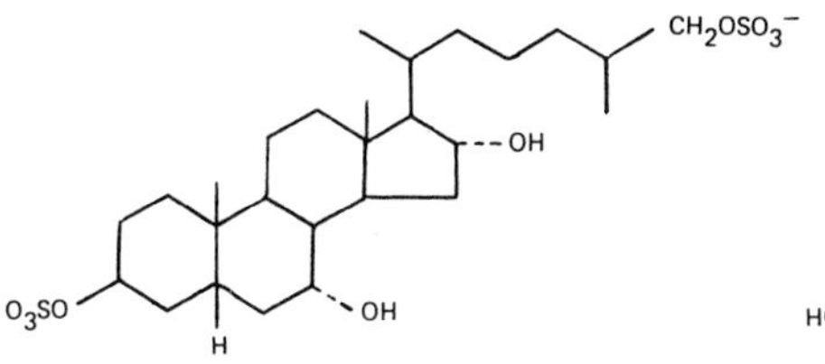

Myxinol Disulfate
(Hagfish)

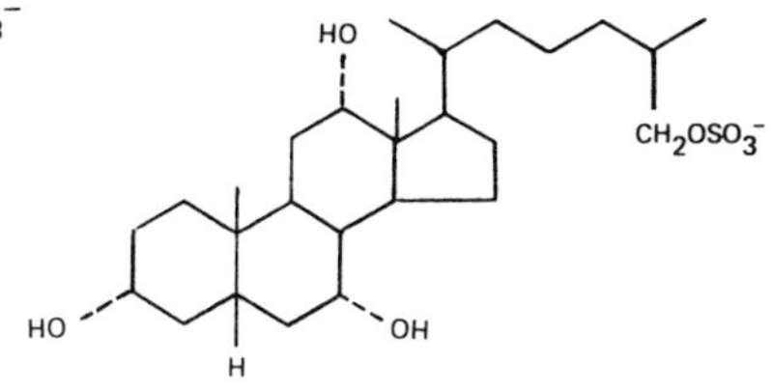

Chimaerol Sulfate
(Chimera)

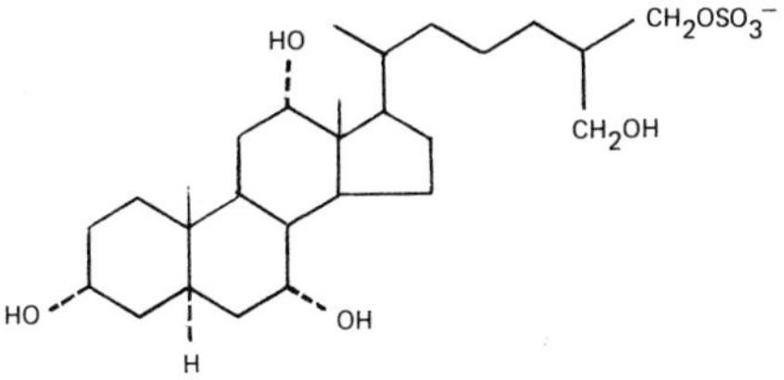

5α -Cyprinol
(Coelacanth)

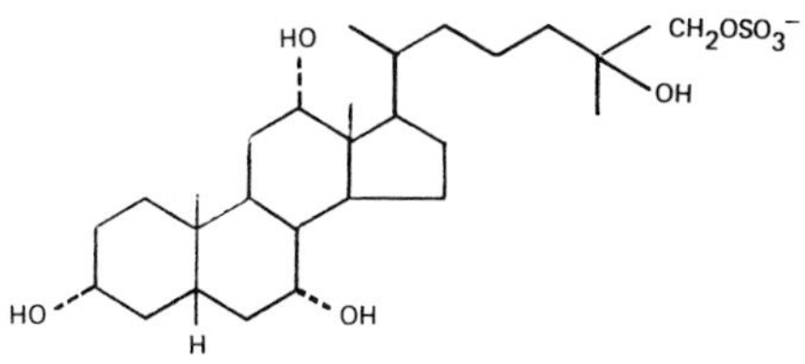

5β -Bufol Sulfate
(Toad)

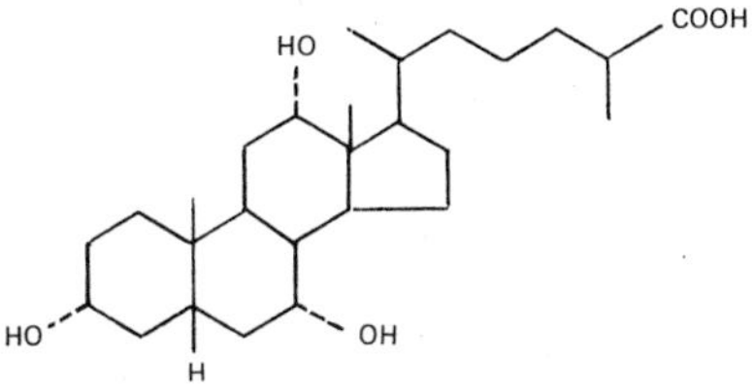

3α , 7α , 12α -Trihydroxy-
coprostanic Acid
(Some reptiles)

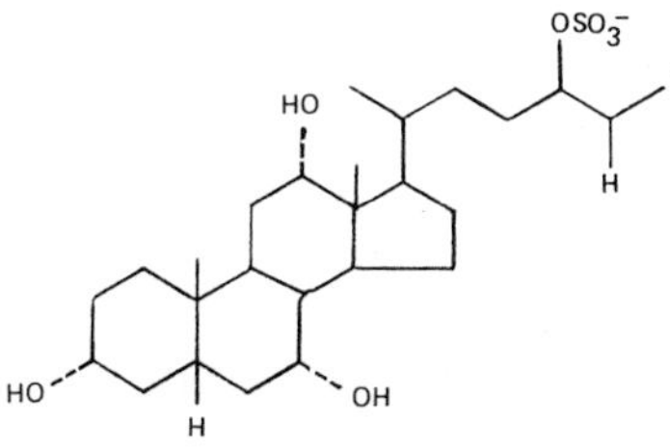

5β -Ranol Sulfate
(Frogs)

Scheme 11.20. Steroids in the bile of vertebrates other than mammals.

diate in structure between those in mammals and the Chondrichthyes (Scheme 11.20). Many reptiles contain cholic acid conjugated to taurine, but the C27 acid, 3α,7α,12α-trihydroxycoprostanic acid (conjugated to taurine), is found in some species. The bile salt pattern in birds seems to be similar to mammals. In conclusion, the general evolutionary trend seems to be from steroids (bile alcohols), which retain the entire cholesterol skeleton occurring as sulfates in primitive vertebrates to C27 acids conjugated to taurine (reptiles), and finally to C24 acids conjugated to taurine and glycine in mammals and birds. For a more thorough discussion of the distribution of bile salts and bile acids the reader is referred to Haslewood (284).

2. Biosynthesis

Bloch, Berg, and Rittenberg (285) were the first to establish that the bile acids are produced from cholesterol. They isolated deuterium-labeled cholic acid from a dog that had been given deuterium-labeled cholesterol. Since that time, much light has been shed on the various steps in the conversion of cholesterol to the bile acids and their conjugation with taurine and glycine forming the bile salts. Modifications of the cholesterol molecule leading to the bile acids include: 1) hydroxylation at the 7α and 12α positions, 2) reduction of the Δ^5-bond, 3) epimerization of the 3β-OH group to 3α-OH, and 4) cleavage of the side chain, yielding a C-24 carboxylic acid. Much of the evidence for the route to the bile acids is derived from experiments with intraperitoneal administration of suspected intermediates to animals with bile fistulas, eliminating the metabolism of intestinal flora.

a. Hydroxylation of Nucleus

1. 7α-Hydroxylation   The first step in the route leading to the bile acids is 7α-hydroxylation of cholesterol to form cholest-5-en-3β,7α-diol (286). 7α-Hydroxylase, a mixed-function oxidase, has been recovered from the microsomal fraction of rat liver (287–289) and the enzyme requires NADPH and molecular oxygen (290). Carbon monoxide and an antibody to NADPH-linked cytochrome c reductase are inhibitory (291, 292), suggesting that the reductase and cytochrome P_{450} participate in the reaction. However, an increase in 7α-hydroxylase activity has been observed when there is a reduction or no change in the concentration of cytochrome P_{450} (287, 291, 296).

7α-Hydroxylation appears to be the rate-determining step in the biosynthesis of the bile acids from cholesterol (286, 294, 296). Biliary drainage or cholestyramine administration stimulates 7α-hydroxylase activity (291–294, 296, 297), but the other enzymes are either unaffected or only slightly stimulated under the same conditions (294, 296).

2. 12α-Hydroxylation 12α-Hydroxylase is also a mixed-function oxidase occurring in the microsomal fraction (290, 298). NADPH is required and there is some evidence that NADPH-cytochrome c reductase and cytochrome P_{450} may participate in the hydroxylation (298, 299). The presence of sterol carrier protein is required for full activity of 12α-hydroxylase (300). 7α-Hydroxycholest-4-en-3-one is the preferred substrate, yielding 7α, 12α-dihydroxycholest-4-en-3-one as the product. Other steroids, such as 5β-cholestane-3α,7α-diol and cholest-5-ene-3β,7α-diol, are hydroxylated at one-half and one-tenth the rate, respectively, of hydroxylation of 7α-hydroxycholest-4-en-3-one (298).

b. Reduction of Δ^5-Bond and Epimerization of 3β-Hydroxyl Group   Reduction of the Δ^5-bond and epimerization of the 3β-hydroxyl group are two steps related via the intermediacy of a Δ^4-3-ketosteroid formed by isomerization of the Δ^5-bond to the Δ^4-position with concomitant oxidation of the

3β-hydroxyl group to a 3-ketone. This step is probably similar to the formation of the Δ^4-3-ketosteroid hormones, and presumably requires the participation of two enzymes, a Δ^5-3β-hydroxysteroid dehydrogenase and a Δ^5-3-ketosteroid isomerase. Reduction of the Δ^4-bond and the 3-ketone yields the A/B *cis* configuration (5β) and 3α-hydroxyl group characteristic of the bile acids. Two enzymes, a Δ^4-3-oxosteroid 5β-reductase and a 3α-hydroxysteroid dehydrogenase, participate in this step.

The enzymes catalyzing the formation of the Δ^4-3-keto functionality are present in the microsomal fraction of rat liver (*301, 302*). Several Δ^5-3β-hydroxysteroids can be converted to Δ^4-3-ketosteroids by the microsomal enzyme system, but cofactor requirements vary for each substrate. NAD is required for the conversion of cholest-5-ene-3β,7α-diol (*301, 302*) and cholest-5-ene-3β,7α,12α-triol (*303*), but NADP is required in the case of cholest-5-ene-3β,12α-diol (*304*). A substrate with a 7β-hydroxyl group, cholest-5-ene-3β,7β-diol, is not metabolized to the corresponding Δ^4-3-ketosteroid (*305*). When the 3β-hydroxyl group is oxidized, the 3α-hydrogen is lost probably as hydride ion that transferred to NAD. About 25% of ^{3}H from [3α-^{3}H]cholest-5-ene-3β,7α-diol is recovered in NAD, but NADH is unlabeled, suggesting a rapid oxidation and turnover of NADH under the experimental conditions (*306*). During the isomerization of the Δ^5-bond of cholest-5-ene-3β,7α-diol to the Δ^4-position, the 4β-H is lost and a small fraction appears at the 6β position (*306*) (Scheme 11.21). In the presence of ^{3}H$_2$O or ^{2}H$_2$O, only small amounts of label are incorporated into the product (*306*).

The enzymes catalyzing the reduction of the Δ^4-3-ketosteroid to the

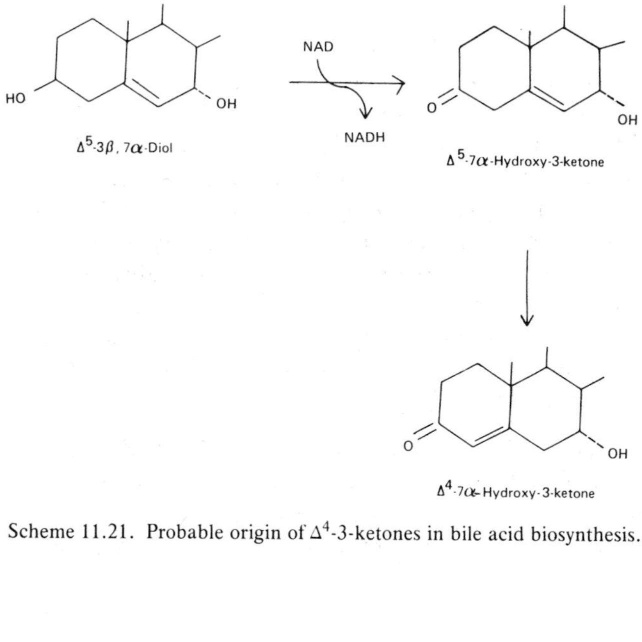

Scheme 11.21. Probable origin of Δ^4-3-ketones in bile acid biosynthesis.

3α-hydroxy-5β-steroid are present in the soluble fraction of rat liver (*307*). Both of the enzymes have been partially purified (Δ^4-3-oxosteroid 5β-reductase, 10-fold purification, and 3α-hydroxysteroid dehydrogenase, 200-fold purification) and their properties investigated (*307, 308*). In the first step, the Δ^4-bond is reduced by *trans* addition of hydride ion from NADPH to the 5β position and of a proton from the medium to the 4α-position by the Δ^4-3-oxosteroid 5β-reductase (*309, 310*) to produce a 3-keto-5β-steroid (Scheme 11.22). Hydride ion is donated from the A face of NADPH (*309,*

Δ^4-3- β Ketosteroid

3 α -Hydroxy-5β-Steroid   3-Keto-5β-Steroid

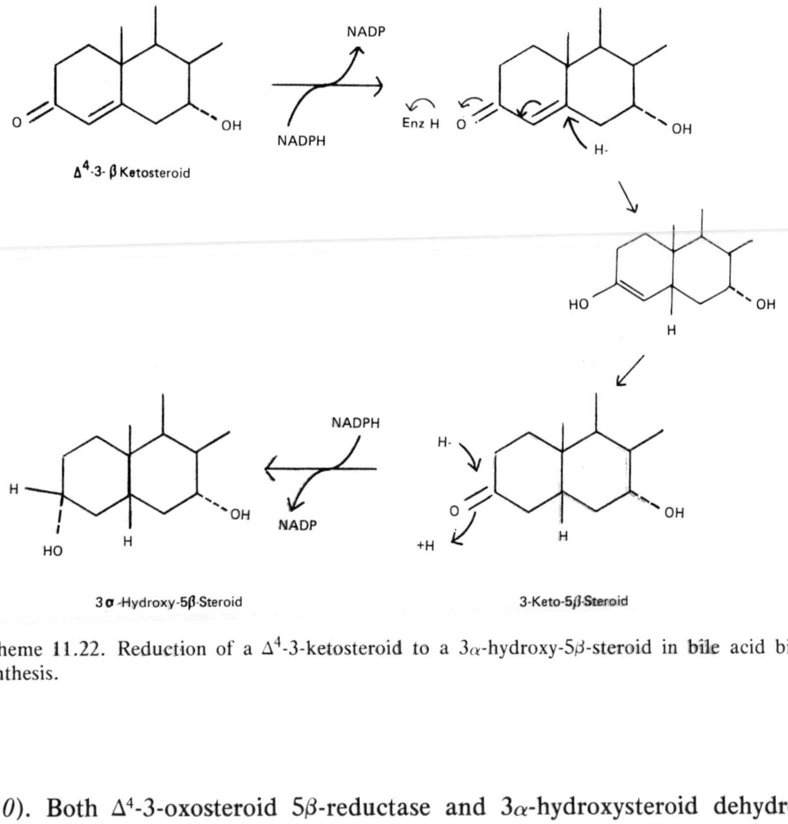

Scheme 11.22. Reduction of a Δ^4-3-ketosteroid to a 3α-hydroxy-5β-steroid in bile acid biosynthesis.

310). Both Δ^4-3-oxosteroid 5β-reductase and 3α-hydroxysteroid dehydrogenase are able to accept a variety of Δ^4-3-ketosteroids as substrates (C_{19}-, C_{21}-, C_{24}-, and C_{27}-steroids) (*307, 311–315*). In the case of the dehydrogenase, the rate of reaction is faster with NADPH and 3-keto-5β-steroids than with NADH and 3-keto-5α-steroids (*307*). One 3α-hydroxysteroid dehydrogenase preparation is also able to catalyze the oxidation of cholest-4-ene-$3\alpha,7\alpha$-diol to 7α-hydroxycholest-4-ene-3-one (*307*). For this preparation, the rate of reduction is about 10 times slower than the rate of oxidation for several substrates (*307*). During reduction, hydride ion is tranferred from the A face of NADPH to the 3β position (*309, 316*), and H^+ from the medium presumably is added to the oxygen atom forming the 3α-hydroxyl group.

c. Oxidation and Scission of Side Chain

1. 27-Hydroxylation   Enzymes catalyzing 27-hydroxylation seem to be present in the mitochondria as well as the microsomal fraction of rat liver (*317–319*). Both hydroxylations are stereospecific, yielding 5β-cholestane-3α,7α,12α,27-tetrol (*320–322*). Moreover, only one of the two *gem*-dimethyl groups is oxidized in 3α,7α,12α-trihydroxy-5β-cholestanoic acid occurring in bile. Independent evidence from two laboratories (*320, 321*) showed that the terminal *gem*-dimethyl carbon atom of the side chain derived from C-2 of MVA is not oxidized. When cholesterol biosynthesized from [2-^{14}]MVA (labeled at C-26) was used for cholic acid biosynthesis, carbon by carbon degradation of the propionic acid fragment (see Section D.2.c.3) revealed that C-3 of propionic acid was derived from C-2 of MVA and that C-1 (the carbon atom which was oxidized before scission) was unlabeled (*321*). In numbering the *gem*-dimethyl carbon atoms of the cholesterol side chain, C-26 is regarded as being derived from C-2 of MVA and C-27 as being derived from C-3′. NADPH is required by both enzymes (*319–324*), but the microsomal fraction in the presence of NADPH exhibits greater hydroxylase activity (*324*). Microsomal 27-hydroxylation is inhibited by carbon monoxide, indicating cytochrome P_{450} participation (*324*). The relative importance of the mitochondrial and the microsomal hydroxylations remains to be assessed.

2. Formation of 27-Carboxylic Acid   Oxidation of the 27-hydroxyl group to the 27-carboxylic acid (Scheme 11.23) occurs in the microsomal or soluble fraction of rat liver in the presence of NAD, but the soluble fraction exhibits the greater activity (*325–327*). A 27-aldehyde, 3α,7α,12α-trihydroxy-5β-cholestane-27-al, is oxidized to the acid by both systems (*328*). The alcohol and aldehyde dehydrogenases from the soluble fraction have been partially purified (*329–331*) and may be identical with ethanol and acetaldehyde dehydrogenases, respectively (*329*). In this connection, horse liver alcohol dehydrogenase will accept the 27-hydroxysteroid as a substrate, but the product of the conversion has not been identified (*332*).

3. Scission of Side Chain   Prior to cleavage of the side chain, the 27-carboxylic acid undergoes hydroxylation at C-24 (Scheme 11.23). A mitochondrial fraction of rat liver, in addition to the supernatant fraction, catalyzes the formation of 3α,7α,12α,24α-tetrahydroxy-5β-cholestanoic acid from 3α,7α,12α-trihydroxy-5β-cholestanoic acid (*333, 334*). The 24α-hydroxysteroid is the only isomer formed (*334, 335*). Cleavage of 3α,7α,12α, 24α-tetrahydroxy-5β-cholestanoic acid to cholic acid or the cholyl coenzyme-A ester is catalyzed by the 100,000 ×g supernatant fraction of rat liver with the release of propionic acid as the coenzyme-A ester (*334*) (Scheme 11.23). This sequence of events is similar to β oxidation of long chain fatty acids, but no comparative studies have been made. The suggestion (*336*) has been made that the enzymes catalyzing the β oxidation of the cholic acid precursor are unique to liver and differ from the enzymes catalyzing the β oxidation of fatty acids.

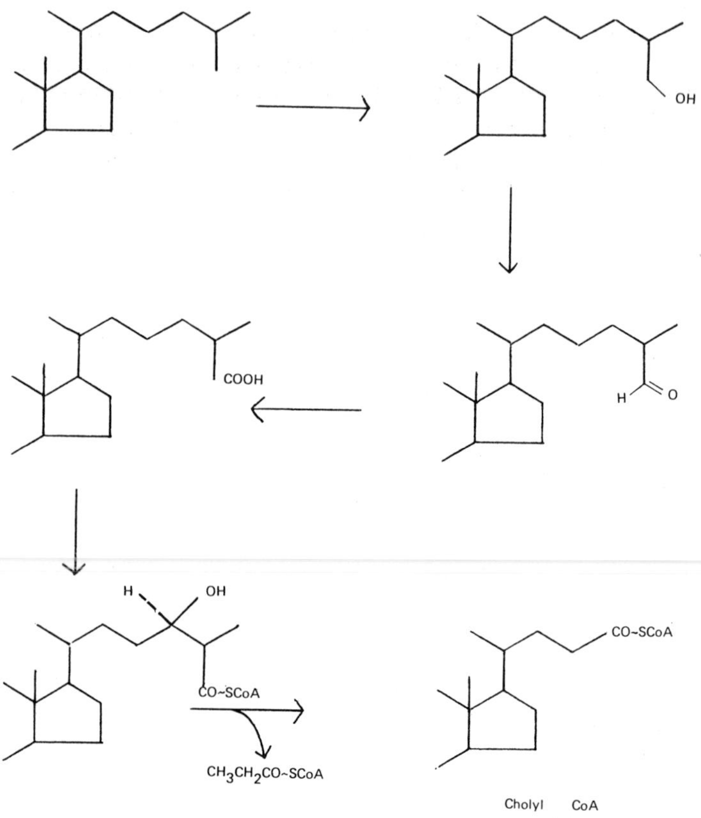

Scheme 11.23. Oxidation and scission of the side chain.

The *gem*-dimethyl group of cholesterol may also be cleaved as acetone by a pathway of uncertain importance. Labeled acetone has been isolated from incubations of rat liver mitochondria with [26-^{14}C]cholesterol (*337, 338*). By analogy to the cleavage of cholesterol to pregnenolone (*339*), a probable precursor for the formation of acetone is a 24,25-dihydroxysteroid. 5β-Cholestane-3α,7α,12α-triol can be hydroxylated at C-24 and C-25 by a microsomal preparation of rat liver (*324*). However, 5β-cholestane-3α, 7α,12α,25-tetrol, 5β-cholestane-3α,7α,12α,24α-tetrol, and 5β-cholestane-3α,7α,12α,24β-tetrol are converted to cholic acid at a slower rate than 5β-cholestane-3α,7α,12α,27-tetrol and 5β-cholestane-3α,7α,12α-triol (*324, 340, 341*).

d. Conjugation of Bile Acids to Taurine or Glycine Bile acids as the coenzyme-A ester are coupled with glycine or taurine in reaction catalyzed by enzymes in the lyposomal fraction of human liver (*342, 343*). Bile acid coenzyme-A esters (cholyl CoA and chenodeoxycholyl CoA), the products of side chain cleavage, undergo direct conjugation (Scheme 11.24, step b). In the case of the free bile acids, absorbed from the small intestine and transported to the liver, conversion of the bile acid to the coenzyme-A ester occurs in the microsomal fraction before conjugation to the amino acid (*344*) (Scheme 11.24, steps a and b). Glycine conjugates have been ob-

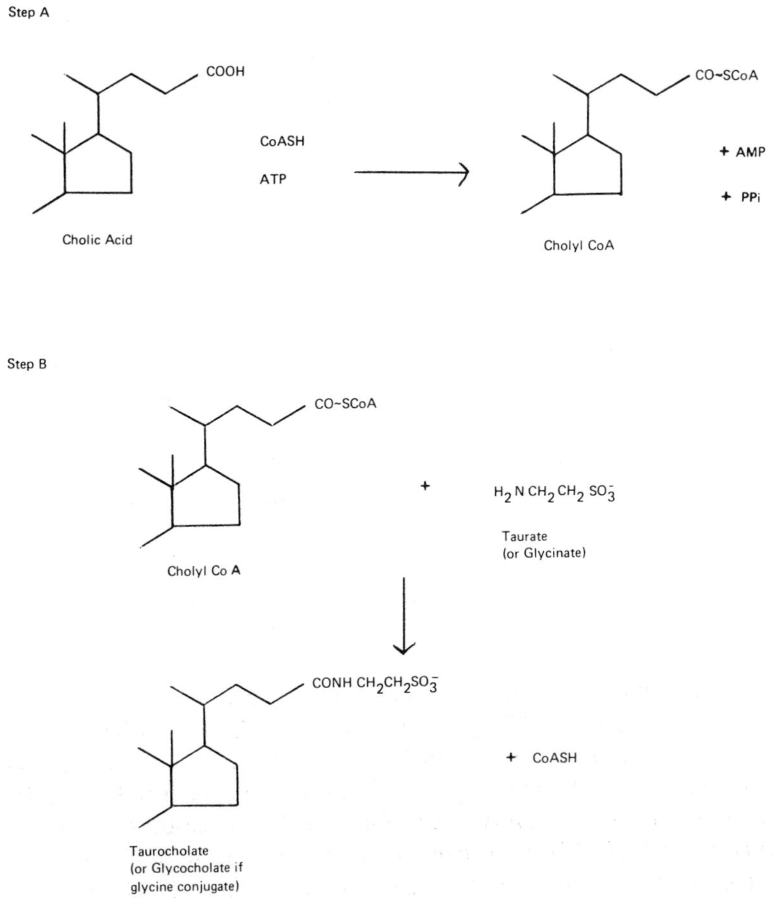

Scheme 11.24. Conjugation of cholic acid with taurine or glycine.

served only in mammals (*284*) (see Section C.1), and the ratio between the taurine- and glycine-conjugated bile acids found in bile varies among species (*284*), with diet, and with the influence of hormones and vitamins (*345, 346*).

3. Sequencing of Bile Acid Biosynthesis

Much of what is known about the sequence of bile acid biosynthesis in mammals is derived from the substrate specificities of the enzymes in the bile acid pathway. It is generally agreed that 7α-hydroxylation is the first step in the modification of cholesterol, and that, moreover, this is the major rate-determining step of bile acid biosynthesis. Several lines of evidence support this conclusion, including a diurnal variation in bile acid secretion in bile fistula rats varying in phase with 7α-hydroxylase activity (*347*), inhibition of 7α-hydroxylase activity by taurocholate (*348, 349*), the lack of inhibition of taurocholate on the conversion of 7α-hydroxycholesterol to the bile acids (*350*), and an increase in 7α-hydroxylase activity in response to cholesterol feeding (*347*).

The second step in the biosynthesis is the conversion of 7α-hydroxycholesterol to 7α-hydroxycholest-4-ene-3-one. At this point, 7α-hydroxycholesterol may undergo 12α-hydroxylation for cholic acid biosynthesis before conversion to the Δ^4-3-ketosteroid. The specificity of the microsomal 12α-hydroxylase indicates that 12α-hydroxylation probably follows formation of the Δ^4-3-ketosteroid, i.e., the rate of 12α-hydroxylation of 7α-hydroxycholesterol is one-tenth the rate of hydroxylation of 7α-hydroxycholest-4-one-3-one (*298*). After 12α-hydroxylation, $7\alpha,12\alpha$-dihydroxycholest-4-ene-3-one undergoes reduction in a stepwise fashion, producing the A/B *cis* ring junction and the 3α-hydroxyl group. Two enzymes are involved, and a study of the substrate specificities of partially purified preparations revealed that reduction of the Δ^4-bond precedes reduction of the 3-ketone (*307, 308*). The product of these steps is 5β-cholestane-$3\alpha,7\alpha$, 12α-triol (*351*). 12α-Hydroxylation may be postponed until rings A and B of cholesterol have been modified, but this occurrence is rendered unlikely again by the substrate specificity of 12α-hydroxylase; i.e., 5β-cholestane-$3\alpha,7\alpha$-diol is hydroxylated at one-half the rate of 7α-hydroxycholest-4-ene-3-one (*298*). The main pathway in the biosynthesis of cholic acid is depicted in Scheme 11.25.

Oxidation, scission, and conjugation of the side chain producing the bile salts occur only after the modifications of the nucleus have been completed (see Schemes 11.23 and 11.24). Rat liver enzyme systems have been prepared that produce 5β-cholestane-$3\alpha,7\alpha,12\alpha$-triol (*352*). In addition, 3β-hydroxy-5-cholenic acid is not an effective precursor of the bile acids (*353*), and 5β-cholestane-$3\alpha,7\alpha,12\alpha$-triol is oxidized by rat liver preparations to the C-27 alcohol and acid, which is subsequently cleaved to form cholic acid (*317, 318*).

Chenodeoxycholic acid, a second primary bile acid of man and many mammals, is biosynthesized by a route similar to cholic acid, with the exception of the omission of 12α-hydroxylation (Scheme 11.26). The sequencing of the other steps seems to be identical to cholic acid biosynthesis. An apparent nonspecificity of the C-27 hydroxylase (*346*) in the

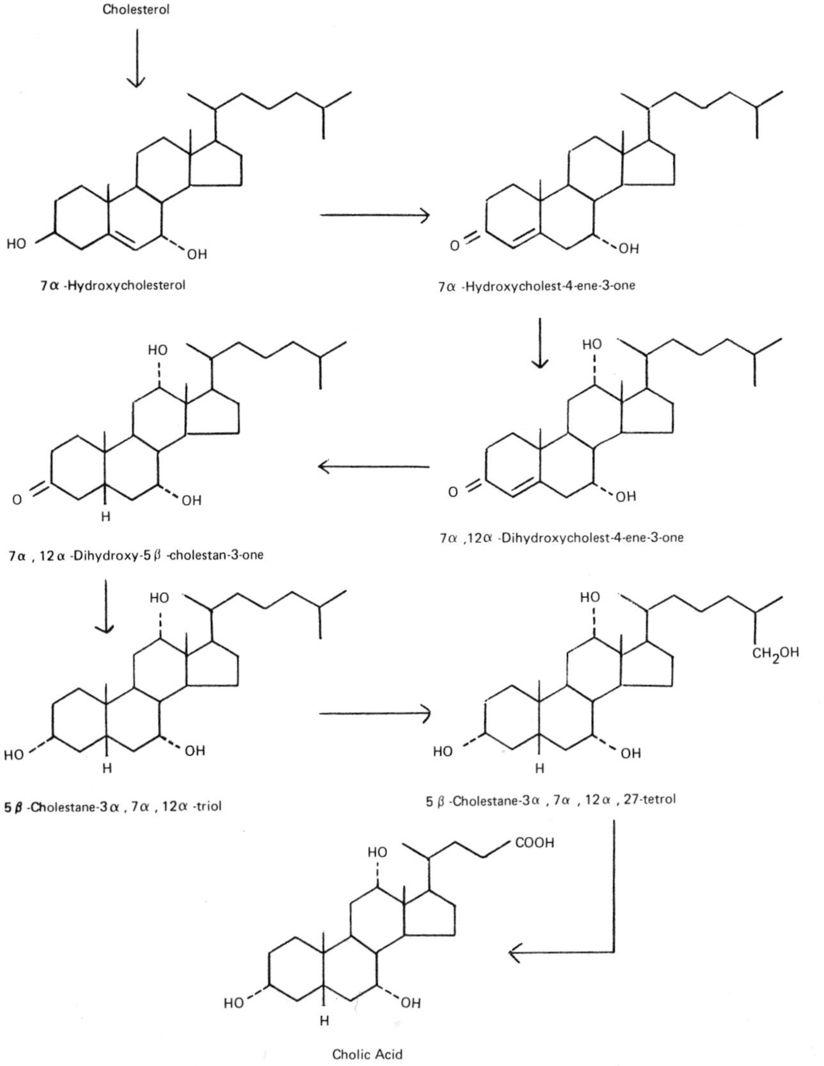

Scheme 11.25. Pathway for the conversion of cholesterol to cholic acid.

chenodeoxycholic acid pathway, which may be able to utilize cholesterol as a substrate, remains to be clarified.

Deoxycholic acid (similar to cholic acid but lacking the 7α-hydroxyl group) is a secondary bile acid of man and many mammals. It is apparently formed from cholic acid. Rat liver homogenates produce only small amounts of a possible precursor, cholest-5-ene-$3\beta,12\alpha$-diol, from cholesterol (304). In man, another possible precursor, 5β-cholestan-3α-ol, is efficiently con-

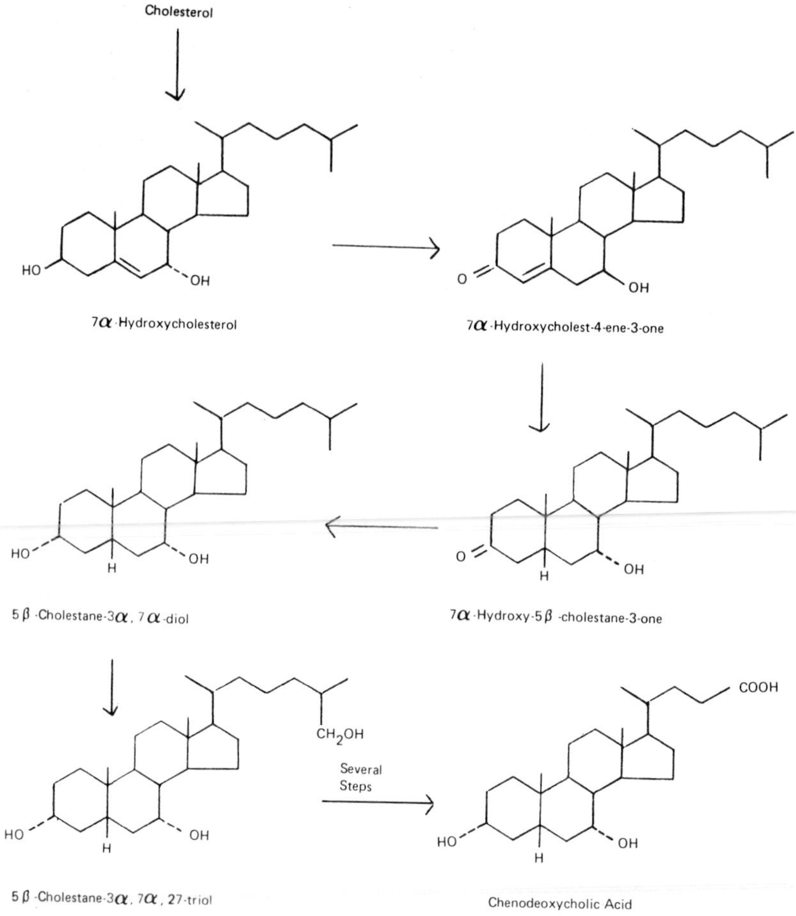

Cholesterol

7α-Hydroxycholesterol

7α-Hydroxycholest-4-ene-3-one

5β-Cholestane-3α, 7α-diol

7α-Hydroxy-5β-cholestane-3-one

CH₂OH

Several
Steps

COOH

5β-Cholestane-3α, 7α, 27-triol

Chenodeoxycholic Acid

Scheme 11.26. Pathway for the conversion of cholesterol to chenodeoxycholic acid.

verted to deoxycholic acid, but there is no evidence for the biosynthesis of 5β-cholestan-3α-ol in liver (354a).

4. Physiology

Bile salts excreted in the bile in conjunction with lecithin act as detergents for the emulsification of ingested fat in the small intestine. The structure of the bile salts is responsible for their detergency property. According to molecular models, there is a clear separation of the polar hydroxyl, carboxyl, and SO_3 groups from the hydrocarbon portion of the molecule. The polar groups lie on the α side of the steroid nucleus. This polar face is easily solvated in the aqueous phase of a fat-water emulsion, whereas the opposite, nonpolar face of the steroid nucleus is solvated in the hydrocarbon phase of the emulsion. At the physiological pH of the small intestine (pH 6.5), the taurine and glycine conjugates of the bile acids exist as a mixture of ions and minor amounts of the free acid (in the case of glycocholic acid). Micelles are easily formed in aqueous solution by molecules with physical properties, such as those of the bile salts in conjunction with other lipids. In the micelles the hydrocarbon portion of the bile salt faces the center for interaction with the lipid phase, whereas the polar portion is exposed to the surface for interaction with the water of the medium. The net effect of the micelle is the uniform dispersion of the nonpolar lipids in an aqueous medium.

The physical properties of detergency and micelle formation briefly described above allow fine dispersions of ingested fat in the aqueous medium of the small intestine. Pancreatic lipase can affect the hydrolysis of the fats only at the interface between the aqueous phase, in which the enzyme is dissolved, and the lipid droplet. The enzyme is activated by bile salts or other surface-tension lowering substances, which would also be capable of dispersing lipid droplets. Bile salts further aid the digestion of fats by a stimulation of peristalsis as well as the stimulation of further bile acid production. In addition, fatty acids liberated by the digestive process also aid the emulsification of ingested fat by acting as soaps at the pH of the small intestine.

Absorption of monoglycerides, fatty acids, cholesterol, and vitamin K is dependent on the bile salts. Fat, and the various detergents (bile salts and the fatty acid soaps) form micelles, which are small and finely dispersed. Fat absorption occurs in man in the jejunum. The small micelles containing bile salts, fatty acid soaps, and mono- and diglycerides may not require any specialized absorption mechanism such as penocytosis to enter the epithelial cells lining the lumen of the jejunum. Bile salts are not absorbed with the other dietary lipids, but are absorbed lower in the small intestine in the ileum.

Biliary excretion of cholesterol is the most important route for the removal of significant amounts of cholesterol from the body. Without such a mechanism to maintain a steady-state relationship in the size of the cholesterol pool, large quantities of cholesterol will accumulate as a direct result of diet and biosynthesis. The rate of turnover of cholesterol to the steroid hormones and its use in membranes is not sufficient, especially in the adult, to compensate for intake and biosynthesis.

The bile contains large amounts of cholesterol, most of which subsequently appears in the feces. The actual amount of cholesterol in the bile varies with diet and the extent of cholesterol biosynthesis in the liver. Bile salts aid in this mode of cholesterol excretion by solubilizing cholesterol in the bile. For a further discussion of the physical properties of the bile acids and their role in fat digestion and absorption, the reader is referred to Haslewood (*284*), Texter et al. (*354b*), and Wiseman (*354c*).

E. VITAMIN D

1. Discovery of Vitamin D

Rickets, a disease of infancy and childhood, was described as long ago as 1650 by Glisson in England. Low blood levels of calcium or phosphorus are typically seen in this condition, resulting in the failure of bone ossification and leading to bone resorption in severe cases. Obvious clinical symptoms include enlarged joints, softening and weakening of the bones, bowed legs, beaded ribs, delayed closure of the fontanelle, and faulty tooth development. Cod liver oil has been used as a therapeutic agent for centuries, but its ability to prevent rickets has only been appreciated more recently. It was only in the 1920s that the curative power of both cod liver oil and sunlight was established by experimental evidence. An antirachitic principle was found in cod liver oil that differed from the previously known vitamin A, and it was discovered that ultraviolet irradiation of certain foods such as cereals, grain, butter, milk, oils, fats, and yeast could introduce an antirachitic principle (355–361). Following these important discoveries, the identity of the antirachitic principle in the fish liver oils and other foods, as well as the mechanism of its production by sunlight and irradiation, was actively sought.

The first clue to the identity of the antirachitic principle was provided by Hess and co-workers (362–364), who found that the substance in vegetable oils, which could be activated by ultraviolet irradiation, was extractable with the nonsaponifiable fraction This fraction was known to contain principally phytosterols; however, phytosterol mixtures themselves were devoid of antirachitic property. Excitingly, antirachitic properties were acquired by phytosterol mixtures upon irradiation. Moreover, cholesterol itself was found to be activatable (364–366). Thus, activatable foods and cholesterol contained a sterol-like provitamin, and cod liver oil contained the fully formed vitamin D.

The search for the identity of vitamin D and its provitamin was accelerated by the development of an optical method that replaced bioassays for the antirachitic principle, which required at least 3–4 weeks. Activatable cholesterol had an absorption band at 282 nm that disappeared when the sterol was rendered antirachitic by irradiation (367, 368). The band at 282 nm was a valuable tool for the identification of the provitamin and formed the basis of an assay for the provitamin that took only 3–4 hours to complete.

Windaus and Hess (369) had the insight to apply the assay to the vitamin D problem and very soon thereafter identified one of the vitamin D provitamins. The provitamin absorbing at 282 nm could not be removed from cholesterol by recrystallization. Only carbon decolorization, partial oxidation with permanganate, overirradiation, or conversion to the dibromide effected removal of the provitamin. The nature of these treatments suggested that the provitamin was more unsaturated than cholesterol. At the same time Windaus and Hess (369) were testing various substances for antirachitic properties after irradiation. A phytosterol with two double bonds failed to develop antirachitic properties, but ergosterol seemed to be a likely candidate. Ergosterol and activatable cholesterol had similar physical properties, including absorption at 282 nm, and the same response to the Lieberman-Buchard reaction. Windaus and Hess (369) concluded that ergosterol or a similar sterol identical to ergosterol in physical properties and ultraviolet absorption was the provitamin. Bioassay data corroborated their conclusion by the demonstration that irradiated ergosterol was more than 1,000 times more antirachitic than irradiated cholesterol.

Investigation turned to the identification of: 1) the products of the irradiation of ergosterol, 2) the cholesterol component that became antirachitic following irradiation, and 3) the antirachitic principle in cholesterol.

Isolation and identification of crystalline products of irradiated ergosterol proved to be exceptionally difficult. A crystalline substance named vitamin D_1, having antirachitic potency, was at long last isolated at about the same time in two laboratories (370, 371). However, vitamin D_1 proved to be a mixture of the antirachitic principle and various inactive components. Vitamin D_2 (also named calciferol), the acitve substance, was isolated and purified subsequently by the same research groups (372, 373). From catalytic hydrogenation data, which indicated four double bonds, and failure to form the Diels hydrocarbon, typically formed by ergosterol and lumisterol (a sterol formed after the irradiation of ergosterol), Windaus and Thiele (374) concluded that vitamin D_2 is formed by the opening of one of the rings of ergosterol. Heilbron and co-workers (375–377) subsequently found that ring B must be opened at the 9,10-position (9,10-secosteroid), the presence of a $\Delta^{7(8)}$-bond, and the presence of a methylene group at C-10. X-ray crystallographic studies of Crowfoot (378, 379) established the structure and stereochemistry of vitamin D_2 as shown in Scheme 11.27.

Discovery of the identity of the provitamin of fish liver oils and the irradiation-induced antirachitic principle of cholesterol arose from investigations of Windaus and Brockmann. Windaus, in an attempt to identify antirachitic substances other than vitamin D_2, synthesized several analogs of ergosterol having the same $\Delta^{5,7}$-diene system but differing in the side chain (380, 381). Of special interest was a sterol with a side chain identical to cholesterol, 7-dehydrocholesterol. Upon irradiation, 7-dehydrocholesterol yielded an oil with an antirachitic potency similar to vitamin D_2. The active principle, named vitamin D_3, was isolated from the mixture as the dinitrobenzoyl ester and the allophanate (382). Brockmann (383, 384) extracted tuna liver oil and obtained a crystalline dinitrobenzoyl ester derivative that, upon hydrolysis, yielded a sterol with antirachitic properties and an

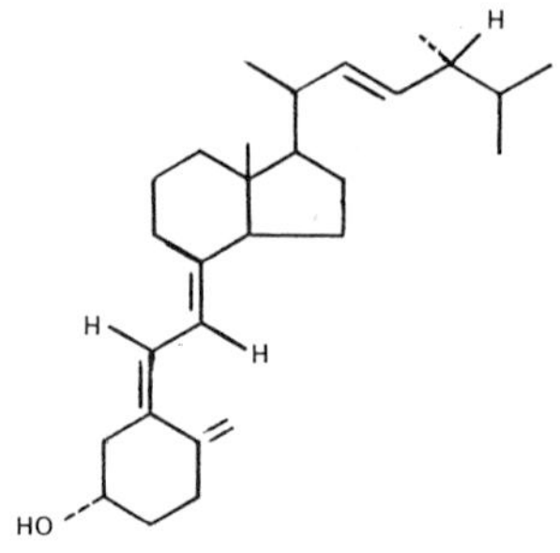

Vitamin D$_2$
(Calciferol)

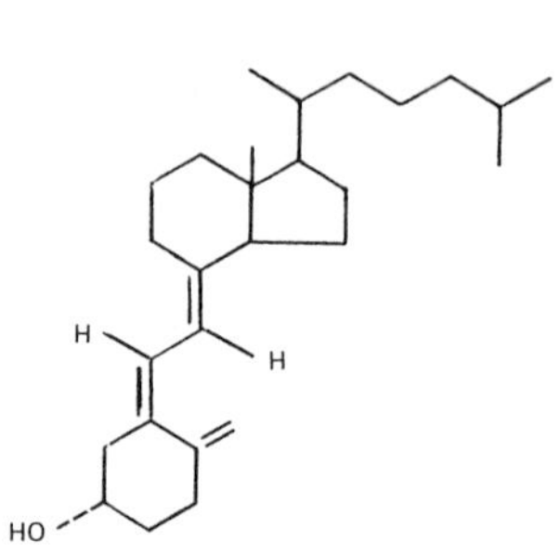

Vitamin D$_3$
(Cholecalciferol)

Scheme 11.27. Structures of vitamin D$_2$ and vitamin D$_3$. Conformations are those in the crystalline state as shown by x-ray data. The use of solid and interrupted lines on ring A is in the general rather than steroid convention, while in the side chain their use conforms to the convention described in Chapter 2.

absorption spectrum similar to vitamin D$_2$ [absorption at 265 nm typical of the triene chromophore (C-19 to C-8)]. The melting point and composition of the crystalline ester differed from vitamin D$_2$, but was identical to the dinitrobenzoyl ester of vitamin D$_3$. Thus, 7-dehydrocholesterol is the provitamin of fish liver oil. The structure of vitamin D$_3$ (cholecalciferol) is shown in Scheme 11.27.

2. Mechanism of Vitamin D Formation

a. Photochemically Induced Formation of D Vitamins With the identity of the antirachitic steroids, calciferol (D$_2$), cholecalciferol (D$_3$), and their provitamins, ergosterol and cholesterol, established, attention turned to the pathway or mechanism of irradiation-induced alterations in the provitamins. Several sterols, isomers of ergosterol, were usually found in the crude mixture, resulting from the irradiation of ergosterol. One of these, lumisterol, can be isolated as a 1:1 complex with vitamin D$_2$ when ergosterol is irradiated at wavelengths above 280 nm (*385*). The physical properties of lumisterol are similar to ergosterol, including three double bonds (*386, 387*), one of which is in the side chain, absorption at 280 nm, formation of the Diels hydrocarbon, and formation of suprasterol I and II (*388*) (compounds without antirachitic potency formed when ergosterol is overirradiated). However, like vitamin D$_2$, lumisterol is not precipitated by digitonin. Another component of the ergosterol irradiation mixture, tachysterol, is similar to vitamin D$_2$ in that it contains four double bonds, one of which is in the side chain, but it does not form the Diels hydrocarbon, and unlike vitamin D$_2$ it is levorotary (*389*). Reduction of an ester of tachysterol affords a mixture of dihydrides (*390*), one of which is identical to dihydrovitamin D$_2$, the reduction product of vitamin D$_2$ (*391*). The similarities of lumisterol and tachysterol to ergosterol and vitamin D$_2$

prompted their inclusion in the sequence ergosterol→lumisterol→tachysterol→vitamin D_2→suprasterol (overirradiation products).

In the early investigations, ergosterol was usually irradiated by an ultraviolet light source that heated the ergosterol solution to about 50° (392). When the temperature was maintained at 20° during irradiation, the irradiated ergosterol solution increased in vitamin D_2 content when subsequently heated. From these experiments resulted the isolation of previtamin D_2, a new ergosterol isomer, by Velluz and his co-workers (393). Upon heating to 65°, approximately 65% of the dinitrobenzoyl ester of previtamin D_2 is converted to vitamin D_2 dinitrobenzoate. In solution, vitamin D_2 reaches an equilibrium with previtamin D_2, with the concentration of the vitamin being favored. In addition to these results, irradiation of 7-dehydrocholesterol under controlled temperature similarly resulted in the isolation of previtamin D_3.

The most striking property of the new ergosterol isomer was the low-intensity absorption at 265 nm (molecular extinction coefficient of 9,000, compared to 18,300 for vitamin D_2). The low-intensity absorption results from the presence of a cis-$\Delta^{6(7)}$-bond. Havinga (394) obtained experimental proof that previtamin D_2 was the cis isomer of tachysterol (trans-$\Delta^{6(7)}$) by treatment of the previtamin with iodine, an isomerization catalyst, and the quantitative recovery of tachysterol. At the same time, Velluz and co-workers (395) found that ultraviolet light could induce the isomerization of previtamin D_2 to tachysterol. After removal of tachysterol from the irradiation mixture, ergosterol and lumisterol remained, indicating that the irradiation process was reversible. With the finding that previtamin D_2 was transformed into ergosterol, lumisterol, and tachysterol, Velluz (396) proposed that previtamin D_3 was the first product of the irradiation of cholesterol. Almost simultaneously, Havinga and co-workers (397) provided experimental proof that previtamin D_2 was indeed the first irradiation product. Irradiation of a mixture of [^{14}C]ergosterol (biosynthesized from [1-^{14}C]acetate), 7-[3-^{14}C]dehydrocholesterol, and unlabeled lumisterol and tachysterol yielded the various products, which differed in specific activity. From the specific activity of lumisterol, it was obvious that lumisterol was not involved in the irradiation sequence and that tachysterol was probably a side product.

A mechanism for the photochemical production of the D vitamins was proposed by Havinga and his associates (397). Structurally, ergosterol and 7-dehydrocholesterol are homoannular conjugated dienes by virtue of the $\Delta^{5,7}$-bond. When it absorbs a photon of ultraviolet radiation, this labile system becomes sufficiently excited to effect homolysis of the doubly activated C-9 to C-10 bond. An activated intermediate (Scheme 11.28) resulting from the excitation then undergoes isomerization to and remains in thermal equilibrium with the actual vitamin. Additional ultraviolet energy is necessary to maintain an equilibrium between the activated intermediate

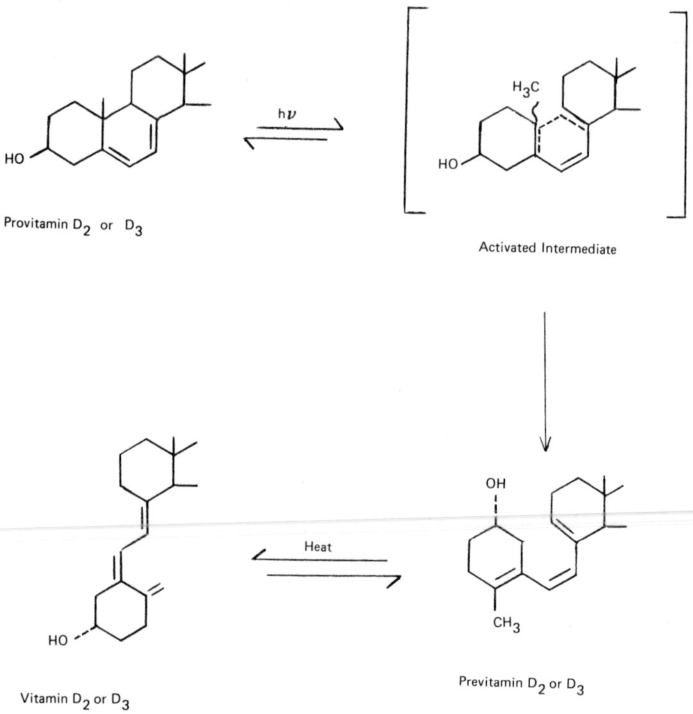

Scheme 11.28. Irradiation-induced conversion of provitamin D_2 or D_3 (ergosterol or 7-dehydro cholesterol) to the D vitamins. See legend to Scheme 11.27.

and the side products, tachysterol and lumisterol (in the case of ergosterol) (Scheme 11.29). Kinetic evidence indicates that more than one excited species may participate in the reaction (*398*).

b. Enzymatic Formation of D Vitamins   The presence of relatively large amounts of the provitamin, 7-dehydrocholesterol, in the skins of higher animals [usually 4% higher than the amount in the internal organs (*399*)] is in agreement with the photochemical conversion of 7-dehydrocholesterol to vitamin D_3. In some species, photochemical means may not be the only method of vitamin D production. Many species of deep-water fish store significant amounts of the D vitamins in their livers, and fish liver oils are in fact the richest source of the vitamin. Ultraviolet radiation of 280 nm, the most effective wavelength for the photochemical production of the D vitamins, cannot penetrate to the depths inhabited by deep-water fish. Diet and/or enzymatic conversion of the provitamin to the vitamin remain the only sources of vitamin D available to the fish. During an investigation of this problem, Bills (*400*) found that ultraviolet radiation does not stimulate vitamin D production in fish and, in fact, exposed fish be-

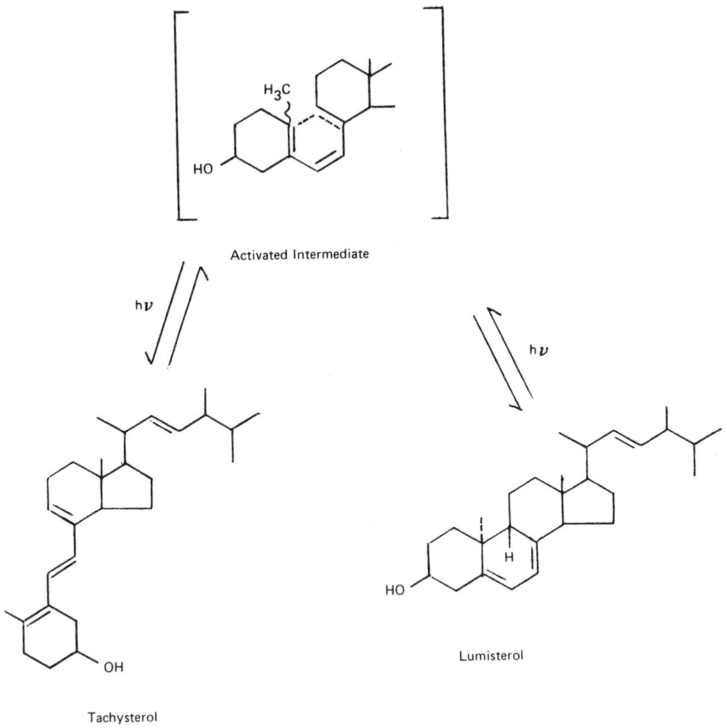

Scheme 11.29. Side reactions of the irradiation of ergosterol (provitamin D₂). See legend to Scheme 11.27.

come ill. In addition, bony fish, such as halibut, catfish, tuna, and cod have very little vitamin D available to them in their diet (*400, 401*). The results prompted the suggestion that vitamin D may be produced in the fish by biosynthesis (*400*).

This hypothesis has been explored by a number of investigators. Various species of fish, including cod, catfish, puffer fish, and possibly pollack, haddock, and tuna, accumulate vitamin D in the liver even though deprived of a vitamin D source for 6 months (*402*). The same researchers noted no conversion of provitamin D to vitamin D. The results of more recent studies also showed slight if any biosynthesis of vitamin D₃ from 7-dehydrocholesterol in sea bass liver homogenates (*403, 404*), and no biosynthesis at all of vitamin D from [2-¹⁴C]mevalonic acid in this species (*404, 405*). Additional evidence against vitamin D biosynthesis was provided by observations that fish reared in total darkness for prolonged periods displayed pathological changes in the skeleton and in calcium metabolism (*406, 407*). The data on the actual amount of vitamin D available in the diet of fish are in conflict (*366, 400–402, 408, 409*). In conclusion, no definitive experimental proof of vitamin D formation is available at this time that would substantiate a hypothesis of vitamin D biosynthesis in fish or other animals without photochemical processes.

3. Physiology

Cholecalciferol, vitamin D_3, is the physiologically important D vitamin. The provitamin, 7-dehydrocholesterol, is found in animal tissue in the greatest concentrations in skin, where it is available for the photochemical transformation. A second important source of cholecalciferol is absorption from the diet. Research has focused on the mode of action of this vitamin rather than of vitamin D_2, calciferol (also called ergocalciferol), which does not seem as important physiologically. Man and rat are able to utilize both vitamins equally well, but in the chick calciferol has only 10% of the activity of cholecalciferol (410).

a. Activation of cholecalciferol (Vitamin D₃)

1. *25-Hydroxylation* After the structural elucidation of the D vitamins, their provitamins, and the route of formation of the vitamins from the provitamins, investigation into the physiology and any further metabolism of the vitamin lagged until the observation by Carlsson (411) of a delay between vitamin D administration and the appearance of a physiological response. This result indicated that the vitamin probably underwent metabolism or activation before any physiological function could be manifested. DeLuca and co-workers were the first to obtain evidence for the existence of a polar metabolite that appeared before the intestinal response of increased calcium transport. This metabolite had very strong antirachitic activity and acted more rapidly than the vitamin to initiate intestinal calcium transport (412, 413). The metabolite was subsequently identified as 25-hydroxycholecalciferol (Scheme 11.30) and prepared synthetically (414, 415). 25-Hydroxycholecalciferol is the major cholecalciferol metabolite in the plasma of man (416), rats (412), and the chick (417).

The liver is the site of the 25-hydroxylation, and the substrate, cholecalciferol, is accumulated in that organ (418). Hepatectomy in the rat abolishes almost completely the appearance of 25-hydroxycholecalciferol in the blood and tissues (419). In the same species, kidney or intestinal homogenates are incapable of 25-hydroxylation (419). However, some 25-hydroxylation may occur in the intestine and kidney of the chick (420). The hepatic 25-hydroxylase is microsomal and requires a cytoplasmic fraction and NADPH (421). Cytochrome P_{450} inhibitors are ineffective in blocking the hydroxylation (421).

2. *1α-Hydroxylation* Not long after the identification of 25-hydroxycholecalciferol, Norman and his colleagues detected a more polar metabolite in the chromatin fraction of intestines (422). This steroid possessed potent biological activity that appeared and disappeared rapidly (423). In Kodicek's laboratory loss of ^{3}H from [4-^{14}C, 1-^{3}H]25-hydroxycholecalciferol with the formation of a more polar metabolite was observed (424). The ^{3}H atom

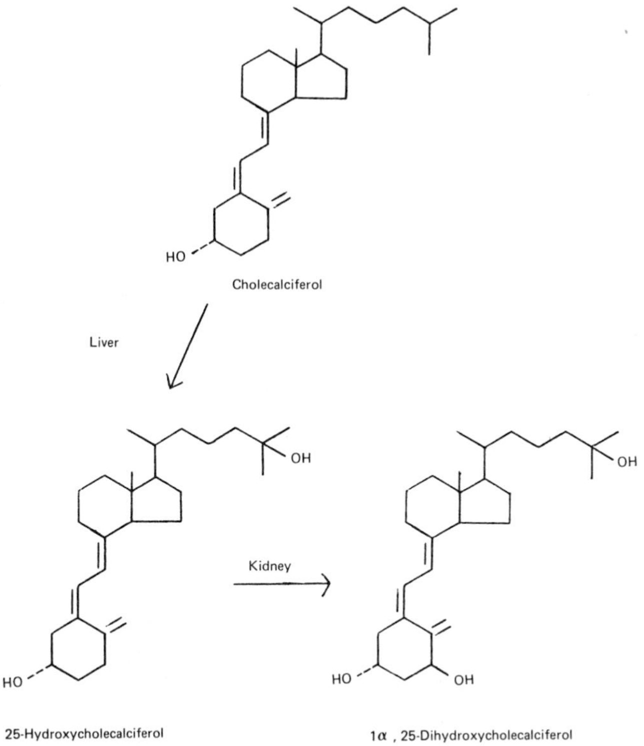

Scheme 11.30. Activation of cholecalciferol (vitamin D_3). See legend to Scheme 11.27.

was recovered in water (*425*). Nephrectomized rats were incapable of transferring the ^{3}H atom from the steroid to water (*425*), indicating that the kidneys were the site of this transformation. It was demonstrated almost simultaneously in three laboratories that this new metabolite was 1α,25-dihydroxycholecalciferol (*425–427*) (Scheme 11.30). The structure has been confirmed by synthesis (*428*).

1α,25-Dihydroxycholecalciferol is the biologically active form of calciferol in four species that have been studied, viz., man (*429, 430*), rat (*431*), dog (*432*), and chick (*431, 433*). Several lines of evidence support these observations. When the vitamin, the monohydroxylated, and dihydroxylated derivatives are administered by various routes, they are concentrated in the intestinal mucosa at rates that increase with increasing functionalization, i.e., 16, 12, or 4 hr, respectively (*434–436*). The only vitamin D_3 derivative that becomes associated with the chromatin fraction of the intestinal mucosal cell is 1α,25-dihydroxycholecalciferol (*410*). 1α,25-Dihydroxycholecalciferol is 100 times more active in isolated bone cultures than 25-hydroxycholecalciferol and infinitely more active than cholecalciferol (437). The typical responses to vitamin D, intestinal calcium (438–441) and phosphate (441) transport, and calcium mobilization in bone (442), are elicited in nephrectomized rats only to 1α,25-dihydroxychole-calciferol and not to 25-hydroxycholecalciferol. These results indicate that in each of the systems investigated 1α,25-dihydroxycholecalciferol is the physiologically active form of the vitamin. The possibility that the vitamin undergoes further metabolism at another site is not excluded by these findings.

The 1α-hydroxylase system, localized in the kidney (see preceding paragraph), is found in the mitochondria (425, 427, 443). NADPH is required for activity (444). Production of 1α,-25-dihydroxycholecalciferol is coincident with cytochrome P_{450} reduction, and is sensitive to the cytochrome P_{450} inhibitors CO and metapyrone (419). Molecular oxygen is the only source of the oxygen atom in the 1α-hydroxy groups, indicating that the enzyme is a mixed-function oxidase (445). An active 1α-hydroxylase system can be reconstituted with a purified NADPH flavoprotein, adrenodoxin from beef adrenal mitochondria, and a soluble cytochrome P_{450} fraction from rachitic chick kidney mitochondria (446).

3. 24-Hydroxylation   25-Hydroxycholecalciferol is further hydroxylated at C-24 (447), and the 24,25-dihydroxy derivative can be further hydroxylated at C-1 (448). The functional significance of the 24,25-functionalization has not yet been elucidated. It is possible that C-24 hydroxylation is the first metabolic step in a degradative pathway. The facts that 24,25-dihyroxycholecalciferol is found in normal animals (449, 450) and that its plasma concentration can be correlated with dietary factors (449) argue against this view. In support of the hypothesis of a physiological function, the 24α-isomer [24α-hydroxycholecalciferol (Scheme 11.31)] mimics 25-hydroxycholecalciferol in its effects on the mineralization of bone, the elevation of serum phosphorus, the mobilization of bone calcium, and intestinal calcium transport, while the 24β-isomer (Scheme 11.31) is much

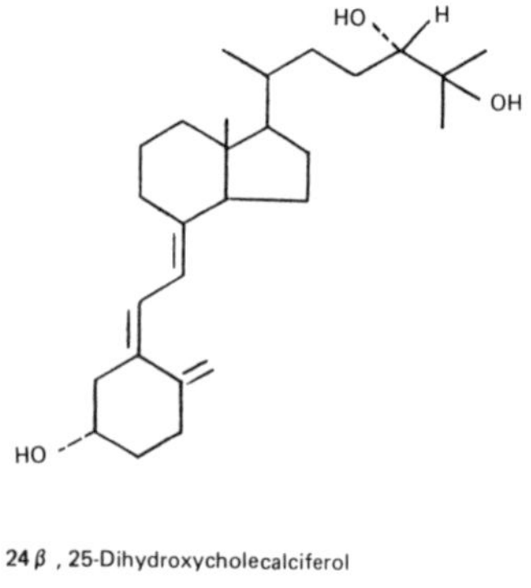

24 β , 25-Dihydroxycholecalciferol

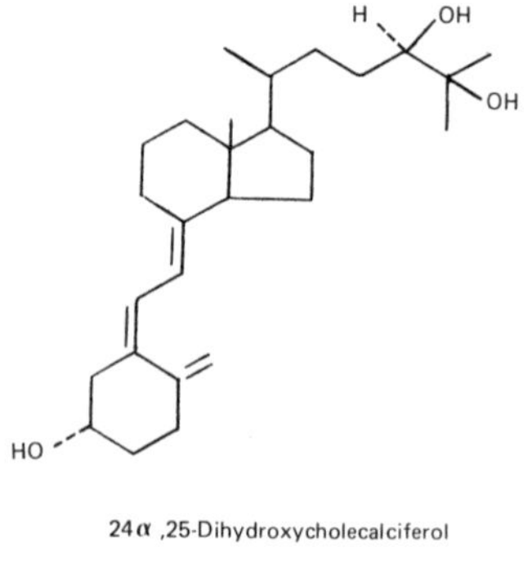

24 α ,25-Dihydroxycholecalciferol

Scheme 11.31. The 24-hydroxy derivatives of 25-hydroxy cholecalciferol. See legend to Scheme 11.27.

less effective in each of these respects, with the exception of intestinal calcium transport (451). On the other hand, the 24,25-dihydroxycholecalciferol is less active than 25-hydroxycholecalciferol in inducing intestinal calcium transport in the chick (452). Correspondingly, in the same animal, 1α,24,25-trihydroxycholecalciferol is less active than 1α,25-dihydroxycholecalciferol.

The C-24 hydroxylase has been isolated and partially purified from chick renal mitochondria (animals raised on high calcium and cholecalciferol-supplemented diet) (453). Oxygen and NADPH are required.

b. Regulation of Cholecalciferol Activation and Metabolism   Many factors interact in a complex fashion to regulate cholecalciferol activation and its action at target sites. These include the hormone parathormone, dietary calcium and phosphate levels, and serum concentrations of calcium and phosphorus. Much research still needs to be done to elucidate fully the interrelationship between these factors. From the results of various experiments, a picture is beginning to emerge.

Biosynthesis of 1α,25-dihydroxycholecalciferol responds directly to dietary levels of calcium; i.e., biosynthesis is repressed by high-calcium diets and stimulated by low-calcium diets (449, 454). Serum calcium concentration is apparently a signal to the kidney for increased or decreased 1α-hydroxylation; e.g., hypocalcemia increases the biosynthesis and hypercalcemia depresses the biosynthesis of 1α,25-dihydroxycholecalciferol. Phosphate serum concentration similarly influences the rate of 1α-hydroxylation (455). Increased biosynthesis of 1α,25-dihydroxycholecalciferol is observed in animals on a low-phosphorus diet accompanied by elevated levels of calcium transport. This effect is seen even in the absence of parathyroid hormone (456).

The regulation of serum levels of 1α,25-dihydroxycholecalciferol is mediated by parathormone. In rats, parathyroidectomy results in decreased production of the 1α,25-dihydroxy compound and increased production of the 24,25-dihydroxy compound. The administration of parathormone (parathyroid hormone) reverses these events (456, 457). Parathormone is not required for 1α,25-dihydroxycholecalciferol stimulation of intestinal calcium transport, but the hormone is necessary for the effect of 1α,25-dihydroxycholecalciferol on bone calcium mobilization (458–460).

The overall picture that emerges is one of a dual role for 1α,25-dihydroxycholecalciferol in calcium and phosphate mobilization. In calcium homeostasis, a system can be visualized (Scheme 11.32) in which parathormone released in response to hypocalcemia stimulates 1α-hydroxylation of 25-hydroxycholecalciferol. The 1α,25-dihydroxy compound stimulates intestinal calcium absorption (parathormone is not required). At the level of bone, both parathormone and 1α,25-dihydroxycholecalciferol act to mobilize calcium from the bone. When the serum calcium levels approach normal as a result of these processes, parathormone secretion is suppressed.

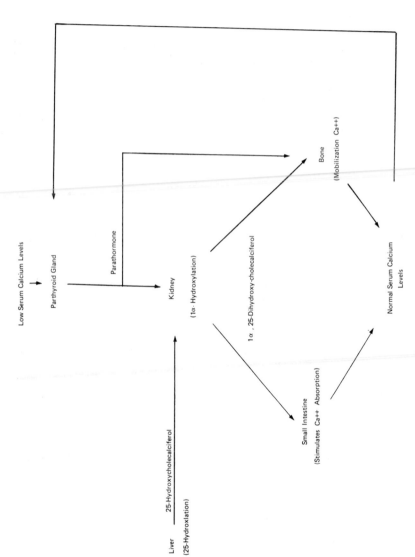

Scheme 11.32. A possible mechanism for the regulation of calcium homeostasis.

c. Molecular Role of 1α,25-Dihydroxylcholecalciferol   The role of 1α, 25-dihydroxycholecalciferol in stimulating intestinal calcium transport has been investigated more intensively than the role of the steroid in bone calcium mobilization. After 1α-hydroxylation in the kidney, the steroid is transported to the epithelial cells lining the lumen of the small intestine. There, it participates in calcium absorption in a process involving induction of a protein [calcium-binding protein (CaBP)]. The intracellular route(s) that calcium takes through the epithelial cell from the lumen of the intestine to blood is not completely understood. Once inside the intestinal cell, 1α,25-dihydroxycholecalciferol becomes associated with a protein that is heat labile, Pronase sensitive, and RNAase or DNAase insensitive (*461*). The association constant for the steroid-protein complex is 2×10^8 M^{-1} and the protein sediments at 3S in a sucrose gradient (*462*). 1α,25-Dihydroxycholecalciferol is also bound to a nuclear protein receptor with the same sedimentation constant (3S). This protein has two binding components with different association constants, 2×10^9 M^{-1} and 5×10^8 M^{-1}, and it is specific only for the natural *cis*-isomer of 1α,25-dihydroxycholecalciferol. 5,6-*Cis*- or 5,6-*trans*-1α-hydroxy- and 5,6-*trans*-25-hydroxycholecalciferol are not bound, but 5,6-*cis*-25-hydroxycholecalciferol is bound to a slight extent (*462*). The function of these steroid-protein complexes is not yet known, but it can be hypothesized that the cytoplasmic protein acts as a cytoplasmic receptor for the steroid, which is then transported to the nucleus in a manner analogous to the steroid hormones. Once in or at the nucleus, the steroid may be transferred to the nuclear receptor.

1α,25-Dihydroxycholecalciferol or the steroid-nuclear protein complex in some manner controls the transcription of mRNA coding for CaBP. With the accumulation of the steroid in the epithelial cell nucleus, biosynthesis of CaBP on large polysomes (*463*) follows in 5–6 hr, and CaBP reaches maximum concentration within 72 hr (*462*). CaBP is the only protein known to be biosynthesized in response to 1α,25-dihydroxycholecalciferol. Other undetected proteins that interact in the calcium transport system may be produced in response to the steroid.

Significant calcium absorption is not detectable until CaBP is biosynthesized. Calcium absorption can be detected 9–10 hr after a dose of cholecalciferol and the rate of absorption increases rapidly up until 24 hr and then increases more slowly until 72 hr. These events parallel increases in the concentration of CaBP (*462*). Chick intestinal CaBP has a molecular weight of 28,000 and four high affinity binding sites for calcium with an affinity constant of 2×10^6 M^{-1} and 20–30 sites with a lesser affinity of ca. 10^2 M^{-1}. A preference is exhibited for calcium over barium, strontium, and magnesium (*464–467*). Intestinal calcium absorption is related to CaBP concentration in a 1:1 relationship (*468*). Further research is needed to establish the role of CaBP and possibly 1α,25-dihydroxycholecalciferol in the passage of calcium across the brush border membrane of the epithelial cell at the intestinal lumen, through the interior of the epithelial cell, and across the serosal/basal membrane of the cell to the blood.

LITERATURE CITED

1. E. Gorter and F. Grendel, J. Exp. Med. 41:439 (1925).
2. J. F. Danielli and H. Davson, J. Cell. Comp. Physiol. 5:495 (1935).
3. J. B. Finean, Circulation 26:1151 (1962).
4. F. A. Vandenheuvel, J. Am. Oil Chem. Soc. 40:455 (1963).
5. F. A. Vandenheuvel, Ann. N. Y. Acad. Sci. 122:57 (1965).
6. J. D. Robertson, Symp. Biochem. Soc. 16:3 (1959).
7. P. Ways and D. J. Hanahan, J. Lipid Res. 5:319 (1964).
8. S. Fleischer and G. Rouser, J. Am. Oil Chem. Soc. 43:594 (1965).
9. G. Dallner, P. Siekevitz, and G. E. Palade, Biochem. Biophys. Res. Commun. 20:142 (1965).
10. R. P. Longley, A. H. Rose, and B. A. Knights, Biochem. J. 108:401 (1968).
11. (a) S. Razin and R. C. Cleverdon, J. Gen. Microbiol. 41:409 (1965); (b) N. L. Gershfeld, M. Wormser, and S. Razin, Biochim. Biophys. Acta 352:371 (1974).
12. G. Hallermayer and W. Newpert, Hoppe-Seyler's Z. Physiol. Chem. 355: 279 (1974).
13. E. Korn, Science 153:1491 (1966).
14. R. L. Conner, F. B. Mallory, J. R. Landrey, K. A. Ferguson, E. S. Kaneshiro, and E. Ray, Biochem. Biophys. Res. Commun. 44:995 (1971).
15. A. J. Clark and K. Bloch, J. Biol. Chem. 234:2583 (1959).
16. (a) A. A. Andreasen and T. J. B. Stier, J. Cell Comp. Physiol. 41:23 (1953); (b) A. A. Andreasen and T. J. B. Stier, J. Cell Comp. Physiol. 43:271 (1954).
17. R. L. Conner, W. J. Van Wagtendonk, and C. A. Miller, J. Gen. Microbiol. 9:434 (1953).
18. H. S. Vishniac and S. W. Watson, J. Gen. Microbiol. 8:248 (1953).
19. R. L. Conner, J. R. Landrey, E. S. Kaneshiro and W. J. Van Wagtendonk, Biochim. Biophys. Acta 239:312 (1971).
20. W. R. Nes, B. Sekula, and J. H. Adler, unpublished observations.
21. W. R. Nes, Lipids 9:596 (1974).
22. D. J. Baisted, E. Capstack, Jr., and W. R. Nes, Biochemistry 1:537 (1962).
23. R. T. van Aller, H. Chikamatsu, N. J. de Souza, and W. R. Nes, J. Biol. Chem. 244:6645 (1969).
24. J. S. O'Brien and E. L. Sampson, J. Lipid Res. 6:537 (1965).
25. P. F. Smith, Advan. Lipid Res. 6:69 (1968).
26. P. F. Smith, The Biology of Mycoplasmas. Academic Press, New York, 1971.
27. M. Freyberg, A. C. Oehlschlager, and A. M. Unrau, Arch. Biochem. Biophys. 160:83 (1974).
28. D. De Kruijff and R. A. Demel, Biochim. Biophys. Acta 339:57 (1974).
29. H. P. Klein, J. Bact. 73:530 (1957).
30. M. Freyberg, A. C. Oehlschlager, and A. M. Unrau, J. Am. Chem. Soc. 95:5747 (1973).
31. S. J. Robbins and A. Miller, J. Lab. Clin. Med. 83:436 (1974).
32. M. Grunze and B. Deuticke, Biochim. Biophys. Acta 356:125 (1974).
33. R. H. Haskins, A. P. Tulloch, and R. C. Micetich, Can. J. Microbiol. 10: 197 (1964).
34. J. W. Hendrix, Science 144:1028 (1964).
35. J. A. Leal, J. Friend, and P. Holliday, Nature (London) 203:545 (1964).

36. W. N. Harnish, L. A. Berg, and V. G. Lilly, Phytopathology 54:895 (1964).
37. C. G. Elliott, M. R. Hendrie, B. A. Knights, and W. Parker, Nature (London) 203:427 (1964).
38. R. A. Woods, J. Bact. 108:69 (1971).
39. S. W. Molzahn and R. A. Woods, J. Gen. Microbiol. 72:339 (1972).
40. L. W. Parks, F. T. Bond, E. D. Thompson, and P. R. Starr, J. Lipid Res. 13:311 (1972).
41. J. Nagai and H. Katsuki, Biochem. Biophys. Res. Commun. 60:555 (1974).
42. F. Karst and F. Lacroute, Biochem. Biophys. Res. Commun. 52:741 (1973).
43. S. Rottem, E. A. Pfendt, and L. Hayflick, J. Bact. 105:323 (1971).
44. P. J. Trocha, S. J. Jasne, and D. B. Sprinson, Biochem. Biophys. Res. Commun. 59:666 (1974).
45. M. Bard, R. A. Woods, and J. M. Haslam, Biochem. Biophys. Res. Commun. 56:324 (1974).
46. D. H. R. Barton, J. E. T. Corrie, D. A. Widdowson, M. Bard, and R. A. Woods, J. Chem. Soc. Perkin I:1326 (1974).
47. J. W. Proudlock, L. W. Wheeldon, D. J. Jollow, and A. W. Linnane, Biochim. Biophys. Acta 152:434 (1968).
48. J. A. Hossack and A. H. Rose, J. Bact. 127:67 (1976).
49. W. R. Nes, J. H. Adler, B. C. Sekula, and K. Krevitz, Biochem. Biophys. Res. Commun. 71:1296 (1976).
50. W. R. Nes, J. H. Adler, J. Joseph, J. R. Landrey, and R. L. Conner, Fed. Proc. 36:708 (1977).
51. G. Zaccai, J. K. Blasie, and B. P. Schoenborn, Proc. Natl. Acad. Sci. U.S.A. 72:376 (1975).
52. D. L. Worcester, in D. Chapman and D. F. H. Wallach (eds.), Biological Membranes. Academic Press, New York, 1976.
53. G. A. Thompson, R. J. Bambery, and Y. Nozawa, Biochemistry 10:4441 (1971).
54. R. L. Conner, F. B. Mallory, J. R. Landrey, and W. L. Iyengar, J. Biol. Chem. 244:2325 (1969).
55. F. B. Mallory and R. L. Conner, Lipids 6:149 (1971).
56. W. R. Nes, A. Alcaide, J. R. Landrey, F. B. Mallory, and R. L. Conner, Lipids 10:140 (1975).
57. W. R. Nes, P. A. G. Malya, F. B. Mallory, K. A. Ferguson, J. R. Landrey, and R. L. Conner, J. Biol. Chem. 246:561 (1971).
58. W. R. Nes, K. Krevitz, S. Behzadan, G. W. Patterson, J. R. Landrey, and R. L. Conner, Biochem. Biophys. Res. Commun. 66:1462 (1975).
59. R. L. Conner, J. R. Landrey, C. H. Burns, and F. B. Mallory, J. Protozol. 15:600 (1968).
60. A. S. Beedle, K. A. Munday, and D. C. Wilton, Biochem. J. 142:57 (1974).
61. K. A. Ferguson, F. M. Davis, R. L. Conner, and J. R. Landrey, J. Biol. Chem. 250:6998 (1975).
62. J. D. Bernal, Nature 129:277 (1932).
63. C. H. Carlisle and D. Crowfoot, Proc. Roy. Soc. (London), Ser. A184:64 (1945).
64. D. Crowfoot, Vitamins and Hormones II:409 (1944).
65. W. L. Duax, C. M. Weeks, and D. C. Rohrer, Rec. Prog. Hormone Res. 32:81 (1976).
66. W. L. Duax and D. A. Norton (eds.), Atlas of Steroid Structure. Vol. I. Plenum, New York, 1975.
67. W. L. Duax, C. M. Weeks, and D. C. Rohrer, in N. L. Allinger and E. L. Eliel (eds.), Stereochemistry. Vol. 9. John Wiley, New York, 1976. p. 271.

68. C. Romers, C. Altona, H. J. C. Jacobs, and R. A. G. de Graff, *in* Terpenoids and Steroids. Vol. 4. The Chemical Society, London, 1974.
69. W. R. Nes, T. E. Varkey, D. R. Crump, and M. Gut, J. Org. Chem. 41: 3429 (1976).
70. W. R. Nes, T. E. Varkey, and K. Krevitz, J. Am. Chem. Soc. 99:260 (1977).
71. J. T. Gordon and T. H. Doyne, Acta Crystallogr. 21(Suppl.): A113 (1966).
72. D. Beach, J. A. Erwin, and G. G. Holz, Jr., *in* A. A. Streikov, K. M. Sukhmanova, and I. B. Raikov (eds.), Progress in Protozology, Abstracts of the 3rd Int. Congress on Protozoology. Nauka, Leningrad, 1969. p. 133.
73. G. G. Holz, Jr., *in* H. Hutner (ed.), Biochemistry and Physiology of Protozoa. Vol. 3. Academic Press, New York, 19 . pp. 199‒242.
74. C. G. Elliott, J. Gen. Microbiol. 51:137 (1968).
75. C. G. Elliott, J. Gen. Microbiol. 72:321 (1972).
76. E. D. Thompson, R. B. Bailey, and L. W. Parks, Biochim. Biophys. Acta 334:116 (1974).
77. J. O. P. Lampen, P. M. Arnow, and R. A. Safferman, J. Bact. 80:200 (1960).
78. S. J. Kim and K. J. Kwen-Chung, Antimicrobial Agenta and Chemotherapy 6:102 (1974).
79. G. H. Rothblat and C. H. Burns, J. Lipid Res. 12:653 (1971).
80. W. B. Heed and H. W. Kircher, Science 149:758 (1965).
81. K. C. Goodnight and H. W. Kircher, Lipids 6:166 (1971).
82. H. M. Chu, D. M. Norris, and L. T. Kok, J. Insect Physiol. 16:1379 (1970).
83. A. Carrington and A. D. McLachlan, Introduction to Magnetic Resonance. Harper and Row, New York, 1967.
84. K. W. Butler, I. C. P. Smith, and H. Schneider, Biochim. Biophys. Acta 219:514 (1970).
85. R. A. Long, F. Hruska, and H. D. Gesser, Biochem. Biophys. Res. Commun. 41:321 (1970).
86. J. B. Leathes, Lancet 208:853 (1925).
87. A. Darke, E. G. Finer, A. G. Flook, and M. C. Phillips, J. Mol. Biol. 63: 265 (1972).
88. M. C. Phillips and E. G. Finer, Biochim. Biophys. Acta 356:199 (1974).
89. B. de Kruyff, P. W. M. van Duck, R. A. Demel, A. Schuijff, F. Brants, and L. L. M. van Deenen, Biochim. Biophys. Acta 356:1 (1974).
90. J. M. Boogs and J. C. Hsia, Biochim. Biophys. Acta 290:32 (1972).
91. R. A. Demel, K. R. Bruckdorfer, and L. L. M. van Deenen, Biochim. Biophys. Acta 255:311 (1972).
92. B. de Kruyff, R. A. Demel, and L. L. M. van Deenen, Biochim. Biophys. Acta 255:331 (1972).
93. R. A. Demel, K. R. Bruckdorfer, and L. L. M. van Deenen, Biochim. Biophys. Acta 255:321 (1972).
94. K. E. Sudsling and G. S. Boyd, Biochim. Biophys. Acta 436:295 (1976).
95. P. A. Edwards and C. Green, FEBS Lett. 20:97 (1972).
96. G. S. Cobon and J. M. Haslam, Biochem. Biophys. Res. Commun. 52:320 (1973).
97. E. D. Thompson and L. W. Parks, J. Bact. 779 (1974).
98. S. Rottem, J. Yashouv, Z. Neeman, and S. Razin, Biochim. Biophys. Acta 323:495 (1973).
99. S. Rottem, V. P. Cirillo, B. de Kruyff, M. Shinitzky, and S. Razin, Biochim. Biophys. Acta 323:509 (1973).
100. R. Bittman, Biochem. Biophys. Res. Commun. 71:318 (1976).
101. J. L. Lippert and W. L. Peticolas, Proc. Natl. Acad. Sci. U.S.A. 68:1572 (1971).

102. B. D. Ladbrooke, R. M. Williams, and D. Chapman, Biochim. Biophys. Acta 150:333 (1968).
103. J. De Gier, J. G. Mandersloot, and L. L. M. van Deenen, Biochim. Biophys. Acta 173:143 (1969).
104. D. Papahadjopoulos, M. Cowden, and H. Kimelberg, Biochim. Biophys. Acta 330:8 (1973).
105. J. De Gier, C. W. M. Haest, J. G. Mandersloot, and L. L. M. van Deenen, Biochim. Biophys. Acta 211:373 (1970).
106. H. Lecuyer and D. G. Dervichian, J. Mol. Biol. 45:39 (1969).
107. D. B. Gilbert, C. Tanford, and J. A. Reynolds, Biochemistry 14:444 (1975).
108. J. Hradec, O. Mach, and Z. Dusek, Biochem. J. 138:147 (1974).
109. W. M. Allen and O. Wintersteiner, Science 80:190 (1934).
110. A. Butenandt, U. Westphal, and W. Hohlweg, Hoppe-Seyler's Z. Physiol. Chem. 227:84 (1934).
111. M. Hartman and A. Wettstein, Helv. Chim. Acta 17:1365 (1934).
112. K. H. Slotta, H. Ruschig, and E. Fels, Chem. Ber. 67:1270 (1939).
113. K. Bloch, J. Biol. Chem. 157:661 (1945).
114. U. Westphal, Hoppe-Seyler's Z. Physiol. Chem. 273:1 (1942).
115. O. Hechter, Fed. Proc. 8:70 (1949).
116. O. Hechter, in R. P. Cook (ed.), Cholesterol. Academic Press, New York, 1958. pp. 309–347.
117. L. Ruzicka and V. Prelog, Helv. Chim. Acta 26:975 (1943).
118. A. Zaffaroni, O. Hechter, and G. Pincus, J. Am. Chem. Soc. 73:1390 (1951).
119. M. Hayano, N. Saba, R. I. Dorfman, and O. Hechter, Rec. Prog. Hormone Res. 12:79 (1956).
120. R. D. H. Heard, E. G. Bligh, M. C. Cann, P. H. Jellinck, V. J. O'Donnell, B. G. Rao, and J. L. Webb, Rec. Prog. Hormone Res. 12:45 (1956).
121. W. S. Lynn, Jr., E. Staple, and S. Gurin, Fed. Proc. 14:783 (1955).
122. E. Staple, W. S. Lynn, Jr., and S. Gurin, J. Biol. Chem. 219:845 (1956).
123. L. T. Samuels, Ciba Coll. Endocrinol. 7:176 (1953).
124. K. F. Beyer and L. T. Samuels, J. Biol. Chem. 219:69 (1956).
125. K. D. Roberts, L. Bandy, and S. Lieberman, Biochemistry 8:1259 (1969).
126. S. Burstein, H. Zamoscianyk, H. L. Kimball, N. K. Chaudhuri, and M. Gut, Steroids 15:13 (1970).
127. S. Burstein, H. L. Kimball, and M. Gut, Steroids 15:809 (1970).
128. S. Burstein, B. S. Middleditch, and M. Gut, J. Biol. Chem. 250:9028 (1975).
129. K. Shimizu, M. Hayano, M. Gut, and R. I. Dorfman, J. Biol. Chem. 236:695 (1961).
130. K. Shimizu, M. Gut, and R. I. Dorfman, J. Biol. Chem. 237:(1962).
131. G. Constantopoulos, P. S. Satoh, and T. T. Tchen, Biochem. Biophys. Res. Commun. 8:50 (1962).
132. G. Constantopoulos and T. T. Tchen, Biochem. Biophys. Res. Commun. 4:460 (1961).
133. S. Ichii, S. Omata, and S. Kokayashi, Biochem. Biophys. Res. Commun. 139:308 (1967).
134. A. C. Chaudhuri, Y. Harada, K. Shimizu, M. Gut, and R. I. Dorfman, J. Biol. Chem. 237:703 (1962).
135. S. Burstein, C. Y. Byon, H. L. Kimball, and M. Gut, Steroids 27:691 (1976).
136. R. J. Kraaipoel, H. J. Degenhart, J. G. Leferink, H. de Leeuw-Boon, and H. K. A. Visser, FEBS Lett. 50:204 (1975).
137. R. J. Kraaipoel, H. J. Degenhart, V. Van Beek, H. de Leeuw-Boon, G. Abelu, H. K. A. Visser, and J. G. Leferink, FEBS Lett. 54:294 (1975).
138. R. J. Kraaipoel, H. J. Degenhart, and J. G. Leferink, FEBS Lett. 57:294 (1975).

139. S. B. Koritz and P. F. Hall, Biochim. Biophys. Acta 93:215 (1964).
140. S. B. Koritz and P. F. Hall, Biochemistry 3:1298 (1964).
141. S. Burstein, Y. Letourneux, H. L. Kimball, and M. Gut, Steroids 27:361 (1976).
142. R. B. Hochberg, P. D. McDonald, M. Feldman, and S. Lieberman, J. Biol. Chem. 249:1277 (1974).
143. E. Caspi, R. I. Dorfman, B. T. Khan, G. Rosenfeld, and W. Schmid, J. Biol. Chem. 237:2085 (1962).
144. L. T. Samuels, M. L. Helmreich, M. Lasater, and H. Reich, Science 113: 490 (1951).
145. W. Ewald, H. Werbin, and I. L. Chaikoff, Steroids 3:505 (1964).
146. H. L. Kruskernper, E. Forchielli, and H. J. Ringold, Steroids 3:295 (1964).
147. W. R. Nes, E. Loeser, R. Kirdani, and J. Marsh, Tetrahedron 19:299 (1963).
148. F. S. Kawahara, S. F. Wang, and P. Talalay, J. Biol. Chem. 1500 (1962).
149. N. M. Drayer, K. D. Roberts, and S. Lieberman, J. Biol. Chem. 239:PC3112 (1964).
150. T. Yoshizawa and Y. Nagai, Japan J. Exp. Med. 44:465 (1974).
151. L. R. Bjorkman, K. A. Karlsson, I. Passcher, and B. E. Samuelsson, Biochim. Biophys. Acta 270:260 (1972).
152. R. Goodfellow and L. J. Goad, Biochem. Soc. Trans. 1:759 (1973).
153. R. Tschesche and G. Snatzke, Ann. Chem. 636:105 (1960).
154. E. Caspi, D. O. Lewis, D. M. Piatak, K. V. Thimann, and A. Winter, Experientia 22:506 (1966).
155. (a) R. D. Bennett and E. Heftmann, Phytochemistry 5:747 (1966); (b) R. D. Bennett and E. Heftmann, Science 149:652 (1965).
156. E. Caspi, and D. O. Lewis, Science 156:519 (1967).
157. H. H. Sauer, R. D. Bennett, and E. Heftmann, Phytochemistry 6:1521 (1967).
158. J. M. H. Graves and W. K. Smith, Nature (London) 214:1248 (1967).
159. (a) M. LeBoeuf, A. Cave, and R. Goutarel, Comp. Rend. Nebd. Séanc. Acad. Sci. (Paris) 259:3401 (1964); (b) A. M. Gawienowski and C. C. Gibbs, Steroids 12:545 (1968).
160. R. Tschesche and G. Lilienweiss, Z. Naturforsch. 19b:265 (1964).
161. E. Caspi and D. O. Lewis, Phytochemistry 7:683 (1968).
162. E. Ramstad and J. L. Beal, Chem. Oil Ind. 177 (1960).
163. E. Ramstad and J. L. Beal, Pharm. Pharmacol. 12:552 (1960).
164. H. Gregory and E. Leete, Chem. Oil Ind. 1542 (1960).
165. E. Leete, H. Gregory, and E. G. Gros, J. Am. Chem. Soc. 87:3475 (1965).
166. J. von Euw and T. Reichstein, Helv. Chim. Acta 47:711 (1964).
167. E. Caspi and G. M. Hornby, Phytochemistry 7:423 (1968).
168. E. Caspi, J. A. F. Wickramasinghe, and D. O. Lewis, Biochem. J. 108:499 (1968).
169. J. A. F. Wickramasinghe, P. C. Hirsch, S. M. Munaralli, and E. Caspi, Biochemistry 7:3248 (1968).
170. H. H. Sauer, R. D. Bennett, and E. Heftmann, Phytochemistry 7:1453 (1968).
171. R. Tschesche and B. Brassat, Z. Naturforsch. 20b:707 (1965).
172. H. Singh, V. K. Kapoor, and A. S. Chawla, J. Sci. Ind. Res. 28:339 (1969).
173. C. H. Gray and A. L. Bacharach (eds.), Hormones in Blood. Vol. 2. 2nd Ed. Academic Press, New York, 1967.
174. V. V. Reddy, H. Balin, and W. R. Nes, Steroids 17:493 (1971).
175. E. B. Astwood and H. L. Feuold, Am. J. Physiol. 127:192 (1938).
176. A. W. Makepeace, G. L. Weinstein, and M. H. Friedman, Am. J. Physiol. 119:512 (1927).

177. G. Pincus, Acta Endocrinol. 23 (Suppl. 28):18 (1956).
178. G. Pincus, Postgrad. Med. 24:654 (1958).
179. C. R. Garcia, G. Pincus, and J. Rock, Am. J. Obst. Gynecol. 75:82 (1958).
180. M. Steiger and T. Reichstein, Helv. Chim. Acta 20:1164 (1937).
181. T. Reichstein and J. von Euw, Helv. Chim. Acta 21:1197 (1938).
182. H. L. Mason, Endocrinology 25:405 (1939).
183. T. Reichstein, Helv. Chim. Acta 20:953 (1937).
184. H. L. Mason, C. S. Myers, and E. C. Kendall, J. Biol. Chem. 114:613 (1936).
185. H. L. Mason, C. S. Myers, and E. C. Kendall, J. Biol. Chem. 116:267 (1936).
186. T. Reichstein, Helv. Chim. Acta 19:1107 (1936).
187. O. Wintersteiner and J. J. Pfiffner, J. Biol. Chem. 116:291 (1936).
188. J. F. Grattan and H. Jensen, J. Biol. Chem. 135:511 (1940).
189. C. N. H. Long, B. Katzin, and E. G. Fry, Endocrinology 26:309 (1940).
190. B. B. Wells, Proc. Staff Meetings Mayo Clinic 15:294 (1940).
191. B. B. Wells, Proc. Staff Meetings Mayo Clinic 15:503 (1940).
192. G. W. Thorn, L. L. Engel, and R. A. Lewis, Science 94:348 (1941).
193. H. L. Mason, W. M. Hoehn, and E. C. Kendall, J. Biol. Chem. 124:459 (1938).
194. P. S. Hench, E. C. Kendall, C. H. Slocumb, and H. F. Polley, Proc. Staff Meetings Mayo Clinic 25:475 (1950).
195. P. S. Hench, Proc. Staff Meetings Mayo Clinic 25:475 (1950).
196. H. L. Mason, W. M. Hoehn, B. F. McKenzie, and E. C. Kendall, J. Biol. Chem. 120:719 (1937).
197. R. Neher and A. Wettstein, Helv. Chim. Acta 39:2062 (1956).
198. V. R. Mattox and H. L. Mason, J. Biol. Chem. 223:215 (1956).
199. V. R. Mattox, H. L. Mason, A. Albert, and C. F. Code, J. Am. Chem. Soc. 75:4869 (1953).
200. R. E. Harman, E. A. Ham, J. J. DeYoung, N. G. Brink, and L. H. Sarett, J. Am. Chem. Soc. 76:5035 (1954).
201. S. A. Simpson, J. F. Tait, A. Wettstein, R. Neher, J. von Euw, and T. Reichstein, Experientia 9:333 (1953).
202. S. A. Simpson, J. F. Tait, A. Wettstein, R. Neher, J. von Euw, O. Schindler, and T. Reichstein, Helv. Chim. Acta 37:1163 (1954).
203. W. R. Nes, in A. Burger (ed.), Medicinal Chemistry. Interscience, New York, 1960. pp. 691-782.
204. A. B. Eisenstein (ed.), The Adrenal Cortex. Little, Brown, Boston, 1967.
205. (a) W. R. Nes, L. Segal, and B. Segal, Fed. Proc. 19:169 (1960); (b) L. Segal, B. Segal, and W. R. Nes, J. Biol. Chem. 3108 (1960).
206. R. C. Puche and W. R. Nes, Endocrinology 70:857 (1962).
207. W. H. Daughaday, J. Clin. Invest. 37:519 (1958).
208. W. R. Slaunwhite and A. A. Sandberg, J. Clin. Invest. 38:384 (1959).
209. W. K. Brunkhorst and E. L. Hess, Arch. Biochem. Biophys. 111:54 (1965).
210. A. A. Sandberg, H. Rosenthal, and W. R. Slaunwhite, J. Clin. Invest 44:1094 (1965).
211. C. N. H. Long, B. Katzin, and E. G. Fry, Endocrinology 26:309 (1940).
212. J. Fried and E. F. Sabo, J. Am. Chem. Soc. 75:2273 (1953).
213. J. E. Herz, J. Fried, and E. F. Sabo, J. Am. Chem. Soc. 78:2017 (1956).
214. I. S. Edelman, R. Bogoroch, and G. A. Porter, Trans. Assn. Am. Physicians 77:307 (1964).
215. H. Selye, Stress. Acta, Inc., Montreal, 1950.
216. D. DeWied, A. M. L. van Delft, W. H. Gispen, J. A. W. M. Weijnen, and

T. B. van Wimersma Greidanus, *in* S. Levine (ed.), Hormones and Behavior. Academic Press, New York, 1972. pp. 135-171.

217. R. K. Sharma, N. K. Ahmed, L. S. Sutliff, and J. S. Brush, FEBS Lett. 45:107 (1974).

218. R. K. Sharma, Biochem. Biophys. Res. Commun. 59:992 (1974).

219. M. K. Mostafapour and T. T. Tchen, J. Biol. Chem. 248:6674 (1973).

220. R. K. Sharma and J. S. Brush, Arch. Biochem. Biophys. 156:560 (1973).

221. R. I. Dorfman and R. A. Shipley, Androgens. John Wiley, New York, 1956.

222. A. Butenandt, Z. Angew. Chem. 44:905 (1931).

223. K. David, E. Dingemanse, J. Freund, and E. Laqueur, Hoppe-Seyler's Z. Physiol. Chem. 233:281 (1935).

224. K. Savard, R. I. Dorfman, and E. Poutasse, J. Clin. Endocrinol. Metabol. 12:935 (1952).

225. E. Steinberger and A. Steinberger, *in* H. Balin and S. Glasser (eds.), Reproductive Biology. Excerpta Medica, Amsterdam, 1972. pp. 144-267.

226. E. Steinberger and M. Ficher, Steroids 11:351 (1968).

227. E. Steinberger and M. Ficher, Biol. Reprod. 1(Suppl.):19 (1969).

228. K. E. Paschkis, A. E. Rakoff, A. Cantarow, and J. J. Rupp, Clinical Endocrinology. 3rd Ed. Harper and Row, New York, 1967.

229. K. W. McKerns (ed.), The Gonads. Appleton-Century-Crofts, New York, 1969.

230. E. L. Rongone, Steroids 7:489 (1966).

231. E. C. Gomez and S. L. Hsia, Biochemistry 7:24 (1968).

232. I. Faredin, A. G. Fazekas, K. Kokai, I. Toth, and M. Julesz, Eur. J. Biochem. 2:223 (1967).

233. W. Voigt, E. P. Fernandez, and S. L. Hsia, J. Biol. Chem. 245:5594 (1970).

234. N. Bruchovsky and J. D. Wilson, J. Biol. Chem. 243:2012 (1968).

235. R. E. Goyna and J. D. Wilson, J. Clin. Endocrinol. 29:970 (1969).

236. K. M. Anderson and S. Liao, Nature (London) 219:277 (1968).

237. A. G. Fazekas and A. Lanthier, Steroids 18:367 (1971).

238. J. M. Davidson, *in* H. Balin and S. Glasser (eds.), Reproductive Biology. Excerpta Medica, Amsterdam, 1972. pp. 877-918.

239. (*a*) E. A. Doisy, C. D. Veler, and S. A. Thayer, J. Biol. Chem. 86:499 (1930); (*b*) A. Butenandt, Hoppe-Seyler's Z. Physiol. Chem. 191:127 (1930).

240. G. F. Marrian, Biochem. J. 24:435 (1930).

241. (*a*) D. W. MacCorquodale, S. A. Thayer, and E. A. Doisy, J. Biol. Chem. 115:435 (1936); (*b*) D. W. MacCorquodale, S. A. Thayer, and E. A. Doisy, Proc. Soc. Exp. Med. Biol. 32:1182 (1935).

242. O. Wintersteiner, E. Schwenk, and B. Whitman, Proc. Soc. Exp. Med. Biol. 32:1087 (1935).

243. N. T. Werthessen, E. Schwenk, and C. Baker, Science 117:380 (1953).

244. R. D. H. Heard, P. H. Jellinck, and V. J. O'Donnell, Endocrinology 57:200 (1955).

245. K. J. Ryan, J. Biol. Chem. 234:268 (1959).

246. A. M. H. Brodie, W. C. Schwarzel, and H. J. Brodie, J. Steroid Biochem., in press.

247. T. Morato, M. Hayano, R. I. Dorfman, and L. R. Axelrod, Biochem. Biophys. Res. Commun. 6:334 (1961).

248. T. Morato, K. Raab, H. J. Brodie, M. Hayano, and R. I. Dorfman, J. Am. Chem. Soc. 84:3764 (1962).

249. J. D. Townsley and H. J. Brodie, Biochemistry 7:33 (1968).

250. J. D. Townsley and H. J. Brodie, Biochem. J. 101:25C (1966).

251. J. D. Townsley and H. J. Brodie, Biochim. Biophys. Acta 144:440 (1967).
252. R. V. Short, Nature (London) 188:232 (1960).
253. H. J. Brodie, G. Possanza, and J. D. Townsley, Biochim. Biophys. Acta 152:770 (1968).
254. H. J. Brodie, K. J. Kripalani, and G. Possanza, J. Am. Chem. Soc. 91:1241 (1969).
255. M. Ganguly, K. L. Cheo, and H. J. Brodie, Biochim. Biophys. Acta 431: 326 (1976).
256. W. C. Schwarzel, W. G. Kruggel, and H. J. Brodie, Endocrinology 92:866 (1973).
257. H. J. Brodie and P. A. Warg, Tetrahedron 23:535 (1967).
258. (a) P. K. Siiteri and P. C. MacDonald, Steroids 2:713 (1963); (b) H. G. Magendantz and K. J. Ryan, J. Clin. Endocrinol. Metab. 24:1155 (1964).
259. C. Longcope, W. Widrich, and C. T. Sawin, Steroids 20:440 (1972).
260. T. M. A. El-Attar and A. Hugoson, Arch. Oral Biol. 19:425 (1974).
261. P. L. Munson, T. F. Gallagher, and F. C. Koch, J. Biol. Chem. 152:67 (1944).
262. K. D. Roberts, R. L. VandeWiele, and S. Lieberman, J. Biol. Chem. 236: 2213 (1961).
263. L. P. Romanoff, R. M. Rodriguez, J. P. Seelye, and G. Pincus, J. Clin. Endocrinol. Metab. 17:777 (1957).
264. S. Ulick and K. K. Vetter, J. Biol. Chem. 237:3364 (1962).
265. M. Stylianou, E. Forchielli, M. Tummillo, and R. I. Dorfman, J. Biol. Chem. 236:692 (1961).
266. F. Ungar, M. Gut, and R. I. Dorfman, J. Biol. Chem. 224:191 (1957).
267. B. P. Lisboa and J. A. Gustafsson, Eur. J. Biochem. 6:419 (1968).
268. H. E. Hadd and R. T. Blickenstaff, Conjugates of Steroid Hormones. Academic Press. New York, 1969.
269. H. Breuer and G. Pangels, Acta Endocrinol. 33:532 (1960).
270. H. Jirku and D. S. Layne, Biochemistry 4:2126 (1965).
271. A. Z. Mehdi and T. Sandor, Steroids 24:151 (1974).
272. J. G. Phillips and P. J. Mulrow, Proc. Soc. Exp. Biol. Med 101:262 (1959).
273. R. Arai, H. Tajima, and B. I. Tamaoki, Gen. Comp. Endocrinol. 12:99 (1969).
274. B. Truscott and D. R. Idler, J. Endocrinol. 40:515 (1968).
275. (a) O. Mancera, A. Zaffaroni, B. A. Rubin, F. Sondheimer, G. Rosenkrantz and C. Djerassi, J. Am. Chem. Soc. 74:3711 (1952); (b) D. H. Peterson and H. C. Murray, J. Am. Chem. Soc. 74:1871 (1952).
276. H. R. Levy and P. Talalay, J. Biol. Chem. 234:2009 (1959).
277. Y. J. Abul-Hajj, Biochem. Biophys. Res. Commun. 43:766 (1971).
278. C. Gual, R. I. Dorfman, and S. R. Stitch, Biochim. Biophys. Acta 49:387 (1961).
279. R. M. Dodsen and R. D. Muir, J. Am. Chem. Soc. 83:4627 (1961).
280. K. Schubert, K. H. Bohme, and C. Hörhold, Hoppe-Seyler's Z. Physiol. Chem. 325:260 (1961).
281. B. W. O'Malley and A. R. Means, in H. Busch (ed.), The Cell Nucleus. Vol. 3. Academic Press, New York, 1974. pp. 379-416.
282. (a) A. Butenandt and P. Karlson, Z. Naturforsch. 9b:389 (1954); (b) W. J. Burdette, Invertebrate Endocronology and Hormonal Heterophylly. Springer-Verlag, New York, 1974.
283. (a) K. Nakanishi, M. Koreeda, S. Sasaki, M. L. Chang, and H. Y. Hsu, J. Chem. Soc. Chem. Commun. 915 (1966); (b) K. Nakanishi, Pure Appl. Chem. 25:167 (1971); (c) M. J. Thompson, J. N. Kaplanis, W. E. Robbins,

and J. A. Svoboda, Advan. Lipid Res. 11:219 (1973); (d) N. J. de Souza, E. L. Ghisalberti, H. H. Rees, and T. W. Goodwin, Biochem. J. 114:895 (1969).

284. G. A. D. Haslewood, Bile Salts. Methuen, London, 1967.
285. K. Bloch, B. N. Berg, and D. Rittenberg, J. Biol. Chem. 149:511 (1943).
286. S. Linstedt, Acta Chem. Scand. 11:417 (1957).
287. S. Shefer, S. Hauser, and E. H. Mosbach, J. Lipid Res. 9:328 (1968).
288. G. Johansson, Eur. J. Biochem. 21:68 (1971).
289. J. R. Mitton, N. A. Scholan, and G. S. Boyd, Eur. J. Biochem. 20:569 (1971).
290. H. Danielsson and K. Einarsson, J. Biol. Chem. 241:1449 (1966).
291. F. Wada, K. Hirata, K. Nakano, and Y. Sakamoto, J. Biochem. (Tokyo) 66:699 (1969).
292. G. S. Boyd, N. A. Scholan, and J. R. Mitton, Advan. Exp. Med. Biol. 4: 443 (1969).
293. S. Shefer, S. Hauser, and E. H. Mosbach, J. Lipid Res. 9:328 (1968).
294. H. Danielsson, K. Einarsson, and G. Johansson, Eur. J. Biochem. 2:44 (1967).
295. W. Voigt, E. P. Fernandez, and S. L. Hsia, Proc. Soc. Exp. Biol. Med. 133:1158 (1970).
296. G. Johansson, Eur. J. Biochem. 17:292 (1970).
297. G. Johansson, Eur. J. Biochem. 21:68 (1971).
298. K. Einarsson, Eur. J. Biochem. 5:101 (1968).
299. M. Suzuki, K. A. Mitropoulos, and N. B. Myant, Biochem. Biophys. Res. Commun. 30:516 (1968).
300. (a) G. A. Grabowski, M. E. Dempsey, and R. F. Hanson, Fed. Proc. 32: 250 (1973); (b) G. A. Grabowski, K. E. McCoy, G. C. Williams, M. E. Dempsey, and R. F. Hanson, Biochim. Biophys. Acta 441:380 (1976).
301. H. R. B. Hutton and G. S. Boyd, Biochim. Biophys. Acta 116:336 (1966).
302. O. Berseus and K. Einarsson, Acta Chem. Scand. 21:1105 (1967).
303. O. Berseus, H. Danielsson, and K. Einarsson, J. Biol. Chem. 242:1211 (1967).
304. K. Einarsson, Eur. J. Biochem. 6:299 (1968).
305. I. Bjorkhem, K. Einarsson, and G. Johansson, Acta Chem. Scand. 22:1595 (1968).
306. I. Bjorkhem, Eur. J. Biochem. 8:337 (1969).
307. O. Berseus, Eur. J. Biochem. 2:493 (1967).
308. O. Berseus, Opuscula Med., Suppl. VI (1967).
309. O. Berseus and I. Bjorkhem, Eur. J. Biochem. 2:503 (1967).
310. I. Bjorkhem, Eur. J. Biochem. 7:413 (1969).
311. G. M. Tomkins, J. Biol. Chem. 225:13 (1957).
312. G. M. Tomkins, J. Biol. Chem. 218:437 (1957).
313. S. S. Koide, Biochim. Biophys. Acta 110:189 (1965).
314. S. S. Koide, Steroids 6:123 (1965).
315. E. Domain and S. S. Koide, Biochim. Biophys. Acta 128:209 (1966).
316. I. Bjorkhem and H. Danielsson, Eur. J. Biochem. 12:80 (1970).
317. H. Danielsson, Acta Chem. Scand. 14:348 (1960).
318. H. M. Suld, E. Staple, and S. Gurin, J. Biol. Chem. 237:338 (1962).
319. K. Okuda and N. Hoshita, Biochim. Biophys. Acta 164:381 (1968).
320. O. Berseus, Acta Chem. Scand. 19:325 (1965).
321. K. A. Mitropoulos and N. B. Myant, Biochem. J. 97:26C (1965).
322. D. Mendelsohn and L. Mendelsohn, Biochem. J. 114:1 (1969).
323. P. P. Shah, E. Staple, and J. L. Rabinowitz, Arch. Biochem. Biophys. 123: 427 (1968).

324. T. Cronholm and G. Johansson, Eur. J. Biochem. 16:373 (1970).
325. K. Okuda and H. Danielsson, Acta Chem. Scand. 19:2160 (1970).
326. T. Masui, R. Herman, and E. Staple, Biochim. Biophys. Acta 117:266 (1966).
327. K. Okuda and N. Takigawa, Biochem. Biophys. Acta 117:266 (1966).
328. K. Okuda and H. Danielsson, Acta Chem. Scand. 19:2160 (1965).
329. K. Okuda and N. Takigawa, Biochem. Biophys. Res. Commun. 33:788 (1968).
330. K. Okuda, N. Takigawa, R. Fukuba, and T. Kuwaki, Biochim. Biophys. Acta 185:1 (1969).
331. E. Staple, Meth. Enzymol. 15:562 (1969).
332. G. Waller, H. Theorall, and J. Sjovall, Arch. Biochem. Biophys. 111:671 (1965).
333. T. Masui and E. Staple, Biochim. Biophys. Acta 104:305 (1965).
334. T. Masui, and E. Staple, J. Biol. Chem. 241:3889 (1966).
335. T. Masui and E. Staple, Steroids 9:443 (1967).
336. P. D. G. Dean and M. W. Whitehouse, Biochem. J. 101:632 (1966).
337. M. W. Whitehouse, J. L. Rabinowitz, E. Staple, and S. Gurin, Biochim. Biophys. Acta 37:382 (1960).
338. M. W. Whitehouse, E. Staple, and S. Gurin, J. Biol. Chem. 236:68 (1961).
339. H. Danielsson, in P. P. Nair and D. Kritchevsky (eds.), The Bile Acids, Chemistry, Physiology and Metabolism. Vol. 2. Plenum Press, New York, 1973. p. 1.
340. K. Shimizu, T. Fujioka, M. Otagaki, and K. Yamasaki, Yonago Acta Med. 3:158 (1959).
341. T. Yamada, Hiroshima J. Med. Sci. 15:375 (1966).
342. T. Schersten, Biochim. Biophys. Acta 141:144 (1967).
343. T. Schersten, P. Bjorntorp, P. H. Ekdahl, and S. Bjorkerud, Biochim. Biophys. Acta 141:155 (1967).
344. W. H. Elliott, Biochem. J. 62:433 (1956).
345. H. Danielsson and K. Einarsson, in E. E. Bittar and N. Bittar (eds.), The Biological Basis of Medicine Vol. 5. Academic Press, New York, 1969. p. 279.
346. H. Danielsson, Advan. Lipid Res. 1:335 (1963).
347. K. A. Mitropoulos, S. Balasubramanian, and N. B. Myant, Biochim. Biophys. Acta 326:428 (1973).
348. H. Danielsson, Steroids 22:567 (1973).
349. S. Shefer, S. Hauser, V. Lapar, and E. H. Mosbach, J. Lipid Res. 14:573 (1973).
350. S. Shefer, S. Hauser, J. Bekersky, and E. H. Mosbach, J. Lipid Res. 11:404 (1970).
351. O. Berseus, H. Danielsson, and A. Kallner, J. Biol. Chem. 240:2369 (1965).
352. D. Mendelsohn and E. Staple, Biochemistry 2:577 (1963).
353. S. Bergstrom, H. Danielsson, and B. Samuelsson, in K. Bloch (ed.), Lipids Metabolism. John Wiley, New York, 1960. pp. 291-336.
354. (a) R. S. Rosenfeld and L. Hellman, Biochemistry 7:3085 (1968); (b) E. C. Texter, C. Chou, H. C. Laureta, and G. R. Vantrappen, Physiology of the Gastrointestinal Tract. C. V. Mosby, St. Louis, 1968; (c) G. Wiseman, Absorption from the Intestine. Academic Press, New York, 1964.
355. E. Mellanby, Lancet 196:407 (1919).
356. K. Huldschinsky, Deutsch. Med. Wschr. 45:712 (1919).
357. E. V. McCollum, N. Simmonds, and J. E. Becker, J. Biol. Chem. 53:293 (1922).
358. A. F. Hess, Am. J. Dis. Child. 28:517 (1924).

359. H. Steenbock, Science 60:224 (1924).
360. H. Steenbock and A. Black, J. Biol. Chem. 61:405 (1924).
361. H. Steenbock and M. T. Nelson, J. Biol. Chem. 62:209 (1924).
362. A. F. Hess and M. Weinstock, J. Biol. Chem. 62:301 (1924).
363. A. F. Hess and M. Weinstock, J. Biol. Chem. 63:297 (1925).
364. A. F. Hess, M. Weinstock, and F. D. Helman, J. Biol. Chem. 63:305 (1925).
365. O. Rosenheim and T. A. Webster, Lancet 1025 (1925).
366. H. Steenbock and A. Black, J. Biol. Chem. 64:263 (1925).
367. R. Pohl, Nachr. Ges. Wiss. Gottingen, Math.-Phys. Kl. 142:185 (1926).
368. R. Pohl, Naturwiss. 15:433 (1927).
369. A. Windaus and A. F. Hess, Nachr. Ges. Wiss. Gottingen, Math.-Phys. Kl. 175 (1926).
370. A. Windaus, A. Luttringhaus, and M. Deppe, Justus Liebigs Ann. Chem. 489:252 (1931).
371. T. C. Angus, F. A. Askew, R. B. Bourdillon, H. M. Bruce, R. K. Callow, C. Fischmann, J. St. L. Philpot, and T. A. Webster, Proc. Roy. Soc. (London), Ser. B 108:340 (1931).
372. A. Windaus, O. Linsert, A. Luttringhaus, and G. Weidlich, Justus Liebigs Ann. Chem. 492:226 (1932).
373. F. A. Askew, R. B. Bourdillon, H. M. Bruce, R. K. Callow, J. St. L. Philpot, and T. A. Webster, Proc. Roy. Soc. (London), Ser. B 109:488 (1932).
374. A. Windaus and W. Thiele, Justus Liebigs Ann. Chem. 521:160 (1936).
375. I. M. Heilbron and F. S. Spring, Chem. Ind. 54:795 (1935).
376. I. M. Heilbron, K. M. Samant, and F. S. Spring, Nature (London) 135:1072 (1935).
377. I. M. Heilbron, R. N. Jones, K. M. Samant, and F. S. Spring, J. Chem. Soc. 905 (1936).
378. D. Crowfoot and J. D. Dunitz, Nature (London) 162:608 (1948).
379. D. Crowfoot Hodgkin, M. S. Webster, and J. D. Dunitz, Chem. Ind. 1149 (1957).
380. A. Windaus and R. Langer, Justus Liebigs Ann. Chem. 508:105 (1934).
381. A. Windaus, H. Lettre, and Fr. Schenck, Justus Liebigs Ann. Chem. 520:98 (1935).
382. A. Windaus, Fr. Schenck, F. von Werder, Hoppe-Seyler's Z. Physiol. Chem. 241:100 (1936).
383. H. Brockmann, Hoppe-Seyler's Z. Physiol. Chem. 241:104 (1936).
384. H. Brockmann and Y. H. Chen, Z. Physiol. Chem. 241:129 (1936).
385. A. Windaus, K. Dithmar, and E. Fernholz, Justus Liebigs Ann. Chem. 493:259 (1932).
386. I. M. Heilbron, F. S. Spring, and P. A. Stewart, J. Chem. Soc. 1221 (1935).
387. K. Dimroth, Ber. Deut. Chem. Ges. 68:539 (1935).
388. P. Setz, Hoppe-Seyler's Z. Physiol. Chem. 215:183 (1933).
389. A. Windaus, F. von Werder, and A. Luttringhaus, Justus Liebigs Ann. Chem. 499:188 (1932).
390. F. von Werder, Hoppe-Seyler's Z. Physiol. Chem. 260:119 (1939).
391. A. Windaus, O. Linsert, A. Luttringhaus, and G. Weidlich, Justus Liebigs Ann. Chem. 492:226 (1932).
392. H. H. Inhoffen, Naturwiss. 43:396 (1956).
393. L. Velluz, G. Amiard, and A. Petit, Bull. Chem. Soc. Fr. 16:501 (1949).
394. A. L. Koevoet, A. Verloop, and E. Havinga, Rec. Trav. Chim. Pay-Bas 74:788 (1955).
395. L. Velluz, G. Amiard, and B. Goffinet, Bull. Chem. Soc. Fr. 22:1341 (1955).
396. L. Velluz, and G. Amiard, Bull. Chem. Soc. Fr. 22:205 (1955).
397. E. Havinga, A. L. Koevoet, and A. Verloop, Rec. Trav. Chim. Pay-Bas 74:1230 (1955).

398. M. P. Rappoldt, J. A. K. Buisman, and E. Havinga, Rec. Trav. Chim. Pay-Bas 77:327 (1958).
399. L. F. Fieser and M. Fieser, Steroids. Reinhold, New York, 1959.
400. C. E. Bills, J. Biol. Chem. 72:751 (1927).
401. A. M. Copping, Biochem. J. 28:1516 (1934).
402. A. F. Hess, C. E. Bills, and E. M. Honeywell, J. Am. Med. Assoc. 92:226 (1929).
403. G. A. Blondin, B. D. Kulkarni, and W. R. Nes, Comp. Biochem. Physiol. 20:379 (1967).
404. G. A. Blondin, B. D. Kulkarni, and W. R. Nes, J. Am. Chem. Soc. 86:2528 (1964).
405. G. A. Blondin, J. L. Scott, J. K. Hummer, B. D. Kulkarni, and W. R. Nes, Comp. Biochem. Physiol. 17:391 (1966).
406. G. W. Harrington, Biol. Bull. 132:174 (1967).
407. P. K. T. Pang, J. Exp. Zool. 178:15 (1971).
408. J. C. Drummond and E. R. Gunther, Nature (London) 126:398 (1930).
409. H. H. Dorby and H. T. Clarke, Science 85:318 (1937).
410. A. W. Norman, Am. J. Med. 57:21 (1974).
411. A. Carlsson, Acta Physiol. Scand. 26:212 (1952).
412. J. Lund and H. F. DeLuca, J. Lipid Res. 7:739 (1966).
413. H. Morii, J. Lund, P. F. Neville, and H. F. DeLuca, Arch. Biochem. Biophys. 120:508 (1967).
414. J. W. Blunt, H. F. DeLuca, and H. K. Schnoes, Biochemistry 7:3317 (1968).
415. J. W. Blunt and H. F. DeLuca, Biochemistry 8:671 (1969).
416. E. B. Mawer, G. A. Lumb, and S. W. Stanbury, Nature (London) 222:482 (1969).
417. D. E. M. Lawson, P. W. Wilson, and E. Kodicek, Nature (London) 222:171 (1969).
418. M. Horsting and H. F. DeLuca, Biochem. Biophys. Res. Commun. 36:251 (1969).
419. H. F. DeLuca, Fed. Proc. 33:2211 (1974).
420. G. Tucker, R. E. Gagnon, and M. R. Haussler, Arch. Biochem. Biophys. 155:47 (1973).
421. M. H. Bhattacharyya and H. F. DeLuca, Arch. Biochem. Biophys. 155:47 (1973).
422. M. R. Haussler, J. F. Myrtle, and A. W. Norman, J. Biol. Chem. 243:4055 (1968).
423. M. R. Haussler, D. W. Boyce, E. T. Littledike, and H. Rasmussen, Proc. Natl. Acad. Sci. U.S.A. 68:177 (1971).
424. D. E. M. Lawson, P. W. Wilson, and E. Kodicek, Biochem. J. 115:269 (1969).
425. D. R. Fraser and E. Kodicek, Nature (London) 228:764 (1970).
426. A. W. Norman, R. J. Midgett, J. F. Myrtle, and H. G. Nowicki, Biochem. Biophys. Res. Commun. 42:1082 (1971).
427. R. Gray, I. Boyle, and H. F. DeLuca, Science 172:1232 (1971).
428. E. J. Semmler, M. F. Holick, H. K. Schnoes, and H. F. DeLuca, Tetrahedron Lett. 40:4147 (1972).
429. A. S. Brickman, J. W. Coburn, and A. W. Norman, N. Engl. J. Med. 287:891 (1972).
430. A. S. Brickman, J. W. Coburn, J. W. Massry, and A. W. Norman, Arch. Intern. Med. 80:161 (1974).
431. A. W. Norman and R. G. Wong, J. Nutr. 102:1709 (1972).
432. A. S. Brickman, C. R. Reddy, J. W. Coburn, E. P. Passero, J. Jowsey, A. W. Norman, Endocrinology 92:725 (1973).

433. J. F. Myrtle and A. W. Norman, Science 171:79 (1971).
434. H. C. Tsai, R. G. Wong, and A. W. Norman, J. Biol. Chem. 247:5511 (1972).
435. M. R. Haussler, J. F. Myrtle, and A. W. Norman, J. Biol. Chem. 243:4055 (1968).
436. M. R. Haussler, and A. W. Norman, Proc. Natl. Acad. Sci. U.S.A. 62:155 (1969).
437. L. G. Raiz, C. L. Trummel, M. F. Holick, and H. F. DeLuca, Science 175: 768 (1972).
438. L. F. Hill, C. J. Van den Berg, and E. B. Mawer, Nature New Biol. 232: 189 (1971).
439. R. G. Wong, A. W. Norman, C. R. Reddy, and J. W. Coburn, J. Clin. Invest. 51:1287 (1972).
440. I. T. Boyle, L. Miravet, R. W. Gray, M. F. Holick, and H. F. DeLuca, Endocrinology 90:605 (1972).
441. T. C. Chen, L. Castillo, M. Korycka-Dahl, and H. F. DeLuca, J. Nutr. 104:1056 (1974).
442. M. F. Holick, M. Garabedian, and H. F. DeLuca, Science 176:1146 (1972).
443. R. W. Gray, J. L. Omdahl, J. G. Ghazarian, and H. F. DeLuca, J. Biol. Chem. 247:7528 (1972).
444. J. G. Ghazarian and H. F. DeLuca, Arch. Biochem. Biophys. 160:63 (1974).
445. J. G. Ghazarian, H. K. Schnoes, and H. F. DeLuca, Biochemistry 12:2555 (1973).
446. J. G. Ghazarian, J. R. Jefcoate, J. C. Knutson, W. H. Orme-Hohnson, and H. F. DeLuca, J. Biol. Chem. 249:3026 (1974).
447. M. F. Holick, H. K. Schnoes, H. F. DeLuca, R. W. Gray, I. T. Boyle, and T. Suda, Biochemistry 11:4251 (1972).
448. M. F. Holick, A. Kleiner-Bossaller, H. K. Schnoes, P. M. Kasten, I. T. Boyle, and H. F. DeLuca, J. Biol. Chem. 248:6691 (1973).
449. I. T. Boyle, R. W. Gray, and H. F. DeLuca, Proc. Natl. Acad. Sci. U.S.A. 68:2131 (1971).
450. R. W. Gray, H. P. Weber, and J. Lemann, Fed. Proc. 32:917 (1973).
451. Y. Tanaka, H. Frank, H. F. DeLuca, N. Koizumi, and N. Ikekawa, Biochemistry 14:3293 (1975).
452. M. F. Holick, L. A. Baxter, P. K. Schraufrogel, T. E. Tavela, and H. F. DeLuca, J. Biol. Chem. 251:397 (1974).
453. J. C. Knutson and H. F. DeLuca, Biochemistry 13:1543 (1974).
454. J. L. Omdahl, M. Holick, T. Suda, Y. Tanaka, and H. F. DeLuca, Nature New Biol. 237:63 (1972).
455. Y. Tanaka and H. F. DeLuca, Arch. Biochem. Biophys. 154:566 (1973).
456. D. R. Fraser and E. Kodicek, Nature New Biol. 241:163 (1973).
457. M. Garabedian, M. F. Holick, H. F. DeLuca, and S. Balsan, Proc. Natl. Acad. Sci. U.S.A. 69:1673 (1972).
458. M. Garabedian, Y. Tanaka, M. F. Holick, and H. F. DeLuca, Endocrinology 94:88 (1974).
459. H. C. Harrison, H. E. Harrison, and E. A. Park, Am. J. Physiol. 192:432 (1958).
460. H. Rasmussen, H. F. DeLuca, C. Arnaud, C. Hawker, and M. von Stedingk, J. Clin. Invest 42:1940 (1963).
461. H. C. Tsai and A. W. Norman, J. Biol. Chem. 248:5967 (1973).
462. D. E. M. Lawson and J. S. Emtage, in R. S. Harris, P. L. Munson, E. Diczfaulsy, and J. Glover (eds.), Vitamins and Hormones. Vol. 32. Academic Press, New York, 1974. pp. 227-298.

463. J. S. Emtage, D. E. M. Lawson, and E. Kodicek, Biochem. J. 140:239 (1974).
464. R. H. Wasserman, R. A. Corradino, and A. N. Taylor, J. Biol. Chem. 243: 3978 (1968).
465. R. H. Wasserman, Biochim. Biophys. Acta 203:176 (1970).
466. R. J. Ingersoll and R. H. Wasserman, J. Biol. Chem. 246:2808 (1971).
467. P. J. Bredderman and R. H. Wasserman, Biochemistry 13:1687 (1974).
468. R. H. Wasserman and R. A. Corradino, in R. S. Harris, P. L. Munson, E. Diczfalusy, and J. Glover (eds.), Vitamins and Hormones. Vol. 31. Academic Press, New York, 1973. pp. 43.

Author Index

Aaronson, S., 464, 465
Abely, G., 560
Abraham, G. E., 138, 140
Abramovich, D. R., 452
Abul-Hajj, Y. J., 588
Acevedo, H. F., 445
Adams, R., 151
Addison, T., 3
Adler, G., 506
Adler, J. H., 337, 338, 343, 383, 421,
   422, 476, 538, 540, 541, 545, 548,
   549, 551, 552
Adler, R. D., 453
Agranoff, B. W., 159, 161, 164, 185
Ahmadjian, V., 479
Ahmed, N. K., 575
Ahrens, E. H., 374, 445, 449, 450, 455,
   456
Akagi, S., 461, 465, 466
Akbar, A. M., 138
Akhtar, M., 328, 333, 337, 339, 351,
   360, 361, 362, 363, 364, 365, 367,
   370, 371, 394, 397
Akagi, S., 256
Akazawa, T., 319
Akazawa, Y., 319
Alais, J., 421, 422
Albert, A., 569
Alberhart, D. J., 371
Albrecht, A., 181
Albrecht, P., 418
Alcaide, A., 340, 350, 352, 371, 375,
   382, 387, 388, 389, 419, 420, 442,
   461, 464, 465, 546
Aldrich, P. E., 151, 152
Alexander, G. J., 328, 332, 333, 394
Alexander, K. T. W., 360, 363, 364,
   365
Ali, E., 515
Allain, C. C., 125
Allais, J. P., 348, 350, 352, 354, 379,
   387, 388, 391, 464, 465
Allee, G. L., 445

Allen, C. M., 184
Allen, E., 26
Allen, W. M., 557
Allsop, I. L., 108
Altman, L. J., 209, 210, 216, 222, 223
Altona, C., 547
Alworth, W., 184
Amarego, W. L. F., 343, 492, 498, 499
Amiard, G., 607
Amir, F., 486
Amdur, B. H., 217
Amoros-Marin, L., 503
Anastasia, M., 367, 394, 398
Andreasen, A. A., 537, 540, 542
Anderson, C. G., 423
Anderson, D. G., 153, 216, 217, 480
Anderson, J. D., 319
Anderson, K. M., 578
Anderson, R. A., 130
Anderson, R. J., 418, 430, 481
Amdur, B. H., 159
Anding, C., 329, 382, 385, 388, 393,
   448, 471, 472
Ando, T., 352, 371, 437
Andre, D., 388, 389
Aneja, R., 515, 516
Angus, T. C., 605
Anitschkow, N., 455
Aplin, R. T., 250
Appel, H. H., 319
Aqurell, D., 277
Arai, R., 587
Archer, B. L., 164, 189
von Ardenne, M., 329
Arditti, J., 370
Arigoni, D., 12, 52, 153, 161, 164, 232,
   234, 237, 238, 248, 249, 250, 300,
   319, 332, 333
Arimura, A., 138
Arison, B. H., 181
Aristotle, 3
Arnaud, C., 613
Arnow, P. M., 552
Arpino, P., 418

Arrequin, B., 149, 150
Arunachalam, T., 424
Aschheim, S., 23
Asenyo, C. F., 503
Ash, L., 222, 223
Askew, F. A., 605
Astwood, E. B., 565
Atallah, A. M., 375, 388, 486, 502, 508, 511
Auda, H., 319
Austern, B. M., 272
Avigan, J., 129, 332, 333, 374, 394, 445
Avivi, L., 420, 471
Avizonis, P. V., 198
Avruch, L., 385
Awata, A., 348, 350, 378, 379
Axelrod, L. R., 583
Ayers, P. J. O., 123

Bacharach, A. L., 564, 569, 582
Bachhawat, B. K., 151
Bachmann, W. E., 19
Bader, S., 332, 333
von Baeyer, A., 15, 16
Bagli, J. F., 369, 374
Bailey, H. H., 450
Bailey, R. B., 335, 384, 552
Baisted, D. J., 153, 154, 155, 257, 331, 480, 481, 515, 516, 517, 538
Baker, C., 582
Baker, G. L., 443
Baker, H., 464, 465
Baker, L. C., 443
Baker, W. H., 458
Balasubramanian, D., 360
Balasubramanian, S., 600
Balin, A. K., 93
Balin, H., 565
Ballauf, A., 328
Balsan, S., 613
Bambery, R. J., 546
Ban, Y., 333
Bandy, L., 558
Banthorpe, D. V., 272, 319
Barbier, M., 333, 337, 340, 347, 348, 350, 352, 354, 371, 375, 376, 378, 379, 380, 381, 382, 387, 388, 389, 391, 429, 430, 435, 437, 442, 461, 464, 465, 501, 504, 510
Bard, M., 339, 371, 544

Barker, N. W., 447
Barksdale, A. W., 424, 425
Barnard, D., 164, 189
Barnes, F. J., 220, 223
Baron, J. M., 184, 186, 188
Barrett, D. A., 125
Bartelt, K., 10
Bartl, Z., 430
Barton, D. H. R., 19, 32, 33, 122, 232, 234, 243, 250, 251, 261, 262, 263, 301, 311, 328, 331, 332, 338, 339, 360, 362, 363, 364, 365, 371, 386, 387, 499, 544
Bataille, J., 160
Bates, R. B., 494
Bates, R. H., 181
Batra, P. P., 315
Battersby, A. R., 272, 274, 277, 278, 283
Bauman, A., 137
Baumann, C. A., 443, 498, 499, 501
Bauslaugh, G., 370
Baxendale, D., 319
Baxter, L. A., 613
Baxter, R. M., 163
Beach, D., 551
Beal, J. L., 561
Beames, C. G., 450
Bean, G. A., 422
Beard, J. W., 415
Beastall, G. H., 210, 262, 263, 343, 388, 392
Bechtold, M. M., 355, 357
Becker, J. E., 604
Beedle, A. S., 350, 351, 420, 546
Beekes, H. W., 129
Beeler, D. A., 153, 217, 314, 480
Beeler, M. F., 455
Beglinger, U., 308, 311, 319
von Behring, H., 416
Behzadan, S., 110, 112, 350, 383, 393, 419, 420, 421, 425, 482, 483, 484, 494, 498, 546
Beiser, S. M., 138
Beisler, J. A., 501
Bekersky, J., 600
Bennett, R. D., 129, 153, 154, 371, 487, 498, 560, 561
Bentley, H. R., 331, 332, 336
Bentley, R., 164, 243
Benveniste, P., 184, 217, 329, 330, 388,

511, 512, 513
Berg, B. N., 594
Berg, L. A., 421, 542
Bergman, J., 329
Bergmann, E. D., 129, 131, 434
Bergmann, W., 86, 346, 347, 377, 425, 428, 429, 434, 436, 439, 441, 472, 474
Bergstrom, B., 450
Bergstrom, S., 52, 600
Berman, M., 445
Bernal, J. D., 47, 547
Bernstein, S., 104
Bernt, E., 125
Berrie, A. M. M., 481, 489, 506
Berthelot, M., 4, 10, 13
Berti, G., 246, 250, 336, 393
Berseus, O., 595, 596, 597, 600
Berson, S. A., 137
Berzelius, J. J. B., 5
Beveridge, J. M. R., 510
Beyer, K. F., 558
Beytia, E., 213, 214, 217, 218, 273, 319
Bhacca, N. S., 110
Bhattacharji, S., 163
Bhattacharya, M. H., 610
Bhattacharyya, A. K., 445, 455, 458
Bhattacharyya, P. K., 319
Biemann, K., 115
Biggs, M. W., 368
Bilezikian, S. B., 138
Billiar, R. B., 154
Bills, C. E., 494, 608, 609
Billy, C. P., 504
Bimpson, T., 371, 372, 379
Birch, A. J., 19, 153, 163, 191, 279, 308, 319, 332, 335
Bird, C. W., 262, 417, 418
Bishop, E. O., 110
Bishop, N. L., 181
Bittman, R., 556
Bjerke, J. S., 194
Bjork, L., 156
Bjorkerud, S., 598
Bjorkhem, I., 416, 417, 443, 595, 596
Bjorkman, L. R., 560
Bjorntorp, P., 598
Black, A., 604, 609
Bladon, P., 101
Blair-West, J. R., 123, 569
Blank, F., 370, 422
Blanke, E., 387, 422

Blasie, J. K., 541
Blickenstaff, R. T., 585
Bligh, E. G., 558
Bloch, K., 13, 30, 31, 32, 148, 149, 150, 154, 159, 160, 161, 184, 210, 217, 218, 230, 231, 232, 235, 241, 243, 249, 250, 262, 263, 328, 329, 332, 333, 347, 355, 370, 375, 379, 384, 419, 433, 434, 458, 460, 537, 540, 542, 557, 594
Block, J. H., 346, 428
Blohm, T. R., 332
Blondin, G. A., 133, 134, 135, 142, 153, 162, 163, 250, 332, 333, 335, 336, 337, 339, 340, 343, 370, 480, 609
Bloom, B. M., 233
Bloomfield, D. K., 154
Bloomfield, G. A., 138
Blunt, J. W., 610
Boar, R. B., 234, 261, 263, 360, 363, 364, 365, 502, 504
Bock, F., 432
Bogdanovsky, D., 435
Bogorad, L., 182
Bogoroch, R., 571
Bohme, K. H., 588
Boid, R., 343
Boiteau, P., 45
Bolger, L. M., 340, 371, 393, 499, 500, 504, 506
Bolker, H. I., 441
Bolla, R. I., 431
Bollinger, J., 138
Bond, F. T., 542, 544
Bonner, J., 149, 150, 153, 154
Boogs, J. M., 555
Booth, M., 140, 569
Borek, F., 138
Boschetti, A., 216
Boswell, G. A., 231, 243, 333
Bottari, F., 246, 250, 336, 393
Bottior, J., 340
Bouchardat, F., 8
Bourdillon, R. B., 605
Bourquin, J. P., 206
Boutry, J. L., 352, 382
Bouden, B. N., 481, 515, 516
Bowers, W. S., 196
Boyce, D. W., 610
Boyd, G. S., 355, 366, 555, 594, 595

Boyle, I. T., 611, 612, 613
Brack, A., 163
Brady, D., 457
Brady, D. R., 355, 357, 395, 396
Brady, R. O., 150
Braithwaite, G. D., 153, 154
von Brand, T., 420
Brandt, R. D., 329, 340, 388, 393, 471, 472, 511, 512, 513
Brante, G., 444
Brants, F., 555
Brassat, B., 191, 561
Bredderman, P. J., 615
Bredenberg, J. B., 307
Breivik, O. N., 387
Brenneisen, K., 52
Breton, L., 503
Brettschneiderova, Z., 196
Breuer, H., 585
Brewer, A. D., 494
Brewik, O. N., 422
Brian, P. W., 272, 308
Brickman, A. S., 611
Brieskorn, C. H., 307
Briggs, L. H., 310, 311, 312
Bright, R. D., 198
Brink, N. G., 569
Britt, J. J., 419
Britton, G., 220, 221, 315, 316, 320
Brockmann, H., Jr., 501, 605
Brodie, A. F., 181
Brodie, A. M. H., 93, 583
Brodie, H. J., 583, 584
Brodie, J. D., 155, 156
Brooks, C. J. W., 89, 116, 119, 130, 136, 262, 417, 418, 436, 437, 443, 458
Brooks, P. W., 418
Brooks, T. J., 378, 431
Brooks, W. A., 362
Brown, J. W., 361, 367
Brown, M. S., 455
Brown, W. H., 435
Bruce, H. M., 605
Bruchovsky, N., 578
Bruckdorfer, K. R., 555
Bruderer, H., 300
Bruhl, J. W., 7
Brundy, S. M., 374
Brunkhorst, W. K., 570
Bruns, K., 294

Brush, J. S., 575
Bruun, T., 362
Bryant, G. D., 138
Bryce, B. M., 347, 433
Bryson, M. J., 154
Buchecker, R., 318
Bucher, N. L. R., 155, 394
Buchi, G., 277, 296, 300
Budzikiewicz, H., 115, 116
Bueding, E., 378
Buisman, J. A. K., 608
Bulbrook, R. D., 93
Burdette, W. J., 589
Burgos, J., 182
Burlingame, A. L., 238, 243
Burnett, J. H., 272
Burns, C. H., 420, 454, 455, 546, 552
Burr, G. O., 481
Burrows, E. P., 191
Burstein, S., 101, 104, 299, 350, 558, 560
Burton, R. B. A., 89
Bush, I. E., 127
Bush, P. B., 515
Buster, J. E., 140
Butenandt, A., 21, 23, 24, 26, 557, 575, 580, 588
Butler, J., 140, 569
Butler, K. W., 554
Butler, V. P., 138, 140
Butsugan, Y., 277
Butterworth, P. H. W., 182
Buu-Hoi, N. P., 458
Buygy, M. J., 220, 221
Buzzelli, N. K., 182
Byon, C. Y., 560

Cabat, G. A., 361
Caglioti, J., 301
Cagnoli-Bellavista, N., 338
Cahn, R. S., 53, 164
Cain, B. F., 311, 312
Cainelli, G., 301
Cais, M., 312
Caldwell, B. V., 138
Calimbas, T., 261
Callow, R. K., 605
Calvin, M., 181, 417
Cambie, R. C., 311, 312
Camerino, B., 301

Campbell, E. A., 445
Campbell, R. V. M., 209, 210, 222
Campbell, W. F., 16
Canfield, R. E., 138
Canonica, L., 361, 362, 364, 366, 367
Cann, M. C., 558
Cannon, J. W., 250, 353, 442
Cantarow, A., 578
Capato, E., 287, 299
Capitaine, H., 7
Capella, P., 460
Capstack, E., Jr., 153, 162, 163, 250, 257, 480, 481, 516, 517, 538
Carlisle, C. H., 547
Carlisle, D. B., 196
Carlson, J. P., 211
Carlsson, A., 610
Carnighan, R. H., 181
Carrier, D. J. R., 338, 423
Carrington, A., 554
Carroll, K. K., 449
Carter, P., 127
Carter, P. W., 458, 461, 465, 466, 467, 472
Caspi, E., 154, 164, 191, 210, 234, 238, 243, 246, 251, 262, 263, 330, 333, 334, 335, 339, 359, 361, 362, 364, 367, 371, 374, 420, 560, 561
Casinovi, G. C., 277
Castelli, W. P., 449, 455, 456
Castillo, L., 612
Castle, M., 134, 332, 333, 335, 336, 337, 339, 340, 343
Castrejon, R. N., 370
Catt, K., 138
Cattabeni, F., 364, 453, 454
Cava, M. P., 311
Cave, A., 561
Cavill, G. W. K., 277
Cawley, R. W., 310
Ceccherelli, P., 338, 401
Černý, V., 196
Chadha, M. S., 484
Chaikoff, I. L., 560
Chakravarti, R. N., 499
Chambaz, E. M., 136
Chan, C. S. G., 135
Chan, J. T., 336, 337, 387, 475
Chandler, R. F., 464, 466, 467
Chang, M. L., 588
Channon, H. J., 148

Chapman, A. C., 18, 148
Chapman, C. B., 450
Chapman, D., 556
Chapman, P. J., 319
Chardon-Loriaux, I., 461, 464, 465, 466
Charlton, J. M., 220, 221
Chaudhuri, A. C., 558
Chaudhuri, N. K., 558
Chawla, A. S., 562
Chaykin, S., 159, 161
Chen, C. S., 515
Chen, T. C., 612
Chen, Y. H., 605
Chen, Y. S., 422
Cheng, A. L. S., 343, 487
Cheo, K. L., 584
Chevallier, F., 447
Chevreul, M. E., 4
Chichester, C. G., 334
Chichester, C. O., 159, 220, 222, 313, 320
Chikamatsu, H., 131, 135, 339, 340, 422, 481, 499, 538
Chou, C., 603
Chu, H. M., 436, 554
Ciereszko, L. S., 428, 429
Cirillo, V. P., 556
Clark, A. J., 262, 347, 379, 434, 437, 537, 540, 542
Clark, K. J., 278
Clarke, H. T., 609
Clarkson, T. B., 457
Claque, A. D. H., 110, 112
Claude, J. R., 129, 131
Clayton, R. B., 125, 132, 133, 134, 163, 164, 231, 234, 238, 332, 357, 358, 369, 374, 375, 379, 395, 398, 433
Cleland, W. W., 161, 164, 218
Cleverdon, R. C., 537, 539
Clifford, K., 165, 209
Clinkenbeard, K. D., 157
Cloud, P. E., Jr., 181
Cmelick, S., 430
Coates, R. M., 209, 210, 216
Cobon, G. S., 555
Coburn, J. W., 611, 612
Cockbain, E. G., 164, 189
Cocker, J. D., 311
Code, C. F., 569

Coggins, C. W., Jr., 315
Coghlan, J. P., 123
Cohen, C. F., 336, 337, 387, 388, 390, 473, 475, 476
Cole, R. H., 108
Cole, R. J., 347, 378, 431
Cole, W., 19
Collins, R. P., 468, 469, 471
Columbus, C., 7
Comai, K., 355, 357
de la Condamine, C., 7
Conner, R. L., 92, 117, 133, 134, 135, 246, 251, 262, 350, 351, 370, 372, 537, 538, 541, 542, 546, 548, 549, 552, 553
Conner, W. E., 455, 458
Constantopoulos, G., 558, 560
Cook, I. F., 348, 350, 370, 379
Cook, J. W., 458
Cook, L. C., 301
Cook, R. P., 368, 369, 446, 449
Coon, M. J., 151
Cooper, A., 238
Copius-Peereboom, J. W., 129, 130, 131
Copping, A. M., 609
Corbella, A., 319
Corcoran, M. R., 308
Corey, E. J., 209, 234, 237, 238, 250, 263, 329
Cori, E., 189
Cori, O., 212, 273, 319
Corley, R. C., 154
Cornforth, J. W., 33, 52, 149, 153, 154, 160, 161, 162, 164, 165, 184, 188, 189, 191, 211, 222, 231, 234, 243, 262
Cornforth, R. H., 34, 153, 154, 160, 162, 164, 165, 189, 210, 211, 222, 231, 243
Corradino, R. A., 615
Corrie, J. E. T., 339, 371, 544
Costes, C., 182
Coughlan, J. P., 569
Counts, M. A., 455
Cox, G. B., 192
Cox, G. E., 455
Cox, J. D., 386, 499
Cox, J. S. G., 110, 503
Cox, L. G., 455
Cowden, M., 557
Coy, U., 157

Crabbe, P., 19, 123, 241, 242, 243, 244, 245, 256, 423
Cram, D. J., 52
Crane, F. L., 181
Cresson, E. L., 151
Crombie, L., 209, 210, 222
Cronholm, T., 597, 598
Cronquist, A., 472, 475
Cross, B. E., 308
Crowfoot, D., 47, 547, 605
Crump, D. R., 254, 547
Cudzinovski, M., 129, 131
Curtis, P. J., 308
Curphey, T. J., 234
Cuzner, M., 447

von Daehne, W., 238
Dahm, K. H., 194
Dallner, G., 537, 539
Dam, H., 25, 26, 86, 416, 417
Damps, K., 234, 261, 263
Dane, E., 458
Danielli, J. F., 536
Danielsson, H., 333, 594, 595, 596, 597, 598, 599, 600
Dankert, M., 181, 193
Dannenberg, H., 458
Daperon, M. R., 515
Darke, A., 554
Das, B. C., 342, 371
Dastillung, M., 418
Datta, J. K., 141
Dauben, W. G., 52, 231, 243, 301, 333
Dauchy, S., 418
Daughaday, W. H., 140, 570
Daves, G. D., Jr., 181, 182
David, K., 576
Davidson, A. G., 368
Davidson, J. M., 579
Davies, B. H., 216, 220
Davis, B. R., 311, 312
Davis, F. M., 546
Davis, J. B., 220
Davison, A. N., 444, 447, 452, 454
Davson, H., 536
Dawber, T. R., 449, 450
Day, A. J., 457
Day, E. A., 455
Dayton, S., 457
Dean P. D. G., 252, 261, 262, 263,

329, 452, 597
Debeljuk, L., 138
Decker, K., 314
Degenhart, H. J., 560
De Gier, J., 557
De Graff, R. A. G., 547
De Kruijff, D., 540
De Kruyff, B., 555, 556
De Luca, H. F., 610, 611, 612, 613
De Luca, P., 346, 377, 427, 432
Delwiche, C. V., 355, 357, 365, 366, 376, 397
Demel, R. A., 540, 555
Dempsey, M. E., 329, 369, 374, 394, 397, 398, 450, 594
Demura, H., 138
Dennick, R. G., 452
Dennis, D. T., 308, 319
Denss, R., 231
Deppe, M., 605
De Rosa, M., 346, 377, 427, 432
Dervichian, D. G., 557
Deshmane, S. S., 486, 502
Deulofeu, V., 443
Deuss, R., 328
Deuticke, B., 542
Dev, S., 486, 502
Devys, M., 337, 340, 347, 352, 354, 371, 375, 387, 388, 389, 391, 429, 430, 437, 442, 464, 465, 504, 510
Dewhurst, S. M., 370, 371
De Wied, D., 574
De Young, J. J., 569
Dhar, A. K., 261, 360, 374, 375, 394, 450
Dialameh, G. H., 182
Diara, A., 311
Dickel, D. F., 52
Dickinson, A. M., 151
Dickson, L. G., 388, 390, 475
Diels, O. P., 17, 19, 30
Dietrich, P., 250
Dietschy, J. M. 446
Digenis, G. A., 378, 470
Dimroth, K., 606
Dingemanse, E., 576
Dithmar, K., 606
Ditullio, N., 129, 131
Dituri, F., 153, 162
Dixon, H., 420
Dixon, P. F., 140, 569

Djerassi, C., 123, 299, 300, 301, 311, 312, 319, 329, 346, 352, 370, 376, 377, 426, 428, 429, 436, 440, 441, 486, 499, 501, 502, 587
Dobbing, J., 444
Dodds, E. C., 27
Dodsen, R. M., 588
Doisy, E. A., 23, 25, 26, 580
Dokusova, O. K., 156
Dolder, F., 308
Dolejas, L., 196, 301
Domain, E., 596
Dominquez, X. A., 487
Don, E., 452
Donabedian, R. K., 138
Donninger, C., 164, 189, 210, 211, 222, 243
Dorby, H. H., 609
Dorée, C., 425, 439
Dorfman, L., 88, 101, 102, 103, 104
Dorfman, R. I., 132, 154, 558, 560, 575, 576, 583, 584, 585, 588
Dorsey, J. K., 218
Dowdy, A., 93
Downey, W. L., 378, 431
Doyle, P. J., 340, 387, 388, 389, 390
Doyne, T. H., 420, 550
Drayer, N. M., 560
Drummond, J. C., 443, 609
Duax, W. L., 547, 548, 549
DuBus, R., 319
Duchamp, D. J., 334
Ducruix, A., 504
Dudowitz, A., 361, 367
Dugan, R. E., 213, 217, 218
Dulit, E., 368
Dunitz, J. D., 605
Dunlap, B. E., 420
Dunn, J., 138
Dunphy, P. J., 182
DuPlessis, J. T., 457
Durr, I. F., 157, 158, 162
Dusek, Z., 557
Dusza, J. P., 101, 104, 428
Dutky, R. C., 154, 347, 434
Dutky, S. R., 336, 337, 340, 347, 387, 388, 389, 390, 431, 473, 474, 475
Dvornik, D., 369, 374

Eberle, M., 161

Eberlein, W. R., 569
Ebersole, R. C., 210, 234, 262
Echenmoser, A., 232, 234, 237, 248, 249, 250
Edel, F., 138
Edelman, I. S., 571
Edlbacher, S., 439
Edmond, J., 209, 210, 213, 214, 222, 301
Edward, D. G. H., 415
Edwards, A. M., 379, 433
Edwards, J. A., 424
Edwards, P. A., 555
Eggerer, H., 153, 155, 157, 159, 161, 162, 164, 184, 185, 208, 217
Eglington, G., 418
Ehrhardt, J. D., 329, 331
Ehrlich, P., 22
Eichenberger, W., 515
Eik-Nes, K. B., 89, 132, 136, 137, 154
Einarsson, K., 594, 595, 599, 600, 601
Eisenbraun, E. J., 319
Eisenstein, A. B., 569, 571, 572, 575
Eisner, T., 272, 277, 278, 319
Ekdahl, P. H., 598
El-Attar, T. M. A., 585
Elbein, A. D., 515
Elden, T. C., 379
Elhafez, A. A., 52
Elkin, Y. N., 421
Ellingboe, J., 130
Elliott, C. G., 421, 542, 551
Elliott, D., 335
Elliott, W. H., 130, 599
Ellis, P. E., 196
Ellouz, R., 341, 342, 371, 372
Elyakou, G. B., 421
Emtage, J. S., 615
Endo, M., 370
Eng, L., 447
Engel, L. L., 127, 568
Engelbrecht, G. P., 457
Engelbrecht, J. P., 429
Engelman, G., 4
English, R. J., 153, 335
Ensminger, A., 418
Entwistle, N., 423, 441
Enwall, E. L., 428
Eppenberger, U., 329
Epstein, W. W., 208, 209, 210, 213, 216, 222, 223, 301, 423

Ercoli, A., 443
Erdman, T. R., 352, 371, 377, 426
Ergenc, N., 494
Erickson, R. E., 181
Erlanger, B. F., 138
Ernst, R., 370
Erwin, J., 419, 551
Eschenmoser, A., 12
Escher, H. H., 6
Etemadi, A. H., 234, 262
Eugster, C. H., 318
von Euw, J., 561, 568, 569
Ewald, W., 560
Eyssen, H., 416, 417, 444

Fagerlund, U. H. M., 332, 343, 352, 374, 380, 381, 392, 439
Faiman, C., 138
Faini, F., 189
Fairbairn, D., 378, 430, 431
Fales, H., M., 196
Fang, T. Y., 515
Fankuchen, I., 47
Faraday, M., 7
Faredin, I., 578
Farkas, T. G., 154
Farrugia, G., 338
Fattorusso, E., 426, 461, 465
Faust, E. S., 430
Fazakerley, H., 246, 250
Fazekas, A. G., 578
Feeney, R. J., 428, 429
Felauer, E. E., 435
Feldbruegge, D. H., 212, 218, 220
Feldman, M., 560
Fels, E., 557
Fennessey, P., 181, 193
Ferezou, J. P., 347, 352, 354, 378, 387, 388, 391, 429, 430, 464, 465
Ferguson, J. J., 156, 162
Ferguson, K. A., 92, 350, 351, 372, 419, 420, 537, 542
Ferin, M., 140
Fernandez, E. P., 578, 594
Ferne, M., 217
Fernholz, E., 498, 606
Ferretti, A., 455
Fetizon, M., 340
Feuold, H. L., 565
Ficher, M., 576

Fiecchi, A., 361, 362, 364, 366, 367, 370, 453, 454, 455
Field, F. E., 182
Fiertel, A., 417
Fieser, L. F., 13, 19, 26, 32, 37, 38, 39, 43, 45, 47, 54, 55, 56, 102, 103, 105, 122, 231, 253, 368, 369, 443, 499, 608
Fieser, M., 13, 19, 32, 37, 38, 39, 43, 45, 47, 54, 55, 56, 102, 103, 105, 122, 231, 499, 608
Fimognari, G. M., 155
Findley, D. A. R., 222
Finean, J. B., 536
Finer, E. G., 554
Fioriti, J. A., 501, 504
Fisch, M. H., 370
Fischer, E., 21, 30
Fischer, E. H., 158
Fischer, F. G., 17, 244
Fischmann, C., 605
Fish, W. A., 332, 374, 443
Fishman, J., 153, 319
Fitzpatric, M. E., 455
Flanagan, V. P., 455
Flegg, H. M., 125
Fleischer, S., 537, 539
Fletcher, K., 162
Flick, B. H., 370
Flood, C., 89, 93
Flook, A. G., 554
Florenzano, G., 460
Folkers, K., 31, 151, 152, 153, 157, 181, 182
Fonken, G. J., 333
Forchielli, E., 164, 243, 560, 585
Ford, D. L., 458
Fornasir, V., 15
Forsee, W. T., 515
Fourcans, B., 364, 367
Fraenkel, G., 433
Frank, H., 613
Franklin, R. M., 415
Frantz, I. D., Jr., 332, 366, 368, 369, 374
Fraser, D. R., 611, 612, 613
Fray, G. I., 278
Frayha, G. J., 378, 430
Frear, D. S., 422
Freeman, C. W., 366
Freeman, N. K., 415

Freund, J., 576
Freundt, E. A., 415
Freyberg, M., 540, 544
Fried, J., 361, 367, 421, 571
Friedell, G. H., 374
Friedland, S. S., 116
Friedman, M. H., 565
Friend, J., 542
Friis, P., 181, 182
Frommhagen, L. H., 415
Frost, D. J., 362, 501, 504
Fry, E. G., 568, 570
Fryberg, M., 338, 339, 352, 367, 369, 370, 384, 385, 386, 394, 397
Fu, P. C., 125
Fuchs, A., 307
Fujimoto, Y., 348, 350, 378, 379
Fujino, A., 277
Fujioka, T., 598
Fukuba, R., 597
Fulch-Pi, J. P., 447
Fumagalli, R., 447, 452, 453, 454
Funahashi, S., 515, 516
Furlenmeier, D., 52
Furst, A., 300
Furuyama, S., 140
Fusco, R., 277

Gadke, W., 19
Gafford, L. G., 415
Gagnon, R. E., 610
Gain, R. E., 361, 364
Galbraith, M. N., 379
Gallagher, B. S., 105, 106
Gallagher, T. F., 585
Galli, G., 116, 117, 119, 361, 362, 364, 366, 367, 370, 394, 398, 444, 453, 454, 455
Galli-Kienle, M., 333, 361, 362, 364, 366, 367, 370, 394, 398, 453, 454
Galskov, A., 138
Galt, R. H. B., 308
Gambacorta, A., 246, 251, 263
Ganapathy, K., 319
Gandy, H. M., 138
Ganguly, M., 584
Garabedian, M., 612, 613
Garbarino, J. A., 277
Garcia, C. R., 565
Gardner, R. C., 331

Gariboldi, P., 319
Garmstom, M., 287
Gaskell, S. J., 418
Gautschi, F., 355, 375
Gawienowski, A. M., 561
Gavey, K., 450
Gaylor, J. L., 332, 335, 355, 356, 357, 365, 366, 370, 376, 384, 395, 396, 397
Gawienowski, A. M., 272
Gelpi, E., 417
Gershengorn, M. C., 388, 467, 468, 469
Gershfeld, N. L., 537, 539
Gesser, H. D., 554
Geus, J. M. C., 516
Gey, K. F., 154, 231, 243
Ghazarian, J. G., 612
Ghetty, G. L., 361
Ghisalberti, E. L., 336, 340, 341, 358, 388, 389, 390, 393, 499, 500, 504, 506, 589
Ghosal, M., 361
Gibbons, G. F., 112, 116, 119, 120, 329, 331, 332, 360, 361, 364, 367, 371, 382, 384, 392, 394, 461, 464, 465, 473, 474, 482, 483, 492, 494, 498, 499, 500, 501, 505, 508
Gibbs, C. C., 561
Gibbs, M. H., 153
Gibson, F., 192
Giessman, T. A., 484, 504
Gilbert, B., 309
Gilbert, D. B., 557
Gilbert, J. D., 436, 437, 458
Giles, J. A., 181
Gilfillian, J. L., 151, 152, 153, 157
Gilkes, J. J. H., 138
Ginger, C., 378
Ginger, C. D., 420
Giordano, F., 346
Giri, V. S., 515
Girgensohn, B., 340, 393
Gispen, W. H., 574
Gjone, E., 457
Gladziatsky, 8
Gloor, U., 153, 181
Glover, J., 153, 369
Glover, M., 369
Goad, L. J., 110, 112, 116, 131, 134, 135, 241, 243, 262, 328, 329, 331,

332, 335, 336, 337, 338, 339, 340, 341, 342, 343, 352, 358, 361, 364, 367, 370, 371, 372, 374, 377, 379, 381, 382, 383, 384, 388, 389, 390, 392, 393, 394, 423, 440, 441, 461, 464, 465, 467, 468, 469, 473, 474, 475, 476, 479, 484, 492, 498, 499, 500, 504, 506, 560
Godtfredsen, W. O., 210, 234, 238, 262
Goffinet, B., 607
Gold, A. M., 300, 333
Goldstein, J. L., 455
Goldzieher, J. W., 104
Gomez, E. C., 578
Gonzalez, A. G., 329, 503
Gooden, E. L., 473
Goodfellow, G., 441
Goodfellow, R. J., 216, 560
Goodfriend, L., 138
Goodman, D. W. S., 29, 98, 129, 211, 212, 217, 218, 262, 332, 374, 394
Goodnight, K. C., 379, 552, 553
Goodnight, K. G., 435
Goodwin, T. W., 116, 131, 134, 135, 153, 154, 164, 189, 210, 216, 220, 221, 222, 241, 243, 252, 262, 263, 272, 274, 313, 314, 315, 316, 318, 320, 329, 331, 332, 335, 336, 337, 338, 339, 340, 341, 342, 343, 348, 350, 351, 360, 361, 364, 367, 370, 371, 372, 374, 376, 377, 379, 382, 388, 389, 390, 392, 393, 394, 420, 461, 464, 465, 467, 468, 469, 471, 473, 474, 476, 479, 484, 485, 492, 498, 499, 500, 501, 504, 506, 589
Gordon, G. S., 455
Gordon, J. T., 250, 251, 420, 550
Gordon, T., 449
Gore, I. Y., 149, 153, 154, 159, 160, 162, 231, 243
Gorter, E., 536
Gosden, A. F., 251, 262, 263
Gosselin, L., 118, 159, 217
Gottlieb, D., 421
Gould, D. H., 425
Gould, R. G., 159, 217, 450
Goulston, G., 328, 339, 384, 387, 388, 423, 467, 468, 469
Goutarel, R., 561
Goyna, R. E., 578

Grabowski, G. A., 594
Graebe, J. E., 184, 308, 319
Graebe, J. W., 217
Grant, P. K., 311
Gratten, J. F., 568
Graves, J. M. H., 561
Gray, C. H., 564, 569, 582
Gray, R. W., 611, 612, 613
Green, C., 555
Green, D. M., 424
Greenwood, F. C., 138
Gregonis, D. E., 220, 221, 222, 223
Gregory, H., 191, 561
Gregson, A., 447
Grendel, F., 536
Grey, C. T., 181
Grieder, A., 238
Grieg, J. B., 243, 246, 251, 262, 263, 333, 339, 367, 371, 420
Grob, E. C., 149, 153, 216, 220, 515
Gros, E. G., 191, 443, 561
Gross, R. A., Jr., 346
Grossi-Paoletti, E., 336, 362, 364, 367, 370, 444, 447, 452, 453, 454, 455
Grove, J. F., 272, 308
Gruber, W., 125
Grundy, S. M., 449, 450, 453, 455, 456
Gruner, J. W., 181
Grunwald, C., 515
Grunze, M., 542
Gual, C., 588
Gueldner, R. C., 198
Guglielmetti, L., 332, 333
Guhn, G., 358, 361, 374, 375, 398
Gunsalus, I. C., 319
Gunter, C. R., 125
Gunther, E. R., 609
Gupta, G. S., 501
Gupta, K., 346
Gupta, K. C., 429
Gupta, N. L., 501
Gupta, P. C., 515
Gurin, S., 150, 151, 152, 153, 154, 155, 162, 558, 597, 598, 600
Gustafsson, B. E., 444
Gustafsson, J. A., 416, 417, 444, 585
Gut, M., 254, 350,547, 558, 560, 585

Haagen-Smit, A. J., 272, 274
Haahti, E. O. A., 134

Haarmann, R., 16
Haber, E., 140
Hadd, H. E., 585
Haest, C. W. M., 557
Hagen, H., 181
Hague, S. M., 151
Haines, T. H., 388
Hale, R., 428
Hale, R. L., 346
Halevy, S., 420, 471
Hall, J., 329, 331, 340, 388, 389, 390
Hall, K., 138
Hall, P. F., 560
Hallermayer, G., 537, 552
Halpaern, A., 370
Halsall, T. G., 246, 250, 311
Ham, E. A., 569
Hamilton, J. G., 262, 370, 458, 460
Hamilton, R. M. G., 449
Hamlow, H. P., 182
Hammerschlag, A., 416
Han, J., 417
Hanahan, D. G., 333
Hanahan, D. J., 537, 539
Handler, P., 239
Hansbury, E., 450
Hansel, W., 154
Hanson, J. R., 308
Hanson, R. F., 594
Hanzlik, R. P., 238, 243
Happ, G. M., 319
Harada, Y., 558
Hardee, D. D.,198
Harel, S., 129, 131
Harland, W. A., 443, 458
Harman, R. E., 569
Harnish, W. N., 421, 542
Harries, C., 16
Harries, P. C., 515, 516
Harries, W. B., 338, 342
Harrington, C. R., 28
Harrington, G. W., 609
Harris, B., 112, 119, 120, 473, 482, 483, 492, 494, 498, 499, 500, 501, 505, 508
Harris, G. C., 312
Harris, W. B., 469
Harrison, D. M., 328, 338, 386
Harrison, H. C., 613
Hart, M. C., 499
Hartman, M., 557

Hartsen, F. A., 6
Harvey, W. E., 370
Hashimoto, S., 457
Hashimoto, Y., 441
Haskins, R. H., 421, 422, 542
Haslam, J. M., 544, 555
Haslewood, G. A. D., 458, 592, 593, 599, 603
Hatefi, Y., 181
Haun, J. R., 153, 154
Haurowitz, F., 428
Hauser, S., 443, 594, 600
Haussler, M. R., 610, 611
Hauth, A., 481, 483
Havinga, E., 607, 608
Hawker, C., 613
Hayaishi, D., 232
Hayano, M., 232, 558, 583, 584
Hayatsu, R., 256, 338, 383, 461, 465, 466, 494, 501
Hayes, E. R., 447
Hayflick, L., 543
Heard, R. D. H., 89, 558, 582
Heble, M. R., 484
Hechter O., 557, 558
Hedin, P. A., 198
Hedlund, M. T., 138
Heed, W. B., 435, 436, 552, 553
Heftmann, E., 127, 129, 153, 154, 272, 308, 371, 421, 487, 498, 560, 561
Heidel, P., 374
Heilbron, I. M., 18, 148, 245, 458, 461, 465, 466, 467, 472, 473, 605, 606
Heilbronner, E., 92
Heintz, R., 330, 388
Helfenstein, A., 18, 148
Heller, M., 101, 104
Hellig, H., 162, 218
Hellman, L., 416, 417, 444, 602
Helman, F. D., 604
Helmreich, M. L., 560
Hemming, F. W., 164, 181, 182, 189, 220
Henbest, H. B., 101
Hench, P. S., 27, 28, 568
Hendrickson, J. B., 272, 274, 277
Hendrickson, L. B., 272, 274
Hendrie, M. R., 421, 542, 551
Hendrix, J. W., 421, 542
Henning, G. L., 315

Henning, U., 153, 155, 157, 159, 161, 162, 164, 184, 185, 208, 217
Henrick, C. A., 308
Henry, J. A., 331, 332, 336
Henze, M., 425
Herman, R., 597
Herout, V., 301
Herz, J. E., 571
Herz, W., 301
Hess, A. F., 604, 605, 609
Hess, E. L., 570
Hesse, A., 181
Hesse, H., 386
Heuser, H., 311
Hewlins, M. J. E., 329, 331
Heyl, F. W., 499
Heys, J. R., 234
Hickey, F. C., 332, 374, 443
Hieb, W. F., 378, 431
Higashi, Y., 181, 182, 193, 194
Higgins, M. J. P., 156, 457
Hill, H. M., 314
Hill, L. F., 612
Hillman, J. R., 481
Hintze-Podufal, C., 196
Hirate, K., 594
Hirayama, K., 466
Hirsch, P. C., 561
Hirth, L., 184, 217, 329, 331
Hochberg, R. B., 560
Hocheder, F., 17, 181, 182
Hodges, R., 311
Hodgkin, D. C., 238, 605
Hoehn, W. M., 568
Hoffman, A., 163
Hoffman, C. H., 151, 152
Hohlweg, W., 557
Holick, M. F., 611, 612, 613
Holliday, P., 421, 542
Holloway, P. W., 161, 184, 186, 187, 188
Holly, F. W., 152
Holmes, W. L., 129, 131
Holt, A. S., 181, 182
Holtz, R. B., 421
Holz, G. G., Jr., 419, 551
Homber, E. E., 486, 501
Homberg, E. E., 486, 501
Honeywell, E. M., 609
Hopkins, J. C., 379
Horak, M., 301

Horbert, E. J., 153
Hörhold, C., 334, 416, 417, 418, 588
Horlick, L., 456, 457
Horn, D. H. S., 379
Horn, L. P., 457
Hornby, G. M., 355, 366, 561
Horning, E. C., 132, 134, 136, 137
Horning, M. G., 136, 231, 243
Horsting, M., 610
Hoshita, N., 597
Hossack, J. A., 545, 546, 551
Houghland, G. V. C., 153
Houser, A. R., 220
Howard, G. A., 206
Howell, J. McC., 444
Howes, C. D., 315
Hradec, J., 557
Hruska, F., 554
Hsia, H. L., 594
Hsia, J. C., 555
Hsia, S. L., 578
Hsiung, H. M., 365
Hsu, H. Y., 588
Hsu, I. N., 428
Huang, R. L., 149
Huff, J. W., 151, 152, 153, 157
Hug, E., 17, 181, 182
Hügel, M. F., 376, 388, 389, 435
Hughes, D. W., 181, 182
Hughes, R. C., 158
Hugoson, A., 585
Huldschinsky, K., 604
Hummer, J. K., 442, 609
Hunek, S., 474
Huni, E., 17
Hunt, P. F., 328, 337, 371
Hunter, G. D., 149
Hunter, K., 422
Hunter, W. M., 138
Huntson, S., 362, 364, 367
Hutchins, R. F. N., 348
Hutchinson, S. A., 422
Hutton, H. R. B., 595
Hutton, T. W., 231, 243
Hyde, P. M., 130
Hygel, M. F., 501, 504

Ichii, S., 164, 243, 558
Idler, D. R., 130, 332, 343, 346, 352, 371, 374, 380, 381, 392, 436, 437,

439, 443, 461, 464, 465, 587
Ikan, R., 129, 131, 460
Ikawa, M., 158
Ikegami, S., 441
Ikekawa, N., 133, 135, 136, 348, 350, 378, 379, 416, 417, 418, 444, 461, 464, 465, 466, 474, 475, 494, 613
Impellizzeri, G., 461, 465
Ingenhousz, J., 4
Ingersoll, R. J., 615
Ingold, C. K., 53, 164
Ingram, D. S., 506, 509
Inhuffen, H. H., 607
Inubushi, Y., 250, 251, 420
Irvine, D. S., 331, 332, 336
Isler, O., 154, 231, 243
Isselbacher, K. J., 374
Isube, K., 250
Itoh, M., 352, 442
Itoh, T., 481, 483, 488, 489, 490, 492, 493, 503, 504
Ittrich, G., 93
Ives, D. A. J., 480
Iwata, I., 181, 182, 474
Iyengar, C. W. L., 117, 133, 134, 135, 370, 419, 420, 546

Jaakonmaki, P. I., 136
Jackman, L. M., 220
Jackson, L. L., 422
Jacob, G., 189, 301
Jacobs, C. S., 129, 131
Jacobs, H. J. C., 547
Jacobsen, N., 378
Jacobsen, O., 6, 181
Jacobsohn, G. M., 154
Jaeger, R., 19, 278
Jaffe, R. B., 138
Jagannathan, S. N., 458
Jakowska, S., 441
Jamen, A. T., 131
Jarman, T. R., 234, 261, 263
Jasne, S. J., 544
Jaurequiberry, G., 338
Jayaraman, J., 153
Jedlicki, E., 189
Jefcoate, J. R., 612
Jefferies, P. R., 308
Jeger, O., 12, 52, 231, 232, 234, 237, 248, 249, 250, 300, 311, 328

Jellnick, P. H., 558, 582
Jenkins, W. T., 158
Jensen, H., 568
Jeong, T. M., 481, 504
Jewers, K., 486
Jirku, H., 585
Johansson, E. D. B., 141
Johansson, G., 594, 597, 598
John J. P., 131, 133, 134, 135, 339, 340, 422, 499
Johnson, D. F., 153, 498
Johnson, D. R., 501
Johnson, M. A., 428, 429
Johnson, M. W., 241, 262, 328
Johnson, P., 370, 379
Johnson, P. R., 198
Jollow, D. J., 540, 545, 546, 551
Jommi, G., 319
Jones, D., 216, 220
Jones, E. R. H., 19, 153, 246, 250, 319
Jones, G., 116, 117, 119, 311
Jones, J. C., G., 374
Jones, R. J., 450
Jones, R. N., 8, 105, 106, 108, 431, 605
Joseph, J., 473, 482, 483, 492, 494, 498, 499, 500, 501, 505, 508, 541, 548, 549
Joseph, J. M., 112, 119, 120
Joshi, V. C., 153
Jowgey, J., 611
Jucker, E., 272, 274
Julesz, M., 578
Juneja, H. R., 319
Jungalwala, F. B., 220
Just, G., 370, 422

Kabara, J. J., 447, 452
Kagan, A., 449, 450
Kahn, A. A., 447
Kahn, S., 357
Kaisin, M., 440, 441
Kajiwara, M., 370
Kalafer, M. E., 355, 357
Kallner, A., 600
Kalnins, K., 468, 469, 479
Kalvoda, J., 300
Kamiya, K., 238
Kamiya, Y., 441
Kamm, E. D., 18, 22, 23, 148

Kammereck, R., 129, 131, 366
Kanazawa, A., 347, 352, 371, 379, 380, 381, 434, 437, 438, 439, 441, 460
Kandel, S. I., 163
Kandutsch, A. A., 184, 368, 369, 498, 499
Kaneshiro, E. S., 419, 537, 546, 552, 553
Kannel, W. B., 449, 450, 455, 456
Kaplanis, J. N., 347, 370, 379, 433, 434, 435, 589
Kapoor, V. K., 562
Karlander, E. G., 476
Karlmar, K. E., 443
Karlson, P., 196, 588
Karlsson, K. A., 560
Karplus, M., 113
Karrer, P., 18, 22, 23, 25, 26, 29, 148, 272, 274, 288
Karrer, W., 175, 179, 272, 274, 275, 279, 284, 299, 301
Karst, F., 542
Kashman, J., 129, 131
Kasper, E., 387, 422
Kasperbauer, M. J., 487
Kasprzyk, A., 343, 367, 371, 372
Kasprzyk, Z., 480, 506
Kasten, P. M., 612
Katan, H., 420
Kates, M., 331, 471, 468, 469
Katsuki, H., 332, 384, 395, 542, 544
Katsumi, M., 308
Katzin, B., 568, 570
Kaufman, G., 334
Kawahara, F. S., 560
Kawalier, A., 6
Kawasaki, T., 494
Kays, W. R., 319
Kayser, F., 418
Keen, G., 361
Kekulé, V. S., 20
Kekwick, R. G. O., 156
Kelch, R. P., 138
Keller, W., 52
Kem, D. C., 140
Kemp, R. J., 480, 510, 511, 514
Kendall, E. C., 27, 28, 29, 568
Kende, H. J., 181, 182
Kennaway, E., 458
Kent, I. S. A., 467, 468, 469
Kepkay, D. L., 457

Kerr, J. D., 182
Kerschbaum, M., 16, 181
Kessel, I., 153, 155, 157, 159, 161, 162, 184, 208, 217
Kentmann, E. H., 89
Keye, W. R.,138
Keys, A., 447, 448, 450
Khalil, M. W., 130, 436, 437
Khan, B. T., 154, 560
Khana, I., 515
Kicherov, V. F., 370
Kieslich, K., 387, 422
Kim, D. N., 456, 457
Kimball, H. L., 558, 560
Kimble, B. J., 418
Kimelberg, H., 557
Kimland, B., 301
Kimura, K., 148
Kimura, S., 378
Kindt, F., 13
King, F. E., 311, 503
King, R. W., 222
King, T. J., 503
Kirby, G. W., 153
Kircher, H. W., 379, 435, 439, 482, 506, 552, 553
Kirdani, R., 560
Kiribuchi, T., 515, 516
Kirk, E., 447
Kirsch, K., 374
Kirschner, K., 216, 220
Kirtley, M. E., 157, 158
Kirvi, K. A., 486
Kliman, B., 123
Klimov, A. N., 156
Kishida, Y., 256, 338, 383, 461, 465, 466, 494
Kita, D. A., 233
Kitchen, P., 445
Klein, H. P., 417, 471, 540
Klein, P. D. 473, 475, 476
Klein, R. M., 472, 475
Kleiner-Bossaller, A., 612
Kliman, A., 368, 369
Klimov, A. N., 156
Kline, W., 444
Klosterman, H. J., 151
Klotsky, M., 472, 474
Klyne, W., 122, 308, 311, 312
Knapp, F. F., 337, 339, 340, 342, 360, 376, 392, 393, 476, 481

Knappe, J., 157, 158, 159, 162
Knapstein, P., 93
Knauss, H. J., 157
Knight, C. A., 415
Knight, J. C., 421, 501
Knights, B. A., 116, 119, 130, 421, 466, 467, 481, 489, 490, 494, 501, 506, 509, 537, 539, 542, 551, 552
Knights, J. G., 376
Knobil, E., 141
Knoche, H. W., 423
Knutson, J. C., 612, 613
Knypl, J. S., 315
Kobayashi, A., 467
Kobayashi, M., 346, 352, 354, 432, 433, 434, 437, 439, 440
Kobayashi, S., 558
Kobel, H., 163
Kober, S., 92
Koch, F. C., 585
Kodicek, E., 181, 193, 610, 611, 612, 613, 615
Koebner, A., 19
Koevoet, A. L., 607
Kofler, M., 181
Kohler, H., 52
Koide, S. S., 596
Koizumi, N., 444, 613
Kok, L. T., 436, 554
Kokai, K., 578
Kolor, M. G., 501, 504
Konyalian, A., 430
Konyalian, J., 378
Koons, C. B., 428, 429
Kording, P., 19
Koreeda, M., 588
Koritz, S. B., 560
Korn, E., 537
Korycka-Dahl, M., 612
Kossell, A., 439
Kostens, J., 490, 498, 515
Kotake, M., 432
Kotze, J. P., 457
Kotzschmar, A., 434
Kowerski, R. C., 209, 210, 216, 222, 223
Koyama, H., 480, 492
Koyama, T., 164, 184, 187, 188
Kraaipoel, R. J., 560
Krakower, G. W., 436, 499, 502
Kramer, J. K. G., 331, 417

Kraml, M., 369, 374
Kraus, R. W., 474, 475
Krevitz, K., 52, 110, 112, 119, 120, 253, 254, 255, 350, 383, 393, 419, 420, 421, 425, 473, 482, 483, 484, 492, 494, 498, 499, 500, 501, 505, 508, 545, 546, 547, 551
Kripalani, K. J., 584
Krishna, G., 212, 218
Krishnaswamy, N. R., 505
Kritchevsky, D., 368, 446, 449, 453
Kruggel, W. G., 584
Krusberg, L. R., 347, 378, 431
Kruskernper, H. L., 560
Kudchodkar, B. J., 456, 457
Kuehl, L., 211
Kuhn, R., 22, 24
Kuhne, M., 387, 422
Kuksis, A., 510
Kulkarni, B. D., 133, 134, 135, 370, 442, 609
Kulshreshtha, M. J., 423
Kumasaka, J., 138
Kupchan, M., 272
Kushwaha, S. C., 314, 320, 331, 417
Kuwaki, T., 597
Kyburz, E., 311

Lablache-Combier, A., 421, 422
Labler, L., 196
Labows, J., 319
Lacoste, L., 421, 422
Lacroute, F., 542
Ladbrooke, B. D., 556
Lal, J., 515
Laine, R. A., 515
Lampen, J. O. P., 552
Landrey, J. R., 117, 133, 134, 135, 246, 251, 262, 350 351, 370, 372, 419, 420, 421, 454, 482, 494, 498, 537, 546, 548, 549, 552, 553
Landon, J., 138
Lane, C. E., 429
Lane, G. H., 116
Lane, M. D., 157
Lang, A., 308
Langdon, R. G., 149
Langemann, A., 181
Langenbach, R. J., 423

Langer, R., 605
Lardon, A., 52
Larsen, B. R., 213, 216, 222, 223
Laseter, J. L., 421, 422
Lanthier, A., 578
Latimer, P. H., 181
Lapar, V., 600
Laqueur, E., 576
Lasater, M., 560
Laureta, H. C., 603
Laves, F., 18
Lavoisier, A. L., 4
Law, C., 431
Law, J. H., 159, 161, 272, 338
Lawrie, W., 503
Lawson, D. E. M., 153, 610, 615
Layne, D. S., 89, 585
Leal, J. A., 421, 542
Leathes, H. B., 554
LeBoeuf, M., 561
Leclercq, J., 346
Lecuyer, H., 557
Lederer, E., 250, 311, 332, 333, 335, 338, 340, 342, 346, 371, 376, 388, 389, 392, 421, 435, 445, 501, 504
Lederberg, J., 115
Lee, K. T., 456, 457
Lee, T., 222
Lee, T. C., 220, 313, 320
Lee, T. H., 222, 313, 320
Lee, W. H., 129, 131, 134, 135, 361, 364, 366, 367
Lees, R. G., 238
Leete, E., 191, 561
de Leeuw-Boon, H., 560
Leferink, J. G., 560
Lefort, M., 471
Lemann, J., 612
Lemin, A. J., 436, 499, 502
Lemmon, R. M., 368
Lenfant, M., 338, 341, 342, 371, 372
Lenton, J. R., 337, 338, 339, 340, 342, 343, 370, 371, 388, 389, 390, 392, 393, 476, 479, 484
LePage, M., 512, 515
Lercker, G., 460
LeRoy, G. V., 450
Lester, D., 346, 428
Lester, R. L., 181
Letourneux, Y., 560
Lettré, H., 605

Leutscher, J. A., 93
Leveille, G. A., 445
Levin, E., 184
Levin, E. Y., 458, 460
Levine, L., 138
Levine, R. A., 138
Levinson, Z. H., 434
Levy, H. R., 160, 587
Lewis, D. O., 560, 561
Lewis, R. A., 568
Lewis, R. W., 481
Lewis, W. H., 447
Lewkowitsch, J., 434
Lezica, R. P., 212
Liao, S., 578
Lichti, F., 308
Liddel, G., 421
Lieberman, M., 138
Lieberman, S., 138, 452, 558, 560, 585
Liebermann, C., 92
Liebig, J., 5
Light, R. F., 387, 422
Lilienweiss, G., 561
Lilly, V. G., 421, 542
Lin, H. K., 423
Lin, K., 238, 241, 263, 329
Lin, J. T., 374, 455
Lin, Y. Y., 444
Lindberg, M., 159, 161, 355
Linde, H., 494
Lindgren, B. O., 181, 329
Ling, N. C., 346, 428
Linn, B. O., 151, 152, 153, 157
Linnane, A. W., 540, 545, 546, 551
Linsert, O., 605, 606
Linstedt, S., 594
Lipke, H., 433
Lippert, J. L., 556, 557
Lisboa, B. P., 585
Littledike, E. T., 610
Liu, L. H., 436, 502
Lloyd-Jones, J. G., 348, 350, 379
Lockard, V. G., 378, 431
Lockley, W. J. S., 348, 485, 501
Loe, J. A., 310
Loebisch, W., 10
Loeser, E., 560
London, R. A., 467, 468, 469
Long, C. N. H., 568, 570
Long, R. A., 554
Longcope, C., 584, 585

Longman, R. T., 116
Longley, R. P., 537, 539, 552
Loomis, W. D., 272, 281
Loomis, W. K., 160
Lord, K. E., 234, 241, 262
Loughron, E. D., 360, 374, 375
Louloudes, S. J., 379, 435
Low, E. M., 425
Lowe, G., 153, 319
Lowry, P. J., 138
Lubich, W. P., 455
Luft, R., 138
Lumb, G. A., 610
Lund, J., 610
Lutsky, B. N., 134, 135, 361, 362, 364, 365, 366, 367
Lüttringhaus, A., 605, 606
Lynch, J. M., 262, 417, 418
Lynen, F., 21, 30, 31, 153, 155, 157, 158, 159, 161, 162, 164, 184, 185, 208, 210, 211, 216, 217, 220, 222
Lynn, W. S., Jr., 558
Lythgoe, B., 458, 461, 465, 466, 467, 472

Maass, W. S. G., 370, 479
Macchia, B., 336, 393
MacCorquodale, D. W., 580
MacDonald, E. F., 346, 436
MacDonald, P. C., 584
Mach, O., 557
Macheboeuf, M. A., 451
Mackie, A. M., 441
MacMillan, J., 272, 308
MacPhillamy, H. B., 498
Macrae, A., 184
MacRae, G. D. E., 151
Maeda, T., 442
Magendantz, H. G., 584
Magiafico, S., 461, 465
Magno, S., 426, 461, 465
Magueur, A. M., 461, 464, 465
Maheshwari, K. K., 358, 361, 374, 375, 398
Majerus, P. W., 155, 156
Makepeace, A. W., 565
Maktoab, A., 467
Malcorn, G. T., 455
Malhotra, H. C., 264, 319, 329, 348, 394

Mallaby, R., 165
Mallory, F. B., 92, 117, 133, 134, 135, 246, 250, 251, 262, 350, 351, 370, 372, 419, 420, 537, 546
Malya, P. A. G., 350, 351, 353, 372, 419, 420, 442, 546
Mancera, O., 587
Mandelbaum, A., 250
Mandersloot, J. G., 557
Mann, G. V., 449
Manning, R. E., 277
Manzoor-I-Khuda, M., 499, 500
Marini, G. B., 277
Markley, F. X., 300
Maroni, S., 116, 117, 119
Marquet, A., 238
Marr, J., 218
Marrian, G. F., 23, 580
Marsh, J., 560
Marsh, S., 371
Marshall, D., 311, 312
Marsili, A., 250, 336, 393, 480
Martin, A. J. P., 132
Martin, J. A., 362, 365
Mascio, O. J., 216
Mason, H. L., 29, 568, 569
Massey-Westropp, R. A., 153, 335
Massry, J. W., 611
Masui, T., 597
Mathieson, A. M., 272
Matsumoto, T., 481, 483, 488, 489, 490, 492, 493, 503, 504
Mattox, V. R. 29, 88, 569
Maudgal, R. K., 231, 243
Maume, B. F., 455
Mawer, E. B., 610, 612
Mayer, E. W., 17
Mayes, D. M., 40
de Mayo, P., 10, 19, 248, 250, 251, 252, 272, 274, 284, 288, 301, 319
Maxwell, J. R., 418
Mazur, Y., 502
Mazzarella, L., 346
McCann, L. M., 192
McCarrahan, K., 155
McCarthy, E. D., 181
McChesney, J. D., 307
McCloskey, J. A., 338, 366
McCollum, E. V., 604
McConnell, J. F., 272
McCorkindale, N. J., 422

McCoy, K. E., 594
McCrindle, R., 301, 329, 486, 502
McDonald, P. D., 560
McElvain, S. M., 198
McEvoy, I. J., 506, 509
McGarrahan, J., 394
McGhie, J. F., 360, 363, 364, 365
McIntyre, N., 374
McKail, R., 481
McKay, P., 506, 509
McKean, M. L., 136, 138, 339, 342, 346, 393, 516, 517
McKenzie, B. F., 568
McKenzie, R. D., 332
McKerns, K. W., 578
McKillican, M. E., 515
McLachlan, A., 554
McLean, M. J., 428
McMahon, P., 420
McMorris, T. C., 424
McNamara, P. N., 449, 455, 456
McNaught, R. P., 501, 504
McReynolds, L. A., 331
McShan, W. H., 194
Meance, J., 515
Means, A. R., 588
Meerman, G., 319
Meerwein, H., 13, 14, 19, 32
Mehdi, A. Z., 587
Meier, H. L., 52
Meinwald, J., 319
Melera, A., 238
Mellanby, E., 604
Mellows, G., 243, 251, 262, 263
Meloche, V. W., 501
Mendelsohn, L., 597
Menke, W., 515
Menozzi, T., 434
Mercer, E. I., 131, 164, 189, 241, 262, 328, 329, 331, 338, 339, 342, 360, 369, 384, 387, 467, 468, 469, 480, 510, 511, 514
Metzger, A. L., 453
Metzler, D. E., 158
Meyer, F., 378
Meyer, H., 378
Meyer, J., 16
Meyer, K., 494
Micetich, R. C., 542
Micetoch, R. G., 421
Michel, G., 422

Mickelsen, O., 447, 450
Middlebrook, R. E., 429
Middleditch, B. S., 262, 417, 418, 481, 490, 506, 558, 560
Middleton, E. J., 379
Midgett, R. J., 611
Midgley, A. R., 138, 140
Mieg, W., 6
Miettinen, T. A., 443
Miglioretto, P., 52
Mikhail, G., 140
Milborrow, B. V., 287
Millardet, A., 6
Miller, A., 542
Miller, C. A., 538, 542
Miller, E. V. O., 447, 450
Miller, J. D. A., 467, 472
Miller, W. L., 355, 357, 396, 397
Mills, J. A., 299, 300
Mills, J. S., 243, 436, 499, 502
Minale, L., 246, 251, 263, 346, 377, 426, 427
Minato, H., 337, 476
Miravet, L., 612
Mitchell, E. D., 198
Mitchell, R. E., 484, 504
Mitchell, W. D., 129, 131
Mitnick, M. A., 138
Mitropoulos, K. A., 360, 594, 597, 600
Mitschner, L., 312
Mitsuhashi, H., 346, 352, 354, 432, 433, 437, 439, 440
Mitton, J. R., 594
Miyake, Y., 355, 357, 396
Miyamoto, M., 238
Miziorko, H. M., 157
Mizunaga, T., 515
Mizuschima, M., 474
Moberley, M. L., 368
Moffet, G. I., 245
Molzahn, S. W., 542
Mondelli, R., 301
Monteiro, H. J., 309
Monroe, R. C., 347
Monroe, R. E., 347, 379, 434
de Montellano, O., 43
Moore, J. T., Jr., 332, 335, 384, 395
Moore, T. C., 319
Mora, M. C. G., 329
Morato, T., 583, 584

Moreau, J. P., 362, 364
Morelli, I., 250, 480
Moreschi, A., 434
Morgan, R. S., 444
Morii, H., 610
Morimoto, A., 250, 251, 420
Morisaki, M., 348, 350, 378, 379, 444, 461, 464, 465, 466
Morisaki, N., 466, 474, 475
Morris, L. J., 129, 131
Morrison, A., 308
Mors, W. B., 309
Morton, R. A., 153, 182, 220, 369
Mosbach, E. H., 443, 594, 600
Mosettig, E., 308, 311, 312, 319, 332, 374, 420, 435
Moskowitz, A., 360
Moslein, E. M., 159, 161, 185
Moss, G. P., 232, 328, 338
Mostafapour, M. K., 575
Motto, J. J., 422
Motzfeldt, A. M., 466
Mueller, J. F., 378
Muhr, A. C., 231, 331, 443
Muir, R. D., 588
Mukerjii, D., 336
Mulheirn, L. J., 110, 112, 119, 238, 243, 333, 359, 498, 508
Mulholland, T. P., 308
Mulrow, P. J., 587
Munaralli, S. M., 561
Munday, K. A., 333, 339, 361, 362, 364, 365, 367, 371, 546
Munson, P. L., 585
Muraca, R. F., 181
von Muralt, A., 149
Murata, T., 238
Murdi, F., 277
Murphy, B. E. P., 140
Murray, H. C., 587
Murray, R. D. H., 501
Muscio, F., 211, 222, 223
Myant, N. B., 594, 597, 600
Myers, C. S., 568
Myhre, D. V., 515
Mylius, F., 5
Myrtle, J. F., 610, 611

Nagai, J., 542, 544
Nagai, Y., 560

Nagasampagi, B. A., 329
Nagler, M. J., 486
Nagy, S., 511
Nakai, C., 417
Nakanishi, K., 105, 106, 370, 588, 589
Nakano, K., 594
Nakata, H., 474
Nakayama, T. O. M., 159, 220
Narayanaswami, S., 484
Nasciemento, C. G., 212
Naudi, D. L., 272
Naya, Y., 432
Nazir, D. J., 457
Neeman, Z., 556
Neher, R., 127, 128, 129, 568, 569
Neill, J. D., 141
Nejad, I., 138
Nelson, A. N., 332, 374
Nelson, A. W., 366
Nelson, E. K., 370
Nelson, J. A., 357
Nelson, M. T., 604
Nes, W. D., 112, 119, 120, 473, 482,
    483, 492, 494, 498, 499, 500, 501,
    505, 508
Nes, W. R., 52, 56, 62, 92, 103, 104,
    106, 110, 112, 130, 131, 133, 134,
    135, 136, 138, 140, 153, 154, 155,
    162, 163, 181, 182, 250, 253, 254,
    255, 257, 262, 264, 319, 328, 329,
    331, 332, 333, 335, 336, 337, 338,
    339, 340, 342, 343, 348, 350, 351,
    353, 370, 372, 374, 382, 383, 393,
    394, 419, 420, 421, 422, 425, 435,
    442, 455, 458, 459, 472, 473, 480,
    481, 482, 483, 484, 492, 494, 498,
    499, 500, 501, 505, 508, 516, 517,
    538, 540, 541, 545, 546, 547, 548,
    549, 551, 552, 560, 565, 569, 570,
    571, 578, 579, 580, 609
Nestel, P. J., 456
Nett, T. M., 138
Neudert, W., 105, 110
Neuhoff, J. S., 457
Neujahr, H. Y., 156
Neville, P. F., 610
Newbold, G. T., 243
Newerly, K., 137
Newpert, W., 537, 552
Newschwander, W. W., 153, 257, 480,
    516, 517

Nicholas, H. J., 153, 272, 360, 375,
    388, 393, 444, 481, 486, 502, 508,
    511
Nicksie, S. W., 501
Nicolaides, N., 18, 445
Nigrelli, R. F., 441
Nikkari, T., 445
Nishikawa, M., 238
Nishino, T., 184, 186, 187, 189
Nishioka, I., 494
Niswender, G. D., 138, 140
Noland, J. L., 434
Nomura, T., 352, 442
Nordby, H. E., 511
Norin, T., 301
Norman, A. W., 610, 611, 612, 615
Norris, D. M., 436, 554
Norton, D. A., 547, 548, 549
Norum, K. P., 457
Norymberski, J. K., 89
Nossel, H. L., 138
Novak, A. F., 151
Novak, V. J. A., 196
Nowicki, H. G., 182, 611
Nozawa, Y., 546
Nugent, C. A., 140
Nusbaum-Cassuto, E., 220
Nyström, E., 130

O'Brien, J. S., 539
Odell, W. D., 138, 140
O'Donnell, V. J., 558, 582
Oehlschlager, A. C., 338, 339, 352,
    367, 369, 370, 384, 385, 386, 387,
    394, 397, 540, 544
O'Grodnick, J. S., 335
Ogura, K., 164, 184, 187, 189
Ohloff, G., 318
Ohotake, H., 350
Ohta, G., 331, 332, 503
Ohtaka, H., 350, 379
Okamoto, M., 93
Okany, A., 163
Okubayashi, M., 350, 379
Okuda, K., 597
Olsen, R. E., 182
Olson, J. A., 355
O'Malley, B. W., 588
Omata, S., 558
Omdahl, J. L., 612, 613

O'Neal, M. J., 116
O'Neill, A. N., 480
Ono, T., 262
Oppe, A., 17
Opute, F. I., 510
Orcutt, D. M., 387, 468, 469, 474
Oriente, G., 461, 465
Oriol-Bosch, A., 154
Oro, J., 417
Orr, J. C., 250, 374
Orme-Johnson, W. H., 612
Ortiz de Montellano, P. R., 209, 234,
    237, 238, 250, 263, 329
Osborn, M. J., 193
Oser, B. L., 92
Osiechi, J., 301
Osske, G., 329, 486
Oster, M. O., 319
Otagaki, M., 598
Ott, W. H., 151
Ourisson, G., 19, 181, 184, 217, 241,
    242, 243, 244, 245, 256, 294, 301,
    329, 331, 336, 382, 385, 388, 393,
    418, 423, 471, 472
Over, J., 441
Overton, K. H., 301
Owades, J. L., 387, 422
Owens, W. M., 18, 148
Oxberry, J., 444
Oxford, A. E., 510

Padieu, P., 455
Page, A. W., 151
Page, H. J., 461
Page, I. H., 447
Pagich, B., 45
Pain, J., 435
Pakrashi, S. C., 515
Palade, G. E., 537, 539
Paliokas, A. M., 129, 131, 370, 371
Palmer, M. A., 481, 515, 516
Pan, M. L., 196
Pang, P. K. T., 609
Pangels, G., 585
Paoletti, C., 460
Paoletti, R., 361, 362, 364, 366, 367,
    370, 447, 452, 453, 454, 455
Papahadjopoulos, D., 557
Park, E. A., 613
Park, R. B., 153

Parker, M. L., 138
Parker, W., 421, 542, 551
Parmentier, G., 416, 417, 444
Parks, L. W., 329, 335, 382, 384, 385,
    542, 544, 552, 556
Parsons, M. A., 368
Parvez, M. A., 328, 337, 370, 371
Paschkis, K. E., 578
Pasedach, H., 328
Passcher, I., 560
Passero, E. P., 611
Pattabhiruman, T., 346, 428
Pattenden, G., 209, 210, 222
Patterson, G. W., 112, 119, 120, 130,
    135, 136, 336, 337, 340, 343, 370,
    387, 388, 389, 390, 392, 401, 419,
    420, 421, 422, 436, 437, 467, 468,
    469, 472, 473, 474, 475, 476, 482,
    483, 492, 494, 498, 499, 500, 501,
    505, 508, 546
Paul, I. C., 364
Paulus, H., 184
Pearson, G., 449
Pelleqrino, J., 309
Pelter, A., 231, 243
Penfold, A. R., 335
Pennock, J. F., 182, 220, 347, 377,
    378, 379, 380, 427, 430, 439
Perkin, W. H., 15
Perkins, E. G., 455
Perkins, H. J., 182
Peron, F. G., 89
Peterson, D. H., 587
Peterson, R. E., 123, 138
Peticolas, W. L., 556, 557
Petit, A., 607
Petrova, L. A., 156
Pettit, G. R., 421
Pettler, P. J., 348, 350, 351, 420; see
    also P. J. Randall
Petzoldt, K., 387, 422
Pfendt, E. A., 543
Pfiffner, J. J., 28, 568
Pharis, R. P., 272, 308
Philip, R. P., 418
Phillips, A. H., 159, 160, 161
Phillips, C. C., 272, 308
Phillips, D. O., 376
Phillips, G. T., 165
Phillips, J. G., 587
Phillips, M. C., 554

Phinney, B. O., 272, 308
Phipers, R. F., 461, 465, 466
Piatak, D. M., 560
Piatelli, M., 461, 465
Pierce, F. T., Jr., 368
Pincus, G., 558, 565, 585
Pinfield, N. J., 516
Pinte, F., 352, 375, 388, 442
Piotrowska, F., 336, 393
Pirt, F. J., 262, 417, 418
Plager, J. E., 140
Plattner, P. A., 54
Pletscher, A., 154, 231, 243
Pohl, R., 604
Polito, A., 453
Pollard, W. O., 420
Polley, H. F., 568
Pollock, J. R. A., 206
Polonsky, J., 338
Polyakova, E. D., 156
Ponsinet, G., 329
Poon, L. S., 125, 457
Popjak, G., 52, 149, 153, 154, 157,
    159, 160, 161, 162, 164, 165, 184,
    186, 187, 188, 189, 209, 210, 211,
    212, 213, 214, 217, 218, 222, 231,
    234, 243, 262, 301
Poretti, G. G., 149
Porter, C. C., 88, 89
Porter, G. A., 571
Porter, J. W., 153, 155, 156, 157, 161,
    164, 212, 213, 214, 216, 217, 218,
    219, 220, 223, 272, 314, 320, 480
Porto, A. M., 191
Possanza, G., 584
Potier, P., 461, 464, 465
Poulter, C. D., 213, 216, 222
Poutasse, E., 576
Powell, S. S., 415
Prange, I., 416, 417
Prasanna, S., 505
Pratt, A. D., 423, 441
Preedy, J. R. K., 93
Pregl, F., 4, 25
Prelog, V., 52, 53, 164, 370, 558
Preston, W. H., Jr., 153, 154
Price, G. H., 198
Priestly, J., 4
Prieto, A., 301
Prost, M., 455
Proudlock, J. W., 457, 540, 545,
    546, 551
Pryce, R. J., 393, 471, 472
Pucke, R. C., 140, 570
Pudles, J., 311, 355
Puliti, R., 346
Purdie, J. W., 181, 182
Pursey, B. A., 422
Pushparaj, B., 460

Quackenbush, F. W., 219
Quilico, A., 301
Quintanilla, J. A., 487
Quintao, E., 449, 450
Quitt, P., 308, 311, 312, 319
Qureshi, A. A., 213, 214, 217, 218,
    220, 223

Raab, K. H., 328, 338, 583, 584
Rabinowitz, J. L., 151, 153, 155, 162,
    597, 598
Rabourn, W. J., 219
Rahimtula, A. D., 333, 351, 355, 356,
    361, 362, 364, 366, 367, 371, 394,
    395, 396, 397
Rahman, R., 358, 395
Raistrick, H., 510
Raiz, L. G., 612
Rakoff, A. E., 578
Rakutis, R. O., 181
Raman, R. S., 182
Ramasarma, T., 153
Ramcharan, S., 89
Ramm, P. J., 361, 362, 364, 367, 371
Ramsey, R. B., 452, 454, 508, 511
Ramsey, R. T., 444
Ramstad, E., 277, 561
Ramstad, J. L., 561
Randall, C. C., 415
Randall, P. J., 348, 350; see also P. J.
    Pettler
Randall, R. J., 342
Rangaswami, S., 515
Rao, M. K., 455
Rao, B. G., 558
Rao, P. R., 415
Rapoport, H., 182
Rappoldt, M. P., 608
Rasmussen, H., 610, 613
Rassat, A., 301
Rastogi, R. P., 423

Ratcliffe, J. G., 138
Rath, F., 386
Ratsimamanga, A. R., 45
Ray, E., 537, 546
Rayford, P. L., 138
Razin, S., 537, 539, 556
Reddy, C. R., 611, 612
Reddy, V. V., 565
Reed, W. D., 157
Rees, H. H., 131, 164, 189, 210, 241,
    243, 262, 263, 329, 336, 340, 341,
    342, 343, 348, 350, 351, 358, 360,
    371, 379, 388, 389, 390, 392, 393, 420,
    485, 499, 500, 501, 504, 506, 589
Rees, L. H., 138
Regnier, F. E., 196, 272
Reich, H., 560
Reichlin, S., 138
Reichstein, T., 27, 28, 29, 30, 52,
    191, 561, 568, 569
Reid, W. W., 262, 417, 418
Reimerdes, A., 492, 499, 500, 506
Reiner, J. M., 456, 457
Reinitzer, F., 4
Reitz, R. C., 262
Reitz, R. G., 458, 460
Resau, C., 11
Resnick, P. R., 301
Retey, J., 157
Revotskie, N., 449, 450
Rey, E., 231, 331, 443
Reynolds, J. A., 557
Riban, J., 13
Rice, L. G., 487
Rice, M. S., 217
Riceberg, L. J., 138
Richards, J. H., 272, 274, 277, 333
Richards, R. E., 110
Richards, R. W., 308
Richardson, B., 387, 474
Richmond, W., 125
Richter, F., 16
Richter, W., 340, 393, 492, 499, 500,
    506
Richter, W. J., 238
Rilling, H. C., 154, 159, 160, 208, 209,
    210, 211, 213, 216, 217, 218, 220,
    221, 222, 223, 261, 301
Rinehart, K. L., Jr., 319
Ringelman, E., 157, 158, 159, 162
Ringold, H. J., 560

Riniker, B., 52, 300, 311
Riniker, R., 300
Ripperger, H., 77
Rittenberg, D., 30, 149, 594
Ritter, F. J., 434
Ritter, M. C., 261, 394, 450
Rizvi, S. A. I., 515
Robbins, P. W., 181, 193
Robbins, S. J., 542
Robbins, W. E., 347, 348, 366, 370,
    379, 431, 433, 434, 435, 443, 589
Roberts, D. L., 301
Roberts, D. P., 485, 501
Roberts, G., 10, 105, 106
Roberts, K. D., 558, 560, 585
Roberts, M. C., 447
Robertson, J. D., 536
Robichaud, C. S., 330, 362
Robinson, D. R., 301, 319, 320
Robinson, F. M., 151, 152, 153, 157
Robinson, J. R., 319
Robinson, R., 13, 19, 26, 33, 148, 230,
    231, 278, 333
Robinson, W. G., 151
Robinson, W. H., 209, 210, 216
Rock, C. O., 450
Rock, J., 565
Rodd, E. H., 13
Rodgman, A., 301
Rodig, O. R., 241, 242, 243, 244, 245,
    256, 423
Rodriquez, R. M., 585
Rodwell, V. W., 155
Roeske, W. R., 163, 164, 358
Roger, B., 435
Rogers, L. J., 314
Rogers, M. T., 110
Rohmer, M., 329, 340, 388, 393, 418
Rohrer, D. C., 547
Rojas, M. P., 487
Röller, H., 194
Romanoff, L. P., 585
Romer, C., 547
Romer, C. R., 502, 504
Romsos, D. R., 445
Rongone, E. L., 578
Röpke, H., 105, 110
de Rosa, M., 246, 251, 263
Röschlau, V. P., 125
Rose, A. H., 422, 537, 539, 545, 546,
    551, 552

Rose, G., 416, 417, 418
Rosenbaum, N., 419
Rosenfeld, G., 154, 560
Rosenfeld, R. L., 564
Rosenfeld, R. S., 416, 417, 444, 602
Rosenheim, S. O., 23, 604
Rosenkrantz, G., 587
Rosenthal, H., 570
Rosin, N., 153, 162, 163, 250, 480
Ross, G. T., 138
Rossipal, E., 89
Rosynov, B. V., 370
Rotchie, E., 331, 332
Roth, L. M., 272, 277, 278
Rothblat, G. H., 454, 455, 552
Rothman, S., 445
Rothschild, M. A., 137
Rothstein, M., 378, 431
Rottem, S., 543, 556
Rouser, G., 537, 539
Rowe, J. W., 329, 494
Rowan, M. G., 252, 262, 263
Rowland, R. L., 181, 301
Rubin, B. A., 587
Rubinstein, I., 110, 112, 339, 340, 352, 382, 383, 392, 440, 468, 469, 473, 475
Ruddat, M., 308
Rudney, H., 151, 154, 155, 156, 157, 158, 162, 182, 457
Ruegg, R., 154, 181, 231, 243
de Ruggieri, P., 443
Rupp, J. J., 578
Ruschig, H., 557
Russell, A. E., 368, 369
Russell, P. T., 92, 133, 134, 135, 257, 332, 394, 435, 516, 517
Russell, S. M., 338
Russey, W. E., 234
Rutledge, P. S., 312
Ruzicka, L., 12, 14, 15, 16, 19, 23, 24, 25, 31, 147, 231, 232, 234, 237, 248, 249, 250, 272, 274, 276, 287, 299, 313, 328, 331, 443, 558
Ryan, K. J., 583, 584
Ryan, R. J., 138
Ryback, G., 119, 210, 211, 222
Ryhage, R., 211
Ryley, J. F., 467, 468, 469, 471

Saba, N., 558

Sabo, E. F., 571
Safe, L. M., 346, 352, 370, 436, 464, 466, 467, 479
Safe, S., 370, 479
Safferman, R. A., 552
Sakai, K., 133, 135, 256, 461, 465
Sakamoto, Y., 594
Sakan, T., 277
Sakurai, E., 476
Sakurai, Y., 181, 182, 474
Sakuri, E., 337
Salen, G., 374, 450, 453, 455, 456
Saliot, A., 347, 378, 380, 381
Salisbury, L. F., 430
de la Salle, P., 4
Salokangas, R. A. A., 93
Salonkangas, A., 154
Salva, A., 301
Salvatori, T., 301
Samant, K. M., 605
Sampson, E. L., 539
Samuel, P., 452
Samuels, L. T., 154, 558, 560
Samuelson, B., 262
Samuelsson, B. E., 560, 600
Sandberg, A. A., 140, 570
Sandermann, W. W., 275, 276, 294, 319
Sanderson, T. F., 312
Sandor, T., 587
Sanghvi, A., 360, 369, 374
Sano, T., 250, 251, 420
Santacroce, C., 426, 461, 465
dos Santos, M. F., 309
Sarett, L. H., 29, 569
Sasaki, S., 588
Sato, Y., 501
Satoh, P. S., 558, 560
Sauer, H. H., 561
Savard, K., 576
Sawin, C. T., 584, 585
Saxena, S. C., 442
Sazena, B. B., 138
Scala, A., 361, 362, 364, 366, 367, 370, 394, 398, 455
Scallen, T. J., 261, 360, 366, 374, 375, 394, 398, 450
Scaramuzzi, R. J., 138
Schaeppi, G., 206
Schally, A. V., 138
Schaloh, D. S., 138

Schanbacher, L. M., 450
Scharf, S. S., 216
Schauble, J. H., 181
Schechter, I., 210, 217, 218, 262, 263, 308, 328
Scheer, I., 103, 104, 106
Schenck, Fr., 605
Schersten, T., 598
Scheuer, P. J., 346, 429
Schiff, J. A., 471
Schiller, H. P. K., 486, 501
Schindler, O., 153, 569
Schinz, H., 206
Schisler, L. C., 421
Schlosser, E., 421
Schmid, W., 154, 560
Schmidt, R. W., 428, 429
Schmitz, F. J., 346, 428
Schneider, H., 554
Schnoes, H. K., 610, 611, 612
Schoenborn, B. P., 272, 541
Schoenheimer, R., 25, 30, 86, 149, 443
Scholan, N. A., 594
Schon, A., 138
Schonfield, J., 191
Schraufrogel, P. K., 613
Schreiber, K., 77, 329, 486
Schreibman, P. H., 445, 456
Schroepfer, G. J., Jr., 129, 131, 134, 135, 210, 211, 222, 360, 361, 362, 364, 365, 366, 367, 368, 369, 370, 371, 397, 398
Schropfer, W. H., 149
Schubert, B., 340, 393, 492, 499, 500, 506
Schubert, K., 334, 416, 417, 418, 588
Schuette, H. A., 501
Schuijff, A., 555
Schulze, E., 231, 443
Schumacher, J. N., 301
Schuppli, O., 17
Schussheim, A., 452
Schuster, M. W., 261, 450
Schuster, W. W., 394, 398
Schwartz, M. A., 213, 214, 216
Schwarz, M., 196
Schwarzel, W. C., 583, 584
Schweers, W., 275, 276, 319
Schweiter, U., 181
Schwenk, E., 328, 332, 333, 394, 580, 582

Sciuto, S., 461, 465
Scolastica, C., 319
Scott, A. P., 138
Scott, J. L., 442, 609
Scott, W. J., 422
Scrikantaiah, M. V., 450
Seaton, J. D., 369, 397, 398
Seebach, J., 460
Seelye, J. P., 585
Seetharam, B., 450
Segal, B., 570
Segal, L., 570
Seidel, C. F., 16
Seifart, K. H., 154
Seiler, N., 244
Sekula, B. C., 422, 538, 540, 541, 545, 546, 551, 552
Selye, H., 28, 574
Semmler, E. J., 220, 223, 611
Semmler, F. W., 10, 14, 15, 16, 181
Serebryakov, E. P., 370
Serougne, C., 447
Seshadri, R., 424
Seshadri, T. R., 515
Seto, S., 164, 184, 186, 187, 189
Setz, P., 606
Shah, D. H., 161, 164
Shah, D. V., 220
Shah, P. P., 597
Sharma, R. K., 191, 367, 372, 575
Sharpless, K. B., 234, 238, 241, 262, 357, 358, 361, 374, 375, 395
Shefer, S., 443, 594, 600
Sheikh, Y. M., 346, 352, 370, 377, 426, 440, 441
Shenk, H. R., 311
Shenstone, W. A., 6
Shewry, P. R., 516
Shimizu, K., 558, 598
Shimizu, Y., 164, 243, 467
Shimuzu, M., 331, 332, 503
Shinitzky, M., 556
Shinohara, M., 238
Shiori, T., 338, 387
Shipley, R. A., 575, 576
Shishibori, T., 163, 164
Shoolery, J. N., 110
Shorb, M. S., 420
Shorland, F. E., 422
Short, R. V., 583
Shortino, T. J., 347, 379

Shriner, R. L., 481
Shull, G. M., 233
Shunk, C. H., 151,152, 153, 157, 181
Sica, D., 426, 461, 465
Siddons, P. T., 220
Siefferd, R. H., 418
Siegenthaler, W., 93
Siekevitz, P., 537, 539
Sieskind, O., 418
Siewert, G., 194
Siiteri, P. K., 584
Simmonds, N., 604
Simolon, A. V., 370
Simon, J. B., 457
Simonsen, J. L., 301
Simpson, I. A., 18, 148
Simpson, K. L., 216
Simpson, R., 329
Simpson, S. A., 29, 569; see also S. A.
  S. Tait
Singh, H., 562
Siperstein, M. D., 455
Sirtori, C. R., 453, 454
Sjövall, J., 130, 444, 597
Skeggs, H. R., 151, 152, 153, 157
Skinner, S. J. M., 339, 371
Skipski, V. P., 451
Sláma, K., 196
Slaytor, M., 335, 370
Slaunwhite, W. R., 140, 570
Sliwoski, J., 480, 506
Sliwowski, S., 330, 343, 362, 367, 371,
  372
Slocumb, C. H., 568
Slopianka, M., 340, 393, 506
Slotta, K. H., 557
Smeltzer, P., 103, 104, 106
Smith, A. G., 352, 381, 382, 383, 440,
  441
Smith, A. R. H., 329, 331, 338, 340,
  342, 367, 371, 372, 388, 389, 390,
  392, 467, 468, 469
Smith, D. C. C., 163
Smith, D. S. H., 441
Smith, E. L., 239
Smith, F., 151
Smith, H., 153, 163, 191, 308, 335
Smith, I. C. P., 554
Smith, L. L., 104, 110, 350, 443, 444
Smith, M., 447
Smith, P. F., 539, 542, 543

Smith, P. L., 415
Smith, T. M., 378, 431
Smith, T. W., 140
Smith, W. K., 561
Snatzke, G., 77, 560
Snell, E. E., 158
Snog-Kjaer, A., 416, 417
Snyder, T. E., 358, 361, 374, 375, 398
Sobel, H., 89
Sobrinho, L. G., 138
Sodano, G., 346, 377, 426, 427, 432
Sodhi, H. S., 456, 457
Sofer, S. S., 208
Soffer, M. D., 16
Soldo, A. T., 419
Sonderhoff, R., 31, 149
Sonheiner, F., 502, 587
Sonnet, P. E., 196
Sorm, F., 196, 272, 274, 301
Soto, H., 138
Souberain, A. E., 7
Soucek, M., 301
de Souza, N. J., 130, 131, 135, 181,
  182, 262, 328, 336, 338, 339, 340,
  358, 422, 458, 481, 499, 538, 589
Spector, A. R., 445
Spencer, E. Y., 319
Spencer, T. A., 357, 358, 361, 374,
  375, 395, 398
Spike, T. E., 364, 365
Spring, F. S., 19, 243, 245, 331, 332,
  336, 503, 605, 606
Sprinson, D. B., 544
Spraggins, R. L., 428
Spyckerelle, C., 418
Srinivasan, R., 319
St. L. Philpot, J., 605
Stabursvik, A., 501
Stanbury, S. W., 610
Standifer, L. N., 337, 510
Stange, O., 443
Stanley, R. G., 153
Stanley, W. H., 27
Stansbury, H. A., 439
Staple, E., 597, 598, 600
Starr, P. R., 542, 544
Starratt, A. N., 484
von Stedingk, M., 613
Steel, G., 443
Steel, W. J., 154
Steele, J. A., 435

Steenbock, H., 604, 609
Steiger, M., 568
Steinberg, D., 129, 332, 333, 374, 394, 445
Steinberger, A., 576, 578
Steinberger, E., 576, 578
Steinfelder, K., 329
Stern, A. I., 471
von Stetton, E., 157
Stewart, P. A., 606
Stewart, P. R., 155, 156, 157
Stier, T. J. B., 537, 540, 542
Stitch, S. R., 588
Stobart, A. K., 516
Stoeckel, M. E., 217
Stokes, W. M., 332, 443, 444
Stokstad, E. L. R., 431
Stone, K. J., 163, 164, 182, 189, 358
Story, J. A., 453
Strecker, A., 5
Strigina, L. I., 421
Strominger, J. L., 181, 182, 193, 194
Stylianou, M., 585
Subbarayan, C., 314, 320
Suchy, M., 301
Sucrow, W., 340, 393, 492, 499, 500, 506
Suda, T., 612, 613
Sudsling, K. E., 555
Suga, T., 163, 164
Suld, H. M., 597, 600
Sullivan, P., 138
Sundeen, J., 424
Sutliff, L. S., 575
Suzue, G., 219, 320, 417
Suzui, A., 277
Suzuki, A., 444
Suzuki, M., 434, 594
Svahn, C. M., 329
Svoboda, J. A., 347, 348, 366, 370, 379, 434, 435, 589
Sweat, F. W., 262, 263, 328
Sweat, M. L., 154
Sweeley, C. C., 132, 181, 182, 183, 193, 194
Swerdloff, R., 140
Swift, A. N., 428, 429
Swindell, A. C., 355, 365, 366, 376, 397
Sykora, V., 301
Sylven, C., 450

Synge, R. L. M., 132
Szent-Gyorgyi, A., 23
Szmant, H. H., 370

Tada, M., 480, 492
Tait, J. F., 89, 93, 123, 569
Tait, S. A. S. (former name: Simpson, S. A.), 89, 93, 123
Tajima, H., 587
Takigawa, N., 597
Takagi, T., 428, 442
Takahashi, T., 370, 480, 492
Takeshita, T., 444
Talalay, P., 560, 587
Tallquist, T. W., 430
Tamaoki, B. I., 587
Tamm, C., 52
Tamura, G., 152
Tamura, S., 441
Tamura, T., 352, 481, 483, 488, 489, 490, 492, 493, 503, 504
Tan, L., 350
Tanabe, K., 461, 465
Tanahashi, Y., 370
Tanaka, S., 219, 417
Tanaka, Y., 613
Tanford, C., 557
Tanret, C., 510
Tarbutton, P. N., 125
Tatchell, A. R., 206
Tavela, T. E., 613
Tavormina, P. A., 153
Taylor, A. J., 467, 468, 469
Taylor, A. N., 615
Taylor, C. B., 450, 455
Taylor, S. I., 370
Taylor, W. C., 331, 332
Tchen, T. T., 159, 160, 161, 162, 231, 232, 243, 250, 558, 560, 575
Teller, R. C., 140
Terada, O., 125
Teshima, S., 347, 352, 371, 379, 380, 381, 434, 437, 438, 439, 441, 460
Teste, J., 461, 464, 465
Texter, E. C., 603
Thampi, N. S., 353, 374, 442, 455
Thayer, S. A., 580
Theorall, H., 597
Thiele, J., 20
Thiele, W., 605

Thiessen, W. E., 301
Thimann, K. V., 560
Thomas, H., 31, 149
Thomas, R., 283
Thomas, R. J., 480
Thomas, W. A., 456, 457
Thompson, A., 18
Thompson, A. C., 198
Thompson, E. D., 335, 384, 542, 544, 552, 556
Thompson, G. A., 546
Thompson, J. V., 431
Thompson, M. J., 196, 332, 340, 347, 348, 370, 374, 379, 387, 388, 389, 390, 420, 434, 435, 439, 443, 473, 474, 589
Thompson, W. R., 447
Thomson, J. A., 379
Thomson, R. H., 352, 371, 377, 426
Thorn, G. W., 568
Thorne, K. J. I., 181, 193
Thorneyeroft, I. H., 138
Thorson, R. E., 378, 430
Threfall, D. R., 153, 182
Threlkeld, S., 508
Tiemann, T., 15, 24
Tilden, W. A., 6, 8, 15
Tilson, S. A., 138
Tiltman, A. J., 374
Tobie, E. J., 420
Todd, N. B., 198
Todd, R. L., 447
Todo, K., 352, 439, 440
Tokes, L., 116, 117, 119
Tomita, Y., 337, 338, 343, 476, 484, 485
Tomkins, G. M., 596
Topham, R. W., 370
Tornabene, T. G., 417, 468, 469
Torres, W. I., 503
Toste, A. H., 329
Toth, I., 578
Touchstone, J., 93
Townsley, J. D., 583, 584
Toyama, Y., 428, 442
Train, K. E., 116
Trave, R., 277
Tregar, G. W., 138
Treharne, K. J., 220
Trenner, N. R., 181
Trocha, P. J., 544

Trockman, R. W., 369, 397, 398
Trost, B. M., 194
Trowbridge, S. T., 360
Troxler, R. F., 182
Trudgill, P. W., 319
Trummel, C. L., 612
Trumpower, B. L., 182
Truscott, B., 352, 587
Truswell, A. S., 129, 131
Tsai, H. C., 611, 615
Tsai, L. B., 343, 473, 475, 476
Tsatas, G., 52
Tscharner, C., 318
Tschesche, R., 191, 231, 443, 560, 561
Tso, T. C., 343
Tsuda, K., 133, 135, 256, 338, 383, 401, 434, 461, 465, 466, 474, 475, 494, 501
Tsuda, T., 256
Tsuda, Y., 250, 251, 420
Tsujimoto, M., 18, 148, 434
Tsukada, K., 219, 417
Tsukamoto, T., 494
Tsuru, R., 352, 439, 440
Tucker, G., 610
Tulchinsky, D., 140
Tulloch, A. P., 421, 542
Tummillo, M., 585
Tummler, R., 329, 416, 417, 418
Tumlinson, J. H., 198
Turnbull, K. W., 319
Turner, A., 104
Turner, A. B., 441
Turner, R. B., 47
Tursch, B., 346, 429

Ubik, K., 435
Uebel, E. C., 196
Uehleke, H., 314
Uhde, G., 318
Ulick, S., 585
Ungar, F., 420, 585
Unraw, A. M., 338, 339, 352, 367, 369, 370, 384, 385, 386, 387, 394, 397, 540, 544
Uomori, A., 337, 338, 343, 476, 484, 485
Upper, C. U., 308, 319
Uritani, I., 319
Uwajima, T., 125

Vacheron, M. J., 422
Vagelos, P. R., 155, 156
Valentine, F. R., 425
Valenzuela, P., 273, 319
Vallisnieri, A., 4
Van Aarem, H. E., 378, 429
Van Aller, R. T., 92, 131, 133, 134,
    135, 332, 339, 340, 394, 422, 481,
    499, 538
Van Beek, V., 560
Van Brand, T., 430
Van Deenen, L. L. M., 555, 557
Van de Kamp, J., 29
Van Delft, A. M. L., 574
Van den Berg, C. J., 612
Vandenheuvel, F. A., 536
Vandenheuvel, W. J. A., 132, 134
Van Den Ord, A., 434
Van der Helm, D., 428
Van Der Horst, D. J., 437, 439
Van Der Merwe, G. J., 457
Van der Molen, H. J., 133
Van De Ruit, J. M., 371, 378, 429, 430
Vande Wiele, R. L., 140, 585
Van Dorsselaer, A., 418
van Duck, P. W. M., 555
Van Duuren, B. L., 151
Vangedal, S., 210, 234, 238, 262
van Inderstine, A., 151
Van Lier, J. E., 443, 444
Van Rheenan, J. W. A., 371, 378, 379,
    429, 430, 432
Van Slyke, D. P., 447
Van Tamelen, E. E., 163, 164, 213,
    214, 216, 234, 238, 241, 243, 262,
    358
Vantrappen, G. R., 603
Van Vanukis, H., 138
Van Wagtendonk, W. J., 419, 537,
    538, 542, 552, 553
Van Wimersma-Greidanus, T. B., 574
Vareune, J., 338
Variharan, V., 515
Varkey, T. E., 52, 253, 254, 255, 547
Varma, K. R., 333, 339, 367, 371
Varma, T. N. R., 159
Vavon, G., 15
Veith, H. J., 435
Vela, B. A., 445
Veler, C. D., 580
Velluz, L., 607

Vendrig, J. C., 516
Vercellone, A., 277
Verloop, A., 607
Vermilion, J., 364, 367
Vesterberg, A., 7, 17
Vetter, K. K., 585
Viala, J., 352, 437, 442
Vidal, G., 421, 422
Villaneuva, V. R., 333
Villetti, R., 436
Villotti, R., 501, 502
Villoutreix, J., 220, 418
Viscontini, M., 52
Vishniac, H. S., 538
Visser, H. K. A., 560
Vogel, W. H., 182
Voigt, W., 578, 594
Volcani, B. E., 468, 469
Vonk, H., 378, 429
Voogt, P. A., 371, 378, 379, 380, 429,
    430, 432, 437, 439, 441
Vorbrueggen, H., 311, 319
Vrkoc, J., 435
Vroman, H. E., 332, 347, 374, 433

de Waard, A., 159, 160, 161
Wachtel, H., 416, 417, 418
Wackenroder, H., 6
Wada, F., 594
Waelsch, H., 428
Wagner, A. F., 152
Wagner, B., 419
Wagner, G., 13, 14, 19, 24, 32
Wagner, W. D., 457
Wagner-Jauregg, J., 23
Wainai, T., 352
Wajda, M., 444, 447
Wakabayashi, N., 196
Wakil, S. J., 333
Wald, G., 22, 272
Walder, S. A., 379
Walens, H. A., 104
Walker, W. E., 301
Wall, M., 104
Wallach, O., 5, 6, 7, 8, 15, 16, 19,
    20, 21, 24, 25, 26, 31, 147, 159
Waller, G., 597
Waller, G. R., 198, 319
Walton, E., 152
Walton, M. J., 347, 377, 378, 379, 380,
    427, 430, 439

Wang, I. H., 364
Wang, S. F., 560
Warburg, O. H., 22
Ward, J. P., 362, 501, 504
Warg, P. A., 584
Wasner, H., 210, 211, 222, 301
Wasserman, R. H., 615
Wasson, G., 155, 156, 157
Watanabe, T., 441
Waters, J. A., 153, 308, 311, 319, 435
Watkinson, I. A., 333, 339, 351, 361,
    362, 364, 365, 367, 371, 394
Watson, H. S., 503
Watson, K. G., 234, 261, 263
Watson, S. W., 538
Ways, P., 537, 539
Webb, J. L., 558
Weber, H. P., 612
Weber, M. M., 181
Webster, M. S., 605
Webster, T. A., 604, 605
Wedner, C. H., 456
Weedon, B. C. L., 220
Weeks, C. M., 547
Weeks, O. B., 220
Weete, J. D., 421, 422
Wehrli, H., 148
Weidlich, G., 605, 606
Weijnen, J. A. W. M., 574
Weiner, I. M., 193
Weinheimer, A. J., 346, 428
Weinstein, B., 311
Weinstein, G. L., 565
Weinstein, P. P., 431
Weinstock, M., 604
Weiss, J. F., 444, 453, 454
Weizmann, A., 502
Wellburn, A. R., 181
Wells, B. B., 568
Welsh, A., 499
Wenkert, E., 283, 312
Werbin, H., 560
von Werder, F., 605, 606
Werner, A., 22
Werner, A. E. A., 243
Werthessen, N. T., 582
West, C. A., 272, 301, 308, 319, 320
Westphal, U., 557
Wetler, F., 432
Wettstein, A., 148, 557, 568, 569
Wheeldon, L. W., 540, 545, 546, 551

Wheeler, R., 422
Whistance, G. R., 182
White, A., 239
White, D. E., 108
White, D. L., 125
White, D. M., 296, 300
White, H. B., Jr., 415
White, J. D., 370
White, M. J., 494
White, R. W., 319
White, W. F., 138
Whitehouse, M. W., 597, 598
Whiting, D. A., 222
Whiting, M. C., 153, 319
Whitlock, H. W., Jr., 212, 218
Whitman, B., 580
Whittingham, C. P., 272
Whittle, K. J., 182
Wickramasinghe, J. A. F., 191, 334,
    561
Widdowson, D. A., 234, 243, 251, 262,
    263, 338, 339, 371, 386, 387, 544
Widmer, C., 181
Widrich, W., 584, 585
Wieland, E., 21
Wieland, H., 5, 19, 21, 30, 328, 386,
    434, 458
Wieland, O., 21
Wieland, P., 370
Wieland, T., 21
Wieland, W., 21
Wientjens, W. H. J. M., 434
Wilds, A. L., 19
Wilkinson, D. I., 376, 501
Willett, J. D., 234, 241, 243, 262, 378,
    431
Williams, B. L., 131, 135, 329, 331,
    467, 468, 469, 471
Williams, C. G., 8, 594
Williams, C. M., 194, 196
Williams, D. H., 110, 115, 116
Williams, R. J. H., 220, 221, 222, 315,
    316, 320
Williams, R. M., 556
Williams, V. P., 209, 210, 213, 214,
    222, 301
Williamson, J., 420
Willix, R. L. S., 108
Willstätter, R., 6, 17, 19, 22, 181, 182,
    461
Willuhn, V. G., 490, 498, 515

Wilson, A. N., 152
Wilson, H., 92
Wilson, J. D., 446, 578
Wilson, P. W., 610
Wilton, D. C., 333, 339, 351, 361, 362, 364, 365, 366, 367, 371, 394, 397, 546
Windaus, A., 4, 5, 11, 19, 21, 23, 30, 86, 231, 443, 481, 483, 499, 604, 605, 606
Winstein, S., 273
Winter, A., 560
Winter, J., 163, 569
Wintersteiner, O., 28, 567, 568, 580
Wirtz-Justice, A., 272
Wiseman, G., 603
Wiseman, P. M., 352, 371, 436, 461, 464, 465
Wiss, O., 153, 181
Wissler, R. W., 450
Wittenaw, M. S., 296, 300
Wittick, J. S., 181
Wittreich, P. E., 151, 152, 153, 157
Wojciechowski, Z. A., 332, 335, 336, 370, 476
Wolff, W., 16
Wolt, D. E., 151, 152
Wong, C. J., 464, 466, 467
Wong, R. G., 611, 612
Wong, S., 209, 210, 213, 214, 222, 301
Wood, B. J., 149, 150
Wood, G. W., 101
Woods, R. A., 339, 371, 542, 544
Woodward, R. B., 13, 32, 101, 102, 230, 231, 232, 235, 241, 249, 300
Wooton, J. A. M., 379, 432
Worcester, D. L., 541
Wormser, M., 537, 539
Worobec, R. B., 138
Worthington, K. J., 452
Wright, A., 181, 193
Wright, B. E., 421
Wright, G., 444
Wright, H. R., 461, 465, 466
Wright, J. J., 243
Wright, L. D., 151, 152, 379, 432
Wriston, J. C., 198
Wu, C. H., 140
Würsch, J., 149, 154, 181, 231, 243

Wyatt, G. R., 196
Wycoff, D. A., 125
Wyllie, S. G., 116, 117, 119

Yagen, B., 334, 335
Yagi, A., 494
Yagi, H., 124
Yalciner, S., 374
Yalow, R. S., 137, 138
Yamada, T., 598
Yamamoto, H., 43, 237, 238, 263
Yamamoto, S., 241, 262, 329
Yamano, T., 355, 357, 396
Yamasaki, K., 598
Yashouv, J., 556
Yasuda, S., 352, 429
Yasumatsu, N., 515, 516
Yasumoto, T., 441
Yengoyan, L. S., 162, 165, 189
Yokoyama, H., 159, 315, 494
Yoshida, T., 466, 474, 475
Yoshizawa, T., 560
Youhotsky-Gore, I., 217; see also I. Y. Gore
Young, I. G., 192
Young, M., 338, 384, 421
Yuan, C., 159, 161
Yudelevich, A., 273

Zabin, I., 150
Zaccai, G., 541
Zaffaroni, A., 89, 127, 558, 587
Zalkow, L. H., 300, 361
Zamoscianyk, H., 558
Zandee, D. I., 378, 379, 380, 429, 432, 434, 442
Zander, J. M., 243, 246, 251, 262, 263, 420
Zak, B., 92
Zeise, W. C., 6
Zeitschel, O., 181
Ziffer, H., 134
Zimmermann, W., 92
Zin, L. H., 499
Zissman, E., 342, 371
Zlatkis, A., 92
Zondek, H., 23
Zscheile, F. P., 219

Subject Index

Abietic acid, 305
  conversion of, to retene, 17
  irregularity of, 10, 11
Abscisic acid, 287, 288
Absolute configuration
  control of, by cyclases, 256-261
  defined, 52
Absorption, infrared
  C—H bending, 106-107
  C=C stretching, 106
  C—H stretching, 105
  C—O stretching, 107-108
  C=O stretching, 106
  O—H stretching, 105
Acansterol, 346
Acanthamoeba, sterols in, 420
Acanthaster planci, 346, 440, 441
Acetate
  C_5 monomer from, expected labeling
    pattern of, 149
  separation factors, 134
  as sterol precursor, 149
Acetoacetate, role of, in isopentenoid
  formation, 150-151
Acetoacetyl-ACP, 156, 157
Acetobacter rancens, triterpenoids of,
  418, 419
Acholeplasma laidlawii, 416
ACP, *see* Acyl carrier protein
Actinidia polygama, 277
Actinidine, 278
Acyclic precursor
  conformations of, 317
  origin of, 313-315
Acylable hydroxyl groups, 86-87
Acylation, 87
Acyl carrier protein
  acetoacetyl, 156, 157
  in biosynthesis of mevalonic acid,
    155-156
Adipose tissue, sterol synthesis in, 445
Adler, K., Nobel Prize of, 30
Adrenal corticoids, 71

Adrenal glands, steroids' effects on, 3
Adrenocortical steroids, 71
  biosynthesis and control, 572-575
  isolation and function of, 568-571
  major pathways to, 573
Adrenocorticoids, 71
Adsorption chromatography, 126
Aerobacter cloacae, 417
Aesculus hippocastanum, 513
Agaricus bisporus, 421
Agaricus campestris, 328, 384, 385
Agaricus sp., 421
Agathic acid, 304
Agathis australis, 310
Agave toumeyana, 329
Aging, and serum cholesterol levels,
  452-453
Agnosterol, 70, 423, 443
Agroclavine, 162-163
Ajmalicine, 284
Alcohols
  separation factors, 134
  see also specific alcohols
Aldehydes, analytical procedures, 93
Aldosterone, 72
  chemical tests for analysis of, 98
  thin-layer chromatography of, 129
  see also Hormones
Alfalfa, sterols in, 493
Algae
  blue-green, 460, 462-463
  brown, 466-467
  cyclolaudenol in, 336
  eukaryotic, 461-479
  golden-brown, 467-471
  green, 472-478
  in lichens, 478-479
  red, 461-466
  sterol biosynthesis in, 387-393
  yellow-brown, 467
  yellow-green, 467-471
  see also species names
Alisols, 238

Alkylase, 394–395
Alkylation
  in blue-green algae, 460
  mechanism of, 335–344
  variations of, 344–346
Alkylation-reduction bifurcation
  discovery of, 332–333
  and organismic type, 331
  shortening of side chain to C_7,
    352–354
24-Alkylidenesterols, 65
Alkylsterols, in coelenterates, 429
24-Alkylsterols, 442
  in bees, 435
  in pathologic states, 455
24α-Alkylsterols, isomerization route to,
    394
"allo," defined, 57
$Allo_h$-arrangement, of polymers, 172
$Allo_t$-arrangement, of polymers, 172
Allocholic acid, 591
Allylic rearrangement, compared with
  homoallylic rearrangement, 296
Alnus glutinosa, 513
Alnusenone, 250, 251
Ambrein, 250, 251–252
Amellus strigosus, 199
Amphora exiqua, 469
Amurensterol, 439, 440
α-Amyrin, 510
  gas-liquid chromatography of, 136
  origin of, 250
β-Amyrin, 164, 510
  formation of, 248–249
  gas-liquid chromatography of, 136
β-Amyroids
  formation, from lupenyl cation, 249
  rearranged, formation of, 250, 251
Anabena cylindrica, 460
  sterols in, 462
Anacystis nidulans, 460
  sterols in, 463
Anaerobes
  facultative, 416
  obligate, 416
  see also species names
Androgens, 72
  biosynthesis and control of, 576–578
  isolation and function of, 575–576
  structure-activity correlations, 578
Andrographolide, absolute configura-
    tion of, 311
Androst-5-en-3β-ol, in bees, 435
Androstan-3-one, ethylene ketal of,
  fragmentation of, 116
5α-Androstan-3,17-dione, gas-liquid
  chromatography of, 138
5α-Androstan-17-one, gas-liquid chromatography of, 138
5α-Androstane, PMR spectra, 111
5α-Androstane-3α,17β-diol, 577
5β-Androstane, PMR spectra, 111
$Δ^4$-Androstene-3,11,17-trione, R_s value
  for, 128
$Δ^4$-Androstene-3,17-dione, R_s value for,
  128
4-Androstene-3,17-dione, gas-liquid
  chromatography of, 138
Androstenediol, 577
Androstenedione, 577
  thin-layer chromatography of, 129
Androsterone, 577
"ane," defined, 61
Anemonia sulcata, 378, 429, 430
Angiosperms
  sterols in, 504–505
  see also species names
Angular methyl groups, 47
Anisomorpha buprestoides, 319
Annelids
  sterols in, 432–433
  see also species names
Anteuphoid, formation, from proto-
  euphoid cation, 246
$Δ^{14}$-Anteuphol, 245
Antetirucallol, 245, 246
Antheridiol, 423, 424
Anthoeidaris crassispina, 560
Anthonomus grandis Boheman, 197
Anthopleura elegantirsima, 428
Anti, defined, 42
Apis mellifera, 197
Apis mellifica, 435
Aplopappus heterophyllus, 361
Aplysterol, 346, 427
Apple, 513
Arenicola marina, 379
Argentation chromatography, 131
Aristotle, 3
Aromadendrene, 297
Aromatic steroids, analytic procedures,
  92–93

Artemia salina, 347
Arachis hypogaea, dominant sterols in, 488
Arteriosclerosis, 455-457
Arthropods
  dealkylation in, 380
  sterols in, 433-436
  see also species names
"Artificial camphor," 13
Ascaris lumbricoides, 431
Ascaris suum, 450
Ascosterol, 70
Aspergillus fenellial, 552
Asperigillus flavers, 422
Aspergillus fumigatus, 179, 182, 371
Aspergillus niger, 362, 367
Aspergillus oryzae, 152
Astacus astacus, 434
Astasia longa, 329, 388, 393
Astasis ocellata, 471
Aster scaber, 480
Asterias amurensis, 439
Asterias pectiuifera, 440
Asterias rubens, 381, 382, 383, 440, 441, 560
Asteroids, sterol biosynthesis in, 382
Asterosaponins, 441
Asterosterol, 440, 441
Aster scaber, sterols in, 492
Astropecten aurantianus, 441
Asymmetric induction, 258
Asymmetry, 258
γ-Atlantone, 286
Atrina fragilis, 380
Aurelia aurita, 429
Avenasterol, 65, 69, 496, 501
  in plants, 483, 486-490, 492-493
Δ^5-Avenasterol, 68
Δ^7-Avenasterol, 69
Avena sativa, 501
Avicularia avicularia, 434
Axinella cannabina, 426
Axinella polypoides, 426
Axinella verrucosa, 426
Azasteroids, 77-79
Azotobacter chroococcum, sterols in, 417, 418

Baboon, cholesterol levels in, 449

Baccharis viminea, 512
Bacillis subtilis, 417
Bacteria
  absence of sterols in, 417, 418
  squalene and sterols in, 417
  sterols in, 416-418
  see also Microorganisms; *species names*
Bactoprenol, 178, 179, 181, 193
Banana, 483
Barley, 339, 484
Barosoma pulchellum, 200
Barton, D. H. R., Nobel Prize of, 32-33
Bathochromic shift, defined, 101
Beans, 491
Bees
  sterols in, 435
  see also species names
Benzenoid systems, spectroscopy of, 103-104
Berthelot, M., 4
Betula alba, 244
Betulafolientriol, 244
Betulaprenols, 177, 181
Betula verrucosa, 177, 181
Beyerene, 307
  absolute configuration of, 311
Bicycle, formation, 301-308
Biddulphia aurita, 469
Bile acids, 74-75
  biosynthesis, 594-599
  sequencing of, 600-602
  conjugation of, to taurine or glycine, 598-599
  discovery of, 5
  mammalian, 591
  mass spectroscopy of, 122
  occurrence, 590-593
  physiological functions of, 602-603
Bile alcohol, 74
Bile salts
  occurrence, 590-593
  physiological functions of, 602-603
Biogenetic isoprene rule, 12
  and Wagner-Meerwein rearrangements, 13-14
α-Bisabolene, 286, 287, 289
  precursors of, 298-299
Bisabolenyl cation, 284
Bisabolol, 286, 299

7,22-Bisdehydrocholesterol, 413
  in sponges, 426
Blakeslea trispora, 424
Blastocrithidia, sterols in, 420
Blatella germanica, 347, 434
Bloch, K., Nobel Prize of, 30-31
Blood cholesterol, 445
Blood-red, 509
Blue-green algae, classification of,
  according to sterol composition,
  462-463
Bombicesterol, 434
Bombyx mori, 347, 348, 350, 434, 588,
  589
Δ^5-Bond, introduction of, 367-371
Δ^{22}-Bond
  introduction of, 371-373
  sterols with, examples of, 66
Bonds
  axial, defined, 48
  double and triple
    nomenclature for, 62
    see also Double bonds
  equatorial, defined, 48
Borneol, 276-277, 279
  stereochemistry of, 281
Botriocephalus latum, 430
Botrydium granulatum, 467
Brain
  cholesterol in, 444
  development, desmosterol in, 452
  human, sterol composition of, 444
  rat, sterol composition of, 444
  tumors, and desmosterol, 453
Brassica campestris, 498
Brassica nigra, 512
Brassica oleracea, 508, 509
  dominant sterols in, 484
Brassica rapa, 499, 508, 509
  dominant sterols in, 489
Brassicasterol, 66, 68, 336, 437, 467,
  468, 495, 499, 506, 508
  in coelenterates, 428
  in Cruciferae, 481
  in green algae, 473
Brittle stars, 439
Brown algae
  sterols in, 466-467
  see also species names
Bryophytes, sterols in, 479-480
Buccineum undatum, 379

Bufalin, 73, 74
Bufanolide, 74
Bufo vulgaris, 73
Bush systems, 127-129
Butenandt, A., Nobel Prize of, 23-24
Butyrate, 333
Butyrospermol, 245
Butyrospermum parkii, 503
  sterols in, 493

C-20, stereochemistry at, 253-256
C-24, dehydrogenation and dealkylation
  at, 346-352
C-24, metabolism, 326, 327
C_6 compounds, absolute configuration
  of, 161-162
C_{30} compounds, 18
  problems of classifying, 39-40
C_{31} compounds, 41
C_5 concept, development of, 7-8
C_{30}-isopentenoids, in gas-liquid chromatography, 136
C_{18} steriods, 73
C_{19} steroids, 72
C_{21} steroids, 72
C_{25}-sterols, in sponge, 426
C_{26}-sterols, 426
  in sponge, 426
C_{27}-sterols
  in fungi, 422-423
  in sponge, 426
C_{28}-sterols, in sponge, 426
C_{29}-sterols, in fungi, 422
C_1 transfer, second, in alkylation,
  339-344
C_5 units
  formation, elimination in, 162
  isomerization of, 162-165
  pair, interconversion, 161
  structure and biosynthesis of,
    159-161
Cabbage, 484, 509
  see also Brassica oleracea
Cadalene, 16, 17
Cadinene, 9, 10
  dehydrogenation of, 16, 17
α-Cadinene, 288, 289, 299
α-Cadinol, absolute configuration of,
  300
β-Cadinol, 288, 289

Cadinyl cation, 288, 289
Caenorhabditis briggsae, 378, 431
Cafestol, 312
  absolute configuration of, 311
Calendula officinalis, 343, 367, 371,
  480, 506
  dominant sterols in, 484
Calliactis parasitica, 347, 378, 429, 430
Callitris glanca, 200
Calluna vulgaris, 513
Camellia japonica, sterols in, 492
Camellia sasangua, sterols in, 492
Camellia sinensis, 367, 372
Campestanol, 68
Campesterol, 64, 68, 495, 498
  in plants, 482–484
  reversed-phase chromatography of,
  131
Camphene, 5, 10, 11, 14, 277, 279, 280
Camphor, 279, 319
α-Camphorene, 301
Cancer pagurus, 434
Carbohydrate carriers, 193–194
Carbons, numbering of, 45–46
Carboxyl dimer, 105
Carcinogens, steroids as precursors for,
  458, 459
Cardenolide, 74
Cardiac-active steroids, 73–74
α-Carene, 279
  biosynthesis of, 276
β-Carene, 280
  biosynthesis of, 276
Carissone, absolute configuration of,
  300
Carneigiea gigantee, 512
Carnosoic acid, 306, 307
Carotene, 5
  first isolation of, 6
α-Carotene, formation of, 316
β-Carotene
  formation of, 316
  precursor of, 314
ζ-Carotene, structure of, 313, 314
Carotenoid cation, 315
Carotenoid rings, formation of,
  315–316
Carotenoids
  in *Acholeplasmas,* 415
  acyclic, biosynthesis of, 313
  cyclic, structure of, 314

  discovery of, 6
  intermediates for biosynthesis of, 191
  Carotenoid stage, enzymology at, 320
  "Carotin," 5
Carpesterol, 69, 501, 502
Carrier proteins, 450–451
  squalene, 264
Carum carvi, 283
Carvacrol, 282
Carvone, 279, 280
  origin of, 283
Caryophyllene, 290, 299, 300
Casbene, 320
  origin of, 301, 302
Cassiopea xamachana, 429
Castaprenol, 181
Castaprenol-10, 177
Castaprenol-11, 177
Castaprenol-12, 178
Castaprenol-13, 178
Castaprenol-13-14, 178
Catnip, 198
Cat's-ear, 513
Cedrela toona, 245
Cedrelone, 245
Cedrenes, 288, 289
Cedrol, 288, 289
Cell-free systems, development of, 155
Celsianol, 69
Cembrene, origin of, 301, 302
Cembrenyl cation, 303
Ceratocystis timbriata, 319
Cerebratulus marginatus, 378
Cerebrosterol, 443, 444
Cerebrotendinous xanthomatosis, 453
Cerianthus membranaceus, 378, 429,
  430
Certonardoa semiregularis, 440
Chaetomorpha crassa, 475, 476
Chain length, regulation of, 187–188
Chalinasterol, 68, 425
Chamaecyparis obtusa, 200
Chara vulgaris, 475
Charophyta, 472–478
Cheiranthus cheri, 481, 509
Chemical shift, defined, 108
Chenodeoxycholic acid, 591
α-Chigadmarene, 292, 293
Chigadmarenyl cation, 292, 293
Chlamydomonas rheinhardi, 474
Chlorella candida, 474

Chlorella ellipsoidea, 388, 390, 473, 474, 475, 476
Chlorella emersonii, 388, 389, 390, 474
Chlorella fusca, 474
Chlorella glucotropha, 474
Chlorella miniata, 474
Chlorella nocturna, 474
Chlorella pringsheimii, 475
Chlorella pyrenoidosa, 178, 474
Chlorella saccharophilia, 475
Chlorella simplex, 474
Chlorella sorokiniana, 474, 476
Chlorella vannilii, 474
Chlorella vulgaris, 474
Chlorophyll biosynthesis, intermediates in, 192
Chlorophyta, 472–478
Cholecalciferol, 610–616
Cholesta-8,14-dien-3β-ol, 66
Cholestan-3β-ol, reversed-phase chromatography of, 131
5α-Cholestane, 543
    PMR spectra, 111
Cholestanol, 68, 442
    chemical test for analysis of, 94
    configuration and conformation of, 53
    polycyclic system of, 39
    scheme of, 40
    in sponges, 426
    in vertebrates, 443
5α-Cholestanol, 53, 68
    enantiomer of, 53
    PMR spectra, 111
5β-Cholestanol, 53, 68
Δ^{22}-Cholestanol, chemical tests for analysis of, 96
Cholestenone, 416
"Cholesterine," 4
Cholesterol, 10, 11, 63, 68, 326, 327, 332, 343, 360, 361, 362, 375, 378, 380, 381, 389, 413, 416, 442, 510, 543
    absolute configuration of, at C-3, 52
    in animals, 446
    in annelids, 432
    and arteriosclerosis, 455–457
    in bacteria, 416, 417
    24-C_1 and 24-C_2, with and without a Δ^{22}-bond, 495
    circulating, 445

    in coelenterates, 428, 429
    conformation, 255
    conversion of, to cholic acid, 601
    derivation of term, 4
    distribution, tissue
        in man, 445–447
        in rat, 445
    in echinoderms, 439
    in fungi, 422
    in green algae, 473
    in insects, 433–435
        need for, 346–347
    isopentenoid character of, 148
    labeling pattern of, after biosynthesis from labeled acetate, 149, 150
    in molluscs, 436
    in nemathelminthes, 431
    NMR absorption, 111
    pathway to progesterone, 559
    in plants, 482–484, 486–490, 498
    in platyhelminthes, 430
    polycyclic system of, 39
    in red algae, 461, 464, 465
    reversed-phase chromatography of, 131
    in sponges, 426
    structure of, importance of to scientific progress, 4
    in vegetable oils, 481
    in vertebrates, 442
    see also Serum cholesterol
Cholic acid, 74, 75, 591
    conjugation of, with taurine or glycine, 599
    polycyclic system of, 39
    taurine and glycine conjugates of, 592
Chondrillasterol, 66, 69, 387, 425, 496
Δ^7-Chondrillastenol, 328
Chondrus crispus, 464
Chromatographic analysis, 124–137
Chromatography
    defined, 126
    see also Adsorption chromatography, Argentation chromatography, Column chromatography, gas-liquid chromatography, Liquid-liquid chromatography, Liquid-solid chromatography, Paper chromatography, Reversed-phase chromatography, Thin-layer chromatog-

raphy, Vapor-phase chromatography
Chrysophyta, 467-471
cis, defined, 42
Citronellal, 181, 279, 280
Citronellic acid, 200
Citronelloic acid, 279
Citronellol, 179, 181
Citrostadienol, 69, 502, 503
Citrullus vulgaris, sterols in, 492, 500
Cladophora flexnosa, 475
Clam, 439
  see also species name
Clerodendrum campbelli, 341, 367, 371, 499, 505, 506
  sterols in, 500
Clerodendrum infortunatum, 499, 505
  sterols in, 500
Clerosterol, 69, 475, 497, 499, 500, 505, 506
Cliona celata, 425, 426
Clionastanol, 68
Clionasterol, 64, 68, 338, 342, 348, 352-353, 425, 495
  in green algae, 473
  in plants, 494
Cocomyxa elongata, 475
Coconut, 487
Cocos nucifera, dominant sterols in, 487
Codisterol, 68, 497
Codium fragile, 475, 476, 477
Coelenterates
  sterols in, 428-430
  see also species names
Coenzyme A, in biosynthesis of mevalonic acid, 155-156
Coffea sp., dominant sterols in, 490
Coffee, 490
Column chromatography defined, 126
Colupulone, 206
Combustion microanalysis, 4
Competitive protein binding, 140-141
Conessine, 77, 78
Configurations
  α, 49-51
  β, 49-51
  A/B *cis*, 47
  absolute, of steroids, 51-54
  cis-anti-trans-anti-trans, 47
  D, 52

L, defined, 52
R, 53, 54
relative, 51
S, 53, 54
trans-anti-trans-anti-trans, 46
Configurational convention for steroids, 50
Configurational isomers, 48
Conformation
  defined, 48
  "up-chair," 316-319
Conformational isomers, defined, 48
Conformers, defined, 48
Conjugated carbonyl groups, spectroscopy of, 103
Conjugated double bonds, ultraviolet spectroscopy of, 101-103
Conjugation, defined, 101
Contraceptives, 565
"copro," defined, 57
Coprostanol, 68, 416
  chemical tests for analysis of, 95
  polycyclic system of, 39
Coreopsis verticillata, 199
Corn, 512
  dominant sterols in, 488
  subcellular organelles of, sterol and steryl ester composition of, 511, 514
Cornforth, J. W., Nobel Prize of, 33-34
Cortexone, thin-layer chromatography of, 129
Corticoids, 71-72
Corticosteroids, biosynthesis of, from mevalonate, 154
Corticosterone, thin-layer chromatography of, 129
Cortisol, 72
  chemical tests for analysis of, 98
  thin-layer chromatography of, 129
Cortisone
  PMR spectra, 111
  thin-layer chromatography of, 129
Corylus avellana, 513, 516
Corynebacterium pseudodiphtheriticum, 417
Cosmene, 199
Cosmos bipinnatus, 199
Cotton, 489
Cotton effect, defined, 123
Cottonwood, 513

Counter current distribution, 124
Coupling constant, 109
Crinosterol, 68
Crithidia, sterols in, 420
Cryptopinon, 304
Ctenophores, 428
Cucumaria elongata, 382, 441
Cucumaria planci, 441
Cucumis melo, sterols in, 492, 500
Cucumis sativus, sterols in, 500
Cucurbita pepo, 319, 501, 506
    sterols in, 492, 500
Culcita schmideliana, 441
α-Curcumene-I, 286, 287
β-Curcumene, 286, 288, 289
γ-Curcumene, 286
Curvularia lunata, 233
Cyanidium caldarium, 460
    sterols in, 462
Cyathula capitata, 343
Cyclases, for squalene, 262–264
Cyclization
    circumventing ion pair, 274
    hydroxylative, 297–298
    of isopentenoids other than squalene,
        rules for, 274
    modes of, 318
    rules of, 234–236
Cycloartenol, 39, 67, 68, 70, 329, 331,
    332, 389, 510
    formation of, 241
    gas-liquid chromatography of, 136
    scheme of, 40
    structure of, 326
Cyclobranol, 70
Cycloeucalenol, 67, 70, 330, 503, 510
Cyclopropane ring, formation of,
    214, 215
1,2-Cyclopentanophenanthrene ring,
    38, 39
1,2-Cyclopentanoperhydrophenan-
    threne, 39
Cyclopentanoterpenoids, 277
Cyclosadol, 70
p-Cymene, 282, 287
α-Cyperone, absolute configuration of,
    300

D, usage of, defined, 52
Δ, significance of, 62

Dam, H., Nobel Prize of, 25–26
Dammaradienol, 243
Dandelion, 513
Darutigenol, absolute configuration of,
    311
DBED salt, 152
Dealkylation
    at C-24, 346–352
    role of 24(28)-expoxides in, 349–350
Dehydration, 116, 117, 119
Dehydroabietic acid, 306, 307
24,28-Dehydroaplysterol, 346
Dehydrocampesterol, 69
Dehydrocholesterol, 63, 69
7-Dehydrocholesterol, 543
    in beetle, 436
    in fruit fly, 435
    in nemathelminthes, 431
    reversed-phase chromatography of,
        131
    in sponges, 426
22-Dehydrocholesterol, 68, 352
    in coelenterates, 428, 429
24,25-Dehydrocholesterol, 326
25(27)-Dehydrochondrillasterol, 499,
    500, 506
Dehydroclionasterol, 70
25(27)-Dehydroclionasterol, 497, 500
7-Dehydrodihydrobrassicasterol, 70
22,23-Dehydrodesmosterol, 348
25(27)-Dehydrodihydrochondrillasterol,
    497, 499, 500
Dehydroepiandrosterone, 65, 577
    chemical tests for analysis of, 95
Dehydroepisterol, 69
7-Dehydro-Δ⁵-ergostenol, 70
Dehydrofungisterol, 69, 496
25(27)-Dehydrofungisterol, 497
Δ⁵-Dehydrogenase, 398
Dehydrogenation, at C-24, 346–352
22-Dehydrohalosterol, in marine
    annelid, 432
Dehydrojuvabione, 197
Dehydrolathosterol, 69
Dehydroporiferasterol, 70
25(27)-Dehydroporiferasterol, 499, 500
Dehydrositosterol, 70, 501
Dehydrostigmasterol, 70
Demethylation
    C-4, 355–360
    C-14, 360–366

23-Demethylgorgosterol, 346
Dennstaedtia punctilobula, dominant sterols in, 482
Deoxychollic acid, 591
Dermestes cadaverinus, 434
Dermestes vulpinus, 347, 433, 434, 537
24-Desalkylsterols, 63
Desmethyl, defined, 44
23-Desmethylgorgosterol, 428
Desmosterol, 68, 332, 343, 347, 348, 352, 374, 380, 442
    in brain development, 451–452
    and brain tumors, 453
    in red algae, 461
    reversed-phase chromatography of, 131
    in vertebrates, 443
Desoxycorticosterone, chemical tests for analysis of, 97
25-Deuterioisofucosterol, 340
24-Deuteriolanosterol, 340
Deuterosteryl acetate, fragmentation of, 117
Development, role of sterols in, 451–452
Dextropimaric acid, 304
    first isolated from rosin, 7
Diastereoisomer, defined, 51
Diatoms, 499, 508
    sterols in, 467–471
    see also species names
Diatomsterol, 66, 68, 433, 499
Dictyostelium discoideum, sterols in, 421
Diels, O. P. H., Nobel Prize of, 30
Diethylstilbestrol, 581
Digitalis lanata, 371, 561
    dominant sterols in, 487
Digitalis purpurea, 73, 76, 560
Digitogenin, 76
Digitonides, defined, 86
Digitonin, 76
Digitonin precipitation, 86–87
Digitoxigenin, 73, 74
Dihydrobactoprenol, 179, 193
Dihydrobrassicasterol, 64, 68, 495, 498
    in green algae, 473
    in plants, 482–484
Dihydrochondrillasterol, 64, 69, 496, 499
22-Dihydrochondrillasterol, 336

Dihydroergosterol, 70
Dihydrogibberellic acid, 310
Dihydrolanosterol, 67
    reversed-phase chromatography of, 131
24,25-Dihydrolanosterol, 326, 331, 332
    gas-liquid chromatography of, 136
Dihydrospinasterol, 69, 496, 498
    in plants, 482–484, 486–490, 492–493
Dihydrosqualene, in bacterium, 417
2,3-Dihydrosqualene, in bacteria, 331
5α-Dihydrotestosterone, 577
$3\alpha,11\beta$-Dihydroxy-5α-androstan-17-one, gas-liquid chromatography of, 137
2,3-Dihydroxy-1,3,5-estratrien-17-one, gas-liquid chromatography of, 137
$3,17\beta$-Dihydroxy-1,3,5-estratriene, gas-liquid chromatography of, 137
17α-21-Dihydroxy-20-keto system, 88–89
$3\alpha,20\alpha$-Dihydroxy-5α-pregnane, gas-liquid chromatography of, 138
$3\beta,21$-Dihydroxy-Δ^5-pregnen-20-one, R_s value for, 128
$11\beta,21$-Dihydroxy-Δ^4-pregnen-3,20-dione, R_s value for, 128
β,β-Dimethylacrylate, in steroid biosynthesis, 149, 154–155
Dimethylacrylic acid, 200
Dimethylallyl pyrophosphate, 161
22,24-Dimethylchola-5-en-3β-ol, 437
24,26-Dimethylcholesterol, in sponges, 427
Dinoflagellate sterols, and gorgonian sterols, 467, 468
Dinosterol, 467, 468
Dioscorea composita, 329
Dioscorea mexicana, 76
Dioscorea spiculifora, 154, 498
Dioscorea tokoro, 343
    dominant sterols in, 485
Dioscorea xanthocarpum, dominant sterols in, 484
Diosgenin, 76
Dipentene, 5, 9, 10
    role in elucidating cyclic terpene structures, 15
Diphyllobotrium latum, 430
Diplopterol, 248, 250, 251, 252, 420
Disease, and sterols, 453–458
Distolaterias sticantha, 440

Diterpenes
  cyclic, 17
  structure of, 17-18
DMA, see β,β-Dimethylacrylate
Doisy, E. A., Nobel Prize of, 25-26
Dolichodial, 278
  origin of, 282
Dolichols, 179, 182
Dominant sterols, 62-71
Double bonds
  analytical procedures, 92
  effects of, on stereochemistry, 47
  nomenclature for, 62
  protons on, 110-114
  UV absorption by, 102
  see also Conjugated double bonds;
    Unconjugated double bonds
Double isotope dilution, 123
Drosophila pachea, 413-414, 435, 552,
  553, 554
Dryopteris noveboracensis, dominant
  sterols in, 482
Dugesia dorotocephala, 378
Dustanin, 250

Eburical, 423
Eburicodiol, 423
Eburicoic acid, 40, 41, 333, 338, 423,
  424
Ecdysones, 588-590
Echinococcus granulosus, 378, 430
Echinoccoccus multilocularis, 430
Echinocystis macrocarpa, 308, 319
Echinoderms
  sterols in, 439-442
  see also species names
Echinus esculentus, 441
Eisenis bicydis, 466
Elaeis guineensis, 512
Elasterol, 69
Eledone aldrovandi, 438
Enantiomer, defined, 51
End apsorption, defined, 100
"ene," defined, 61
Enhydra fluctuans, 505
Enteromorpha intestinales, 474
Enteromorpha linea, 388
Enteromorpha linza, 474
Enzyme assays, 123-124
Enzymes, 394-399

  for demethylation at C-4, 395-397
  polymerizing, 184
Eperuic acid, 302, 311, 312
Epibrassicasterol, 433, 495
3-Epicholestanol, chemical test for
  analysis of, 94
3-Epi-5β-cholestanol, 53
20-Epi-5α-cholestanol, 53
Epidehydrofungisterol, 69
Epidermophyton floccosum, sterols in,
  422
Epiergosterol, 66, 70
  in plants, 482
Epifungisterol, 64, 69, 496
Epiikshusterol, 501
Epimer, defined, 51
Epischottenol, 496, 499
Episterol, 64, 69, 338, 385, 386
24(28)-Epoxides, role of, in dealkylation, 349-350
Equilenin, 41, 73, 581
Eremophilone
  absolute configuration of, 300
  methyl migration in biosynthesis of,
    295
Eremophilyl cation, 295
Ergostatetraenol, 338
Ergostanol, 68
Δ⁵-Ergostenol, 68
Δ⁷-Ergostenol, 69
Ergosterol, 66, 70, 328, 332, 333, 336,
  337, 338, 346, 347, 362, 370-371,
  385, 386, 543, 551
  in beetle, 436
  chemical tests for analysis of, 97
  in fungi, 421, 422
  in plants, 482-483
  in protozoa, 420
  reversed-phase chromatography of,
    131
Escherichia coli, sterols in, 417, 418
Estradiol, 581
  thin-layer chromatography of, 129
Estriol, 581
Estrogens, 72-73
  biosynthesis of, 582-584
  fragmentation of, 121
  isolation and function of, 578-580
  polarity of, 129
  structure-activity correlations,
    580-582

Estrone, 10, 11, 41, 73, 581
  chemical tests for analysis of, 99
  fragmentation of, 121
  thin-layer chromatography of, 129
24-Ethylcholestanol, 342
24α-Ethylcholestanol, 68
24β-Ethylcholestanol, 68
24-Ethylcholesterols, 64
24α-Ethylcholesterol, 413
  in housefly, 435
  see also Sitosterol
24ξ-Ethylcholesterol, 421
  in coelenterates, 428, 429
  in plants, 483
24-Ethylidenecholesterol, 328, 442
24-Ethylidenelanosterol, gas-liquid
  chromatography of, 136
Ethylidenelophenol, 510
24-Ethylidenelophenol, 340, 343
24-Ethylidenesterols, $\Delta^{24(28)}$ routes to,
  341
24-Ethylidine-7-lanosten-3β-ol, reversed-
  phase chromatography of, 131
24a-Ethyllanosterol, 436
24-Ethyllathosterol, in fungi, 422
24a-Ethyllathosterol, 498, 499
  in plants, 482
24α-Ethylsterols
  routes to, 397
  $\Delta^{24(28)}$-routes to, 341
24β-Ethylsterols
  possible sequences to, 391
  $\Delta^{24(28)}$-routes to, 341
  $\Delta^{25(27)}$-route to 342
Eucalyptus microcorys, 503
Euchinaster sepositers, 441
Eucoelomates, sterols in, 432-458
α-Eudesmol, 292
β-Eudesmol, 291, 292
  absolute configuration of, 300
Euglena gracilis, 329, 388, 393, 471,
  472
Euglenaphyta, 471-472
Euglenoids
  alkylation in, 340
  sterols in, 471-472
  see also species names
Eugoria ampla, 428
Eukaryotic algae
  red algae, 461-466
  sterols in, 461-479

see also specific kinds
Eukaryotic organisms
  brown algae, 466-467
  diatoms, 467-471
  euglenoids, 471-472
  golden-brown algae, 467-471
  green algae, 472-478
  yellow-brown algae, 467
  yellow-green algae, 467-471
Eupatorium perfoliatum, dominant
  sterols in, 487
Euphoid
  formation, from protoeuphoid cation,
  245
  vs. steroids, 38
Euphol, 39, 243
  configuration at C-20, 256
  scheme of, 40
Euphorbia obtusifolia, 503
Euphorbia peplus, 331
Euphorbia polygonifolia, dominant
  sterols in, 484
European alder, 513
Eurycotic floridana, 434
Eusteroids, defined, 43-44
Evodia rutaecarpa, 199
Exocyclic, defined, 102

Farnesene, 199
α-Farnesene, 291
β-Farnesene, 291
Farnesoic acid, 200
Farnesol, 9, 10, 81, 176, 181, 192
  in bacterium, 417
  structure of, 16
  synthesis of squalene from, 18
Farnesyl pyrophosphate
  cyclization of, 291, 297
  as γ-bisabolene precursor, 298-299
  as squalene precursor, 208, 211-216
Farnesyl pyrophosphate synthetase, 184
Fasciola hepatica, 430
Feces, sterols of, 444-445
Fecosterol, 70, 338, 385, 386
Felinine, 175, 198
Fenchol, 279
Fenchone, 279
Fern
  Christmas, 482
  cinnamon, 482

Fern—*continued*
  hay-scented, 482
  New York, 482
Fernene, 251
Ferruginol, 306, 307
Ficus elastica, 7
Fieser convention, in side chain
  nomenclature, 54
Finger print region, defined, 104–105
Firebrat, 347
Fish, sterol biosynthesis in, 442
Fluorescence, 104
Fomes applanatus, 421
Formate, 333
Fowlpox virus, sterols in, 415
Fragilaria sp., 469
Fragmentation, process of, 115–116,
  117, 118, 119, 121, 122
Framingham Study, 449, 450
Fremyella diplosiphon, 460
  sterols in, 463
French breakfast, 509
Friedelin, 250, 251
  formation, mechanism of, 257
Fucosterol, 65, 68, 338, 340, 347,
  348–349, 495
  in brown algae, 466–467
  reversed-phase chromatography of,
  131
Fucus spiralis, 338, 340, 360, 367, 388
Fucus vesiculosus, 466
Fundulus heteroclitus, 587
Fungi
  alkylation in, 337–339
  lanosterol pathway in, 329
  in lichens, 478–479
  sterol biosynthesis in, 383–387
  sterols in, 421–425
  see also Microorganisms; *species
    names*
Fungisterol, 64, 69, 336, 421, 496
  in green algae, 473
Furostane, 77
Fusarium moniliforme, 308
Fusidic acid, 238–239, 359, 423, 424
  formation, 240
Fusidium coccineum, 234, 359

Galactosides, 515
Gallstones, 453

Garnegiea gigantea, 388
Garryfoline, 312
  absolute configuration of, 311
Gas-liquid chromatography, 87, 126,
  131–137
Gelidium amansii, 464
Gelidium japonicum, 464
Genistein, 581
Gentiobiosides, 515
Gentiopicroside, 283, 285
Geranial, 197, 200
Geranioic acid, 200
Geraniol, 6, 14, 15, 82, 175, 181, 197,
  319, 543
Geranoic acid, 197
Geranylgeraniol, 177, 302
Geranylgeranyl pyrophosphate syn-
  thetase, 184
Geranyllinalool, 302, 304
Gibberella fujikara, 308, 319
Gibberellic acid, 308, 309, 310, 516
Gibberellins
  biosynthesis of, 308–310
  structural relationship of, to kaurenes,
    308–310
  structures of, 309
Ginkgo biloba, dominant sterols in, 482
Glioblastoma, 453, 454
Globulol, biosynthesis of, 296–297
Glucocorticoids, 72, 570
  secretion of, 572–575
Glucose, 515
Glyceraldehyde, absolute configuration
  of, 52
Glycine max, 516
  dominant sterols in, 483
Glycocholic acid, 592
Golden algae, alkylation in, 339
Golden-brown algae
  sterols in, 467–471
  see also species names
Gonads, and steroids, 3
Gonyaulax tamarensis, 467
Gorgonia tamarensis, 467
Gorgonia flabellum, 428
Gorgonia ventitian, 428
Gorgosterol, 346
  from coelenterates, 428
Gossypium hirsutum, dominant sterols
  in, 489
Gradient elution, 127

Granisterol, 69, 502, 503
Grantia compressa, 377, 427
Graphidostreptus tumuliporus, 434
Green algae
    alkylation in, 339
    sterols in 472-478
    see also species name
Guajazulene, 293
δ-Guajene-I, 292, 293
δ-Guajene-II, 292
Guajenyl cation, 292, 293
Guajol, 293

Haliclona coerulescens, 425
Haliclona (Chalina) oculata, 425
Haliclona permollis, 426
Haliclona rubens, 425
Haliclonasterol, 69, 256
Halimeda incrassata, 474, 475
Halobacterium cutirubum, 331
    sterols in, 417
Halocynthia roretzi, 352, 437, 442
Halosterol, 437, 442
Haplopappus heterophyllus, 560
Hartmannella, sterols in, 420
Hassel, O., Nobel Prize of, 32-33
Hazel, 513
Heartsease, 512
Heather, 513
Helianthus annus, 501, 513
    dominant sterols in, 486
Helminthosporum sativum, 319
Hench, P. S., Nobel Prize of, 28-29
Henrica sanguinolenta, 381, 441
Hepatomas, 454-455
Heracleum mantegazzianum, 199
Herpetomonas, sterols in, 420
Heteroannular, defined, 102
Heteroannular diene, in resin acid
    formation, 305
Hevea brasiliensis, 7, 159, 178
Hevea guianensis, 7
Hexahydropolyprenols, 179
αψω-Hexahydropolyprenol, 182
Hibiscus abelmoschus, 176
Hinokiol, 307
Hinokion, 306, 307
Hiochic acid, 152
Historia Animalium, 3
HMG, *see* β-Hydroxy-β-methylglutarate

Holarrhenna floribunda, 561
Holothuria tabulosa, 441
Homarus grammarus, 434
Homoallylic rearrangements, cyclization
    with, 295-296
Homoannular, defined, 102
Homoannular diene, in resin acid
    formation, 305
Hopene-b, 251
Hopenyl cation, formation of, 247
Hordeum vulgare, 339, 340, 343
    dominant sterols in, 484
Hormonal steroids, separation of,
    136-137, 138
Hormones, 557-590
    effects of, on target cell nuclei, 588
    fragmentations of, 119-122
    mammalian, metabolism of, 584-585
    metabolism of, by microorganisms,
        587-588
    nonmammalian, metabolism of, 587
    radioimmunoassay for, 140
    thin-layer chromatography of, 129
Human
    approximate cholesterol content in,
        446
    surface lipids of, 445
Humulene, 290, 299
Humulenyl cation, 289, 290
Humulus lupalus, 199
Hydrodictyon reticulatum, 474
Hydrophyllum capitatum, 513
3α-Hydroxy-5α-androstan-17-one, gas-
    liquid chromatography of, 137, 138
3α-Hydroxy-5β-androstan-17-one, gas-
    liquid chromatography of, 137, 138
3α-Hydroxy-5β-androstan-11,17-dione,
    gas-liquid chromatography of, 137
11β-Hydroxy-Δ⁴-androstene-3,17-dione,
    R_s value for, 128
17β-Hydroxy-Δ⁴-androsten-3-one, R_s
    value for, 128
3β-Hydroxy-5-androsten-17-one, gas-
    liquid chromatography of, 137, 138
17β-Hydroxy-4-androstene-3-one, gas-
    liquid chromatography of, 138
22-Hydroxycholesterol, 69
24β-Hydroxycholesterol, 443
26ξ-Hydroxycholesterol, in humans, 443
Hydroxyeremophilone, absolute con-
    figuration of, 300

3-Hydroxy-1,3,5-estratrien-17-one, gas-
liquid chromatography of, 137
Hydroxylation, in bile acid biosynthesis,
594
7α-Hydroxylation, 594
12α-Hydroxylation, 594
β-Hydroxy-β-methylglutarate
formation of, 156–157
reduction of, to mevalonic acid,
157–158
role of, in isopentenoid formation,
151
in steroid bionsynthesis, 154–155
Hydroxymethylglutarate CoA, 156–157
17α-Hydroxypregnenolone, 577
17α-Hydroxyprogesterone, 577
3α-Hydroxy-5α-pregnan-20-one, gas-
liquid chromatography of, 138
3β-Hydroxy-5α-pregnan-20-one, gas-
liquid chromatography of, 138
3α-Hydroxy-4-pregnen-20-one, gas-
liquid chromatography of, 138
3β-Hydroxy-Δ⁵-pregnen-20-one, R_s
value for, 128
17α-Hydroxy-Δ⁴-pregnene-3,20-dione,
R_s value for, 128
18-Hydroxy-Δ⁴-pregnene-3,20-dione, R_s
value for, 128
20α-Hydroxy-Δ⁴-pregnene-3,20-dione,
R_s value for, 128
21-Hydroxy-Δ⁴-pregnene-3,20-dione,
R_s value for, 128
6β-Hydroxy-Δ⁴-pregnene-3,20-dione,
R_s value for, 128
11β-Hydroxy-Δ⁴-pregnene-3,20-dione,
R_s value for, 128
20β-Hydroxy-Δ⁴-pregnene-3,20-dione,
R_s value for, 128
Hymeniacidon perleve, 426
Hymenolopsis diminuta, 430
Hypnea japonica, 464
Hypochaeris radiata, 513

I₃ bicycles, 287–295
I chains, bound through C—C links,
180
I classification, 80–82
I₁ compound, 81
I₂ compounds
bicyclic, origins of, 293

cyclized, metabolism of, 282–284
I₃ compound, 81
absolute configurations of, 300
I₃-I₃ compound, 81
I₄ compounds
tetracyclic, 307
tricyclic, 308–310
I nomenclature, 172–174
I₂ stage
cyclization at, 273–284
mechanism of, 273–279
stereochemistry of, 279–282
enzymology at, 319
I₃ stage
cyclization at, 284–301
mechanism, 284–287
enzymology at, 319
stereochemistry at, 298–301
I₄ stage
bi- and tricycles at, probable origin
of, 304
cyclization and metabolism at,
301–313
enzymology at, 319–320
stereochemistry at, 310–313
I₃ Tricycles, 287–295
Ikshusterol, 501
Imino derivatives, 88
Indosterol, 70, 501, 502
Influenza virus, cholesterol in, 415
Inlet temperature, 117
Insects
dietary sterols in, 433, 434
ecdysone action in, 588–589
need for cholesterol in, 346–347
nuclear double-bond transformations
by, 381
see also Arthropods; *species names*
Intestine, sterol synthesis in, 445
Invertebrate route, of sterol biosynthesis, 377–383
Invertebrates
annelids, 432–433
arthropods, 433–436
echinoderms, 439–442
molluscs, 436–439
sterols in, 432–442
Ips confusus, 197
Iresin, 297, 298, 299, 300
Iridodiol, 278, 283
Iridomyrmecin, 277, 278

Iridomyrmex humulis, 277
Isoborneol, 281
Isocaproic acid, 558
Isofucosterol, 65, 68, 340, 343, 348,
    466, 495, 499, 501, 510
    in plants, 483, 485, 486-491
Isoguajenyl cation, 292, 293
Isohelenalin, 293
Isokaurene, 308
Isomenthone, 279, 280
Δ^8-Isomerase, 397-398
Isopentane, 82
Isopentanol, 82
Isopentenoid
    classification of, 80-81
    first chemical isolation of, 4
    formation, role of mevalonic acid in,
        153-155
    role of acetoacetate in formation of,
        150-151
Isopentenoid polymers, *see* Polymers
Isopentenoid precursors, absolute con-
    figuration of, 161-162
Δ^2-Isopentenol, 81, 175
Δ^3-Isopentenol, 175
Isopentenylation, 191-192, 206
Isopentenyl pyrophosphate
    cis-conformer of, 163-164
    stereochemistry of formation of, 165
Δ^3-Isopentenyl pyrophosphate
    conversion of mevalonate to, 159-161
    interconversion with Δ^2-isopentenyl
        pyrophosphate, 161
Isophyllocladene, 308
Isoprene, 199
Isoprene rule, 147-148
    proposal of, 8
    statement of, 9
    ways in which compounds follow, 9
Isoprenoid, 147-149
    defined, 9
Isopropyl cation, tricyclic, 305
Isopropylidene hydrocarbon, in resin
    acid formation, 305
IUPAC, systematic nomenclature of,
    57-71

Jervine, 79, 80
Juniperus utahensis, 512
Jurubidine, 77, 78

Juvabione, 196, 197
Juvenile hormone, 194-196

Kalanchoe daigremontiana, 499, 505,
    506
    sterols in, 500
Kalmia latifolia, dominant sterols in,
    483
Karrer, P., Nobel Prize of, 22
Kaurene, 257, 258, 307, 308, 312
    enantiomers of, 310
    structural relationship of, to
        gibberellins, 308, 310
Kaurenol, 307, 308
Kaurenyl cation, 307, 308
Kendall, E. C., Nobel Prize of, 27-28
11-Keto-androstan-17β-ol, chemical
    tests for analysis of, 99
12-Ketocholanic acid acetate, PMR
    spectra, 111
20,21-Ketol system, 89
Ketones, 88-92
Δ^4-3-Ketones, 111
    fragmentation of, 122
3-Ketones, PMR spectra, 111
17-Ketones, 89-92
Kiganene, 288, 289
Kiganol, 288, 289
Kiganyl cation, 288, 289
Krebs cycle, 354
Kuhn, R., Nobel Prize of, 22-23

L, usage of, defined, 52
Labdanolic acid, 302, 304, 311, 312
Labyrinthula vitellina, 538
Lactaroviolin, 293
Lactobacillic acid, 346
Lactobacillus acidophilus, 151, 152,
    162, 416
Lactobacillus bulgaricus, 417
Lactobacillus casei, 179, 181
Lactobacillus heterohiochi, 152
Lactobacillus homohiochi, 152
Lactuca sativa, dominant sterols in, 490
Laister leachii, 381, 441
Lanceol, 286, 299, 300
    origin of, 287
Lanostanol, 68
Lanosterol, 39, 67, 70, 164, 355, 360,
    361, 367, 374, 385, 386, 443

Lanosterol—*continued*
formation of, 241
gas-liquid chromatography of, 136
in nemathelminthes, 431
in photosynthetic plants, 328
reversed-phase chromatography of, 131
scheme of, 40
in squalene formation, 231
structure of, 326
Lanosterol-cycloartenol bifurcation, 328–331
and organismic type, 329–330
Larix decidua, 342, 371
Lathosterol, 63, 69, 328, 368, 369, 375, 389, 442
in fruit fly, 435
in molluscs, 436
in plants, 482, 492, 498
in vertebrates, 443
reversed-phase chromatography of, 131
24-C_1 and 24-C_2, with and without Δ^{22}-bond, 496
Laurel, 483
Lavandulol, 206
Leaves, as source of sterols, 508
Lecithin-cholesterol acyltransferase, 457
Lepidochitona cinerea, 438
Leptomonas, sterols in, 420
Leptosphaeria typhae, 421
Lettuce, 490
Levopimaric acid, 305
Liagosterol, 461
Lichens, sterols in, 478–479
Lichesterol, 479
Limonene, 5, 15, 197, 257, 258, 273, 279, 280
Linalool, 6, 15, 176, 181
Linckia multiflora, 441
Linderina pennispora, 421
Linoleic acid, 511, 515
Linolenic acid, 515
Linseed, 490
Linum usitatissimum, dominant sterols in, 490
Liolophura japonica, 379, 438
Lipidosis, 453
Lipoprotein, 450, 451
Liquid-liquid chromatography, 127–129
Liquid phases, nature and effect of, 132–133
Liquid-solid chromatography, 129–131
Liriodendron tulipifera, dominant sterols in, 483
Lissodendoryx noxiosa, 426
Liver
sterol synthesis in, 445
tumors, and sterols, 454–455
Lobaria pulmonaria, 479
Lobaria scrobiculata, 479
Locusta migratoria L., 348, 350
Loganic acid, 278, 284
Loganin, origin of, 283, 284
Lombardy poplar, 513
London-rocket, 512
Longifolene, metabolism of, 294
Lophenol, 67, 69, 375, 382, 502, 503
Lophocereus schottii, 413, 436, 499, 502
Lophocolea heterophylla, 480
Lumbricus spencer, 432
Lumbricus terrestris, 379, 432
Lumisterol, 606–607, 608
Lupeol, formation of, 248
Lupenyl cation, 248–250
Lupinus albus, 248
Lycopene, 6
cyclization of, 313–319
products of, 314
Lycopersene, biosynthesis of, 220
Lycopodium clavatum, 252
Lycopodium complanatum, 494
dominant sterols in, 482
Lynen, F., Nobel Prize of, 31
Lymnaea stagnalis, 438
Lysastrosoma anthostictha, 440

Maaliol, 296
absolute configuration of, 300
Macdougallin, 41, 70, 375, 501
Macrocycle, 14-membered, probable origin of, 302
Magnetogyric ratio, 108
Malonate, in mevalonate biosynthesis, 156
Malus sylvestris, 513
Mammalian hormones, metabolism of, 584–585
Mammalian route, of sterol biosynthesis, 374–376
Mammals, lanosterol pathway in, 329

Manduca sexta, 348, 434
Mannosides, 515
Manool, 302
  absolute configuration of, 311
  tricycle from, 303, 304
Manoyl cation, 302
Manoyl oxide, 302, 304
Marathasterone, 440
Marrubin, 304
Marthasterias glacialis, 441
Matricaria chamomilla, 299
Matricaria indora, 199
May apple, 483
Mayorella, sterols in, 420
Medicago sativa, 343
Melampsora lini, 422
Membranes
  isolation of steroids from, 538–539
  sterols in, 537–557
Menthofuran, 282
Menthol, 281–282, 283
Menthone, 279, 280, 282, 283
Δ^{24}-Metabolase, 332
Methionine, 333
2-Methoxy-3-hydroxy-1,3,5-estratrien-
  17-one, gas-liquid chromatography
  of, 137
3-Methyl-Δ^3-butenyl pyrophosphate, *see*
  Δ^3-Isopentenyl pyrophosphate
24α-Methylcholestanol, 68
24β-Methylcholestanol, 68
24-Methylcholesterols, 64, 339, 510
  in vegetable oils, 481
24α-Methylcholesterol, 498
  in housefly, 435
24β-Methylcholesterol, 336
24ξ-Methylcholesterol
  in coelenterates, 428–429
  in fungi, 421
  in plants, 483–485, 486–491
24ξ-Methyl-22-dehydrocholesterol, in
  coelenterates, 428, 429
β-Methylcrotonate, *see* β,β-Dimethyl-
  acrylate
β-Methylcrotonic acid, 200
24-Methylene-5-cholestene-3β-ol, reversed-phase chromatography of, 131
24-Methylenecholest-4-en-3-one, in
  sponge, 426, 427
Methylenecholesterol, 68, 495, 510
  in plants, 486, 490

24-Methylenecholesterol, 339, 340, 348,
  351, 442
  in bees, 435
  in coelenterates, 428, 429
  in sponge, 426
Methylenecycloartanol, 67, 503
24-Methylenecycloartanol, 331, 332,
  340
  gas-liquid chromatography of, 136
24-Methylene-8-lanosten-3β-ol, reversed-phase chromatography of, 131
24-Methylenelanosterol, 503
  gas-liquid chromatography of, 136
Methylenelathosterol, in plants, 486,
  492–493, 496
Methylenelophenol, 510
24-Methylenelophenol, 340
4α-Methylergosta-8,24(28)-dien-3β-ol,
  338
Methyl groups
  elimination from C-4, 355–360
  elimination from C-14, 360–366
  nuclear magnetic spectroscopy of,
    110
29-Methylisofucosterol, 346
Methyl isohexyl ketone, 11, 12
Methyllathosterol, in plants, 498
24-Methyllathosterols, 64
24ξ-Methyllathosterol, in plants,
  482–484, 486, 492
Methyl migration, cyclization at I_3
  stage with, 295
Methylococcus capsulatus, 262
  sterols in, 417, 418
4α-Methyl sterols, in higher plants, 330
24α-Methylsterols, route to, in tracheophytes, 396
24β-Methylsterols, $\Delta^{24(28)}$ route to, 338
24ξ-Methylsterols, in bacterium, 417
L-Methyl-succinic acid, 280
Metridium senile, 378, 429, 430
Mevaldic acid, 157–158
Mevalonate
  biosynthesis of corticorsteroids from,
    154
  conversion of, to Δ^3-isopentenyl
    pyrophosphate, 159–161
  biosynthesis of, 155–158
  discovery of, 151
  reduction of hydroxymethyl glutarate
    to, 157–158

Mevalonate—*continued*
    structure and properties of, 152
Mevalonic kinase, 160
Micrococcus lysodeikticus, 178, 181,
    184, 193, 194
Micromonospora sp., sterol mixture in,
    417
Microorganisms, hormone metabolism
    by, 587–588
Micropterus salmoides, 442
Microsporum, steroids in, 422
Mineralocorticoids, 72, 571
Mirene, 312
Mirror image, defined, 51
Mobile phase, defined, 126
Molar extinction coefficient, 101
Molds, *see specific names*
Molecular ion, 114
Molecular weight, determination of, 98
Molluscs
    sterols in, 436–439
    see also species names
Molting hormone, 196
Monocycles, formation of, 301
Monodonta turbinata, 438
Monodus subterraneus, 338, 342, 467
Mosses, 479–480
Mucor pusillus, 337, 423
Mule fat, 512
Muricea appressa, 428
Musa sapientum, 393
    dominant sterols in, 483
Musca domestica, 347, 435
Musca vicina, 434
Mussel, 439
Mustard, 512
MVA, *see* Mevalonic acid
Mycobacterium bovis, 417
Mycobacterium smegmatis, 334, 417
Mycobacterium tuberculosis, 417
Mycobacterium sp., 223, 224
Mycophenolic acid, 335
Mycoplasma arthritidis, sterol
    requirements of, 543
Mycoplasma gallinarum, 415
Mycoplasma mycoides, 556
Mycoplasmas
    sterols in, 415–416
    sterol requirements of, 543
Myeloblastosis virus, chlolesterol in,
    415

Myocarpus fronsosus, 176
Myrcene, 199, 291
Myrospernum erythroxylon, 176
Mytilus californianus, 380
Mytilus edulis, 380, 381, 439

Naphthalene acetic acid, and sterol bio-
    synthesis, 516
Nardoa varilata, 441
Narthecium ossifragum, 501
Nasutitermes rippertii, 435
Natica cataena, 439
Navicula pelleculosa, 469
Nematodes, dietary sterol requirement
    of, 347
Nemathelminthes
    sterols in, 431
    see also species names
Neoabietic acid, 305
    absolute configuration of, 311
Neodiprion pratti, 434
Nepetalactone, 198
Nepta cataria, 198
Nereis diversicolor, 379, 432
Nereis pelagica, 379
Neral, 200
Nerol, 82, 176, 181, 273, 319
Nerolidol, 176, 299, 302
    "α-form," 176
Nerolidyl pyrophosphate, 211, 304
    biosynthesis, 212
    as γ-bisabolene precursor, 298–299
    cyclization of, 290–291
Neurospora crassa, 220, 421
Neurosporene
    cyclization of, 313–319
    structure of, 313, 314
New York fern, 498
Nicotiana langsdorffii, dominant sterols
    in, 487
Nicotiana suaveolens, dominant sterols
    in, 487
Nicotiana tabacum, 329, 331, 338, 340,
    343, 344, 371, 387
    dominant sterols in, 484
Nippostrongyllus brasiliensis, 431
Nitella flexilis, 475
Nitzschia alba, 468, 469
Nitzschia closterium, 469
Nitzschia frustulum, 469

Nitzschia longissima, 468
Nitzschia ovalis, 468, 469
Nonphotosynthetic organisms
  less advanced
    bacteria, 416–418
    coelenterates, 428–430
    fungi, 421–425
    mycoplasmas, 415–416
    nemathelminthes, 431
    protozoa, 419–420
    slime molds, 421
    sponges, 425–427
    sterols in, 415–431
    viruses, 415
  more advanced
    annelids, 432–433
    arthropods, 433–436
    echinoderms, 439–442
    invertebrates, 432–442
    molluscs, 436–439
    sterols in, 432–458
    vertebrates, 442–458
Nor, defined, 46
24-Norcholesterol, 352
30-Norcycloartenol, 330
30-Norcyclolaudenol, 330
Nostoc commune, 460
  sterols in, 462
Nystatin, 540

Obtusifoliol, 67, 70, 338, 340, 503, 510
Occelasterol, 432, 437
Ochromonas danica, 372, 388, 469
Ochromonas malhamensis, 263, 329,
  331, 338, 339, 340, 342, 343, 344,
  367, 371, 372, 388, 389, 390, 469
Ocimene, 199, 291
Ocimum gratissimum, 199
Octopus vulgaris, 438
"oic," defined, 61
Oil palm, 512
"ol," defined, 61
Olea europaea, dominant sterols in,
  489
Oleate, 510
Olefin alkylation, 184
Oleic acid, 510, 515
Oligoprenols, 181, 192
  natural, 200
Oligoprenyl hydrocarbons, natural

acyclic, 199
Olive, 489
Omphalea diandra, 200
"one," defined, 61
α-Onocerin, 252
Ononis spinosa, 252
Oocystis polymorpha, 387, 474
Optical antipode, defined, 51
Optical rotatory dispersion, 100, 122
Osmunda cinnamomea, dominant
  sterols in, 482
Ostrea gryphea, 347, 381
Ostrea sp., 380
Ostreasterol, 65, 68, 425, 461, 495, 501

Palm, dominant sterols in, 488
Palmitic acid, 515
Palmitoleic acid, 510
Palythoa tuberculosa, 492
Panagrellus redivivus, 378, 431
Panulirus japonicus, 434
Paper chromatography, defined, 126
Paramecium aurelia, 538, 552, 553, 554
  sterol requirement of, 419
Parent systems, in nomenclature, 57–61
Parkeol, 70, 503
Parthenium argentatum, 149
Partition, 124
Partition coefficient, 124
Patchouliol, 292, 293
Patinosterol, 437
Pea, 483
  see also species names
Peanut, dominant sterols in, 488
Pelargonium hortorum, 508
Penaeus japonicus, 347, 434
Penicillium claviforme, 421, 422
Peniocereus fosterianus, 501
Peniocereus macdougalli, 501
Peniocerol, 70, 501, 502
Peptidoglycan, 193
Peposterol, 501
  in plants, 486, 492
Peranema trichophorum, 471
Perezone, 286, 287
Perilla alcohol, 279
Perilla aldehyde, 279
Perivine, 284
Persea gratissima, 481
Phaeodactylum tricornutum, 339, 469

Phaeophyta, 466–467
Phaseolus aureus, 516
Phaseolus vulgaris, 329, 511
  dominant sterols in, 491
Phellandral, 279
Phellandrene, 5
α-Phellandrene, 279, 280
β-Phellandrene, 279
Phenanthrene, polycyclic system of, 39
Pheromones, 196–200
  aggregating, 196
  alarm, 196, 197, 198
  insect, 197–198
  recruiting, 196, 197, 198
  sex, 197
Phleum pratense, 512
Phormidium luridum, 458–459, 460
  sterols in, 462
Phosfon, 320
Phosphomevalonic kinase, 160
Photosynthetic organisms
  less advanced
    euglenoids, 471–472
    eukaryotic algae, 461–479
    green algae, 472–478
    lichens, 478–479
    prokaryotic organisms, 458–460
    sterols in, 458–479
  more advanced
    bryophyta, 479–480
    sterols in, 479–517
    tracheophytes, 480–517
Phycomyces blakesleeanus, 224, 320,
  328, 338, 384, 385, 423
Phyllocladene, 307, 308, 312
  absolute configuration of, 311
Physalia physalis, 429
Physarum polycephalum, sterols in, 421
Physostigma venenosum, 481
Phytanic acid, 200
Phytoene, 313, 316
  biosynthesis of, 219–224
    enzymology of, 222
    stereochemistry of, 222–224
  structure of, 313, 314
Phytoene synthetase, 222
Phytofluene, structure of, 313, 314
Phytol, 17, 179, 181, 192, 333
Phytophthora cactorum, 551
Pieris brassica, 434
"Pill," 565, 567

Pimenta acris, 199
Pincsterol, 68
Pinene, 5
α-Pinene, 197, 257, 258, 279, 280
  biosynthesis of, 275–276
  role in elucidating cyclic terpene
    structures, 15
  Wagner-Meerwein rearrangement
    of, 14
β-Pinene, 15, 16, 279
"Pinene hydrochloride," 13
Ping pong mechanism, 158
Pinus longifolia, 319
Pinus mugo, 513
Pinus nigra austriaca, 275
Pinus pinea, 328, 329, 331, 332, 338,
  339, 340, 342, 394, 499
  dominant sterols in, 483
Pinus radiata, 273
Pinus sylvestris, 513
Piper cubeba, 7
Piperitone, 279, 280
  metabolism of, 282
Piperitenone oxide, 282
Pisum sativum, 319, 331, 480, 515
  dominant sterols in, 483
Pithophora sp., 475
Placopecten magellanicus, 346, 352,
  436
Placosterol, 426, 437
Planobarius corneus, 438
Plants
  category I-A, 486–491, 505, 508
  category I-B, 492–493, 506
  category II, 500, 508
  category II-A, 505–506
  category II-B, 506
  category III, 506, 507
  gibberellins in, 308
  sterol features at different develop-
    mental stages, 506–509
  see also; Photosynthetic organisms,
    Nonphotosynthetic organisms,
    specific names
Plasmodiophora brassicae, 421
Plastoquinone-n, 180
Platinopecten yessoensis, 437
Platyhelminthes
  sterols in, 430–431
  see also species names
Platysamia cecropia, 194

Plexaura flexuosa, 428
Plexaura sp., 428
PMR, *see* Proton magnetic resonance
Podocarpic acid, 306, 307
Podocarpus ferrugineus, 310
Podocarpus nakii, 588
Podophyllum peltatum, dominant
    sterols in, 483
Polar, defined, 127
Polarimetry, 122-123
Pollen, sterol composition of, 510,
    512-513
Pollinastanol, 68, 387, 389, 503, 504
Polygonum sp., 512
Polymerization
    mechanisms, 184-187
        alternative, 186
Polymers
    biochemical role of, 191-200
    biosynthesis of, 182-191
    formation, 183
    isopentenoid, relationship to other
        polymers, 174
    naturally occurring, 174-182
    "normal arrangement," 172
    stereochemistry, 188-191
    structure and nomenclature, 171-174
Polypodium vulgare, 251, 336, 359,
    360, 379, 393
Polyporenic acid C, 423, 424
Polyprenols, 180
Polystichum acrostichoides, dominant
    sterols in, 482
Populus balsamifera, 199, 299
Populus fremontii, 513
Populus nigra, 513
Poriferastanol, 68
Poriferasterol, 66, 68, 338, 342, 387,
    388, 425, 495, 499, 506
    in green algae, 473
Porphyridium cruentum, 388, 464
Porter-Silber reaction, 88
Portunus trituberculatus, 434
Poststeroid, formation of, 242
Prefixes, in nomenclatures, 62
Pregnanediol, thin-layer chromato-
    graphy of, 129
Δ^4-Pregnene-3,11,20-trione, R_s value
    for, 128
Δ^4-Pregnene-3,20-dione, R_s value for,
    128

Prephytoene pyrophosphate, as caro-
    tenoid precursor, 224
Persqualene pyrophosphate, 223
    as squalene intermediate, 208-211,
        212-216
Previtamin D, 75
Progesterone, 71, 543
    in animals, 557-560
    in bees, 435
    chemical tests for analysis of, 96
    function of, 562-568
    mammalian metabolism of, 566
    NMR absorption, 111
    in plants, 560-562
    thin-layer chromatography of, 129
Progestogens, 71
Prokaryotic organisms
    sterols in, 458-460
    see also species names
(E)-24-Propylidenecholesterol, 437
(Z)-24-Propylidenecholesterol, in
    sponge, 426
Prosopis spicigera, dominant sterols in,
    486
Protoeuphoid, formation of, from
    protoeuphoid cation, 244
Protoeuphoid cation, 243-246
    formation of, 244
Proton magnetic resonance, 254-255
    absorption, of steroidal methyl
        protons, 113
    spectra
        effect of changes in steroid struc-
            ture on, 111
        of common sterols, 112
Protons
    on carbon atoms bearing a hydroxyl
        group, 114
    on double bonds, 110-114
    steroidal methyl, PMR absorption of,
        113
Protoreaster lincki, 441
Protoreaster nodosus, 441
Protosteroid cation
    defined, 42
    evidence for, 238-239
    formation of, 236-238
    origin of, 260
    steroid formation from, 239-242
        evidence for, 242-243
Protosteroids, defined, 43

Protosterols
  in fungi, 423–424
  defined, 43
Protozoa
  sterols in, 419
  see also species names
Provitamin D, 75, 608–610
Pseudomonas testosteroni, 587
Pseudopotamilla occelata, 432
Pseudopterogorgia americana, 428
Puccinia grammis, 422
Puccinia striiformis, 422
Pulegone, 280, 282, 283
Pullularia pullulous, 421
Pumpkin, 506
  see also species names
Pyrophosphomevalonic anhydrodecar-
  boxylase, 161
Pyrrhyophyta, 467

Quinine, 284, 285
Quinone cofactors, 191–192

Radioactive assay, 123
Radioimmunoassay, 137–140
Rapeseed, 489, 509
  see also Brassica rapa
Radical ion, 115
Raphanus sativus, 509
Red algae
  sterols in, 461–466
  sterols of (table), 465
  see also species names
Red clover, 512
Δ⁷-Reductase, 398
Δ²⁴-Reductase, 394–395
Reduction, mechanism of, 333–335
Refsum's disease, 200
Reichstein, T., Nobel Prize of, 29–30
Reinitzer, F., determination of formula
  for cholesterol by, 4
Reserpine, 284, 285
Resin acids, probable origin of, 305
Resonance, defined, 108
Resonance frequency, defined, 108
Retene, 17, 18
Retention time
  defined, 132
  relative, defined, 133
Reversed-phase chromatography, 126,
  130

Rhesus monkey, cholesterol level in,
  449
Rhizostoma sp., 378, 429
Rhodophyta, 461–466
Rhodospirillum rubrum, squalene in,
  417
Rhodymenia palmata, 354, 387, 388,
  391, 464
Rice, dominant sterols in, 488
Ricinus communis L., 301
Ricinus communis, 319
Rimuene, 10, 11, 304
  metabolites of, 304–305, 306
Rings, letter designations of, 44–45
Robinson, R., Nobel Prize of, 26–27
Robinson hypothesis, for cyclization of
  squalene, 230
Roccus saxtilis, 442
Rotational isomers, defined, 48
Δ²⁴⁽²⁸⁾-Route, to 24β-methylsterols, 338
Δ²⁵⁽²⁷⁾-Route, to 24β-methylsterols,
  336–337
R, S notation, 53
Rubber, 178
  discovery of, 6–7
  pyrolysis of, 8
Ruzicka, L., extension of isoprene rule
  by, 12–13
Ruzicka, L., Nobel Prize of, 24–25
Rye, 512
Rytiphlea tinctoria, 464

SAM, see S-Adenosylmethionine
S-Adenosylhomocysteine, 335
S-Adenosylmethionine, in alkylation,
  335
Sabinene, 279
Saccharomyces cerevisiae, 328, 421, 422
Saccharomyces sp., 384, 385, 386
Saccharum officinarum, 501
  dominant sterols in, 486
Saguaro cactus, 512
Salix sp., 513
Salmo gairdneri, 587
Salmonella, 178, 181
Salmonella anatum, 193
Salvia sclarea, 199
Samandarine, 77, 80
Sandaracopimaradiene, 304
Santene, 10, 11

Santonin, 291
  absolute configuration of, 300
Sapogenins, 76-77
Sargassum ringgoldianum, 466
Sargasterol, 69, 256, 466
Saringasterol, 69
Saxidomus gigantea, 381
Saxidomus giganteus, 439
Scallops
  sterols of, 436-437, 438
  see also species names
Scarelinius erythrophthalmus, 442
Scenedesmus obliquus, 332, 335, 336, 474
Schistosoma mansoni, 430
Schottenol, 64, 69, 436, 496, 498, 499
Scilla maritima, 74
Scillirosidin, 74
Scinaia sp., 461
Sclareol, 302, 304
Scleroderma aurantium, 423, 441
Scotch pine, 513
Screening parameter, 108
Scymnol, 74, 75
Sea cucumbers, 439
Sea lilies, 439
Sea urchins, 439
  Δ^7-sterols in, 441
Sebum, sterols in, 445
Secale cereale, 512
Secologanin, 283, 285
Second Law of Thermodynamics, 182
Selinene
  eremophilyl cation derived from, 295
  metabolism of, by hydroxylation, 292
α-Selinene, 291
  absolute configuration of, 300
β-Selinene, 291, 299
Selinyl cation, 291
Selinyl ring system, origin of, 291
Senecio kaempferi, 200
Sepia officinales, 378, 438
Sequence Rule, 53
Serine, 333
Serpentine, 284
Serratene, 250
Serum cholesterol
  and arteriosclerosis, 455-457
  and diet, 449-450
  levels
    age dependence of, 447, 448,

452-453
    effect of weaning on, 449
    normal, 447
Seseli indicum, 501
Sesquibenihiol, 291, 292
Sesquiterpene structure, 16
Sesquiterpenes, first discovery of, 7
Side chain
  configurational nomenclature for, 54-56
  fragmentations of, 119
  oxidation and scission of, 597-598
Siloxanes, 132
Sisymbrium irio, 512
Sitostanol, 68
Sitosterol, 64, 68, 338, 343, 347, 348, 350, 371, 378, 380, 416, 481-494, 495, 498, 504, 508, 510, 543
  β-sitosterol, 495
  γ-sitosterol, 442-443
  in bees, 435
  in coelenterates, 428
  in plants, 482-485, 486-491
  reversed-phase chromatography of, 131
  structure of, 18-19
  in vegetable oils, 481
Skytanthine, 277, 278
Skytanthus actus Meyen, 277
Slime mold
  alkylation in, 341-342
  sterols in, 421
  see also species names
Sobrerol, 279
Soladulcidine, 77, 79
Solanesol, 177, 181, 543
Solanidine, 77, 79
Solanum dulcamara, 498
  dominant sterols in, 490
Solanum melongeana, 481
Solanum tuberosum, 243, 498
Solanum xanthocarpum, 501
Solasodine, 77, 78
Solaster papposus, 383
Solvent systems, 127-129
Sorghum vulgare, 516
  dominant sterols in, 486
Soybean, 483
Spanish moss, 486, 502
Spatial convention of solid and interrupted lines, 51

Spectroscopy
  infrared, 98
    principles of, 104-105
  mass, 98
    principles of, 114-115
  nuclear magnetic resonance, 98
    principles of, 108-110
  ultraviolet, principles of, 100-101
Spermatogenesis, 578
Spinacea oleracea, 340, 343, 498, 499
  sterols in, 492
Spinasterol, 66, 69, 340, 343, 371, 474,
    496, 499, 506, 500
  in plants, 492-493
  reversed-phase chromatography of,
    131
Spirocodon saltatrix, 429
Sprioketals, 76
Spirostanes, 56, 76
Spirulina platensis, Mao I and Mao II,
    sterols in, 462
Spirulina sp., sterols in, 462
Sponges
  sterols in, 425-427
  see also species names
Spongesterol, 425
Squalene, 162, 164, 333, 543
  asymmetric conformation of, 258-260
  in bacteria, 416, 417
  biosynthesis of, 208-218
  mechanism of condensation and
    reduction, 211-216
  as I_3-I_3 compound, 81
  cyclization of
    enzymology of, 262-264
    hydroxylation in, 232-234
    Robinson hypothesis, 230
    rules of, 235-236
    summary of, 264-267
  direct cyclization of, 250-251
  discovery of, 18
  folding pattern, 231
  gas-liquid chromatography of, 136
  isopentenoid character of, 148
  from [2-^{14}C] MVA, 153
  mono- and bicyclic metabolism of,
    251-253
  in nemathelminthes, 431
  in sponge, 427
Squalene synthetase, in squalene
    formation, 217-219

Squalene oxide
  asymmetric conformation of, 260-261
  cyclization of, 326
    to euphol and sterols, 254,
      255-256
  role of, in cyclization of squalene,
    232-234
Squalene oxidase, 262
Stanols, fragmentation of, 118
Staphylococcus aureus, 219
Staphylococcus sp., squalene in, 417
Starfish, 439
  sterols in, 440
Stationary phase, defined, 126
Stearic acid, 515
Stella clarella, steroids in, 426
Stereochemistry, 46-56, 161-165
  of elimination to form C_5 units, 162
  of isomerization of C_5 units, 162-165
Steroids
  absolute configuration of, 51-54
  activities of, in capon's comb assay,
    578, 579
  adrenocortical, 71, 568-575
  biological classification of, 71-75
  biosynthetic relationship of, to other
    isopentenoids, 147-150
  C_{18}, 73
  C_{19}, 72
  C_{21}, 72
  as carcinogen precursors, 458, 459
  chemical analysis, 85-97
  cis-anti-trans-anti-trans structure of,
    549
  classification
    biosynthetic basis for, 42-44
    structural basis for, 37-42
  configurational convention, 50
  defined, 42
  derivation of term, 37-38
  difficulty in synthesizing, 18-19
  dominant, structure of, 326, 327
  Fiesers' definition of, 38
  hormonal, separation of, 136-137,
    138
  intermediates for biosynthesis of, 191
  isopentenoidal, role of, in adrenal
    and gonadal function, 3
  membraneous, elongation of,
    548-550
  naming, 57-71

nomenclature of, 57–71
  double and triple bonds, 62
  parent systems, 57–61
  prefixes, 62
  suffixes, 61–62
relative configuration of, 51
of sponges, 425–427
stereochemistry at C-20, 253–256
trans-anti, structures of, 548
x-ray diffraction patterns, 47
$\Delta^{5,7}$-steroids, and Vitamin D, 75
Steroid nucleus, 51
Steroid skeleton, flat condition of, 46–47
Steroid transition, defined, 42
Steroidal alkaloids, 77–79
Steroidal ethers, behavior of, in gas-liquid chromatography, 137
Sterols
  absence of, in bacteria, 417, 418
  absorption of, from diet, 450
  acetate as precursor of, 149
  24-alkenyl, 331
  biosynthesis of
    in algae, 387–393
    in fungi, 383–387
    in invertebrates, 377–383
    in mammals, 374–376
    in tracheophytes, 393
  in blue-green algae, 462–463
  chromatographic behavior of, in reversed-phase system, 131
  defined, 44
  in development, 451–452
  and disease, 453–458
  dominant, 62–71
  fragmentations of, 116–119
  fungal, 421–425
  inter-organismic distribution of, 413–414
  isolation of, from membranes, 538–539
  as membraneous components, 536–557
  in membranes
    model system structure-activity correlation, 554–557
    in vivo structure-function correlation, 539–554
  4α-methyl, 330
  PMR spectra of, 112

retention time, influence of carbonyl groups and double bonds on, 134–135
separation of, in gas-liquid chromatography, 133–136
structure, influence of, on retention time, 134–135
trivial names of, 68–70
C_{26}-Sterols, 352
  in molluscs, 437
Δ^{0}-Sterols, trivial names of, 68
Δ^{5}-Sterols
  bond angles in, 547
  in echinoderms, 439
  mass spectra of, 120
  separation factors, 134
  structure of, 326–328
  trivial names of, 68–69
$\Delta^{5,7}$-Sterols
  fragmentation of, 121
  trivial names of, 69–70
Δ^{7}-Sterols
  in echinoderms, 439
  mass spectra of, 120
  origins and role of, in lanosterol and cycloartenol metabolism, 366–367
  trivial names of, 69
Δ^{8}-Sterols, trivial names of, 70
$\Delta^{9(11)}$-Sterols, trivial names of, 70
$\Delta^{25(27)}$-Sterols, 497
Steryl esters, of fatty acids, 510
Steviol, 307, 308
  absolute configuration of, 311
Stichopus japonicum, 440
Stichopus regalis, 441
Stigmastanol, 68
$\Delta^{7,9(11),24(28)}$-Stigmastatrienol, in plants, 487
Stigmasterol, 66, 68, 343, 348, 371, 378, 495, 499, 505, 506, 510, 543
  as first tracheophyte sterol, 481
  in plants, 482–485, 486–491, 494
  reversed-phase chromatography of, 131
Δ^{7}-Stigmastenol, 69
Stomolophus sp., 429
Stone pine, 483
Streptomyces olivaceus, cholesterol in, 417, 418
Strophanthus kombé, 561
Strychnine, 284

Subcellular organelles, sterol and steryl ester composition of, 511, 514
Suberites domuncula, 377, 425, 427
Succinea putris, 438
Suffixes, in nomenclature, 61-62
Sugar cane, 486
Sugiol, 306, 307
Sulfuric acid spectra, 104
Sunflower, 486, 513
Suriana maritima, 504
  dominant sterols in, 484
Surianol, 504
Sweet chestnut, 513
Sweroside, 283, 285
Swietenia mahagoni, 503
Sylvestrene, 5
syn, defined, 42
Synura petersenii, 468, 469, 470

Taenia hydatigena, 378, 430
Taenia saginata, 430
Taenia taeniaeformus, 430
Tailing, defined, 127
Tapes philippinarum, 437
Taraxacum dens leonis, 388
Taraxacum officinale, 513
Taraxerol, 250, 251
Taurine, 74
Taurocholic acid, 592
Temperature, influence of, in fragmentation of sterols, 117-119
Tenebrio molitor, 348, 350
Tenulin, 293
Terpene, derivation of term, 5
Terpene structures, cyclic, elucidation of, 15
Terpenes, discovery of, 5-6
Terpinene, 5
α-Terpinene, analog, 286
γ-Terpinene, analog, 286
Terpinenol-4, 279
α-Terpineol, 279, 280
  analog, 286
α-Terpineyl cation
  as cyclic terpene precursors, 276
  formation of, 274-275
  skeletal rearrangement of, 277
Terpinolene, 5
Testosterone, 72, 73, 543, 577
  chemical tests for analysis of, 99

thin-layer chromatography of, 129
Tethya aurantia, 346, 426
Tetracycles, 40
  C_{18}, 41
  C_{28}, 41
  C_{31}, 40, 41
  formation, 301-308
Tetracyclic skeleton, 46-47
Tetrahydrosqualene, in bacterium, 417
22,23-Tetrahydrosqualene, 331
Tetrahymanol, 251, 252, 259, 420
  formation, 246, 247
  gas-liquid chromatography of, 136
Tetrahymena pyriformis, 246, 248, 251, 350, 351, 369, 372, 379, 413, 419, 420, 537, 545, 546, 551
  pentacycles in, 420
Thallasiosira pseudonana, 469
Thea sinensis, sterols in, 493
Thermobia domestica, 347, 433
Thin-layer chromatography, 129-131
  defined, 126
Thuja occidentalis, 276
Thujene, biosynthesis of, 276
Thujone, 319
Thujopsis dolabrata, 200
Thymoquinone, 286, 287
Tillandsia usneoides, 502
  dominant sterols in, 486
Timothy, 512
Tirucallol, 245, 256
Tobacco, 329, 484
  see also species name
α-Tocopherylquinone, 180
Tomatidine, 77, 79
Tomatillidine, 77, 78
Tracheophytes
  cyclolaudenol in, 336
  sterol biosynthesis in, 393, 480-517
trans, defined, 42
22-*trans*-Dehydrohalostanol, 437
Transfer, defined, 126
Transition definition, explained, 42-43
Trebouxia declorans, 479
Trebouxia sp., 332, 335, 336, 337, 476, 477
Trentepohlia aurea, 473
Tribonema aeguale, 467
Trichothecium roseum, 319
Trichophyton, sterols in, 422
Tricycle, formation of, 301-308

Tricyclic character, and irregularity, 9, 10
Tricyclic ethyl cation, 304, 305
Trifolium pratense, 512
3,16α,17β-Trihydroxy-1,3,5-estratriene, gas-liquid chromatography of, 137
Triparanol, 348, 374
  as cholesterol biosynthesis inhibitor, 332
Triple bonds, nomenclature for, 62
Trisdesmethylsterol, 328
Trisporic acid C, 301
Triterpenes, structure of, 18-19
Triterpenoids
  acyclic, 81
  in bacterium, 418, 419
  classification, biosynthetic basis for, 42-44
  pentacyclic, 81
Triterpenoid transition, 44
  defined, 42
Triticum vulgare, dominant sterols in, 489
Trivial names
  defined, 57
  table of, 68-70
Trough, defined, 123
Trypanosoma evansi, 420
Trypanosoma gambiense, 420
Tulip tree, 483
Tumors, and sterols, 453-455
Tumulonic acid, 423
Turbatrix aceti, 378, 431

Ubiquinone-n, 180
Ulva lactuca, 388, 474
Ulva pertussa, 474
Ultraviolet spectroscopy, 87
Unconjugated carbonyl group, ultraviolet spectroscopy of, 101
Unconjugated double bonds, ultraviolet spectroscopy of, 101
Urine, cholesterol in, 445
Uromyces phaseoli, 423
Usnea longissima, 479
Ustilago maydis, 422

Vapor-phase chromatography, 126
Velella spirans, cholesterol in, 428

Veratramine, 77, 78-79, 80
Verbena officinales, 277
Verbenalin, 277
Vernonia anthelmintica, 362, 501, 506
Vernosterol, 70, 502
Vernosterol, 501
Verongia aerophoba, 427
Vertebrates
  sterols in, 442-458
  steroids in bile of, 593
Vinca rosea, 278
Vinhaticosic acid, 306
Viperidinone, 501
Viruses
  fowlpox, 415
  influenza, 415
  myeloblastosis, 415
  sterols in, 415
  see also species names
Visible spectra, 104
Vitamin D, 75
  discovery of, 604-606
  formation of
    enzymatic, 608-610
    mechanism of, 606-610
    photochemically induced, 606
Vitamin D$_2$, 605-607, 610
Vitamin D$_3$, 610-616
Vitamin K$_1$, 180
Voucapenic acid, 306
Voucapenol, 306
Voucapenyl cation, 306

Wagner-Meerwein rearrangements, 13-14
Wallach, O.,
  first purification of terpene hydrocarbons by, 5-6
  Nobel Prize of, 20
  proposal of isoprene rule by, 8-9
Waterleaf, 513
Wave number, 105
Wheat, 489
Wilcoxia viperina, 501
Wieland, H., Nobel Prize of, 20-21
Willow, 513
Windaus, A., Nobel Prize of, 21
Withania somnifera, 501
  dominant sterols in, 485
Woodward, R. B., Nobel Prize of, 32

Woodward-Bloch conformation, for
squalene, 230, 231–232
Wormwood diterpene, 301

"X-group mechanism," 189, 190
X-ray crystallography, in determining
steroidal configuration, 51
Xanthoria parietina, 479
Xanthorrhoea preissii, 179
Xanthoxylum piperitum, 200
Xylaborus ferrugineus, 435–436, 554
Xysmalobium undulatum, 560

Yeast
anaerobic, sterol requirements of,
545, 546
sterols of, 544

Yellow-brown algae, sterols in, 467
Yellow-green algae
sterols in, 467–471
see also species names
"yne," defined, 61

Zaffaroni systems, 127–129
Zea mays, 329, 331, 480, 510, 511,
512, 514
dominant sterols in, 488
Zeorin, 250
Zerumbone, 290
Zoanthus convertus, 429
Zoanthus proteus, 429
Zygacine, 79, 80
Zymosterol, 70, 386
in bacterium, 417
in fungi, 421

DATE DUE